Educational Neuroscience

The field of educational neuroscience uses new insights about the neural mechanisms of learning to improve educational practices and outcomes. The first volume to bring together the latest knowledge on the development of educational neuroscience from a life-span perspective, this important text offers state of the art, authoritative research findings in educational neuroscience before providing evidence-based recommendations for classroom practice.

Thomas, Mareschal, Dumontheil, and the team of expert international contributors assembled in this volume thoroughly explore four main themes throughout the book. The first theme is individual differences, or what makes children perform better or worse in the classroom. The second theme is the nature of individual differences at different stages in development, from early years into adulthood. The third theme addresses cognitive enhancement, summarizing research that has investigated activities that might give general benefits to cognition. And the fourth theme considers the translation of research findings into classroom practices, discussing broader ethical issues raised by educational neuroscience, and what teachers need to know about neuroscience to enhance their day-to-day practice. Specific topics explored include neuropsychological perspectives on socioeconomic disparities in educational achievement, reading difficulties, phonological skills, executive function, and emotional development.

Educational Neuroscience is essential reading for researchers and graduate students of educational psychology, developmental science, developmental psychology, and cognitive psychology, especially those specializing in emotion regulation.

Michael S. C. Thomas obtained his PhD from the University of Oxford and completed a postdoctoral fellowship at the UCL Institute of Child Health. His research in developmental cognitive neuroscience focuses on the origins of cognitive variability, including developmental disorders. He is Director of the University of London Centre for Educational Neuroscience, UK.

Denis Mareschal is Director of the Centre for Brain and Cognitive Development, University of London, UK. He has published extensively on all aspects of learning and development across infancy and childhood, and is a recipient of the Marr Prize (Cognitive Science Society, USA), the Young Researcher Award (International Society on Infant Studies, USA), and the Margaret Donaldson Prize (British Psychological Society, UK).

Iroise Dumontheil obtained a PhD from the University of Paris VI and then was a postdoctoral fellow in labs in London, Cambridge and Stockholm. She is a recipient of the Spearman Medal (British Psychological Society, UK) and the Elizabeth Warrington Prize (British Neuropsychological Society, UK). Her research focuses on the typical development of the brain, cognition and behaviour during adolescence, and on the implication of these findings for education.

Frontiers of Developmental Science
Series Editors: Martha Ann Bell and Kirby Deater-Deckard

Frontiers of Developmental Science is a series of edited volumes that aims to deliver inclusive developmental perspectives on substantive areas in psychology. Interdisciplinary and life-span oriented in its objectives and coverage, the series underscores the dynamic and exciting status of contemporary developmental science.

Social Cognition
Development Across the Life Span
Jessica A. Sommerville and Jean Decety

Executive Function
Development Across the Life Span
Sandra A. Wiebe and Julia Karbach

Emotion Regulation
A Matter of Time
Pamela M. Cole and Tom Hollenstein

Reach-to-Grasp Behavior
Brain, Behavior, and Modelling Across the Life Span
Daniela Corbetta and Marco Santello

Educational Neuroscience
Development Across the Life Span
Edited by Michael S. C. Thomas, Denis Mareschal and Iroise Dumontheil

For more information about this series, please visit: www.routledge.com/Frontiers-of-Developmental-Science/book-series/FRONDEVSCI

Educational Neuroscience
Development Across the Life Span

Edited by Michael S. C. Thomas,
Denis Mareschal and Iroise Dumontheil

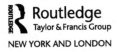

Routledge
Taylor & Francis Group

NEW YORK AND LONDON

First published 2020
by Routledge
52 Vanderbilt Avenue, New York, NY 10017

and by Routledge
2 Park Square, Milton Park, Abingdon, Oxon, OX14 4RN

Routledge is an imprint of the Taylor & Francis Group, an informa business

Library of Congress Cataloging-in-Publication Data
A catalog record for this book has been requested

ISBN: 978-1-138-24034-6 (hbk)
ISBN: 978-1-138-24035-3 (pbk)
ISBN: 978-1-003-01683-0 (ebk)

Typeset in Goudy
by Apex CoVantage, LLC

Theme	Chapters focused on that theme
Atypical development	Chapters 1, 5, 6, 7, 11, 14, 15, 18, 19, 20
Cognition	All chapters
Communication/language	Chapters 1, 2, 3, 4, 5, 6, 8, 15, 16, 18, 19, 20
Computational modeling	None
Continuity/discontinuity	Chapters 1, 2, 8
Cross species	None
Cultural context	Chapters 1, 2, 4, 5, 8, 10, 15, 17, 18
Developmental robotics	None
Emotion/affect	Chapters 1, 2, 4, 9, 10, 12, 13, 17, 19, 20
Family/parenting	Chapters 1, 4, 5, 10, 13, 16, 19, 20
Gene-environment	Chapters 1, 3, 4, 13, 16, 18, 19, 20
Individual differences	Chapters 1, 3, 4, 5, 6, 7, 8, 9, 10, 13, 14, 16, 17, 18, 20
Intergenerational transmission	Chapters 3, 4
Mechanisms of developmental change	Chapters 1, 2, 4, 5, 6, 7, 8, 9, 10, 12, 13, 14, 15, 16, 17, 18, 19, 20
Neuroscience	All
Ontogeny	All
Plasticity/repair	Chapters 1, 2, 4, 5, 6, 7, 14, 15, 17, 18, 19, 20
Sensory/Motor	Chapters 1, 2, 4, 5, 6, 8, 11, 13, 14, 16, 17, 18, 20
Social	Chapters 1, 2, 4, 5, 8, 9, 10, 12, 13, 16, 17, 18, 19, 20

Contents

Contributors

Irene Altarelli, Department of Psychology, Paris Descartes University, Paris, Île-de-France, France

Daniel Ansari, Department of Psychology, University of Western Ontario, Canada

Ruth Bailey, School of Education, University of Bristol, Bristol, UK

Daphne Bavelier, Faculty of Psychology and Educational Sciences, University of Geneva, Switzerland

Derek Bell, Director of Learnus, Visiting Research Associate, UCL Institute of Education, University College London, London, UK

Helen M. Darlington, Faculty Progress Leader: Science, South Wirral High School, Birkenhead, Wirral, UK

Bert De Smedt, Faculty of Psychology and Educational Sciences, University of Leuven, Belgium

Georgina Donati, Department of Psychological Sciences, Birkbeck, University of London, London, UK

Iroise Dumontheil, Centre for Educational Neuroscience, Department of Psychological Sciences, Birkbeck, University of London, London, UK

Selma Dündar-Coecke, Department of Psychology and Human Development, UCL Institute of Education, University College London, London, UK

Roberto Filippi, Centre for Educational Neuroscience, Department of Psychology and Human Development, UCL Institute of Education, University College London, London, UK

Usha Goswami, Centre for Neuroscience in Education, Department of Psychology, University of Cambridge, Cambridge, UK

Rebecca J.M. Gotlieb, Rossier School of Education; Brain & Creativity Institute, University of Southern California, Los Angeles, California, USA

C. Shawn Green, Department of Psychology, University of Wisconsin, Madison, USA

Daniel A. Hackman, USC Suzanne Dworak-Peck School of Social Work, University of Southern California, Los Angeles, California, USA

Christopher-James Harvey, Faculty of Medicine, Imperial College London, London, UK

Paul Howard-Jones, School of Education, University of Bristol, Bristol, UK

Gaby Illingworth, Nuffield Department of Clinical Neurosciences, University of Oxford, Oxford, UK

Mary Helen Immordino-Yang, Rossier School of Education; Brain & Creativity Institute; Department of Psychology; Neuroscience Graduate Program, University of Southern California, Los Angeles, California, USA

Konstantina Ioannou, School of Education, University of Bristol, Bristol, UK

Tim Jay, Sheffield Institute of Education, Sheffield Hallam University, Sheffield, UK

Heidi Johansen-Berg, Wellcome Centre for Integrative Neuroimaging, University of Oxford, Oxford, UK

Douglas Kennedy, Earl E. Bakken Center for Spirituality and Healing, University of Minnesota, Minneapolis, USA

Victoria Knowland, Department of Psychology, University of York, York, UK

David J. M. Kraemer, Department of Education, Dartmouth College, Hanover, New Hampshire, USA

Denis Mareschal, Centre for Educational Neuroscience, Department of Psychological Sciences, Birkbeck University of London, London, UK

Catherine McBride, Freiburg Institute for Advanced Studies (FRIAS), University of Freiburg, Germany; Department of Psychology, The Chinese University of Hong Kong, Hong Kong

Emma Meaburn, Centre for Educational Neuroscience, Department of Psychological Sciences, Birkbeck University of London, London, UK

Sabine Peters, Department of Developmental and Educational Psychology, Leiden University, the Netherlands; Leiden Institute for Brain and Cognition, the Netherlands

Jacqueline Phelps, Department of Psychology, University of Cambridge, UK

Jayne Prior, School of Education, University of Bristol, Bristol, UK

E. Glenn Schellenberg, Department of Psychology, University of Toronto Mississauga, Mississauga, Canada

Andrei D. Semenov, Institute of Child Development, University of Minnesota, Minneapolis, USA

Rachel Sharman, Nuffield Department of Clinical Neurosciences, University of Oxford, Oxford, UK

Michael S. C. Thomas, Centre for Educational Neuroscience, Department of Psychological Sciences, Birkbeck University of London, London, UK

Andy Tolmie, Centre for Educational Neuroscience, Department of Psychology and Human Development, UCL Institute of Education, University College London, London, UK

Xiuhong Tong, Department of Psychology, The Educational University of Hong Kong, Hong Kong

Thomas Wassenaar, Wellcome Centre for Integrative Neuroimaging, University of Oxford, Oxford, UK

Catherine Wheatley, Wellcome Centre for Integrative Neuroimaging, University of Oxford, Oxford, UK

Shu Yau, School of Education, University of Bristol, Bristol, UK

Philip David Zelazo, Institute of Child Development, University of Minnesota, Minneapolis, USA

Introduction

1 Educational Neuroscience

Why Is Neuroscience Relevant to Education?

Michael S. C. Thomas and Daniel Ansari

Educational neuroscience is an emerging field whose goal is to translate new insights, garnered from the study of neural mechanisms underpinning learning, into practical applications in the classroom in order to improve educational outcomes. The field began in the 1990s, the so-called 'decade of the brain' (Jones & Mendell, 1999), when technological advances in brain imaging spurred progress in the scientific understanding of how the brain supports the mind and its facility to learn. The field is also referred to as 'mind, brain, and education' and as 'neuroeducation', and now supports a range of societies, research centres, conferences, and journals. It falls under the broader banner of the 'Science of Learning'.

While educational neuroscience is founded on the intuition that new findings on the neural mechanisms of learning may be helpful for teachers in the classroom, educational neuroscience is not intended to be reductionist—it does not maintain that brain-level explanations are the best, nor seek to reduce education from its intrinsic nature as a societal and cultural enterprise. The contribution of educational neuroscience is intended to be more modest: an understanding of mechanisms of learning may help improve some learning outcomes.

As we believe the diverse contributions contained within this volume show, educational neuroscience has great potential to propel advances in educational practices. However, the current cultural context presents challenges. Teachers are often enthusiastic about techniques that are 'brain-based', but some of these techniques are advocated by companies where the neuroscience is only window dressing for a commercial product, and the techniques are not supported by scientific data (Simons et al., 2016). In amongst a public understanding of how the brain works there have appeared myths (e.g., that we only use 10% of our brains, or that some children are left brain learners while others are right brain learners[1]). These 'neuromyths' have frequently led to classroom practices, again without scientific support (e.g., visual-auditory-kinaesthetic learning styles; Pashler, McDaniel, Rohrer, & Bjork, 2009). In addition, while educational policymakers have proved keen to inform their decisions with neuroscience evidence (e.g., Thomas, 2017; Willetts, 2018), researchers must be careful to ensure that recommendations do not exceed the current level of scientific understanding (Bruer, 1999). Moreover, while it is important to educate the public about neuromyths or ineffective educational approaches, it should also be acknowledged that despite knowledge translations, ineffective methods may continue to be used.

This volume presents the latest research in educational neuroscience. Across seventeen chapters, there are four main areas of focus. The first is on individual differences: what makes children perform better or worse in the classroom? Note this is a slightly different question to the theoretical puzzle of how education-relevant skills are acquired. It is the distinction between asking, say, what makes children better or worse at mathematics, compared to asking how can humans learn something like mathematics at all. The second focus is to consider this question at different stages in development—from the early years, through mid-childhood, adolescence, and into adulthood. Each age range can pose different challenges for teachers and offers different opportunities to modify approaches. Our consideration of individual differences considers their respective origins in genetic and environmental causes (the latter particularly focusing on the contribution of socioeconomic status). The chapters following address individual differences in *discipline-specific abilities*, including literacy, numeracy, and science, and then in *discipline-general abilities*, including executive functions and social and emotional development.

The third focus of the book, represented by a collection of six chapters, considers *cognitive enhancement*, summarising research that has investigated activities that might give general benefits to cognition. These include action videogame playing, mindfulness training, the role of sleep in learning, aerobic exercise, learning a second language, and learning a musical instrument. These chapters assess which of these activities (if any) have proven to have widespread benefits that extend to educational achievement.

The fourth focus of the book is on the translation of research findings into classroom practices, and broader ethical issues raised by educational neuroscience. Offering the teachers' perspective, one of our contributors argues:

> we are the professionals, and understanding learning and the implications it has for our teaching should be the basis of our practice. Just as we would expect doctors to understand how the body works and keep up to date with new techniques, for example in treating cancer, teachers need to understand how learning takes place.
>
> (Bell & Darlington, Chapter 19)

Yet what exactly do teachers need to know about neuroscience that will actually change their day to day practice—for example, how they plan a lesson? Do teachers need to know how a brain scanner works? What neurotransmitters do? How the brain consolidates memories? The final section of the book seeks to answer this question.

How Does Educational Neuroscience Work?

Neuroscience interacts with education via two routes, shown in Figure 1.1. It can interact indirectly via psychology, whereby evidence from neuroscience

Routes from neuroscience to education

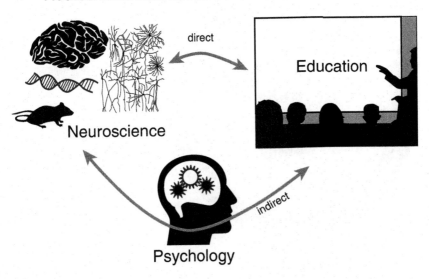

Figure 1.1 Two Bi-directional Routes Linking Neuroscience and Education
Source: Reproduced with permission from Thomas et al., 2019.

is used to advance psychological theory. Under this view, as an isolated discipline, psychology produces theories of learning that are too unconstrained, speculating on how cognitive systems *might* work rather than focusing on how our actual cognitive system works given the constraints of delivering it in real-time through brain function (Thomas, Ansari, & Knowland, 2019). Neuroscience and education can also interact directly, by virtue of the fact that the brain is a biological organ and therefore subject to metabolic constraints. Factors such as energy supply, nutrition, response to stress hormones and environmental pollution can potentially influence brain function, including learning. Thus, while educational neuroscience generally places psychology at its centre, research on the impact of non-psychological factors on educational outcomes, such as aerobic fitness, diet, and air quality, also falls within its remit. The direct route can be thought of in terms of 'brain health'—placing the organ in the optimal condition to maximise the individual's learning when he or she enters the classroom.

Even if educational neuroscience can offer insights into mechanisms of learning, it should also be recognised that learning is only one part of education. Educational outcomes need to be thought of in terms of the nested constraints that encompass the individual, classroom, school, family, and society. For example, the effect of home conditions is often more powerful in influencing educational outcomes than what occurs in school, suggesting that school practices are not always the limiting factor on performance. Figure 1.2 borrows

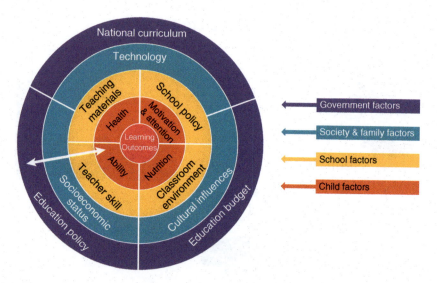

Figure 1.2 Proximal and Distal Factors That Support and Constrain Change in Learning Outcomes, Following the Layered Influences on Behavioural Change Proposed by Michie, van Stralen, and West (2011), and the Interactive Relationships Between an Individual and His or Her Environment as Proposed by Bronfenbrenner (1992). The white arrow reflects bidirectional influences between layers.

Source: Reproduced with permission from Thomas et al., 2019.

from Bronfenbrenner's ecological systems theory (Bronfenbrenner, 1992) to identify some of the nested factors constraining educational outcomes. It places learning outcomes at the heart of education, but illustrates the range of other factors—child-internal, societal, institutional, and governmental— which make up the broader picture. In line with Bronfenbrenner's view, the factors that influence a child's learning outcomes operate at vastly different degrees of proximity to the learning process and should be seen as an interactive, interconnected system. The potential impact of educational neuroscience is to improve educational outcomes by changing the most proximal factors to learning outcomes as shown in Figure 1.2: ability, motivation and attention, health and nutrition. However, its scope to do so depends on the range of barriers to change that may be encountered beyond learning itself.

The Job of Educational Neuroscience Is a Difficult One

Part of the challenge of educational neuroscience is that translation from basic science to practical application is difficult, even for a mature discipline such as psychology. Roediger (2013) observed that despite a hundred years of psychological evidence on learning and memory, there were still techniques used in the classroom despite the existence of a body of evidence showing that they are ineffective (e.g., highlighting/underlining text to aid memorisation), and techniques with good evidence of their effectiveness that were not used in the classroom (e.g., learning through testing) (see Dunlosky, Rawson, Marsh, Nathan, & Willingham, 2013). It is not straightforward to translate an understanding of how learning occurs in the brain into ways to improve learning outcomes through instruction. Such translation requires investment into structures and mechanisms that can facilitate it.

A second challenge is that even though 'learning' may seem like a unitary construct—something that hopefully happens in the classroom, or through study—its realisation in the brain is highly complex. As a product of evolution, the human brain has a number of priorities. Its first is to support motor movements by integrating perceptual information. Its second is to purse basic goals built into its very structure in the systems that support emotions, in what one might call the eight Fs (fear, fight, flight, freeze, feed, fun, frolic, and forty-winks).[2] As the brain of a social primate, its third priority is other people, be they parents, siblings, mates, friends, or enemies. The brain dedicates many systems to processing other people's identities, actions, emotions, and intentions. Its fourth priority—*only* the fourth—is high-level cognition, the kind of knowledge and reasoning skills that are the target of education. There is much, then, that could get in the way of learning.

Learning itself is the interplay of perhaps eight different neural systems (Thomas et al., 2019[3]). These are depicted schematically in Figure 1.3 (see Chapter 2 of this volume for an overview of actual brain regions and functional networks). The eight are:

1. A system for memorising individual moments, which produces *episodic or autobiographical memory*. This is realised by the hippocampus and the structures around it. This system can change its connections very quickly to record snapshots.

2. A system for learning *concepts*. The brain learns associations between perceptual information and motor responses, spotting complex spatial and temporal patterns. This happens within the cortex, where changing connections takes seconds, minutes, and hours.

3. A system for *classical conditioning*. Some associations are unconscious and involve the emotion (limbic) structures further inside the brain. These are associations between stimulus and response, such as when a particular food made you sick and puts you off it thereafter. These associations can form over seconds and minutes.

4. A system for *control*. The brain learns to control content-specific systems in the posterior cortex so that they are activated in the appropriate contexts. This system learns strategies and when to apply them. Control involves the prefrontal cortex, which also interacts with limbic structures to integrate planning with emotion.

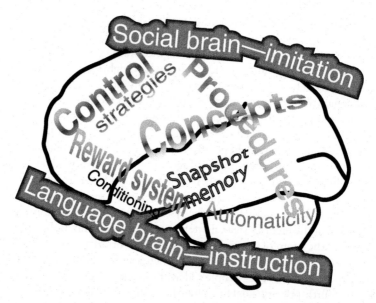

Figure 1.3 A Schematic of Eight Neural Systems for Learning, Whose Interplay Pro-
duces the Phenomenon of 'Learning' in the Classroom (From the Centre for
Educational Neuroscience Resource www.howthebrainworks.science). See
Chapter 2 of this volume for overview of actual brain regions and networks.

5. A system for learning how to get *rewards*. This system works out what
    we have to do to get what we want, to make nice things happen and
    avoid bad things happening. It operates over seconds and minutes. The
    system is based deep within the brain (the ventral tegmental area in the
    midbrain), where neurons release a neurotransmitter called dopamine
    that tracks the presence or absence of rewards and in turn influences the
    operation of other systems.
6. A *procedural learning* system for learning activities that we perform fre-
    quently and often unconsciously, such as tying shoelaces, reading or driv-
    ing a car. These automatic skills can take tens or hundreds of hours to
    learn through practice. The structures involved are the cerebellum and
    the looping outer-to-inner circuits connecting the cortex through the
    basal ganglia to the thalamus and back again.
7. The *social-learning system*. The brain can take advantage of its widespread
    circuits for perceiving, understanding, and imitating other people, so that
    skills can be learned simply by watching other people do them.
8. The *language system*. The brain can take advantage of its widespread cir-
    cuits for using language to construct new concepts and plans, so that skills
    can be learned through instruction.

In addition to these multiple systems, a broader principle operates: *make all processes automatic*, so they occur quickly, smoothly and without need for cognitive effort or even awareness. The more knowledge/skills are used, the more they become automatic. With automatized skills, there is increasing involvement of basal ganglia and cerebellar structures and decreasing involvement of prefrontal cortex. In contrast, the less often skills or knowledge are used, the more likely they are to be lost. Forgetting happens at a different pace in different learning systems: for instance, factual knowledge crumbles more quickly than motor skills, such as riding a bicycle.

All of these systems work in an integrated fashion. They respond differently over time and prefer different regimes of training. And they can be differentially modulated by factors such as motivational and emotional states. In face of this complexity, understanding the implications of this constellation of mechanisms for the term 'learning' as construed by educators represents a huge challenge.

Educational Neuroscience Is Still Controversial

Educational neuroscience remains controversial in some quarters. Some researchers feel that neuroscience data are simply too remote from the classroom to be of educational value, and approaches that focus more overtly on behaviour, such as psychology, are more appropriate (e.g., Bowers, 2016). Some feel that claims that neuroscience data can be of use in diagnosing developmental disorders or predicting individual outcomes are overstated, and these methods are not currently practical or viable (e.g., Bishop, 2014). There have been recent, lively debates on these issues in leading psychology journals (e.g., a critique by Bowers, 2016, and a response by Howard-Jones et al., 2016, in *Psychological Review*; or a critique by Dougherty and Robey, 2018, and a response by Thomas, 2019, in *Current Directions in Psychological Science*).

Educational neuroscience is a fledgling field, and there are indeed legitimate criticisms that can be made of it. For example, educational neuroscience must amount to more than a re-labelling of phenomena already well known from behavioural psychology with the names of brain structures—such as re-labelling 'executive function' with 'prefrontal cortex', or 'episodic memory' with 'hippocampus'. Educational neuroscience must progress psychological theory, and it must point to ways to improve brain health.

Bishop (2014) is correct to argue that neuroscience methods are still limited in their sensitivity and specificity as screening or diagnostic tools for deficits. They can only complement more traditional behavioural and social markers of risk. However, some neuroscience measures may be available earlier, such as infant electroencephalographic measures of auditory processing to predict later dyslexia risk (Guttorm, Leppänen, Hämäläinen, Eklund, & Lyytinen, 2009); or, in the future, available-at-birth DNA measures to predict possible educational outcomes (Plomin, 2018). Early availability increases the opportunity for intervention or simply more targeted monitoring of traditional risk markers in tracking the progress of individual children.

Lastly, educational neuroscience needs to improve the quality of the dialogue between teachers, psychologists, and educators to ensure that the discussion is genuinely bidirectional, for example, through co-designing studies with teachers to improve the relevance of research and increase the chance of changing practices in the classroom. It is imperative that the dialogue be as much about teachers stimulating research directions and thinking about how new findings may be useful in the classroom as it is about researchers communicating the findings of their cognitive neuroscience studies.

There are also distracting but spurious criticisms. One is that to contribute to education, the insights of neuroscience must be brand new and revolutionary (otherwise the retort is, 'But we already knew that!'). While there may be pre-existing folk theories about, say, the importance of sleep ('my old granny always said a good night's sleep was good for you!'), this does not undermine the possible contribution that the neuroscience of sleep can bring through, for example, its investigation of consolidation effects on learning during the interactions between hippocampal and cortical structures (see Sharman, Illingworth & Harvey, this volume). Neuroscience can tell us not only that sleep is good but how much sleep is required (e.g., Wild, Nichols, Battista, Stojanoski, & Owen, 2018). Even when behavioural effects are already known, they can be improved by understanding mechanisms at lower levels of description.

Another spurious criticism is that neuroscience explanations are dangerous because they have a 'seductive allure' (Weisberg, Keil, Goodstein, Rawson, & Gray, 2008), that is, they make psychologists and teachers more likely to believe new proposals for teaching techniques irrespective of supporting evidence. While that may be true (unfortunately), when neuroscience is used merely as window dressing, it is a contextual framing effect, not a reflection on the progress of the discipline of educational neuroscience itself (Farah & Hook, 2013; Scurich & Shniderman, 2014).

An Overview of the Chapters

The volume unfolds as follows. For those who are coming to this volume unfamiliar with neuroscience, the next chapter by Dumontheil and Mareschal gives an introduction to key concepts and methods within neuroscience—the broad anatomy and functioning of the brain, how it changes across development, the main regions that are referred to in subsequent chapters, as well as the leading brain imaging methods such as magnetic resonance imaging and electrophysiology. This is the place to familiarise yourself with the key terminology and what abbreviations like MRI and EEG mean.

Section 1 includes two chapters on *Genetic and Environmental Factors*, tackling genetic and environmental contributions to individual differences in educational achievement. In Chapter 3, Donati and Meaburn explain how genetic methods have been increasingly applied to educational abilities. The focus here is on emphasising that not all differences between children and adults are environmental in origin. Educational achievement, intelligence, and personality dimensions run in families to some extent—as revealed by the traditional behavioural genetic method of twin studies, yielding the heritability of these traits. Breakthroughs in molecular genetics now allow measurements of actual DNA variations between individuals, and how these correlate with variations in high-level abilities such as reading or mathematics. Donati and Meaburn discuss how the results of these so-called genome-wide association studies can be used in education, such as using DNA to predict educational outcomes via polygenic risk scores. Notably, they declare that genetic outcomes are not inevitable (genetic effects may change in magnitude in different environments) and that 'genes for education simply do not exist' (p. 70)!

In Chapter 4, Hackman and Kraemer consider the nurture side of the equation, and how environmental factors contribute to individual differences in educational outcomes. One of the most predictive and readily available measures of the environment is the socio-economic status (SES) of the families in which children are raised. Hackman and Kraemer review current research on the effects of SES on brain and cognitive development. They conclude that 'many of the same aspects of neurocognitive performance that are associated with SES are also predictive of educational outcomes' (p. 99). Although these are individual-level factors, Hackman and Kraemer emphasise how the findings point to the centrality of social and systemic factors in education. However, SES is a proxy for multiple potential causal pathways of environmental influence, and the chapter carefully unpacks how SES effects might operate on educational outcomes—stressing that even though their impact is measurable in the brain, SES effects are by no means immutable or deterministic.

Section 2, *Discipline-Specific Abilities*, considers the contribution of educational neuroscience to understanding abilities relevant to particular disciplines. These include literacy, numeracy, and science. Chapters 5 and 6 both address reading. In Chapter 5, Tong and McBride-Chang give a broad overview of how reading develops in the brain—given that as a recent cultural invention, reading must involve re-purposing other neural systems for object recognition, oral language, and meaning to fashion a system dedicated to literacy. Tong and McBride-Chang show how different imaging methods have been used to reveal these brain pathways. They show how both structure and function differ in cases of dyslexia, and how brain pathways may be modified by the language (and script) that children are learning, such as in a comparison of English and Chinese. Notably, measures of electrical brain activity in infants in response to auditory stimuli are able to predict language and literacy skills some eight years later, indicating the early origin of differences in literacy skills.

In Chapter 6, Goswami takes a deep dive into one skill underlying language and literacy, one that is particularly implicated in dyslexia: phonology. Understanding the brain mechanisms that underpin this skill points to an unexpected possible avenue of remediation for dyslexia: practising playing on the bongo drums, and reciting poetry. How can this be? The child's early learning of phonology—via a home or pre-school environment rich in language—involves constructing a hierarchy of the linguistic information available in the speech stream. Much of the key information involves rhythm. The brain's processing of rhythm can be investigated through the auditory system's tendency to entrain its activity to the different rhythms present in language input. Neurons actually fire in tune with different beats! In dyslexia, there appears to be a particular problem in detecting the rhythmic 'envelope' not just of words but whole sentences, compromising the child's later ability to match phonology to the written form of language. Goswami argues that interventions which focus on metrical language activities, such as nursery rhymes and rhythmic music, may aid the brain's construction of the appropriate phonology to prepare for reading acquisition. Since these activities are appropriate for pre-school, they permit an early intervention for children who are flagged as at risk of developing literacy problems.

In Chapter 7, de Smedt focuses on mathematics and asks why learning mathematics is so easy for some but so hard for others. De Smedt considers the virtues and disadvantages of understanding school-taught skills at the biological level. Mathematics involves the integration of many different mechanisms in the brain, and mathematics problems frequently involve many steps. This makes mathematical skills difficult to study with current brain imaging methods, which either average together activity over several seconds or pull it apart into milliseconds. De Smedt focuses on arithmetic development—adding, subtracting, multiplying and dividing whole numbers. Here, it turns out that different strategies are available to solve the same problem, and the strategies that children have available depends on the way that they are taught, as well as individual preferences. Often it appears that strategy, not problem type (e.g., single digit vs. multidigit arithmetic), modulates the brain regions that are correlated with doing arithmetic. But there is also developmental change—for example, fact retrieval is mediated by temporal-parietal cortex in adults (conceptual) but is more hippocampal (episodic) in children. De Smedt considers whether there are particular core skills that serve as constraining factors in learning arithmetic, and concludes that symbolic magnitude processing (that is, understanding how numerical symbols, such as Arabic numerals, represent numerical quantities/sets of objects), 'is as important to arithmetic as phonological awareness is to reading' (p. 176).

In Chapter 8, Tolmie and Dündar-Coecke consider science education, and the lifespan development of the conceptual skills that underpin scientific knowledge, from the early years, mid and late childhood, adolescence and into adulthood. They note that in childhood, perceptual knowledge of how the physical world behaves seems separate from conceptual knowledge: 'by the time they have reached the age of 11 children show acute perceptual awareness of variables that genuinely affect outcomes, even if this is conflated with false beliefs about other factors' (Chapter 8, p. 197). They argue that talk in science class is essential, because language is key in closing the gap between perceptual and conceptual understanding—language-provoked mechanistic ideas focus attention on relevant perceptual properties to understand how physical systems work. However, elaborated concepts emerge at different rates in different areas (e.g., freezing versus sublimation), depending on the extent and nature of environmental input. Adolescence is marked by the addition of detail, the linking up of knowledge and the connection to procedures and application. In adulthood, there are multiple systems of knowledge, flexibly used, but expertise is now more important than age. Notably, prediction and explanation skills can still separate—one study of undergraduates described by Tolmie and Dündar-Coecke on the path of rotating objects found the correlation between prediction and explanation was close to zero. The implication is that science skills and knowledge are fractured, and a key aspect of science learning is integrating knowledge and correctly applying it.

Section 3, *Discipline-General Abilities*, focuses on individual differences in abilities that may affect performance *across disciplines*. In Chapter 9, Peters considers executive functions, and how they develop across childhood and adolescence. She considers the main components of cognitive control, including working memory, inhibition, and flexibility and the extent to which these skills are trainable. Peters argues that the brain substrates underpinning executive functions take a long time to mature, which explains the poor executive function skills of young children. Importantly, she argues that not all classrooms and education programmes are currently well tailored for the level of neural development and executive function skills that children possess at that age. In adolescence, by contrast, executive function skills are more advanced, but pubertal changes impact decision making around risk taking, particularly in a social context, with associated adverse health outcomes. However, Peters also identifies opportunities in adolescence, including the heightened sensitivity of reward systems to feedback and to social environments. The teenage years may be a window of opportunity for learning, but also a time when individual differences are exaggerated since the brain is more influenced by affective and social context.

In Chapter 10, Immordino-Yang and Gottleib focus on the emotions. They address the question of why learning is such an emotion-dependent process, and what this means for teachers and schools. They answer:

> students' abilities to recognise, understand and manage their emotions; to build and maintain a sense of interest and curiosity; to persist through challenges and uncertainty; to embrace new experiences; to imagine alternative futures for themselves and their communities; and to feel purposeful . . . all of these powerfully influence personal and academic success.
>
> (p. 242)

Despite the key role of emotion in learning—and indeed recent government focus on Social Emotional Learning—Immordino-Yang and Gottleib argue that the message is frequently misconstrued by teachers; for example that focusing on emotions in the classroom is a luxury when time affords, or is simply about ensuring students are 'having fun'. They argue that emotions are key to learning but need to be relevant to what is being learned, otherwise they will interfere with learning outcomes (for instance, as is the case with anxiety around mathematics). Immordino-Yang and Gottlieb explain how brain systems for sensing the gut (including the insula) are co-opted for emotional experiences, but that 'gut feelings' reflect extensive learning rather than naïve intuitions. Even when people experience a complex emotion like admiration, this still appears to involve activation of the insula! Finally, the authors consider cross-cultural differences, in particular to how individuals report feelings of emotionality in response to otherwise equivalent activation of body sensory systems in the brain.

Section 4, *Leading Methods for Cognitive Enhancement*, contains six chapters that evaluate various forms of *cognitive enhancement*. On the whole, training cognition produces what is called 'near transfer'—gains on the task that is trained on, smaller gains on similar tasks, but little or no improvement on very different tasks, referred to as far transfer (e.g., Sala et al., 2019). However, researchers continue to seek evidence for techniques that confer general benefits across cognition. This section uniquely brings together in one place evaluations of several such approaches, including action videogame playing, mindfulness training, the role of sleep in learning, aerobic exercise, learning a second language, and learning a musical instrument, each of which, at one time or another, has been claimed to produce either general benefits for cognition or improved educational outcomes.

One must be cautious in this area: some researchers have reservation about the very notion of 'cognitive enhancement', both in the goal that it implies and the necessity of measurement of aspects of education that are not readily quantifiable (Cigman & Davis, 2009). For example, Cigman (2009, p. 174) argues that

> the enhancement agenda is not simply about getting children to perform better. It is about getting them to *feel* better—more motivated, more confident, happier—and about the idea that feeling good in these ways leads to success at school and in life generally.

but Cigman notes that 'it is not obvious that one can identify particular feelings as unconditionally good, so that more is necessarily better' (p. 174). Nevertheless, to the extent that cognitive abilities can be measured, education as a whole can be said to act as a cognitive enhancer, with one meta-analysis reporting a gain of approximately one to five IQ points for each additional year of education attended (Ritchie & Tucker-Drob, 2018).

In Chapter 11, Altarelli, Green and Bavelier consider the impact of sustained playing of *action video computer games* on cognition. These games are fast paced and engaging, involving rapid motor responses to fast changing visual scenes. Some teenagers and young adults spend a great deal of time playing these games, and games have been found to have the capacity to powerfully alter brain and behaviour. Meta-analyses reveal uneven effects on cognition, mostly influencing top-down attention, spatial cognition and visual attention. Altarelli and colleagues reveal the key properties that these games must have to be effective: fast pacing to force decision making under time constraints, pressure to divide attention and monitor multiple sources of information, a requirement to switch flexibly between divided attention and focused attention states, adaptive tailoring of difficulty (not too easy, not too hard), and rich and variable experiences. Because action video games are so engaging, it has been an ambition among educators to exploit these properties for educational purposes—to 'gamify' education. However, Altarelli and colleagues comment that most educational games focus on content and are unsuccessful in capturing the game mechanics that trigger engagement. They also note that there is as yet little evidence base for cognitive effects of action video games in younger children (where there is also a risk of age-inappropriate content, such as violence). Yet there remain intriguing findings, such as the possibility that action video game playing can improve the reading skills of some children with dyslexia.

In Chapter 12, Semenov, Kennedy and Zelazo consider mindfulness training in children and adolescents, and its potential impact on executive function skills in the classroom. Meditation is often connected to religious practice, most notably Buddhism, but it has recently been exploited as a secular method to enhance health and wellbeing. As Ven. Ajahn Sumedho says, within Buddhism 'all the teachings are for encouraging and directing our attention, investigating and examining experience in the present moment. To do this, you need to be fully awake. You have to pay attention to life as it happens' (Panawong Green, 2001, p. 8). Semenov and colleagues consider the role of mindfulness training for improving both hot (emotion regulation) and cold (cognitive control) aspects of executive function such as attention. They emphasise its potential to improve internal regulation by preventing bottom-up influences (such as emotional responses) overriding and interfering with goals and attention. While cognitive training usually only produces near transfer, Semenov and colleagues argue mindfulness training has the potential for far transfer because it supports metacognition through reflection: metacognitive awareness of skills and their range of application can be a vehicle for far transfer. The neuroscience of mindfulness training—mostly in adults—points to the importance of the anterior cingulate cortex (ACC), a brain system that monitors current performance against goals. Notably, studies report that the ACC is *more* active when expert meditators are practising mindfulness, but *less* active than non-meditators during regular cognition—suggesting that the filtering out of distractions may become automatic with practice. In an educational context, Semenov, Kennedy and Zelazo consider the potential benefits of mindfulness not only for children but also for teachers, where it may aid wellbeing in a stressful job.

In Chapter 13, Sharman, Illingworth and Harvey consider the neuroscience of sleep and its relation to educational outcomes. They review how sleep works in the brain—how cycles of sleep are revealed by electrical brain activity—and how sleep is linked to the circadian rhythm. Particular attention is paid to the shift in circadian rhythm in adolescence of around three hours, with teens staying up later at night and waking later in the morning. As yet, the cause of this shift is unknown. But later bedtimes combined with the same fixed start time for school translates to reduced amounts of sleep for teenagers. Sleep is associated with psychosocial functioning and emotional/behavioural regulation, and so reductions in sleep may influence students' wellbeing, their ability to get on with their peers and teachers, and their behaviour at school (though the direction of causality has not yet been completely clarified). Not only may teenagers be more 'tired and emotional', cognition may be impacted and so too quality of learning. Sharman and colleagues consider the role of sleep in memory and learning in the brain, with cycles of replay, consolidation, reorganisation, and integration of memories. They note that sleep efficiency may turn out to be more important than duration—children need to sleep well! The authors then evaluate the parallel possibilities of altering school start times to fit better with adolescent circadian rhythms, or of sleep education, improving students' understanding of behaviours that encourage good sleep (such as avoiding use of screen-based media devices close to bedtime; see e.g., Mireku et al., 2019) in order to maximise sleep efficiency.

In Chapter 14, Wheatley, Wassenaar and Johansen-Berg consider the possible benefits of aerobic exercise for improving educational outcomes. It seems a no-brainer that exercise is good for you, in this age of concerns around obesity. But the focus here is less on health benefits and more on potential effects on cognition, particularly on executive function skills such as attention. Wheatley and colleagues carefully consider cross-sectional studies, evaluating whether those undertaking more aerobic exercise have better educational outcomes, and then intervention studies, where the target is to improve existing fitness levels. The story becomes complex: is exercise about 'acute', immediate improvements so that, say, children perform better in a mathematics class after a PE lesson? Or about 'chronic' improvements, acting via sustained improvements in fitness? Are improvements to do with cardiovascular fitness or better motor skills (e.g., better flexibility, balance and speed)? What are the brain mechanisms underpinning observed improvements? Animal studies point to the involvement of improved brain connectivity, growth of new blood vessels, greater expression of chemical 'growth factors' such as Brain Derived Neurotropic Factor (BDNF), and even the generation of new neurons in the hippocampus. What kind of exercise is better? Moderate to vigorous physical activity (MVPA) seems a favourite. There are suggestions that aerobic fitness activity may be more effective in the primary years than for teenagers, and there may be diminishing returns for children who are already fit. 'On balance,' Wheatley and colleagues conclude, 'young people's executive functions can be improved by physical activity' (p. 376), before they turn to consider the practicalities of how this activity can be fitted into the school day, and who should be in charge (turns out specialist PE teachers aren't required!).

Chapter 15 turns to consider the possible cognitive benefits (and disadvantages) of bilingualism and multilingualism. Phelps and Filippi address this question both for children and also across lifespan—given suggestive evidence that learning a second language could be a protective factor against the cognitive decline associated with ageing. Research on bilingualism and cognition seems like a rollercoaster—in the first half of the 20th century, bilingualism was deemed to have a negative effect on IQ; in the latter half of the century, it was thought to enhance cognition. This conclusion is now contested; meanwhile, in the educational sector (at least in the UK) English as an Additional Language (EAL) is viewed as a risk factor for poorer outcomes with such pupils in need of support. The picture is confused by a lack of random allocation to condition. Because it is not randomly decided who will be monolingual and who bilingual, there may be systematic differences between these groups that depend on historical and cultural factors—for example, in some country or region, bilingual groups may have higher (or lower) SES than monolingual groups; as we have seen, SES is itself associated with differences in cognition. Phelps and Filippi sift the behavioural and brain evidence: There is stronger evidence that bilingualism produces benefits for attention in processing language, while the evidence is more mixed that the demands of controlling two language systems produce general benefits for cognition. Part of the problem is that bilinguals are so variable in their abilities and experiences, and wider benefits may only surface in children and ageing populations, rather than in young adults whose cognitive skills are at their strongest. This diversity prompts Phelps and Filippi to argue that it is time for a new theoretical framework. Their strongest messages are that there is no evidence for 'mental overload' for children learning two languages (even for children with autistic spectrum disorder or attention deficit hyperactivity disorder)—indeed, the wider cultural contact afforded by two languages offers greater opportunities for support. And that the EAL profile is not atypical—it is not like developmental language disorder—and educators should abandon the negative connotations associated with EAL status.

In Chapter 16, the final chapter in the cognitive enhancement section, Schellenberg considers whether music training can raise IQ levels. He asks whether music training has systematic consequences that extend beyond music knowledge and ability to non-musical cognitive abilities. Once more, a frequent lack of random allocation to condition poses problems. Schellenberg observes that children who take music lessons are a select group, and randomly allocating children to a music lesson group in an intervention study is not realistic, since children need to commit to practise beyond the classroom to progress in musical training. Schellenberg views the positive claims made for music training in the face of these experimental challenges as a 'kind of radical environmentalism' (p. 414): a focus on brain plasticity has led researchers and educators to ignore pre-existing individual differences between children who do and don't undertake musical training, and has encouraged a tendency to interpret correlational findings as evidence of causation. In this, he views educational neuroscientists as particularly guilty. Since they are studying the brain—a mechanism—it is all too easy for these researchers to see correlational evidence as causation. But Schellenberg points out that common factors may cause children to both persist with musical training and to have higher IQs: for example, supportive middle-class families, or genetic differences in intelligence and willingness to persist with practise. Schellenberg reviews the evidence and finds little convincing support for improvements in cognition from music training. However, there are intriguing findings, such as the possibility of improvements in speech processing and in reading for dyslexics—a hypothesis we saw put forward by Goswami (see Chapter 6). At the end of the chapter, we come full circle to reservations about the cognitive enhancement agenda. Why should the goal be to achieve measurable improvements in IQ?, asks Schellenberg. Music training improves musical skills, music promotes social bonding, 'music listening often makes us feel good, and making music often makes us feel good together. Isn't that enough?' (p. 432).

Section 5, *Into the Classroom*, enters the classroom. Up to this point in the volume, teachers might legitimately say, 'this research is all very interesting but . . . how do I use it in the classroom?' In Chapter 17, Howard-Jones, Ioannou, Bailey, Prior, Jay and Yau attempt to answer this question. Their focus is on the quality of teaching, pointing out that 'a teacher in the top 16% of effectiveness, compared with an average teacher, has been estimated to produce students whose level of achievement is somewhere between 0.2 and 0.3 standard deviations higher by the end of the school year (p. 443).' However, they argue that good teaching is not simply about applying best practice, but knowing how and when to apply each practice. They argue that the sciences of mind and brain enrich education by informing the processes by which teachers critically reflect upon and develop an understanding of their own practice. The goal of these authors is to select core scientific concepts that will aid in this reflection, and to demonstrate their relation to established educational practices. Howard-Jones and colleagues settle on three key categories of the learning process: (1) Engagement with Learning, (2) Building of New Knowledge, and (3) Consolidation of Learning, characterised in terms of the key brain systems involved. These concepts are then systematically linked to published 'Principles of Instruction' and 'Principles for Emotion and Learning' within education. The authors ground this cycle in examples such as classroom instruction and teacher emotions, guiding student practice, and daily review. Crucially, the utility of these concepts for teachers is road tested in a postgraduate course for teachers being developed at the authors' own university.

In Chapter 18, Knowland tackles the ethical issues raised by classroom research in educational neuroscience, given that the targets of its interventions are usually children. Within neuroscience and psychology, the ethical bar is set higher in considering research with children. Yet one could argue that education as a whole concerns authority figures changing children's brains. The issues are potentially emotive. For example, in the context of how much discretionary screen time children should have, Sigman (2019) argued for the precautionary principle: until we know the full impact of screen time on children's health and development, health care professionals should err on the side of caution and advise low limits. To ignore the precautionary approach of child health professions, Sigman says, 'promotes a hubristic picture of psychology and 'educational technology' researchers knowing better than the many paediatric and public health professionals what is best for protecting child health' (p. 926). Knowland takes a hypothetical but stark example to consider the question of cognitive enhancement. If we knew that neuromodulation was effective in enhancing cognition (e.g., via psychostimulants, such as Ritalin used to treat attention deficit hyperactivity disorder; or via transcranial electric stimulation of the brain) should we use it on children? Don't we have a duty to improve educational outcomes for kids? Out of fairness, shouldn't we then target such interventions to the least advantaged in society, to level the playing field? What of possible side effects? What of the fact that these kinds of interventions work for some kids but not for others? What age should we intervene—should we be using neuromodulation with infants, because their brains are more plastic? Or perhaps the pre-school years shouldn't be within the remit of educational neuroscience at all? The issues here are complex, as are our intuitions. In one study probing the attitudes of adults, any pharmacological enhancement to improve academic endeavours, employment, and personal relationships was deemed to be morally unacceptable—yet participants judged a hypothetical 'smart pill' to improve intelligence to be more morally wrong than taking a 'motivation pill' that would improve an individual's ability to work hard. The brain systems that the hypothetical pills targeted altered people's judgement of their moral worth!

Chapter 19 presents the view of teachers practising in the classroom. Bell and Darlington offer their view on all the preceding chapters. They consider why teachers should try to understand learning in the first place: 'the first reason for understanding learning and teaching,' say Bell and Darlington, 'is that we are the professionals; the people who have responsibility for a significant part of children's education . . . [we] need to keep up to date with new evidence on ways of improving the learning experience for all students' (p. 500). They step through how an understanding of learning might better inform practice, addressing the environment and context of learning, the process of learning, as well as emotional welfare and mental health. On the lifespan perspective, they say 'each setting and age range requires approaches based on sound principles and evidence . . . understanding the developmental changes that take place across the lifespan potentially has differing implications for individual teachers at each stage of education' (p. 498). They embrace Howard-Jones and colleagues' three categories of the learning process: engage, build, and consolidate, but also emphasise a fourth, the application and transfer of learning. Although the general pattern of near transfer does not augur well for automatic application of learning to new situations, the authors emphasise the potential of developing metacognitive skills alongside the domain-specific knowledge and skills, and identify a role for teachers in modelling transfer skills. They seek to identify concrete classroom activities that would capture the (now) four categories of learning. And finally, they identify half a dozen features of learning, and list questions for teachers to consider guiding reflection on practice.

In the concluding chapter, Chapter 20, the editors pull out the main themes of the volume, and look to the future of educational neuroscience. They in particular address two questions.

What's the Added Value of Neuroscience?

Part of the debate around the field of educational neuroscience is the added value of the neuroscience itself. Isn't behaviour the most important feature of education, that is, children's learning outcomes? How does the understanding of brain mechanisms help? What more does neuroscience add than is contributed by psychology? All the contributors to this volume were asked to finish their chapter with a consideration of just this question.

What's the Concrete Implication of Research for the Classroom?

Given that educational neuroscience is an intrinsically translational field, the second challenge posed to the authors was to identify the concrete implications of research and opportunities for translation in the classroom.

How well the authors answer these two questions is a good indicator of current progress in the field of educational neuroscience.

Notes

1. www.educationalneuroscience.org.uk/resources/neuromyth-or-neurofact/
2. Forty-winks = sleep. It turns out that there are few synonyms for sleep beginning with F!
3. www.howthebrainworks.science

References

Bishop, D. V. M. (2014). *What is educational neuroscience?* Retrieved from https://figshare.com/articles/What_is_educational_neuroscience_/1030405

Bowers, J. S. (2016). The practical and principled problems with educational neuroscience. *Psychological Review, 123*, 600–612.

Bronfenbrenner, U. (1992). Ecological systems theory. In U. Bronfenbrenner (Ed.), *Making human beings human: Bioecological perspectives on human development* (pp. 106–173). Thousand Oaks, CA: Sage Publications Ltd.

Bruer, J. T. (1999). *The myth of the first three years.* New York: The Free Press.

Cigman, R. (2009). Enhancing children. In R. Cigman & A. Davis (Eds.), *New philosophies of learning* (pp. 173–190). Oxford: Wiley-Blackwell.

Cigman, R., & Davis, A. (2009). The enhancement agenda. In R. Cigman & A. Davis (Eds.), *New philosophies of learning* (pp. 171–172). Oxford: Wiley-Blackwell.

Dougherty, M. R., & Robey, A. (2018). Neuroscience and education: A bridge astray? *Current Directions in Psychological Science, 27*(6), 401–406.

Dunlosky, J., Rawson, K. A., Marsh, E. J., Nathan, M. J., & Willingham, D. T. (2013). Improving students' learning with effective learning techniques: Promising directions from cognitive and educational psychology. *Psychological Science in the Public Interest, 14,* 4–58.

Farah, M. J., & Hook, C. J. (2013). The seductive allure of "seductive allure". *Perspectives on Psychological Science, 8*(1), 88–90.

Guttorm, T. K., Leppänen, P. H. T., Hämäläinen, J. A., Eklund, K. M., & Lyytinen, H. J. (2009). Newborn event-related potentials predict poorer pre-reading skills in children at risk for dyslexia. *Journal of Learning Disabilities, 43,* 391–401.

Howard-Jones, P., Varma, S., Ansari, D., Butterworth, B., De Smedt, B., Goswami, U., . . . Thomas, M. S. C. (2016). The principles and practices of educational neuroscience: Commentary on Bowers. *Psychological Review, 123,* 620–627.

Jones, E. G., & Mendell, L. M. (1999). Assessing the decade of the brain. *Science, 284,* 739.

Michie, S., van Stralen, M. M., & West, R. (2011). The behaviour change wheel: A new method for characterising and designing behaviour change interventions. *Implementation Science, 6,* 42.

Mireku, M. O., Barker, M. M., Mutz, J., Dumontheil, I., Thomas, M. S. C., Röösli, M., . . . Toledano, M. B. (2019). Night-time screen-based media device use and adolescents' sleep and health-related quality of life. *Environment International, 124,* 66–78.

Panawong Green, S. P. (2001). *A handful of leaves.* Bangkok, Thailand: Mental Health Publishing.

Pashler, H., McDaniel, M., Rohrer, D., & Bjork, R. (2009). Learning styles: Concepts and evidence. *Psychological Science in the Public Interest, 9*(3), 105–119.

Plomin, R. (2018). *Blueprint: How DNA makes us who we are.* London: Allen Lane.

Ritchie, S. J., & Tucker-Drob, E. M. (2018). How much does education improve intelligence? A meta-analysis. *Psychological Science, 29*(8), 1358–1369. doi:10.1177/095 6797618774253

Roediger, H. L. (2013). Applying cognitive psychology to education: Translational educational science. *Psychological Science in the Public Interest, 14,* 1–3.

Sala, G., Aksayli, N. D., Tatlidil, K. S., Tatsumi, T., Gondo, Y., & Gobet, F. (2019). Near and far transfer in cognitive training: A second-order meta-analysis. *Collabra: Psychology, 5*(1), 18. https://doi.org/10.1525/collabra.203

Scurich, N., & Shniderman, A. (2014). The selective allure of neuroscientific explanations. *PLoS One, 9*(9), e107529. doi:10.1371/journal.pone.0107529

Sigman, A. (2019, June). Invited commentary on "prospective associations between television in the preschool bedroom and later bio-psycho-social risks": Erring on the wrong side of precaution. *Pediatric Research, 85*(7), 925–926. doi:10.1038/s41390-019-0357-0. Epub March 5, 2019.

Simons, D. J., Boot, W. R., Charness, N., Gathercole, S. E., Chabris, C. F., Hambrick, D. Z., & Stine-Morrow, E. A. L. (2016). Do "brain-training" programs work? *Psychological Science in the Public Interest, 17,* 103–186.

Thomas, M. S. C. (2017). A scientific strategy for life chances. *The Psychologist, 30,* 22–26.

Thomas, M. S. C. (2019). Response to Dougherty and Robey (2018) on neuroscience and education: Enough bridge metaphors—interdisciplinary research offers the best hope for progress. *Current Directions in Psychological Science, 28*(4), 337–340. https://doi.org/10.1177/0963721419838252

Thomas, M. S. C., Ansari, D., & Knowland, V. C. P. (2019). Annual research review: Educational neuroscience: Progress and prospects. *Journal of Child Psychology and Psychiatry*, 60(4), 477–492. doi:10.1111/jcpp.12973

Weisberg, D. S., Keil, F. C., Goodstein, J., Rawson, E., & Gray, J. R. (2008). The seductive allure of neuroscience explanations. *Journal of Cognitive Neuroscience, 20*, 470–477.

Wild, C. J., Nichols, E. S., Battista, M. E., Stojanoski, B., & Owen, A. M. (2018, December). Dissociable effects of self-reported daily sleep duration on high-level cognitive abilities. *Sleep, 41*(12), zsy182. https://doi.org/10.1093/sleep/zsy182

Willetts, D. (2018). *A university education*. Oxford: Oxford University Press.

2 An Introduction to Brain and Cognitive Development

The Key Concepts You Need to Know

Iroise Dumontheil and Denis Mareschal

Educational Neuroscience asks how our understanding of brain function can inform our understanding of how pupils learn in the classroom and what lessons educational practitioners can take away from this. The following chapters will make reference to many concepts from the cognitive neurosciences. The aim of this chapter is to provide a quick primer of what the different parts of the brain are, how these work together and the factors that influence the way the brain develops, and consequently how behaviour emerges. We begin with an overview of the structural components of the brain. This is then followed by a concise summary of how different cognitive functions are implemented in the brain.[1] Next we discuss the early development of the brain and the neuroimaging methods that can be used to assess how functions emerge in the brain as an individual learns a new skill. Finally, we present a leading theoretical framework, called *Neuroconstructivism*, which encapsulates the key dimensions of brain and cognitive development.

What Is The Brain?

The brain is not the largest organ in our bodies; however, it is the organ that consumes the most energy, at 20% of the body's total energy use. The overall function of the brain is to take in information from our environment and our bodies and produce actions. At the small scale, the brain is composed of different types of cells, which communicate through electrical and chemical signals. At the large scale, the brain is divided into five lobes and the cerebellum.

Brain Cells

The most important brain cell type for cognition and learning is neurons. Although there are various types of neurons, their structure is relatively similar. The cell body contains the nucleus and is surrounded by branches called dendrites. A long arm called an axon allows the neuron to send information, in the form of an electrical signal called the action potential, to other neurons, which can be quite far away in a different part of the brain (Figure 2.1).

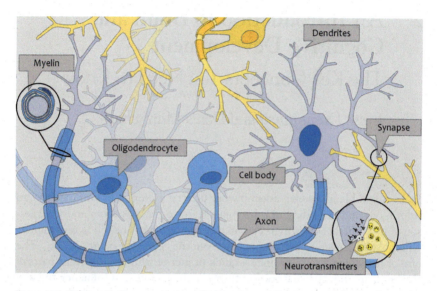

Figure 2.1 Schematic Representation of a Neuron and Supporting Oligodendrocytes.

The axon divides into branches, which end in synapses. At synapses, the cell membranes of two neurons are very close together—20–40 nanometres apart (for reference, the width of a human hair is 50,000 nanometres!). The incoming electrical signal from the presynaptic neuron leads to the release of neurotransmitters into the synaptic cleft. These neurotransmitters then bind to receptors on the membrane of the post-synaptic neuron and a series of chemical reactions leads to changes in the membrane potential of the dendrite of the post-synaptic neuron. Each neuron can receive input from thousands of other neurons, through on average 7,000 synaptic connections. If they pass a certain threshold, the changes in membrane potential occurring in the ensemble of dendrites of a neuron can lead to an action potential being sent into the axon.

Neurons make up 50% of brain cells. The other type of brain cells are glial cells, which support neurons through the provision of nutrients, maintenance of the ion balance outside the cells, repair, removal of damaged neurons or synapses, and removal of infectious agents. Oligodendrocytes and Schwann cells are glial cells that provide support and insulation to axons in the central (brain) and peripheral (body) nervous system respectively. Oligodendrocytes do this by wrapping axons in several layers of a myelin sheath (Figure 2.1), which is made of 80% lipid, i.e., fat. This insulates the neurons and allows a faster conduction of the electrical signals along the axons. As fat is white, this leads to the distinction between white matter and grey matter. White matter contains axons covered in myelin and some glial cells; grey matter contains neuronal cell bodies and glial cells. Grey matter is also called the cortex and is

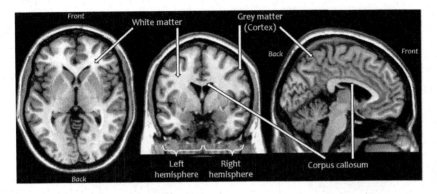

Figure 2.2 Brain Images. From left to right: axial, coronal and sagittal slices through an example structural magnetic resonance imaging scan.

the folded surface of the brain (Figure 2.2). Subcortical structures are located deeper in the brain, underneath the cortex.

Neurotransmitters

Information at the synapses is exchanged via neurotransmitters. More than 200 neurotransmitters have been identified. Most neurotransmitters are small chemical molecules. Neurotransmitters have been classified as *excitatory*, i.e., they make it more likely that the post-synaptic neuron will fire an action potential along its axon, or *inhibitory*, i.e., they make it less likely that the post-synaptic neuron will fire. The most common neurotransmitter is glutamate, which is excitatory at more than 90% of the synapses of the human brain. Next is gamma-aminobutyric acid (GABA), which is inhibitory at more than 90% of the synapses that do not use glutamate. Other neurotransmitters have often been studied in the context of cognition. Dopamine is involved in the reward system, in the control of movement and in the release of various hormones. Serotonin regulates mood, appetite and sleep and is involved in memory and learning. Norepinephrine (sometimes called noradrenaline) increases arousal and alertness, promotes vigilance and focused attention, can enhance memory and increase restlessness and anxiety.

Structural Organisation of the Brain

The folding of the cortex allows its large surface to fit within our skulls. A bump is called a gyrus; a trough is called a sulcus. While the folds of the cortex are unique in each individual, major folds and subdivisions of the brain are broadly consistent across humans. On the basis of these folds, each hemisphere of the brain has been divided into five lobes; each lobe is in turn

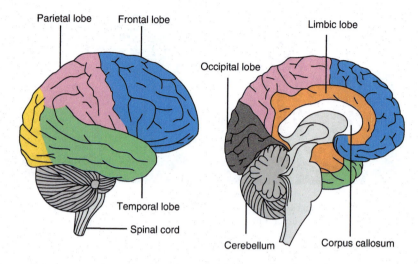

Figure 2.3 Division of the Brain Into Five Lobes and the Cerebellum. On the left is a view of the right side of the brain, on the right is a view of the middle of the brain, where it is split into two hemispheres, connected by a large white matter tract, the corpus callosum.

divided into major gyri and sulci (Figure 2.3). For example, the temporal lobe is divided into the superior, middle and inferior temporal gyri by the superior temporal sulcus and inferior temporal sulcus. These terms allow researchers to share an atlas of the brain and common terminology to compare and discuss their findings. The cortical regions of each hemisphere are connected by a number of white matter tracts (like bundles of cables). In addition, the left and right hemispheres are connected by the corpus callosum, a white matter tract that contains 200 million axons (Figures 2.2 and 2.3). Below the back of the two hemispheres lies the cerebellum. This brain structure has a different aspect and its neurons are organised differently from the rest of the brain.

How Are Behavioural Functions Organised in the Brain?

A key finding of neuropsychology and later cognitive neuroscience is that brain regions and networks of brain regions are specialised for particular cognitive functions. For example, a key function of the cerebellum is motor control—the regulation of movements, allowing us to perform precise, coordinated and timely actions but also to regulate our balance. Major brain networks that have been identified support social cognition, cognitive control, emotions and motivation, memory and language. Brain imaging techniques indicate that these networks show greater activation during experimental tasks involving these functions than during rest or when participants are asked to look at a fixation cross on the screen, and will be discussed in turn. Another network, which will not be discussed in detail, is the so-called default mode network, which tends to show greater activation during rest, or fixation, than during experimental tasks. The default mode network includes the ventral (underneath) and dorsal (on top) medial (middle) prefrontal cortex; the posterior (back) cingulate cortex and adjacent precuneus; and part of the lateral (side) parietal cortex. The function of this network is still debated but it may reflect the monitoring of bodily sensations and internal thoughts, including mind-wandering and self-referential mental activity, as well as the recollection of prior experiences (Raichle, 2015).

Social Cognition

The "social brain" is the network of brain regions supporting social cognition—how we process, store and use information about other people to influence our behaviour, feelings and social interactions (Frith & Frith, 2010; Van Overwalle, 2009). Social cognition includes the processing of faces, supported in part by the fusiform face area (FFA), a region located in the inferior temporal cortex at the bottom of the brain. The FFA is part of the visual processing stream and allows us to recognise the identity of human faces. More broadly the FFA is thought to support expert recognition of stimuli that have similar configurations. For example, the FFA has been found to be activated when car and bird experts identify cars and birds, respectively. Living bodies and movements are recognised by the posterior superior temporal sulcus (pSTS) (Figure 2.4).

The amygdala, part of the emotions and reward network discussed in the following, is involved in the recognition of emotion from faces. The medial prefrontal cortex and superior temporal sulcus (STS) receive input from visual and auditory cortices, which process sights and sounds respectively, and can read a person's feelings regardless of whether the emotional cues come from a face, body or voice. The medial prefrontal cortex and temporo-parietal junction are more broadly involved in mentalising, which is our ability to infer other people's thoughts, feelings and intentions based on their actions, utterances, tones and facial and body expressions. For example, having seen another child snatch a toy from our daughter, and seeing our daughter's mouth tremble, we can infer that she is distraught because of what happened. Another child may instead stand up and head towards us and we may infer they would like us to help them get their toy back.

Cognitive Control

Cognitive control is the ability to flexibly adapt one's behaviour in the pursuit of an internal goal by coordinating cognitive processes. Executive functions—as the "executive" in a company, who takes the important decisions—is another term for the cognitive processes we engage when we are faced with novel or unexpected situations where routine behaviours or automatic

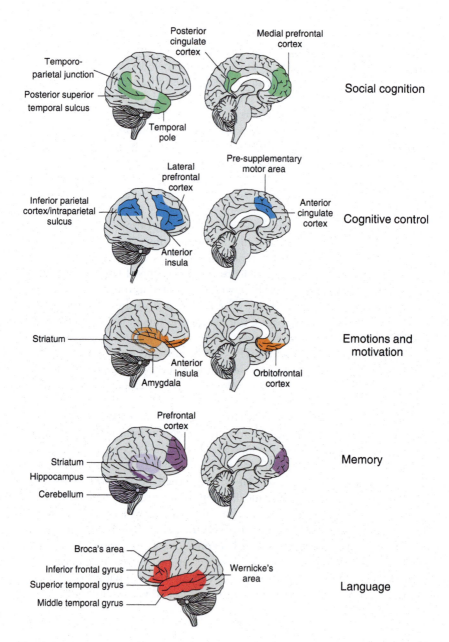

Figure 2.4 Brain Networks Supporting Broad Domains of Cognition: Social Cognition, Cognitive Control, Emotions and Motivation, Memory and Language. On the left: side views of the right hemisphere. On the right: view of the medial side of the left hemisphere. Note that these networks tend to show bilateral activation (i.e., symmetrical in both hemispheres), except the language network, which tends to be dominant in the left hemisphere (shown here is a side view of the left hemisphere).

thoughts are not appropriate. Whether cognitive control is a unique cognitive function or divided into a subset of functions is the subject of debate—perhaps there is a board rather than a single executive running the company (Duncan, 2010; Friedman & Miyake, 2017; Shallice, Stuss, Picton, Alexander, & Gillingham, 2008). A common network including the lateral prefrontal cortex, anterior insula, superior parietal cortex and intraparietal sulcus, and along the medial wall of the brain, the pre-supplementary motor area and anterior cingulate cortex (Figure 2.4) all show greater activity whenever people are asked to perform a challenging task than when they are asked to perform an easier task. Part of the role of this system is to maintain the current goals (e.g., the rules of the task) in mind, focus attention over a sustained period, and allow quick shifts of attention between different stimuli or task rules. It also allows a greater engagement of resources, and focus, when it is not clear what the response should be and more processing of the stimuli is needed.

Three basic executive functions have been proposed. *Inhibitory control* is the ability to stop an inappropriate dominant or automatic response and ignore distractions. Inhibitory control helps us stop crossing a road when a car is suddenly arriving, or ignore chatter when trying to read a book on the bus. *Working memory* is the ability to temporarily monitor, maintain and manipulate information in a mental workspace. It allows us to perform mental arithmetic and remember the start of a long sentence when we reach its end. *Shifting* is the ability to shift between mental states, rule sets or tasks, and to think flexibly. Shifting allows us to speak differently to our boss or our child. The respective abilities to sustain, divide or selectively orient attention are closely related cognitive processes, also implemented by the fronto-parietal network described earlier. More complex executive functions involve a combination of basic executive functions, for example planning or multitasking.

Emotions and Motivation

How do we decide on what goals we want to achieve? What distracts us from achieving our goals? Emotions and motivation come into play (Goschke & Bolte, 2014). There are various types of motivation: some are driven by physiological needs, like thirst and hunger, or the desire to interact socially with others. This type of motivation is associated with primary rewards. In addition, a distinction has also been proposed between *intrinsic motivation*, whereby the activity being performed is enjoyable in itself (e.g., gardening as a hobby), and *extrinsic motivation*, whereby an activity is performed to obtain a reward that is separate from the activity itself (e.g., mowing the lawn to get pocket money). A key driver of behaviour in humans and most animal species is to approach and maximise contact with rewarding stimuli and avoid harmful stimuli. The striatum, deep in the brain, and in particular the ventral striatum, is a vital element of the circuitry for decision making and reward-related behaviour (Figure 2.4). The striatum appears to act as a selector of the most appropriate behaviour to maximise gains/rewards/pleasurable outcomes, and minimise loss/harmful outcomes. One key neurotransmitter involved in reward-based decision making is dopamine; the striatum has the highest concentration of dopamine receptors in the brain.

The limbic system is a region of the brain underneath the cortex, comprised of several specialised structures, that deals with three key functions: emotions, memories and arousal/stimulation. The amygdala is a small structure within the limbic system that connects to the ventral striatum and can drive motivation towards rewarding stimuli. The amygdala also shows strong responses to stimuli that are associated with avoidance behaviours, such as fearful or angry faces, or pictures of snakes. The anterior insula, also part of the limbic system, is thought to play a role in the body experience associated with emotions (so-called "gut" feelings), as well as our self-awareness and our subjective experience of a wide range of emotions—e.g., maternal and romantic love, disgust, sadness, trust, empathy. Finally, the orbitofrontal cortex, which is located just above the eyes and connected to the striatum, may represent a mapping of the associations between actions and their expected emotional/reward outcomes in specific contexts (Stalnaker, Cooch, & Schoenbaum, 2015).

Memory

Memory is the retention of information over time to influence future actions. Research distinguishes between *declarative* or *explicit memory*, which can be consciously recalled, and *non-declarative* or *implicit memory*, which is unconscious. Declarative memory includes *semantic memory*, which corresponds to memories with specific meaning such as words, concepts, and their definitions. For example, I remember the word whale, and that it refers to a large sea mammal that was heavily hunted a few centuries ago. Declarative memory also includes *episodic memory*, which is the memory of events situated in time and space in a rich context. For example, I remember that I saw a whale on a boat off the coast of Iceland a few years ago, that I was slightly seasick on the way out and struggled to take good pictures of the whale. The hippocampus (Figure 2.4) within the limbic system is a key brain region supporting the formation of explicit memory. Memories themselves are stored throughout the cortex, with specific types of information stored in specialised brain regions. For example auditory memories are stored in the auditory cortex, which processes sounds; visual memories in the visual cortex, which processes sight; and spatial memories in the temporal lobes. The prefrontal cortex is involved in memory retrieval, and maintenance of the retrieved information in working memory for further processing. The prefrontal cortex, hippocampus and distributed cortical areas are further involved in memory consolidation, when a memory is revisited. The amygdala can be added to this system as providing an emotional component to memories and facilitating the formation of memories that have a high emotional content.

Non-declarative memory includes *priming*, when information we have unconsciously processed can influence our later actions, and *procedural memory*. Procedural memory refers to the slow and gradual learning of skills. Typical examples are learning how to drive a car or a bicycle. Once the skills have been mastered they are difficult to verbalise and are automatic in that they take very little conscious thought. Novice drivers consciously focus on changing gears, pressing the clutch at the right time, checking the mirrors and finding the indicators; they typically cannot hold a conversation at the same time. In contrast, expert drivers unconsciously perform all these actions and can talk or eat at the same time as they drive. The cerebellum, which we previously described as allowing fine control of movements, plays a key role in implicit memory formation (Figure 2.4).

Language

Broadly speaking, the language network includes both relatively functionally specialised brain regions and brain regions typically considered to be part of the cognitive control network (Fedorenko & Thompson-Schill, 2014; Thompson-Schill, Bedny, & Goldberg, 2005). A distinction has been made between three types of brain regions. Sensory language regions in the auditory and visual cortices respond both to stimuli that are meaningful (e.g., hearing or reading a word, like "boat") and stimuli that are meaningless (e.g., a pseudo-word, like "boak"). Overt speech articulation regions similarly can show activation when participants are asked to repeat non-words—in particular in the premotor cortex along the precentral gyrus (Price, 2010). Finally "higher-level" language-processing regions are those involved in phonological, lexical and combinatorial (e.g., syntax) processing (Fedorenko & Thompson-Schill, 2014). Within the language network some specialisation of function is observed. The middle temporal gyrus and angular gyrus show greater activation for words than non-words. Sentence comprehension shows activation in the middle temporal gyrus along the superior temporal sulcus. The resolution of semantic or syntactic ambiguity shows activation in the inferior frontal cortex and in the posterior superior temporal sulcus, in Wernicke's area. Finally, the inferior frontal cortex, including a region named the Broca's area, is also recruited during word retrieval (see Price, 2010 for review, and Figure 2.4).

Two key pathways have been proposed to support language processing. The dorsal pathway connects Wernicke's area and Broca's area via the premotor cortex through a long-range white matter tract called the arcuate fasciculus and through part of the superior longitudinal fasciculus; this pathway is assumed to support auditory-to-motor mapping that would, for example, allow you to repeat a word you have heard without understanding it. The ventral pathway connects the primary auditory cortex in the middle part of the superior temporal gyrus to the anterior superior temporal gyrus and then the inferior frontal cortex, via the uncinate fasciculus white matter tract, allowing auditory sentence comprehension (Friederici, 2012; Friederici & Gierhan, 2013).

Imaging Brain Development

Structural Brain Imaging

Magnetic resonance imaging (MRI) allows the non-invasive study of the human brain. Participants are asked to lie down inside a scanner shaped like a vertical doughnut, with their head in the hole of the doughnut and their body mostly out of it. Through a system of mirrors participants can see a screen displaying stimuli and are given buttons to answer. The doughnut is in fact a superconductive magnet with a strength of 1.5 to 7 teslas, ~ 100 times the strength of the Earth's magnetic field. MRI is completely safe as long as participants do not have metal in or on their body (e.g., braces, insulin pump). It can therefore be used with participants of all ages, and the same participants can be scanned several times. This allows, for example, to track the structural development of the brain over time, including changes in grey and white matter volumes, in children, adolescents and young adults, but also in aging. One key constraint of MRI is that participants need to stay very still while they are being scanned, which is very difficult for 2–5-year olds—infants can be trained to stay still by sleeping through a scanning session. This means there is limited MRI data on toddlers. Two main approaches have been used to study brain structure development across the lifespan. The first method, structural MRI, provides information about grey and white matter, the thickness and folding of the cortex and the volume of sub-cortical region. The second method, diffusion tensor imaging (DTI) is a different MRI technique, which allows a more detailed study of the structural properties of white matter tracts, as it were, the cabling of the brain.

Structural MRI data can be collected in a single scan taking 5–10 min. Participants do not have to do anything apart from keeping their head still; they can close their eyes and relax or watch a short movie. Structural MRI records changes in the orientation of protons in the brain when the surrounding magnetic field is repeatedly changed during scanning. The changes in orientation of the protons depend on the tissue they are in, which allows researchers to distinguish and study the properties of white and grey matter and subcortical structures (see Figure 2.2 for an example structural image). Coincidentally on these images white matter appears white, and grey matter grey. These images can be acquired at a resolution of $1 \times 1 \times 1$ mm^3, the size of a grain of sugar, and new types of scanners and scanning sequences can give an even higher spatial resolution, i.e., the ability to see smaller details. Various statistical techniques can be used to separate grey and white matter to calculate their respective volume, or to measure the thickness and surface area of the cortex. However, one significant hurdle in MRI research is that, although the general organisation of the brain previously described is consistent between people, there are significant differences in the shape and size of the brains of different individuals. This is in part due to the fact that the brain pretty much fills up the space within the skull, so if someone has an overall larger skull, their brain is likely to be larger, but if their skull is narrow and high, or very round, the shape of the brain will also differ. This means that for statistical analyses to be performed on groups of participants, or compared between studies, the structural brain images need to be stretched or shrunk to match a common template. Unfortunately, these transformations are not perfect, which means that some degree of spatial detail is lost.

Post-mortem studies have shown that in the first few months and years after birth, brain volume and the number of dendrites and synapses increase rapidly (Huttenlocher & Dabholkar, 1997). Structural MRI data has shown that the thickness of the cortex, or the amount of grey matter in the cortex, then decreases during childhood, adolescence and early adulthood (Mills et al., 2016), and that the timing of this decrease is region-specific. Notably, the frontal lobes, which support cognitive control, and the temporal lobes, which support social cognition (Figure 2.4), undergo the most protracted development, with significant changes occurring during adolescence (Gogtay et al., 2004; Shaw et al., 2008). These changes are thought to reflect in part the process of synaptic pruning, whereby infrequently used connections between neurons are eliminated, allowing the developing brain to fine-tune to the individual's experiences and their environment, optimising the circuits of most use. While cortical thinning is thought to be adaptive, leading to more efficient brain functioning, anomalies in this neural developmental process may underlie developmental disorders such as attention deficit and hyperactivity disorder (ADHD), where delayed cortical thinning is observed, especially in the frontal lobes (Shaw et al., 2007) and schizophrenia, which is associated with accelerated cortical thinning during adolescence and early adulthood (Penzes, Cahill, Jones, VanLeeuwen, & Woolfrey, 2011). While most studies have focused on studying developmental changes in the cortex, the development of subcortical regions involved in the processing of emotions and rewards, and aspects of memory, has also been investigated (Figure 2.4). The amygdala and hippocampus increase in volume during adolescence, while regions of the striatum show decreases in volume during adolescence; importantly, these developmental changes have been found to be driven by a combination of age and pubertal stage, suggesting that the hormonal changes associated with puberty during adolescence impact the development of subcortical structures (Goddings et al., 2014).

While structural MRI can provide information about total or regional white matter volume, diffusion tensor imaging can provide more detailed information about white matter tracts. Diffusion tensor imaging measures the predominant direction of movement of protons in the brain. As axons are covered in myelin, a fatty substance, protons from water molecules are less likely to move across axons and white matter tracts (think of oil vs. vinegar) than to move along them. If protons move very consistently in one direction, this indicates that the white matter tracts in this region have high axonal diameter and/or high myelination. In addition, diffusion tensor images can be analysed to reconstruct the white matter tracts of an individual's brain. Longitudinal structural MRI and DTI studies have shown that there is an increase in white matter volumes until the mid-twenties, reflecting increases in axon diameter and myelination (Lebel & Beaulieu, 2011; Mills et al., 2016). These changes allow faster exchange of information across brain networks with increasing age, for example, as shown in faster motor responses from childhood to adulthood. Like grey matter changes, white matter changes are region- or tract-specific, with some tracts showing more prolonged increases in *fractional anisotropy*—a DTI measure thought to reflect increased myelination—into the twenties, than other tracts which stabilise earlier (Lebel & Beaulieu, 2011). White matter developmental structural changes also show significant variation between individuals (Lebel & Beaulieu, 2011). However it is not clear at this point what would be the characteristics of "optimal" brain development, if this exists.

Beyond development, structural MRI studies have also investigated whether differences in grey and white matter volumes or cortical thickness are associated with individual differences in cognitive skills. There is, for example, evidence of lower grey matter volumes in the intraparietal sulcus, the brain region supporting numerical magnitude comparison and arithmetic discussed earlier, in children with developmental dyscalculia (Ansari, 2008). While there are a number of studies investigating such individual differences, it is still unclear at present whether more or less grey matter is optimal (Kanai & Rees, 2011). Less grey matter may reflect a more efficient, mature cortex, while more grey matter may reflect increased processing power. As another example, although previous research is inconsistent (Moreau, Stonyer, McKay, & Waldie, 2018), a recent study has shown that pre-school children who later develop dyslexia show pre-reading white matter anomalies in the left arcuate fasciculus—the tract connecting Wernicke's area, which supports language comprehension, in the posterior temporal lobe and Broca's area, which supports language expression, in the inferior frontal lobe (Figure 2.4, Vanderauwera, Wouters, Vandermosten, & Ghesquière, 2017).

Functional Brain Imaging

Functional MRI (fMRI) uses the same scanner as structural MRI and can be collected during the same testing session. fMRI allows the study of brain activity, recorded while participants are performing a task while they lie in the scanner. fMRI is an indirect measure of brain activity in that it measures changes in blood oxygenation and blood flow associated with changes in neural processing of nearby neuronal populations. When neurons receive more synaptic input via their synapses, the post-synaptic chemical reactions and changes in electrical potentials in the dendrites consume energy, i.e., glucose and oxygen. As the brain does not store any oxygen and very little glucose, a series of signals lead to increases in local blood flow to bring more glucose and oxygen to the activated neuronal populations. Unfortunately, the changes in blood flow and oxygenation are slow and peak around 5 seconds after the neuronal activity. This means that while fMRI has a very good spatial resolution (data is typically recorded for units, called voxels, of $3 \times 3 \times 3$ mm^3), it has poor time resolution: it cannot easily identify the order in which brain regions are activated after a stimulus is presented.

fMRI has been used to study most cognitive functions and helped identify the networks introduced earlier (Figure 2.4). In terms of development, the pattern of changes in activation during childhood and adolescence is mixed and depends on the experimental task used and the aspect of cognition investigated. Similar to structural MRI, it is not clear whether lower or higher activity in a brain region in a specific task reflects more optimal, or more mature, functioning. fMRI can be used with a wide range of participants as long as they are able to stay still for 5–10 minutes at a time while they are carrying out a cognitive task. However, the conditions inside the scanner can be claustrophobic and scary for young children or individuals with mental health problems. Even though movement is minimised, differences in movement between age groups (e.g., children and adults, or children with ADHD and typical children) can still impact on our ability to interpret brain activity differences between these groups.

While fMRI has predominantly been used to study brain activation in specific regions in different tasks, more recently novel approaches have been used to assess the extent to which these brain regions work together, their *functional connectivity*. This has been studied during the performance of experimental tasks, but mostly during rest, i.e., when participants are asked to not think about anything in particular and keep their eyes on a fixation cross or just close them. *Resting state functional connectivity* studies which brain regions seem to show similar fluctuations in activation over a period of 5–10 minutes during rest. Networks of regions where activity increases and decreases in concert can be identified. Interestingly, these analyses reveal the networks found to be activated during task performance (Figure 2.4), as well as the default mode network. The assumption is that brain regions that are part of a functional network and have strong structural (white matter tracts) connectivity will tend to show similar fluctuations of activity over time. Resting state functional connectivity has been used to study the development of brain functional networks and overall suggests that there is an increase in long-range functional connectivity and a decrease in short-range functional connectivity, giving rise to broader networks encompassing different lobes (e.g., Vogel, Power, Petersen, & Schlaggar, 2010). One issue, however, is that functional connectivity measures are affected by movement, so careful analyses need to be performed to make sure that differences—e.g., between age groups—are not due to differences in movement inside the scanner (Satterthwaite et al., 2012).

Electroencephalography (EEG) is another non-invasive cognitive neuroscience approach allowing the measurement of brain function. In contrast to fMRI, EEG has poor spatial resolution but a good temporal resolution, of the order of milliseconds, which means it allows researchers to identify the temporal sequence of cognitive processes. For example, using EEG can tell us how quickly people can distinguish between words and non-words (random combination of letters). EEG measures the electrical potential at the surface of the scalp using electrodes enclosed in something resembling a bathing cap, or arranged in a net for high density recordings (e.g., with 128 electrodes—channels—or more). Electrical potential on the scalp reflects the sum of the membrane potentials along dendrites of a particular type of neurons, pyramidal neurons, which are aligned and perpendicular to the cortex. As these neurons are aligned, their electrical potentials are summed over many neurons, which leads to a signal large enough to be detected on the scalp (albeit measured in microvolts).

Two main approaches have been used to study brain function using EEG. The first one separates the fluctuations of the electrical signal over time into different frequencies (alpha, beta, etc.)— "brainwaves"— and assesses which frequencies are dominant (i.e., have greater power) when participants are carrying out specific cognitive functions (e.g., attending to movements or locations) or in different states of arousal (e.g., alert, distracted, asleep). These frequencies are taken to reflect the concerted signalling between populations of neurons.

The second approach involves the identification of event-related potentials (ERPs). ERPs are calculated by averaging the fluctuations in the electrical signal after stimulus presentation, or a response, across many trials to maximise detection of a consistent neural response and remove noise. EEG has been recorded for close to a century and over the years specific fluctuations in ERPs—"components"—have been associated with specific cognitive processes. For example, a negative inflection in the ERPs around 170 milliseconds after presentation of a stimulus (called the N170) has been associated with the processing of faces compared to other visual stimuli, and is sensitive to whether faces are upright or inverted, or to their emotional expression. When EEG data are collected in many electrodes, statistical analyses can allow some limited inferences regarding where the signal being measured comes from. The source of the N170 is in the posterior temporal lobe, including the fusiform gyrus, where the fusiform face area is located (see *Social brain* section above). EEG is significantly cheaper than MRI and is more mobile. It can therefore be used with infants, toddlers (who can sit on their parents' lap) and children, as well as older participants. Comparisons between age groups, however, is not easy because the EEG signal is affected by the size of the brain and the size and thickness of the skull, in addition to any developmental changes in neural processing. In part because of the low levels of myelination, neural processing is slower in children, which makes it difficult to identify and link findings to ERP patterns observed in adults.

Brain Stimulation

fMRI and EEG allow researchers to track activity in the brain, to study associations between brain and behaviour and to assess the temporal nature of these relationships. However, these studies are correlational, and cannot provide any certainty regarding whether activity in a particular brain region *causes* a particular cognitive function. This limits our ability to understand the mechanisms of brain and cognitive functions. Neuropsychology, the study of the impact of brain lesions on cognition, has a long history and was instrumental in building our early understanding of brain organisation, such as the left lateralisation of the language network (e.g., Broca's and Wernicke's brain regions were identified in 1861 and 1874, respectively). However, there are a number of limitations to lesion studies, most of all the fact that patients are rare and there is very little control over the location of brain damage. In addition, brain plasticity can lead to compensation, whereby a cognitive function initially lost because of a brain lesion is later recovered. By contrast, brain stimulation techniques use magnetic or electrical stimulation in healthy people to interfere or enhance electrical neuronal processing in specific brain regions to study consequences on cognition. Two non-invasive stimulation techniques are transmagnetic stimulation (TMS) and transcranial direct current stimulation (tDCS).

TMS uses a figure of eight magnetic coil positioned above a specific brain region to induce a local electric field and interfere with neural processing in the underlying cortex. This technique can be used on a trial-by-trial basis and be implemented at very specific times after the presentation of a stimulus, to assess when a particular brain region may be necessary for cognitive processing. Alternately, TMS can be used in a repetitive manner for 5–15 minutes before participants perform an experimental task. TMS has been used, for example, to demonstrate that the visual cortex is organised in a modular manner, with specific regions specialised for the recognition of objects, faces, and bodies (Pitcher, Charles, Devlin, Walsh, & Duchaine, 2009). One limit of TMS is that the equipment is costly and not easily transportable. A recently developed alternative, tDCS, is still in its relatively early days, but is advantageous because it is much cheaper and more portable than TMS. tDCS uses constant, low direct current delivered via electrodes on the head and leads to changes in the resting membrane potential of neurons. This can change neuronal excitability and has been proposed to lead to long-term changes in neuronal function. tDCS has been used to treat depression and for cognitive enhancement. However, at this stage the evidence is inconclusive regarding whether it is useful in healthy people (e.g., Horvath, Forte, & Carter, 2015), or in certain disorders, and there are likely significant individual differences in the effect of electric stimulation (Fertonani & Miniussi, 2017).

The Developing Brain

In this section, we provide an overview of the factors involved in brain development. A more detailed account can be found in Johnson and De Haan (2015) or Mareschal et al. (2007). We first describe how the brain develops in the uterus, before turning our attention to the forces that help shape the postnatal development of brain functions.

The events that go toward building our brains are very similar to those observed in other mammals except that the time schedule over which these events occur is significantly slower in humans. This slower timetable has two major consequences. The first of these is that there is a prolonged period of brain development postnatally, so that the latter stages of brain development can be influenced by the individual's interaction with their environment. The second consequence is that changing the timetable of neural development also changes the relative size of different parts of the human brain as compared to other species. In general, the more delayed the time course of development is in a given species, the larger the relative volume of the late developing structures (such as the cerebral cortex, and particularly the frontal cortex). Consequently, the slowed rate of development in humans leads to the emergence of a relatively larger volume of cortex, and an especially large frontal cortex, compared to other species.

Very early brain development can be summarised in terms of three stages in the life-course of a single neuron. First, neurons are *born*. Second, they travel, or *migrate*, from the place of their birth to their final locations in the brain. Third, they *differentiate*, or take up their final form/shape. A few weeks after conception the human embryo develops a structure called the neural tube that will eventually transform into the different parts of the human brain. Neurons are born along the inner surface of the tube and then need to migrate to their final locations in the developing brain. Cells that will contribute to the cerebral cortex are formed around 6–18 weeks after conception. Neurons migrate from the location where they are born to arrive at the particular region where they will be used in the mature brain. In the cerebral cortex, neurons find their way to the correct position by moving along the long fibres of radial *glial cells*. This process is called active migration and creates an "inside-to-outside" pattern in which the newest cells move past older cells towards the surface of the brain to find their appropriate position. This pattern of migration eventually creates the distinctive layered structure of the cerebral cortex. Some other parts of the brain are formed by passive migration in which the most recently born neurons simply push their older cousins further away from the location where they were all born.

Once neurons have migrated to their final positions, they begin to differentiate or take on their mature shape and form. One aspect of differentiation is growth and branching of dendrites. The dendrites of a neuron are like antennae that pick up signals from many other neurons and, if the circumstances are right, pass the signal down the axon and on to other neurons (Figure 2.1). The pattern of branching of dendrites is important because it affects the amount and type of signals the neuron receives. During development, one change that occurs is an increase in size and complexity of neurons' dendritic trees. For example, by adulthood the length of the dendrites of neurons in the frontal cortex can increase over thirty times their length at birth. A second aspect of differentiation that occurs in most neurons is myelination. As discussed in the opening sections of this chapter, a myelin sheath forms around the axons of neurons. This occurs before birth and continues for many years, even into adulthood in some areas of the cortex. When formation of myelin is delayed, it can cause a delay in development. For example, in the motor cortex, delayed myelination is associated with delayed acquisition of motor milestones such as crawling and walking. The generation of synapses (synaptogenesis) occurs at different times in different cortical areas. For example, the maximum density of synapses is reached at about 4 months in the visual cortex but not until about 24 months in the prefrontal cortex (Huttenlocher & Dabholkar, 1997).

At the same time that the brain is growing and increasing in size and complexity, regressive events are also occurring. For example, it is estimated that 20–50% of neurons die during development in a process called programmed cell death (Cowan, Fawcett, O'Leary, & Stanfield, 1984; Oppenheim, 1991). Such neuronal death occurs prenatally during migration and during differentiation as part of a gene-expression–related program. Neurons may die during normal prenatal development because of errors in cell division, because they were only temporarily needed, or to eliminate surplus neurons. Broadly, however, humans are born with all of the neurons that will serve them throughout life, with the exception of some limited generation of new neurons in the hippocampus (the functional consequences of which are still debated). Neurons can live as long as the individual, but can also die through diseases (e.g., Parkinson's, Huntington's, Alzheimer's), blows to the brain, or spinal cord injury.

Another regressive event that occurs during brain development is the elimination of synapses. During the process of synapse formation, the number of synapses increases beyond the level observed in adults and remains at this level for some time. Then, synapses are eliminated until the typical adult number of synapses is reached. For example, in certain parts of the visual cortex, the density of synapses per neuron reaches a peak of around 150% of the adult level at about 4 months, then starts to decrease at the end of the first year of life to reach the adult level by about 4 years (e.g., Huttenlocher, 1990). The timing of this process is different for different areas of cortex. In the frontal cortex, the peak level is reached at about 1 year, and then slowly declines to reach adult levels sometime in adolescence. This loss of synapses does not cause a loss of behaviours but instead is thought to be related to the development or stabilization of behaviours.

In adults, the brain has a very specific pattern of branching of dendrites and synapses between cells. This involves a larger number of cells and connections—there are about 10^{11} neurons that make up the brain, each with 10^3 connections. This specificity is achieved partly through selective "pruning", allowing useful connections to remain and eliminating surplus ones. This is how the experience can influence the specialisation of the brain. This type of learning is thought to happen only at certain points in development—in adults, learning is usually related to an increase or modification of existing synapses rather than a loss of synapses.

While some developmental processes can be traced from pre- to postnatal life, in postnatal development there is obviously more scope for influence from the world outside the infant. This need not be a passive process, but rather may reflect the actions of the infant within her environment. A striking feature of human brain development is the comparatively long phase of postnatal development, and therefore the increased extent to which the later stages of brain development can be influenced by the environment of the child.

A controversial issue is the extent to which the differentiation of the cerebral cortex into areas or regions with particular cognitive, perceptual, or motor functions can be shaped by postnatal interactions with the external world. This issue reflects the debate in cognitive development about whether infants are born with domain-specific "modules" for particular cognitive functions such as language, or whether the formation of such modules is an activity-dependent process (discussed in more detail next). Recent advances in brain imaging techniques have provided us with an unprecedented window into the functional development of the brain.

Brodmann (1908) was one of the first to propose a scheme for the division of the cortex into structural areas assumed to have differing functional properties. A century of neuropsychology has taught us that the majority of normal adults tend to have similar functions within approximately the same regions of cortex (e.g., Figure 2.4). However, we cannot necessarily infer from this that this pattern of differentiation is intrinsically pre-specified (the product of genetic and molecular interactions), because most humans share very similar pre- and postnatal environments. In developmental neurobiology, this issue has emerged as a debate about the relative importance of neural activity for cortical differentiation, as opposed to intrinsic molecular and genetic specification of cortical areas. Supporting the importance of the latter molecular and genetic processes, Rakic (1988) proposed that the differentiation of the cortex into areas is due to a protomap or blueprint. The hypothesised protomap either involves pre-specification of the tissue that gives rise to the cortex during prenatal life or the presence of intrinsic molecular markers specific to particular areas of cortex. An alternative viewpoint, advanced by O'Leary and Stanfield (1989) among others, is that genetic and molecular factors build an initially undifferentiated "protocortex", and that this is subsequently divided into specialised areas as a result of neural activity, as regions compete to take on functions and when successful, inhibit their competitors. This activity within neural circuits need not necessarily be the result of input from the external world, but may result from intrinsic, spontaneous patterns of firing within sensory organs or subcortical structures that feed into the cortex, or indeed from activity within the cortex itself (e.g., Katz & Shatz, 1996).

Although the neurobiological evidence is complex, and probably differs between species and regions of cortex, overall it tends to support the importance of neural activity-dependent processes (see Mareschal et al., 2007, and described in the next section). With several exceptions, it seems likely that activity-dependent processes contribute to the differentiation of functional areas of the cortex, especially those involved in higher cognitive functions in humans. During prenatal life, this neural activity may be largely a spontaneous intrinsic process, while in postnatal life it is likely also to be influenced by sensory and motor experience. However, it is unlikely that the transition from spontaneous intrinsic activity to that influenced by sensory experience is a sudden occurrence at birth, for in the womb, the infant can process sounds and generate movement, and in postnatal life the brain maintains spontaneously generated intrinsic electrical rhythms (EEG).

Turning to education-relevant skills, it is worth noting that the developmental processes that produce the specialised functional networks described here were shaped over the course of evolutionary time. Properties were selected to permit adaptive functions in the environments of those times, such as allowing members of the species to act to obtain rewarding goals and avoid harm, to remember their previous experiences and to interact with each other. Very recent cultural changes have led to the teaching and learning of literacy and numeracy during schooling in what are, from this perspective, evolutionarily novel environments. Interestingly, brain activations when people are reading words or solving simple arithmetic problems are remarkably consistent across the population, even though our brains have not evolved to read or do mathematics. Instead we capitalise on the particular strengths and connectivity of specific brain regions to carry out reading or mathematics, in what has been called "neuronal recycling" (Dehaene & Cohen, 2011). The circuits with the most appropriate functions are repurposed through practice to take on these new cultural abilities.

In the case of literacy, reading requires the fast recognition of small visual stimuli. Across various scripts it has been shown that adults show increased activity in a region of the fusiform gyrus named the visual word form area when they are processing words, apparently recycling brain areas that had evolved to process objects and faces (Dehaene & Cohen, 2011). The intraparietal lobule is thought to support the conversion from orthography to phonology and semantics, while the rest of the reading network encompasses language-related regions in the left hemisphere supporting semantic representation (middle temporal gyrus), phonological representation (superior temporal gyrus) and semantic, syntactic and phonological processing (inferior frontal gyrus) (Cao, 2016).

In the case of numeracy, current theories suggest that cultural number symbols ("2", "two") acquire their meaning by being mapped on non-symbolic representations of numerical magnitude that are also observed in infants and in other species such as chimpanzees, in the intraparietal sulcus (Ansari, 2008). The visual number forms themselves, similarly to words, are thought to be processed in both hemispheres in the fusiform gyrus, before being transformed into numerical magnitudes in the intraparietal sulcus, which supports comparison and subtraction processes. Simple multiplications, which are learned by heart, are stored as verbal representations in the left angular gyrus, a brain region associated with complex language function (Dehaene, Molko, Cohen, & Wilson, 2004).

Neuroconstructivism: A Framework for Understanding Brain and Cognitive Development

Neuroconstructivism (Mareschal et al., 2007; Westermann et al., 2007) is a relatively recent theory that unifies a Piagetian, constructivist approach to cognitive development with our current understanding of functional brain development. It views the development of functional brain systems as heavily constrained by multiple interacting factors that are both intrinsic and extrinsic to the developing child. In other words, cognitive development occurs in the context of the constraints operating on the development of the brain that span multiple levels of analysis: from genes and the individual cell to the physical and social environment of the developing child.

By taking seriously constraints on all levels, from the gene to the environment, neuroconstructivism integrates different views of brain and cognitive development such as (1) probabilistic epigenesis, which emphasises the interactions between experience and gene expression in shaping development (Gottlieb, 1992), (2) neural constructivism, which focuses on the experience-dependent elaboration of small-scale neural structures (Quartz, 1999; Quartz & Sejnowski, 1997), (3) the *interactive specialisation* view of brain development, which stresses the role of interactions between different brain regions in functional brain development (Johnson, 2000), (4) embodiment views, which highlight the role of the physical body in cognitive development (e.g., Clark, 1999), (5) the constructivist approach to cognitive development (Piaget, 1955), with its focus on the proactive acquisition of knowledge, and (6) approaches focusing on the role of the social environment for the developing child. We briefly discuss each of these constraints in turn, to give a sense of how the theory seeks to integrate our understanding of cognitive development with neuroscience and biology.

Genes

The traditional view of gene function holds that there is a one-directional flow of cause and effect from genes (DNA) to RNA to the structure of proteins they encode.[2] From this perspective, development consists in the progressive unfolding of information that is laid out in the genome. However, more recent research presents a subtler picture by showing that environmental and behavioural influences play a fundamental role in triggering the expression of genes. This probabilistic epigenesist view of development (Gottlieb, 1992) emphasises that gene activity, instead of following a strictly pre-programmed, deterministic schedule, is regulated by signals from the external and internal environment. Development is therefore subject to bidirectional interactions between gene activity, neural activity, behavior, and the environment. For example, in canaries and zebra finches, a gene involved in regulating synaptic plasticity and learning has been found to be closely related to experience. The motor activity involved in singing has been shown to lead to a rapid increase of expression of this gene in motor areas, whereas hearing song induces expression of the same gene in parts of auditory areas (Jarvis et al., 1997). Furthermore, researchers found the amount of expression varied with the specific songs that were experienced: it was greatest when birds heard songs of their own species and lower for songs from other species (Mello, Vicario, & Clayton, 1992). These results show that gene expression can be influenced in very specific ways by experience with the environment.

Encellment

The development of a neuron is constrained by its cellular environment throughout development. Even at the earliest stages of foetal development, the way in which a particular cell develops is influenced by molecular interactions with its neighbouring cells (Jessell & Sanes, 2000). At later stages of development, neural activity, either spontaneously generated or derived from sensory experience, begins to play an important part in the formation of neural networks. Neural activity is responsible both for the progressive elaboration of neural connection patterns, as well as for their subsequent stabilisation and loss (neural constructivism; Quartz & Sejnowski, 1997). The remodelling of axonal and dendritic branches can occur rapidly with progressive and regressive events occurring in parallel (Hua & Smith, 2004). A higher rate of structural elaboration compared with retraction leads to a gradual overall increase in network complexity. The specific role of neural activity in the formation of neural networks has been extensively studied in the development of ocular dominance columns (ODC). ODC are areas of primary visual cortex (arranged in stripes or patches) where neurons selectively respond to inputs from only one eye. The initial formation of these columns is likely to be dependent on pre- and postnatal spontaneously generated neural activity (Feller & Scanziani, 2005). During a subsequent critical period, altered visual experience can lead to changes in ODC organisation. For example, transiently closing one eye during early postnatal development over several days results in shrinking of the columns responding to the closed eye and expansion of the columns responding to the open eye (Antonini & Stryker, 1993; Hubel & Wiesel, 1963). These results suggest that activity-based competition between neurons for synaptic connections is a driving mechanism in the establishment of precise connection patterns (Stryker & Strickland, 1984).

Embrainment

As the brain is embedded in a body (embodiment), so an individual functional brain region is embedded in a brain where it co-develops with other brain regions. This embrainment view contrasts with a modular perspective, which focuses on the development and functioning of specialised brain areas in isolation. It is supported by neuroimaging studies suggesting that the functional properties of a brain region are strongly context sensitive and constrained by its interactions with other regions, for example through feedback processes and top-down interactions (Friston & Price, 2001). Examples for the importance of interregional interactions in brain development can be found in studies with people who lack one sensory modality. For example, in people blind from an early age, the cortical area activated by Braille reading corresponds to the primary visual cortex in sighted people (Sadato et al., 1996). Therefore, brain regions that normally process visual information can take on a different functional role in the absence of visual input. This *interactive specialisation* view (Johnson, 2000) implies that cortical regions might initially be non-specific in their response but gradually sharpen their responses as their functional specialisation restricts them to a narrower set of circumstances.

Embodiment

The mind exists within a body that is itself embedded in a physical and social environment. This fact both constrains and enhances the experiences of a developing child. Neural activation patterns are generated by sensory inputs, and therefore the functioning of the sensory organs has a highly constraining effect on the construction of representations in the mind. In this sense the body acts as a filter for information from the environment. Two examples for this body-as-filter aspect of embodiment are the limited visual acuity and the limited motor control of the young infant. These restrict the infant's possible sensory experiences (what is looked at, what is seen) and thus limit the potential complexity of representations at this developmental stage. It has been argued that the gradual loosening of physical restrictions might be beneficial to allow for an orderly developmental trajectory with a gradual increase in the perceived complexity of the environment and resulting progressively complex representations (Turkewitz & Kenny, 1982).

However, the developing body not only serves as a filter for information, but also as a means to manipulate the environment and to generate new sensory inputs and experiences. For example, even newborn infants will intentionally move their arm into a light beam, resulting in an illuminated spot on the limb that is not visible unless the limb is moved to the correct location (van der Meer & van der Weel, 1995). The reward for seeing the light spot completes a feedback loop between the infant and her environment, changing this environment to generate specific sensory inputs. At later ages, infants use their increased mobility and sensorimotor coordination to explore and manipulate their environment further, generating ever more sensory inputs which in turn lead to the modification of neural networks and to the construction of more complex representations

The embodiment view emphasises that a proactive approach to exploring the environment is a core aspect of development: The child does not passively absorb information, but through manipulating the environment, selects the experiences from which to learn. It also shows that what can be called the "classic" model of cognition—the mind acquiring rich representations of the external world, operating off-line on these representations, and generating an output—neglects the important aspect of real-time interactions with a changing world. An embodied alternative to the classic view emphasises multiple real-time adjustments to the coupled brain—body—environment system to coordinate between inner and outer worlds (Kleim, Vij, Ballard, & Greenough, 1997).

Ensocialment

The specific environment in which the developing child is situated has a highly constraining effect on the emergence of neural representations because it restricts the possible experiences of the child and offers to her certain ways in which it can be manipulated. These constraints refer mainly to the physical properties of the environment. Another source of constraints concerns the social aspects of the environment, for example the interactions between a caregiver and her child. It has long been recognised that synchronous interactions between mother and child have a strong effect on the development of a secure attachment, the expression of emotions, social and cognitive development (Harrist & Waugh, 2002). By contrast, disrupting a normal mother–infant relationship and exposure to early stressors such as death of a caregiver, child abuse or neglect can have profound effects on the neural and behavioural development of the infant (Cirulli, Berry, & Alleva, 2003; Kaufman, Plotsky, Nemeroff, & Charney, 2000).

Conclusion

Brain function and development is a highly complex and interactive process where constraints operating at multiple levels of description all come together. Although a biological level of description can sometimes be very far from the behaviour that an educational practitioner is interested in, understanding the systems that underlie this behaviour can also help us understand how they are shaped by the many sources of constraints that exist in the child's environment.

External resources

White matter tracts: www.dtiatlas.org/
Video about TMS: www.youtube.com/watch?v=XJtNPqCj-iA
Prof. Michael S. C. Thomas's online resource giving a brief, non-technical overview of how the brain works for a general audience: http://howthe brainworks.science/
The brain from top to bottom online resource: http://thebrain.mcgill.ca/ avance.php

Notes

1. For a non-technical introduction to how the brain works, see here: www.howthe brainworks.science/
2. The chapter by Donati and Meaburn offers an excellent introduction to the key principles of genetics.

References

Ansari, D. (2008). Effects of development and enculturation on number representation in the brain. *Nature Reviews Neuroscience, 9*(4), 278–291. https://doi.org/10.1038/nrn2334

Antonini, A., & Stryker, M. P. (1993). Rapid remodeling of axonal arbors in the visual cortex. *Science, 260*, 1819–1821.

Brodmann, K. (1908). Beitraege zur histologischen Lokalisation der Grosshirnrinde. VI. Mitteilung: Die Cortex-gliederung des Menschen. *Journal Psychology and Neurology. (Lzp), 10*, 231–246.

Cao, F. (2016). Neuroimaging studies of reading in bilinguals. *Bilingualism: Language and Cognition, 19*(4), 683–688. https://doi.org/10.1017/S1366728915000656

Cirulli, F., Berry, A., & Alleva, E. (2003). Early disruption of the mother—infant relationship: Effects on brain plasticity and implications for psychopathology. *Neuroscience and Biobehavioral Reviews, 27*(1–2), 73–82.

Clark, A. (1999). An embodied cognitive science? *Trends in Cognitive Sciences, 3*(9), 345–351.

Cowan, W. M., Fawcett, J. W., O'Leary, D. D., & Stanfield, B. B. (1984). Regressive events in neurogenesis. *Science, 225*, 1258–1265.

Dehaene, S., & Cohen, L. (2011). The unique role of the visual word form area in reading. *Trends in Cognitive Sciences, 15*(6), 254–262. https://doi.org/10.1016/J.TICS.2011.04.003

Dehaene, S., Molko, N., Cohen, L., & Wilson, A. J. (2004). Arithmetic and the brain. *Current Opinion in Neurobiology, 14*(2), 218–224. https://doi.org/10.1016/j.conb.2004.03.008

Duncan, J. (2010). The multiple-demand (MD) system of the primate brain: Mental programs for intelligent behaviour. *Trends in Cognitive Sciences, 14*(4), 172–179. https://doi.org/10.1016/j.tics.2010.01.004

Fedorenko, E., & Thompson-Schill, S. L. (2014). Reworking the language network. *Trends in Cognitive Sciences, 18*(3), 120–126. https://doi.org/10.1016/j.tics.2013.12.006

Feller, M. B., & Scanziani, M. (2005). A precritical period for plasticity in visual cortex. *Current Opinion in Neurobiology, 15*(1), 94–100.

Fertonani, A., & Miniussi, C. (2017). Transcranial electrical stimulation. *The Neuroscientist, 23*(2), 109–123. https://doi.org/10.1177/1073858416631966

Friederici, A. D. (2012). The cortical language circuit: From auditory perception to sentence comprehension. *Trends in Cognitive Sciences, 16*(5), 262–268. https://doi.org/10.1016/J.TICS.2012.04.001

Friederici, A. D., & Gierhan, S. M. (2013). The language network. *Current Opinion in Neurobiology, 23*(2), 250–254. https://doi.org/10.1016/J.CONB.2012.10.002

Friedman, N. P., & Miyake, A. (2017). Unity and diversity of executive functions: Individual differences as a window on cognitive structure. *Cortex, 86*, 186–204. https://doi.org/10.1016/j.cortex.2016.04.023

Friston, K. J., & Price, C. J. (2001). Dynamic representations and generative models of brain function. *Brain Research Bulletin, 54*(3), 275–285.

Frith, U., & Frith, C. (2010). The social brain: Allowing humans to boldly go where no other species has been. *Philosophical Transactions of the Royal Society of London: Series B, Biological Sciences, 365*(1537), 165–176. https://doi.org/10.1098/rstb.2009.0160

Goddings, A.-L., Mills, K. L., Clasen, L. S., Giedd, J. N., Viner, R. M., & Blakemore, S.-J. (2014). The influence of puberty on subcortical brain development. *NeuroImage, 88,* 242–251.

Gogtay, N., Giedd, J. N., Lusk, L., Hayashi, K. M., Greenstein, D., Vaituzis, A. C., . . . Thompson, P. M. (2004). Dynamic mapping of human cortical development during childhood through early adulthood. *Proceedings of the National Academy of Sciences of the United States of America, 101*(21), 8174–8179.

Goschke, T., & Bolte, A. (2014). Emotional modulation of control dilemmas: The role of positive affect, reward, and dopamine in cognitive stability and flexibility. *Neuropsychologia, 62,* 403–423. https://doi.org/10.1016/j.neuropsychologia.2014.07.015

Gottlieb, G. (1992). *Individual development and evolution.* Oxford: Oxford University Press.

Harrist, A. W., & Waugh, R. M. (2002). Dyadic synchrony: Its structure and function in children's development. *Developmental Review, 22*(4), 555–592.

Horvath, J. C., Forte, J. D., & Carter, O. (2015). Evidence that transcranial direct current stimulation (tDCS) generates little-to-no reliable neurophysiologic effect beyond MEP amplitude modulation in healthy human subjects: A systematic review. *Neuropsychologia, 66,* 213–236. https://doi.org/10.1016/J.NEUROPSYCHOLOGIA.2014.11.021

Hua, J. Y. Y., & Smith, S. J. (2004). Neural activity and the dynamics of central nervous system development. *Nature Neuroscience, 7*(4), 327–332.

Hubel, D. H., & Wiesel, T. N. (1963). Shape and arrangement of columns in cat's striate cortex. *Journal of Physiology, 165,* 559–568.

Huttenlocher, P. R. (1990). Morphometric study of human cerebral cortex development. *Neuropsychologia, 28*(6), 517–527.

Huttenlocher, P. R., & Dabholkar, A. S. (1997). Regional differences in synaptogenesis in human cerebral cortex. *Journal of Comparative Neurology, 387,* 167–178.

Jarvis, C. R., Xiong, Z.-G., Plant, J. R., Churchill, D., Lu, W.-Y., Macvicar, B. A., & MacDonald, J. F. (1997). Neurotrophin modulation of NMDA receptors in cultured murine and isolated rat neurons. *Journal of Neurophysiology, 78,* 2362–2371.

Jessell, T. M., & Sanes, J. R. (2000). The induction and patterning of the nervous system. In E. R. Kandel, J. H. Schwartz, & T. M. Jessell (Eds.), *Principles of neural science* (4th ed., pp. 1019–1040). New York and London: McGraw-Hill.

Johnson, M. H. (2000). Functional brain development in infants: Elements of an interactive specialization framework. *Child Development, 71*(1), 75–81.

Johnson, M. H., & de Haan, M. (2015). *Developmental cognitive neuroscience* (3rd ed.). Oxford, UK: Wiley-Blackwell.

Kanai, R., & Rees, G. (2011). The structural basis of inter-individual differences in human behaviour and cognition. *Nature Reviews Neuroscience, 12*(4), 231–242. Retrieved from www.nature.com/nrn/journal/v12/n4/abs/nrn3000.html

Katz, L. C., & Shatz, C. J. (1996). Synaptic activity and the construction of cortical circuits. *Science, 274,* 1133–1138.

Kaufman, J., Plotsky, P. M., Nemeroff, C. B., & Charney, D. S. (2000). Effects of early adverse experiences on brain structure and function: Clinical implications. *Biological Psychiatry, 48*(8), 778–790.

Kleim, J. A., Vij, K., Ballard, D. H., & Greenough, W. T. (1997). Learning-dependent synaptic modifications in the cerebellar cortex of the adult rat persist for at least four weeks. *Journal of Neuroscience, 17*, 717–721.

Lebel, C., & Beaulieu, C. (2011). Longitudinal development of human brain wiring continues from childhood into adulthood. *Journal of Neuroscience, 31*(30), 10937–10947.

Mareschal, D., Johnson, M., Sirios, S., Spratling, M., Thomas, M. S. C., & Westermann, G. (2007). *Neuroconstructivism: How the brain constructs cognition.* Oxford: Oxford University Press.

Mello, C. V., Vicario, D. S., & Clayton, D. F. (1992). Song presentation induces gene expression in the songbird forebrain. *Proceedings of the National Academy of Sciences, 89*(15), 6818–6822.

Mills, K. L., Goddings, A.-L., Herting, M. M., Meuwese, R., Blakemore, S.-J., Crone, E. A., Dahl, R. E. et al. (2016). Structural brain development between childhood and adulthood: Convergence across four longitudinal samples. *NeuroImage, 141*, 273–281.

Moreau, D., Stonyer, J. E., McKay, N. S., & Waldie, K. E. (2018). No evidence for systematic white matter correlates of dyslexia: An activation likelihood estimation meta-analysis. *Brain Research, 1683*, 36–47. https://doi.org/10.1016/J.BRAINRES.2018.01.014

O'Leary, D. D. M., & Stanfield, B. B. (1989). Selective elimination of axons extended by developing cortical neurons is dependent on regional locale: Experiments utilizing fetal cortical transplants. *Journal of Neuroscience, 9*, 2230–2246.

Oppenheim, R. W. (1991). Cell death during development of the nervous system. *Annual Reviews of Neuroscience, 14*, 453–501.

Penzes, P., Cahill, M. E., Jones, K. A., VanLeeuwen, J.-E., & Woolfrey, K. M. (2011). Dendritic spine pathology in neuropsychiatric disorders. *Nature Neuroscience, 14*(3), 285–293.

Piaget, J. (1955). *The child's construction of reality.* London: Routledge & Kegan Paul.

Pitcher, D., Charles, L., Devlin, J. T., Walsh, V., & Duchaine, B. (2009). Triple dissociation of faces, bodies, and objects in extrastriate cortex. *Current Biology, 19*(4), 319–324. https://doi.org/10.1016/j.cub.2009.01.007

Price, C. J. (2010). The anatomy of language: A review of 100 fMRI studies published in 2009. *Annals of the New York Academy of Sciences, 1191*(1), 62–88. https://doi.org/10.1111/j.1749-6632.2010.05444.x

Quartz, S. R. (1999). The constructivist brain. *Trends in Cognitive Sciences, 3*(2), 48–57.

Quartz, S. R., & Sejnowski, T. J. (1997). The neural basis of cognitive development: A constructivist manifesto. *Behavioral and Brain Sciences, 20*(4), 537–596.

Raichle, M. E. (2015). The brain's default mode network. *Annual Review of Neuroscience, 38*(1), 433–447. https://doi.org/10.1146/annurev-neuro-071013-014030

Rakic, P. (1988). Specification of cerebral cortical areas. *Science, 241*(4862), 170–176.

Sadato, N., Pascual-Leone, A., Grafman, J., Ibañez, V., Deiber, M.-P., Dold, G., & Hallett, M. (1996). Activation of the primary visual cortex by braille reading in blind subjects. *Nature, 380*, 526–528.

Satterthwaite, T. D., Wolf, D. H., Loughead, J., Ruparel, K., Elliott, M. A., Hakonarson, H., . . . Gur, R. E. (2012). Impact of in-scanner head motion on multiple measures of functional connectivity: Relevance for studies of neurodevelopment in youth. *NeuroImage, 60*(1), 623–632. https://doi.org/10.1016/j.neuroimage.2011.12.063

Shallice, T., Stuss, D. T., Picton, T. W., Alexander, M. P., & Gillingham, S. (2008). Mapping task switching in frontal cortex through neuropsychological group studies. *Frontiers in Neuroscience, 2*(1), 79–85. https://doi.org/10.3389/neuro.01.013.2008

Shaw, P., Eckstrand, K., Sharp, W., Blumenthal, J., Lerch, J. P., Greenstein, D., . . . Rapoport, J. L. (2007). Attention-deficit/hyperactivity disorder is characterized by a delay in cortical maturation. *Proceedings of the National Academy of Sciences of the United States of America, 104*(49), 19649–19654.

Shaw, P., Kabani, N. J., Lerch, J. P., Eckstrand, K., Lenroot, R., Gogtay, N., Greenstein, D. et al. (2008). Neurodevelopmental trajectories of the human cerebral cortex. *Journal of Neuroscience, 28,* 3586–3594.

Stalnaker, T. A., Cooch, N. K., & Schoenbaum, G. (2015). What the orbitofrontal cortex does not do. *Nature Neuroscience, 18*(5), 620–627. https://doi.org/10.1038/nn.3982

Stryker, M. P., & Strickland, S. L. (1984). Physiological segregation of ocular dominance columns depends on the pattern of afferent electrical activity. *Ophthalmological Visual Science, 25*(Suppl.), 278.

Thompson-Schill, S. L., Bedny, M., & Goldberg, R. F. (2005). The frontal lobes and the regulation of mental activity. *Current Opinion in Neurobiology, 15*(2), 219–224. https://doi.org/10.1016/j.conb.2005.03.006

Turkewitz, G., & Kenny, P. A. (1982). Limitations on input as a basis for neural organization and perceptual development—a preliminary theoretical statement. *Developmental Psychobiology, 15*(4), 357–368.

van der Meer, A. L. H., & van der Weel, F. R. (1995). Move yourself, baby! Perceptuomotor development from a continuous perspective. In P. Rochat (Ed.), *The self in infancy: Theory and research* (pp. 257–275). Amsterdam, North Holland: Elsevier Science Publishers.

Van Overwalle, F. (2009). Social cognition and the brain: A meta-analysis. *Human Brain Mapping, 30*(3), 829–858. https://doi.org/10.1002/hbm.20547

Vanderauwera, J., Wouters, J., Vandermosten, M., & Ghesquière, P. (2017). Early dynamics of white matter deficits in children developing dyslexia. *Developmental Cognitive Neuroscience, 27,* 69–77. https://doi.org/10.1016/J.DCN.2017.08.003

Vogel, A. C., Power, J. D., Petersen, S. E., & Schlaggar, B. L. (2010). Development of the brain's functional network architecture. *Neuropsychology Review, 20*(4), 362–375. https://doi.org/10.1007/s11065-010-9145-7

Westermann, G., Mareschal, D., Johnson, M. H., Sirois, S., Spratling, M. W., & Thomas, M. S. C. (2007). Neuroconstructivism. *Developmental Science, 10,* 75–83.

Section 1

Development and Variation

Genetic and Environmental Factors

3 What Has Behavioural Genetic Research Told Us About the Origins of Individual Differences in Educational Abilities and Achievements?

Georgina Donati and Emma Meaburn

Chapter Overview

The purpose of education is to prepare students for adult life by equipping them with the knowledge, character, and skills required to contribute to society and navigate their way in the world (Department for Education, 2015). However, as any teacher or parent can attest, children show remarkable differences in their appetite for learning, academic progress, and educational achievements. Why is it, for example, that some children in a classroom find learning to read so much harder than their peers, despite being taught by the same teacher in the same school, with access to the same learning resources and support? **Behavior Genetics** is a field of Psychology that uses genetic methods to query the origins of these individual differences. To what extent are the differences we observe in learning and academic outcomes between children due to genetic (nature) or environmental (nurture) factors? We each share a set of genetic instructions that are similar enough to build—from scratch—a highly complex organism that is characteristically human. Yet we differ in important and meaningful ways, including at the genetic level; if you were to pick any two unrelated individuals at random and examine their DNA sequence you would find that they differ at roughly 1 in every 1,200–1,500 **DNA** bases (or 'letters') (Auton et al., 2015). Given that the human genome is 3 billion DNA base pairs in length, this represents a substantial amount of genetic variability. How important are these genetic differences in accounting for the differences we observe between students? And how do they stack up against the importance of environmental influences such as the school the child attends, their home environment, neighborhood, and wider social and cultural factors? Several decades of behavior genetic research has robustly demonstrated that it is both nature *and* nurture and their interplay, and the focus now is on understanding the *specific* causes—which genes and which environments— that drive variability in traits and behaviors related to education (Knopik, Neiderhiser, DeFries, & Plomin, 2016). Charting the developmental dance between stable inherited DNA differences and dynamic environments will be critical for understanding the cellular, structural and functional mechanisms by which DNA shapes our learning, and will aid the identification of relevant educational environments and practices that cater to and accommodate our differences. Given that how well a child does at school is predictive of a wide range of important social, economic, and physical and mental health outcomes, understanding the specific contributions to individual differences in academic success is of fundamental importance both for the individual and for society (Cutler, Lleras-Muney, & Vogl, 2008; Ross & Wu, 1995).

The aim of this chapter is to introduce teachers and educational neuroscience students to how behavior genetic research has contributed to our understanding of the genetic contributions to individual differences in educationally relevant traits and outcomes. We focus primarily on intelligence (or general cognitive function; 'g'), how long you stay in education ('educational attainment'), and how well you do ('educational achievement') as these are the areas where the majority of research has been conducted, and the most progress has been made. We also limit our focus to cognitive and academic traits within the normal range of function; readers interested in the genetic basis of marked intellectual disability, or specific learning disabilities such as dyslexia and specific language impairment are referred to excellent recent reviews (Bishop, 2015; Reader, Covill, Nudel, & Newbury, 2014). During the course of the chapter we highlight what we consider to be the three key areas of progress, the immediate implications of these insights, and how they might practically be used to improve children's learning and educational experiences. Along the way we hope to highlight some of the current issues or debates in the field before finally considering likely future directions for behavior genetic research in education. Where possible we have minimized the use of jargon, but some terminology is unavoidable: Terms in **bold** are defined in the glossary at the end of this book.

Educational Phenotypes

Before we jump to what we consider to be the most robust scientific findings, we first provide a brief overview for the uninitiated of how intelligence and educational outcomes are typically operationalized in behavior genetic research. If you are already familiar with the concept of intelligence and psychometric testing of cognitive functions, you may wish to skip this section.

One of the main **phenotypes** used by behavior genetic researchers is intelligence, also known as general cognitive ability or 'g' (Spearman, 1904). Intelligence or 'g' is a statistical construct that captures what is in common between diverse ability tests; that is, it describes the fact that if you do well on a specific cognitive test (e.g., a test of numerical reasoning or memory), you also *tend* to do well on other cognitive tests (e.g., vocabulary or spatial awareness). A nuanced discussion of what intelligence might represent both at the cognitive and neurological level is beyond the scope of this chapter, but broadly speaking it can be thought of as a general measure of problem-solving ability and information processing (Carroll, 1993; Deary, 2012). As you might well expect, intelligence and educational outcomes are closely interconnected. The relationship is not perfect, but in general people who score higher on intelligence tests tend to stay in school longer, and vice versa (Deary, Strand, Smith, & Fernandes, 2007). As we shall see in later sections, this relationship is at least partly explained by shared genetic effects (Johnson, Deary, & Iacono, 2009). More recently there has been a move to studying educational attainment (length of time spent in formal education), and educational achievement (typically, the highest academic qualification achieved) directly (Rietveld et al., 2014a). One critical benefit of studying very broad social phenotypes such as these is that they are easily measured in very large samples of individuals for relatively low cost, which is necessary to detect specific genetic influences. However, how well you do in school is undoubtedly influenced by facets of cognitive function other than intelligence, in addition to emotional behaviors, personality, creativity, motivation, resilience, and social and economic circumstance. All of these more specific phenotypes have been studied in a behavior genetic framework (although typically on a smaller scale), and we touch on them where appropriate.

Twin Studies: Dissecting the Origins of Individual Differences in Educational Phenotypes

When considering the origins of individual differences in educational phenotypes, how do we know if genetic influence is important? Fundamentally, we can infer genetic effects by contrasting the phenotypic similarity between related individuals with their genetic similarity; if genes contribute to a trait we can predict that the resemblance between pairs of relatives will increase with increasing genetic relatedness. However, familial resemblance could also be due to shared environmental exposures and experiences (e.g., the number of books in the home, parenting style) as well as shared genes. Fortunately, twin studies are able to tease apart the relative influence of genetic (variation in DNA sequence) and non-genetic factors (variation in environments) by exploiting the fact that identical twins (monozygotic or MZ) and non-identical or fraternal twins (dizygotic or DZ) share the same family environmental experiences but differ in their genetic similarity. Specifically, MZ twins develop from one egg (or zygote) and share 100% of their DNA sequence, while DZ twins develop from two separately fertilized eggs and share on average only 50% of their segregating genes (just like regular siblings with the same parents). Working under the assumption that within twin pair prenatal and postnatal environmental variation is similar for both MZ and DZ twins (the 'equal environments assumption'), genetic influence can be quantified by the extent to which MZ twins are more similar for a trait than DZ twins by virtue of their greater genetic similarity (Knopik et al., 2016); doubling the difference between MZ and DZ correlations for a measured phenotype (such as educational attainment) provides an estimate of genetic influence known as twin **heritability**.

Twin studies of many hundreds of families use the principle just described and structural equation models to partition observed variance in the phenotype being studied into a) additive genetic effects (heritability), b) shared (or common) environmental effects and c) non-shared (or unique) environmental effects (Neale & Cardon, 1992). Within the twin model framework, shared environmental effects are considered to be any non-genetic influences that are shared by twins in the same family and *serve to make them more similar*, such as characteristics of the home environment (e.g., number of books or social-economic status), prenatal environment, and neighborhood. In contrast, non-shared environmental factors are taken to be any aspects of the environment that are experienced differently by twins in the same family and *serve to make them different*, and includes idiosyncratic events such as individual-specific illnesses, random biological noise, differential treatment (either real or perceived) by teachers, parents or peer group members, and good old-fashioned luck (Plomin, 2011). Like all research paradigms, twin studies come with important qualifications and assumptions and these have been extensively tested and critically discussed elsewhere (e.g., see (Rutter, 2006; Kendler, Neale, Kessler, Heath, & Eaves, 1993)).

Individual Differences in Educational Phenotypes Are Heritable

So what do twin studies tell us about the importance of genes in explaining the relative gaps that we see between students' abilities and educational achievements? One of the most consistent and replicable findings to emerge is that individual differences in educationally relevant traits and behaviors—whether measured in childhood or adulthood—are heritable (Plomin & von Stumm, 2018). Figure 3.1 provides a roadmap of the key research papers published in the last 12 years that have been critical to our understanding of the nature and magnitude of genetic contributions to educationally relevant traits. Whilst exact heritability estimates vary across twin studies, they all find that a sizable proportion of the differences we see between students can be attributed to genetic differences that exist between them. For example, intelligence or 'g' has a heritability estimate of ~40% in childhood, rising to ~60% in adulthood (Haworth et al., 2010; Trzaskowski, Yang, Visscher, & Plomin, 2014). Twin study research has also demonstrated that academic achievement is heritable, whether considering standardized achievement scores during childhood, or high-stakes exam outcomes in late adolescence. For example, a large representative UK-based study of ~10,000 twin pairs (Haworth, Davis, & Plomin, 2013) has reported heritability estimates of 68% for literacy and 66% for numeracy at age 7 (Kovas, Harlaar, Petrill, & Plomin, 2005; Kovas et al., 2013), 52–58% for performance in core General Certificate of Secondary Education (CGSE) exams at the end of compulsory education at age 16 (Shakeshaft et al., 2013), and 59% for average performance in A-level exams at age 18 (Rimfeld, Ayorech, Dale, Kovas, & Plomin, 2016; Smith-Woolley, Ayorech, Dale, von Stumm, & Plomin, 2018). The Rimfeld et al. study also

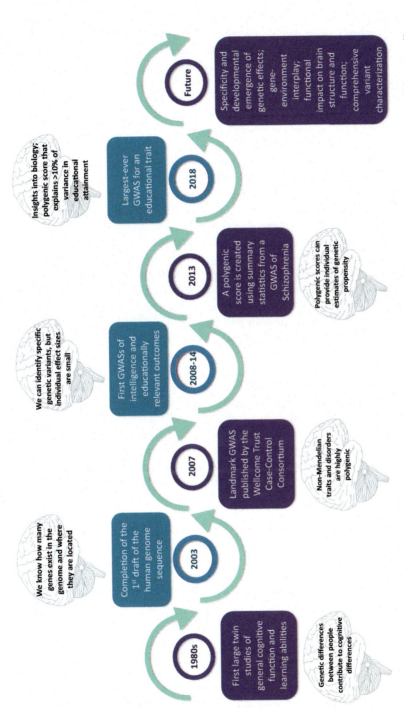

Figure 3.1 A Roadmap of Key Behavior Genetic Studies That Have Provided Critical Insights Into Genetic Contributions to Educationally Relevant Traits; Thought Bubbles Describes the Insights Provided by Each Study.

demonstrated that genetic influence extends beyond achievement and influences the choice of academic *subject* studied; the authors reported heritability estimates of 50–80% for A-level subject choice, suggesting that a reciprocal relationship exists across development between ability, previous achievement, and academic interests. Similarly high heritability estimates have also been reported in non-UK twin cohorts (e.g., (Schwabe, Janss, & van den Berg, 2017), and a recent meta-analysis of 61 studies reported a heritability estimate of 66% for educational achievement (de Zeeuw, de Geus, & Boomsma, 2015). Notable genetic influence has also been found for psychological and behavioral correlates of academic achievement such as self-efficacy (Krapohl et al., 2014; Waaktaar & Torgersen, 2013), personality traits such as neuroticism (Docherty et al., 2016; Power & Pluess, 2015), and perseverance for long-term goals ('grit'; (Rimfeld, Kovas, Dale, & Plomin, 2016) in addition to well-being (Bartels, 2015) and behavior problems in childhood (Cheesman et al., 2017).

In the past few years, advanced statistical methods have been developed that allow researchers to estimate relatedness between individuals directly from their DNA, enabling heritability estimates to be derived from very large samples of unrelated people and side-stepping the requirement for twin cohorts (Bulik-Sullivan et al., 2015; Yang et al., 2010; Yang, Lee, Goddard, & Visscher, 2011). The assumptions and limitations of DNA-based heritability estimates differ from twin study estimates in important ways (e.g., see (Mayhew & Meyre, 2017; Wray et al., 2014), but broadly speaking the results are similar insofar as they too demonstrate a marked genetic component to individual differences in cognitive and educational traits. For example, for educational attainment and achievement the proportion of variance explained by common **DNA variants** is typically ~20–30% (Lee et al., 2018; Rimfeld et al., 2018), but rises to ~60% in more environmentally homogenous cohorts (Morris, Davies, Dorling, Richmond, & Smith, 2018). To conclude, it transpires that your grandmother was right and the apple does not fall far from the tree—the genes we inherit from our parents play an important role in shaping our educational journeys.

A Note on How to Interpret Heritability

Encouragingly, a recent study of UK-based primary school teachers demonstrated that teachers intuitively understand the importance of genetic factors in explaining differences in intelligence and educational performance between children (Crosswaite & Asbury, 2019). What this study highlighted however, is that what is less clear to teachers is how heritability (or genetic influence) relates to malleability, as illustrated by debates around growth mindset. For this reason, we feel it prudent to detail how heritability can (and cannot) be interpreted, as it is a statistic open to misunderstanding.

Heritability is a descriptive statistic that is concerned with what makes people in a population different from each other; if what we are interested in is universal and does not tend to vary in the population (for example, the number of fingers on one hand or the ability to use speech to communicate), heritability will be zero—even if the outcome is entirely genetically determined. Furthermore, because it is focused only on variance, it does not provide any information on genetic effect sizes for an individual. For example, finding a heritability of 70% for phonological decoding ability at age 7 (Harlaar et al., 2014) is *not* the same as saying 70% of a child's word decoding skill is due to their genetic makeup, and the remaining 30% is topped up by the environment. It simply tells us that 70% of the differences in phonological decoding that we see between individuals in that *specific study* are explained by naturally occurring genetic differences that exist between the children. It is also worth emphasizing that identification of a genetic component to cognitive and academic abilities is not unexpected, nor does it make unusual. Several decades of twin studies have demonstrated that no matter where we look, genetic influence can be found. Genes contribute to variance in liability for mental health disorders, behaviors harmful to health (e.g., smoking or alcohol consumption), physical traits (e.g., height and body mass index) and 'environmental' measures such as social economic status (SES) (Polderman et al., 2015).

It would also be a mistake to arrive at the unpalatable conclusion that children who don't do well in school just have 'bad' genes, and nothing can be done to help them as their DNA sequence is fixed from birth. Finding genetic influence does *not* mean that outcomes are predetermined, as no necessary relationship exists between heritability and malleability. To illustrate this point, let's consider human height. About 80% of individual differences in height are due to genetic differences, but average height in developed countries has increased by 10–15 cm during the past 150 years (Jelenkovic et al., 2016; Wood et al., 2014). Genes have not evolved substantially in this time frame; rather what has changed is the environment. On the whole, children are eating more nutritious diets and have better access to good quality medical care. Consequently, everyone has gotten a little taller (the population mean has increased), but differences in stature between people are still evident and are largely for genetic reasons. Similarly, we know that formal education (which can be conceptualised as an environmental intervention on a population-scale) increases cognitive abilities (Ritchie & Tucker-Drob, 2018), and we each know from personal experience that we can improve at something with training, effort, and practice. By extension, finding low heritability for a cognitive domain does not mean that it is more amenable to training or intervention than a trait with high heritability. Even if phonological decoding ability were 100% heritable and the genes responsible operated entirely at the level of brain function, it is plausible that a new environmental 'reading training' intervention program would improve everyone's performance.

A final important point when thinking about how behavior genetic findings might be utilized in an academic setting is that we cannot gauge from heritability estimates alone how the rank order of individuals might change in response to a blanket environmental intervention, such as a change in classroom discipline, or implementation of a new cognitive training or behavior management program. In our previous hypothetical example, the reading intervention might improve the average performance of the population and the rank order of individuals remains the same (everyone gets a little bit better)—but the students that were doing well before are still the ones doing well after, and vice versa. However, it is also possible for the average performance to increase, but the rank order of individuals changes—some people who were doing well before do less well after, some show improvements, and/or some people remain unaffected (Haworth & Davis, 2014). If we want to be able to explore this relationship, we first need a much better understanding of the genes involved and how they work.

Genetic Influences Are Context Dependent and Dynamic

You may have noted at this point that whilst heritability estimates are not zero, they differ depending on the cohort and phenotype studied. This is because genetic influences on a trait (and by extension, heritability estimates) are not fixed; they are dependent on environmental context, developmental stage, and the degree of variability in the environment (Visscher, Hill, & Wray, 2008). Heritability quantifies the contribution of genetic differences to measurable differences between people in a population, *at that point in history, at that age, in that country, and within that cultural and societal context*. Consequently, heritability estimates for academic traits fluctuate as environmental influences (such as diet, access to technology and medical care, educational curricula, and societal factors) change, and has even been demonstrated to vary by geographical region within a population (Davis, Haworth, Lewis, & Plomin, 2012). A general pattern to emerge is that greater genetic influence is observed in populations with higher quality and more uniform educational systems and egalitarian societies. In their meta-analysis of 61 twin studies, de Zeeuw et al. noted that heritability of reading comprehension, mathematics, and language in primary-aged school children differed by country; heritability was uniformly high for the Netherlands (64%, 71%, and 66% respectively), but more variable for the US (67%, 26%, and 32%)—a country that has a more decentralized educational system and greater socioeconomic inequality.[1] Similarly, in their study of US students, Taylor, Roehrig, Hensler, Connor, and Schatschneider (2010) observed greater heritability estimates for reading ability when teacher quality was good (Taylor et al., 2010). Social systems and social inequality also impact genetic influence, with reported heritability estimates for IQ being lower in impoverished (as compared to affluent) US families (Turkheimer, Haley, Waldron, D'Onofrio, & Gottesman, 2003). This pattern might seem contradictory, but it is likely that widely available (and good quality) educational and socioeconomic environments will maximize learning and educational opportunities for all and minimize environmental variance. If environmental variance is restricted, then the relative differences that remain between students are more readily explained by their genetic differences, which will result in higher heritability estimates. Conversely, in a uniformly 'bad' educational environment no one is able to reach their potential and heritability estimates will be lower (Thomas, Kovas, Meaburn, & Tolmie, 2015).

A second somewhat surprising finding to emerge from twin studies is that heritability for intelligence increases across the course of development, despite DNA sequence being stable from birth (Plomin & Deary, 2015). For example, in a cross-sectional study of 11,000 twin pairs Haworth et al. (2010) reported a linear increase in heritability from 41% in childhood (age 9), to 55% in early adolescence (age 12), and 66% in young adulthood (age 17), a finding mirrored in DNA-based analyses (Trzaskowski et al., 2014). The exact mechanism underpinning this observation is unclear, but it is likely that as we develop in our cognitive capacities and progress through the educational system we are better able to seek out, select, and modify our learning environments and experiences so that they best suit our genetic propensities; a process known as active **gene-environment correlation** (Rutter, 2006; Tucker-Drob, Briley, & Harden, 2013). In an educational context this might be accentuated by class ability streaming, as this process will encourage children who excel at certain subjects or activities to pursue them and foster their development in these areas.

What Does This Mean for Education?

The main message from twin and DNA-based studies is that whether we measure general intelligence, specific learning abilities or exam outcomes, there is clear and consistent evidence for genetic influence. However, in isolation these studies don't tell us about how easy (or how hard) it might be to change mean levels of educational attainment, or individual trajectories, or indeed how we might go about it. What are the most effective and salient pedagogical methods? What we do know is that if we ever want to fully account for why children differ academically, then we need to jointly consider both genetic and environmental influences. So, what does this mean for education right now? On its own, it has no direct policy or practical implications other than to tell us that if a child is struggling (or excelling) at school, the reasons are complex and inter-related; children don't fail or succeed solely due to parental, social or educational failings or advantages. Importantly, we should not feel pessimistic about genetic influence as even highly heritable phenotypes can be altered with environmental manipulation. In the future, twin research may be useful in modelling how genes and environments interact with each other over time, within different educational contexts and in evaluating educational interventions. For example, comprehensive cross-cultural twin studies could be used to identify populations that show maximal heritability estimates, providing useful clues as to teaching practices and policies that foster greater environmental equality and support educational development (Rodic et al., 2018).

Arguably, one of the most important sequelae of finding genetic influence has been the mobilization and coordination of large-scale molecular genetic efforts (i.e., the study of DNA) focused on identification of the contributory genetic variants. Twin studies tell us that—in aggregate—DNA differences are important, but do not tell us where in the genome these DNA sequence variants reside or how they work. Are they in genes, or the spaces between genes? How many variants are we looking for if we wish to explain the heritability estimates (10, 100, or 10,000+?). What is their mechanism of action? Arguably, the holy grail for translation is to identify specific genetic variants as this will provide the crucial starting point for understanding the neurobiology of individual differences in cognitive functions, learning processes, and academic behaviors. Identification of specific genes will also aid prediction (who might struggle or excel based on their genetic profile), along with a greater understanding of what might be the most relevant environmental contexts, and how they work in concert with genetic factors. The following section summarizes what contemporary molecular genetic studies have told us about the genetic architecture of educational traits and outcomes.

Molecular Genetic Studies: Identification of Specific Genetic Variants

It has long been recognised that rare and severe disorders that show clear-cut inheritance patterns within families (termed **Mendelian disorders**) are the result of alterations in a single **gene**. Typically, the alterations—or mutations—are so severe that they disrupt normal functioning of the gene. In this situation **molecular genetic** strategies for the identification of the mutation (and gene) responsible are well-established, and typically involve the analysis of family-based data (e.g., see (Gilissen, Hoischen, Brunner, & Veltman, 2011; Teare & Santibanez Koref, 2014)). They have also been enormously successful; as of April 2018, 5,222 Mendelian phenotypes have been described where the molecular basis is known (http://omim.org/statistics/geneMap). Single gene causes of intellectual disability—defined as an IQ below 70 with associated deficits in adaptive behaviors—form part of this group, with mutations in ~800 genes identified to-date (Chiurazzi & Pirozzi, 2016). However, while these alterations in DNA sequence have severe cognitive effects on the affected individual, they do not explain meaningful amounts of population-level variation in intelligence. Put simply, they do not contribute to the heritability observed for variability in cognition function in the general population.

Early efforts to hunt for the specific genetic variants that contribute to the normal range of cognitive function were largely ineffective and marred by a lack of replication (e.g., see (Chabris et al., 2012)). The breakthrough came in 2006, with the development and application of **genome-wide association studies** (GWAS—pronounced 'gee-woz'). GWASs became feasible following developments in three keys areas (Kruglyak, 2008): (1) the completion of the Human Genome Project provided us with the **human genome** sequence (the consensus sequence of 3 billion nucleotide base pairs); (2) large-scale international projects such as HAPMAP developed comprehensive catalogues of common **genetic variation** in major human populations (areas of the genome that differ from one person to the next); and (3) the development of new technologies that are able to measure many hundreds of thousands of genetic variants in large numbers of individuals quickly and cost effectively (**SNP genotyping arrays**). See Figure 3.1.

In the GWAS approach, 1+ million common genetic variants distributed throughout the human genome—typically **single nucleotide polymorphisms** (SNPs; single base changes in the DNA sequence)—are **genotyped** in very large samples of unrelated individuals, and each SNP is systematically tested for association with the measured trait or outcome using standard statistical methods (Balding, 2006; Hardy & Singleton, 2009). Because the SNP tested has been mapped to a specific position on a **chromosome**, identification of a statistically significant signal immediately indicates the location of the genetic variant(s) that are associated with the trait and allows researchers to home in on specific biological pathways and functions (Spain & Barrett, 2015). Crucially, this approach requires no prior hypotheses or assumptions about the chromosomal location or biological function of DNA sequence variants that influence the trait or disorder, and instead allows researchers to systematically search the entire genome in an unbiased manner, searching for the independent contribution of each variant. However, this 'a-theoretical' approach comes at a cost; due to the large number of genetic variants being tested for association in a GWA study, a stringent p value of $p \leq 5 \times 10^{-8}$ has been established as the threshold for statistical significance (Dudbridge & Gusnanto, 2008). The adoption of this standard has helped guard against chance findings that fail to replicate in subsequent studies and largely mitigated the proliferation of 'false positive' results that have plagued other areas of research (Open Science Collaboration, 2015). The landmark GWAS was published in 2007, and demonstrated for the first time that the approach can robustly and reliably identify modest-to-small genetic association signals for common diseases and disorders (Wellcome Trust Case Control Consortium, 2007). GWASs rapidly become the molecular genetic research paradigm of choice, identifying for the first time the *specific* DNA variants that are common in the population and contribute to the observed heritability of a human phenotype.[2]

Educational Phenotypes Are Highly Polygenic

The first wave of GWA studies of reading disability and ability (Meaburn, Harlaar, Craig, Schalkwyk, & Plomin, 2008), receptive language (Harlaar et al., 2014), maths (Docherty et al., 2010), and general cognitive ability (Benyamin et al., 2014; Davies et al., 2011; Davis et al., 2010) were united in one critical finding—they were unable to robustly identify individual DNA variants that replicated in independent samples. Associations that were spotted in one study would not be found in a second study using an independent sample. These studies were conducted on samples of up to ~18,000 individuals and were statistically well-powered enough to have detected genetic variants of large to modest effect—yet none were identified. What they starkly demonstrated was that cognitive and learning abilities are **polygenic** ('poly' meaning many, and 'genic' meaning genes), with thousands of common DNA variants contributing to their heritability (see (Visscher, Brown, McCarthy, & Yang, 2012) for a review). Unlike Mendelian diseases, where variation in a single gene is both necessary and sufficient for the development of the disorder, each gene (or DNA sequence variant) explains only a fraction of the differences observed between individuals. This led to the prediction that much larger sample sizes would be able to reliably identify genetic signals of small effect, and there was a subsequent explosion in the number of individuals examined in a GWAS framework.

The first very large GWAS of educational outcomes was published by the Social Science Genetics Association Consortium (SSGAC[3]) in 2013 and contained over 100,000 individuals, which at that time was one of the largest GWASs ever conducted (Rietveld et al., 2013). Gathering together such a large number of individuals for whom both educationally relevant measures and genome-wide genetic data were available was not straightforward and required unprecedented levels of collaboration between researchers from around the world. It also posed significant analytical problems, one of which was characterization of the phenotype. Typically, as in the earlier GWA studies, researchers interested in cognitive performance and learning abilities employ a battery of detailed, well characterized, reliable, and validated psychometric tests. This was simply not feasible for the SSGAC because each contributing research group had typically used different measures of cognitive ability. The consortium instead centered on two measures that had been collected across all cohorts as a standard demographic variable: years in education (an individual's number of years of schooling; 'Edu-Years') and college completion (did the individual complete university—yes/no; 'College'). The resulting GWAS identified three independent genome-wide significant SNPs—two for 'College' and one for 'Edu Years'—that replicated in 12 independent cohorts. Just three years later the SSGAC performed a follow-up study consisting of 293,723 individuals, which identified a further 71 SNPs associated with 'Edu-Years' (Okbay et al., 2016). Most recently, the consortium analyzed ~1.1 million individuals and characterized 1,271 SNPs that each contribute to the number of years of schooling (Lee et al., 2018). A similar pattern of results was observed for GWASs of cognitive functions, with specific DNA variants identified once samples sizes exceeded 30,000 participants, and an increasing number of genome-wide significant 'hits' as the sample size increased. The largest published GWAS of general intelligence to-date consisted of 78,308 individuals and identified 18 independent genetic regions (Sniekers et al., 2017). What has rapidly transpired is that cognitive and educational phenotypes are highly polygenic and genetic influences tapped by twin studies are due to the aggregate effects of *thousands* of genetic variants; each individual DNA variant exerts only a small influence on outcome and current GWASs are powered to detect only the strongest of (very small) genetic signals.[4]

While GWASs have been hugely successful at identifying specific genetic variants associated with educationally relevant traits, statistical significance alone is not very informative. If the findings are to have any immediate practical or predictive value then what we really need to know is the magnitude of effect and mechanism of action. In the context of individual differences research, **effect size** is usually reported as a proportion of variance explained in the outcome variable (such as a score on a cognitive test) by the other variable (here, the genotype). One key finding to emerge is that each individual genetic variant identified in a GWAS confers only a *very* small effect on a polygenic phenotype. For example, the median effect size of the SNPs identified in the 2018 Lee et al. study of 'Edu-Years' corresponds to 1.7 weeks of schooling per allele (Lee et al., 2018). More sobering still, it transpires that these might in fact be overestimates; a recent family-based analysis suggests that effect size estimates for Edu-Years SNPs are biased upwards due to the contribution of 'genetic nurture', whereby parental genotype influences behavior and the rearing environments that parents provide for their children (Kong et al., 2018). That is, more educated parents provide a rearing environment more conducive to educational achievement, irrespective of whether the child has inherited the alleles for higher academic achievement from their parents.

So what practical use is this information? If the *strongest* individual genetic variant explains only a tiny fraction of differences in educational achievement between individuals, it precludes its use as a predictor of educational risk and resilience. The discovery of such small individual effects sizes was unexpected, and initially undermined the primary purpose of genome-wide association studies. However, researchers quickly realized that GWAS data could be interrogated in other ways, and methods were developed that moved beyond the identification of individual trait-associated DNA variants (Maier, Visscher, Robinson, & Wray, 2018; Wray et al., 2014).

Polygenic Scores

One such method recently developed is the construction of genetic 'scores' for individuals using the summary statistics from a well-powered GWAS. Even though DNA sequence variants that are identified in a GWAS individually have very little effect on outcome, they act independently and additively and can be aggregated into a single genetic score that can explain useful amounts of variance and have a wide range of research applications. The creation of a composite measure of genetic signal using the results of a GWAS has been termed **polygenic scoring (PGS)**, and construction of a PGS for an individual is now briefly outlined.[5]

Creation of Individual-Specific Polygenic Scores

Polygenic scores are constructed in the following way: Firstly, SNPs from a 'discovery' GWAS (i.e., the original GWAS of the phenotype of interest) are ranked for evidence of association, usually by p-value. Then in a second independent 'target' dataset, a PGS is calculated for *each individual* as a sum of each 'risk' allele carried by the individual for the selected SNPs, with each SNP weighted by the effect size in the discovery GWAS (Wray et al., 2014). For example, suppose we identify 100 SNPs in a GWAS that each accounts for 0.1% of the variance of reading ability. The two **alleles** (A_1 and A_2) for each of the 100 SNPs are each assigned a value of zero or one, with the allele associated with higher reading scores (A_1 in this example) given the higher score ($A_1 = 1$, $A_2 = 0$). This results in the three possible genotype combinations of A_1/A_1, A_1/A_2 and A_2/A_2 that have a respective genotype score of 2, 1, and 0. These scores are then 'weighted' based on evidence of association and the process is repeated for all 100 SNPs. For each individual in the target dataset the scores for all 100 SNPs are summed so that the maximum polygenic score for any individual is 200 (i.e., they carry all the alleles associated with better reading performance) and the lowest value is zero (they carry none of the alleles). The PGS now collectively accounts for ~10% of the variance in reading ability ($100 × 0.1\%$), which opens up the possibility of using it as a measure—or predictor—of individual genetic propensity.

Polygenic Scores for Educational Attainment

A PGS created from the 53 genome-wide significant SNPs to emerge from the 2016 SSGAC study of ~300,000 individuals explained 0.3–0.6% of the variance in educational attainment in a second 'target' sample (Okbay et al., 2016). What was interesting was that including all 9.3 million SNPs assayed in the discovery GWAS—including those that failed to show any statistical evidence of association with years spent in education—resulted in a *better* polygenic predictor that explained 2.7–3.8% of the variance. This indicated that educational attainment is extremely polygenic and a large percentage of the DNA sequence that varies between individuals contributes to the length of time spent in formal education. The first PGS for educational attainment was quickly superseded by a polygenic score based on the 2018 SSGAC GWAS of 1,131,881 individuals that (depending on how the PGS was constructed) explained ~11–13% of the variance in educational attainment in independent samples of both adolescents and adults. To put the size of this explanatory power into context, the authors highlighted that this makes it a better predictor of educational attainment than household income, although not quite as good as the current gold standard of maternal education (Lee et al., 2018). Most importantly, because polygenic scores are specific for an individual, they can be used to identify individuals with extreme polygenic scores who might be more likely to struggle in school (i.e., individuals with a low PGS) and those who might flourish (with a high PGS). For example, when a US sample of adults were ranked for the 2018 Edu-Years PGS, the mean percentage completing college (the UK equivalent of graduating from university) was 10% for the bottom quintile as compared to 55% in the top quintile (Lee et al., 2018). A similar pattern was observed in polygenic predictions of childhood learning abilities in a UK sample (Selzam et al., 2017a). Additionally, polygenic scores can differentiate between children in the same family in a way that standard demographic predictors—such as household income, or level of parental education—cannot. This benefit was exemplified in a sibling study that found that siblings with higher Edu-Years polygenic scores went on (on average) to complete more years of education than their sibling with a lower PGS (Domingue, Belsky, Conley, Harris, & Boardman, 2015).

Since their conception, polygenic scores for Edu-Years have been used extensively in the social science and behavior genetic communities to explore a range of research questions (Anderson, Shade, DiBlasi, Shabalin, & Docherty, 2019). Most notably, polygenic scores have been used to query the genetic relationship between years spent in education and a diverse array of conceptually related outcomes such as intelligence and cognitive abilities (Hagenaars et al., 2016; Rietveld et al., 2014b), educational achievement (even after accounting for IQ (Selzam et al., 2017b)), psychiatric disorders (de Zeeuw et al., 2014; Hill, Harris, & Deary, 2019), brain-related measures (Cullen et al., 2018; Elliott et al., 2018), personality and well-being (Smith-Woolley, Selzam, & Plomin, 2019), and other phenotypes such as socioeconomic status (Krapohl & Plomin, 2016) and life outcomes (Belsky et al., 2016). It is perhaps not surprising to discover that a polygenic score for educational attainment explains a significance amount of variance in adult intelligence (Sniekers et al., 2017), but it might be surprising to know that it also explains variance in social deprivation indices (Hill et al., 2016), risk for psychiatric diseases (Hill et al., 2019) and behavior problems in childhood (Krapohl et al., 2016). So far, the published studies that use polygenic scores derived from the series of SSGAC GWAS results have universally demonstrated that traits or outcomes that correlate or co-occur with time spent in education, do so partly for shared genetic reasons. This biological phenomenon is termed **pleiotropy**, and can generally be interpreted in one of two ways: (1) the DNA variants affect both trait 1 (Years in Education) and trait 2 (a correlated outcome such as mental health) independently so that the two traits have shared biological pathways ('biological pleiotropy') or (2) the DNA variants affects trait 1, which in turn affects trait 2 ('mediated pleiotropy') (Solovieff, Cotsapas, Lee, Purcell, & Smoller, 2013). When pleiotropy of polygenic scores is observed, establishing which scenario is the likely explanation is not always obvious but statistical and methodological approaches are actively under development to address this issue (Pickrell et al., 2016). The widespread prevalence of pleiotropy between educational attainment, mental health outcomes, cognitive function, and personality—coupled with very small effect sizes that are distributed throughout the entire human genome —has sparked discussion and debate about plausible biological links between genetic variation and specific outcomes (for example, the **Omnigenic model** (Boyle, Li, & Pritchard, 2017; Wray, Wijmenga, Sullivan, Yang, & Visscher, 2018).

In summary, our understanding of the genetic architecture of educationally relevant traits and abilities is still evolving, but we finally have undisputable scientific evidence that the cumulative impact of common genetic variation plays a central role. Furthermore, we can robustly identify a fraction of the variants that contribute to differences in educational outcomes by recruiting and analyzing extremely large samples of unrelated individuals within a GWAS framework. The approach works! The next question then, is how are GWAS findings of relevance to educators and educational neuroscientists? Is the identification of specific genetic variants of practical use? Does it offer insights into the molecular mechanisms of learning, or how the brain works to process information? Do the current polygenic scores for educational attainment have utility for individual genetic prediction? What implications does genetic work have for environmental research? We address these questions in the following sections.

What Does This Mean for Education?

Polygenic Scores for Prediction of Educational Outcomes

Polygenic scores that account for a proportion (~10%; (Lee et al., 2018) of heritability allow the identification of individuals with extreme (very high or very low) scores, which may in turn be of practical use in an educational setting. For example—as has been suggested elsewhere—polygenic scores for educational attainment could be used to identify children who might be prone to learning or behavioral difficulties long before the emergence of overt cognitive or behavioral symptoms (see Asbury & Plomin, 2014). This would provide parents and teachers with the opportunity to allocate additional support and resources, put early interventions in place, or simply monitor the child more closely before difficulties arise. In theory, this would not only address the learning problems, but also help alleviate the collateral emotional, social, and familial damage frequently experienced by those who struggle at school. Sidestepping for a moment the very real ethical and societal issues raised by the potential to cause harm with polygenic prediction, there are some important caveats to consider when thinking about the use of polygenic scores for prediction of educational risk and resilience. As discussed, the educational attainment PGSs capture and predict a wide range of cognitive, non-cognitive, and environmental traits and therefore they currently have no specificity; at present we are unable to differentiate between children who will struggle at reading, or math, or exhibit behavior problems or experience some combination of all of these, making the task of selecting appropriate interventions complex. On the other hand, given that these traits tend to be moderately genetically correlated, one could argue that it is prudent to use polygenic scores to identify individuals for earlier (or more frequent) monitoring, or select interventions that aim to generally enrich a child's learning opportunities, such as those offered by Sure Start. However, it is worth remembering that polygenic prediction also only realistically caters for the smaller fraction of individuals at the extremes of the distribution of polygenic scores, i.e., those with very low scores or those with very high scores, and so has no immediate applicability to the majority of the general population. Furthermore, with the exception of those individuals at the very extreme tails of the distribution—polygenic scores contain tens of thousands of genetic variants and their composition will differ between people; that is, two individuals might both have low polygenic scores, but for different genetic reasons. Quite possibly, this means a universal 'one size fits all' intervention will not be effective, and a much more personalized approach (with associated logistical and cost issues) will be required. It is also worth pointing out that the majority of polygenic research in education has focused on adult or adolescent populations, and we lack a full understanding of the developmental timing or specificity of polygenic scores. There are also practical barriers to the use of polygenic scores for prediction, namely that it requires the availability of genetic data for the individual. In the future, it is plausible that DNA sequence data might be generated for children at birth as a routine part of healthcare (Robert Plomin, n.d.), but it remains unclear quite who would be responsible for interpreting this information (and re-interpreting it as more powerful PGSs are developed), and under what circumstances an individual's genetic data might be shared with educators and parents (Palk, Dalvie, de Vries, Martin, & Stein, 2019). It is also important to note that the vast majority of genome-wide association studies have been performed using European populations, and current polygenic scores do not appear to work as well in non-European samples (Duncan et al., 2018). Consequently, if they are to have broad applicability in education and mitigate (rather than exacerbate) educational and social inequality, large-scale GWASs of populations with diverse ancestral histories are urgently required (Martin et al., 2019).

Finally, it may have occurred to you that a polygenic score for educational attainment is fundamentally uncoupled from biological mechanisms—it doesn't tell you which specific DNA variants are influencing school performance, or how. Arguably polygenic scores for prediction will remain of limited value until we know what the relevant environments to change are, or what type of intervention will help mitigate risk. For that, we need a better understanding of molecular and biological mechanisms and the developmental interplay between genes and the environment.

What Might This Mean in the Future?

Insight Into Biological Mechanisms

In the future, as GWAS sample sizes expand to ever greater numbers, they will detect a greater number of associated genetic variants, but their individual effect sizes will be even smaller than the ones already identified—we will see diminishing returns in terms of variance explained by common genetic variation alone. However, the insights from genome-wide association studies will remain highly valuable, as they have the potential to shed light on the neurobiological mechanisms of cognitive performance and understanding mechanisms will be critical for the effective translation of research to the classroom (Thomas, Ansari, & Knowland, 2019).

It is perhaps worth stating that genes that directly encode 'for' education or educational behavior do not exist; rather, genetic variants operate at the level of the cell to create subtle biochemical, structural, and functional differences between people that (over the course of development) act in a probabilistic way to influence brain development, cognition, and exposure to environments. For example, having a high polygenic score for intelligence might translate to more effective communication between neurons, or more efficient myelination of axons during adolescence. Or it might operate on neurophysiological pathways that act to make you slightly more resilient to hardship, or better able to remain focused in the presence of visual or aural distractors. Tracing the causal paths from DNA sequence, to biological pathways, to the structure and function of the brain, and educational behaviors and outcomes—all within a developmental context—is an incredibly complex task. An immediate complicating factor is that genetic variation in the same physical location on a chromosome is correlated (i.e., it tends to be inherited together), making it difficult to pinpoint the exact causal DNA variant (or variants) that are responsible for the association signal identified in the GWAS (Wang et al., 2010). That is, while we get an instant chromosomal location, the signal is often 'spread out' over multiple variants in the immediate neighborhood and identifying the true causal variant requires additional experiments. Furthermore, even when we are confident of the precise location of the genetic variant(s) driving the association signal, it turns out that they *tend* to be located in regions of the genome that do not encode for protein sequences (in 'non-coding' regions). In fact, an overwhelmingly consistent finding across GWASs from psychology, psychiatry, and the social sciences is that the majority of trait-associated variants are not located in genes, but rather in the non-coding spaces between the genes (Zhang & Lupski, 2015). This is not an insurmountable problem however, and statistical and functional interrogation of the SSGAC educational attainment GWAS datasets resulted in a prioritized list of genes that carry out neurophysiological brain functions such as neurotransmitter secretion, activation of ion channels, synaptic plasticity, and are expressed in neural tissue pre- and postnatally (Lee et al., 2018). Interestingly, the consortium failed to find evidence for the involvement of glial cell function, suggesting that either common genetic variation does not contribute to *individual differences* in cell firing rate, or that this is not a core mechanism underpinning variability in speed of cognitive processing (although note that this does not rule it out in having a universal role in human learning). In parallel, while the majority of SNPs identified in the 2017 GWAS of intelligence are located in non-coding regions of the genome, many are linked to the regulation of genomic activities and expression of (nearby) genes, and the authors detected enrichment for genes regulating cell development (Sniekers et al., 2017).

To conclude, while the timeline to translation is likely to be measured in years, we predict that comprehensive interrogation of GWAS data and its integration with additional biological datasets will provide greater understanding of the causal paths between genes, the brain, and educationally relevant behaviors, as recent biological insights from psychiatric research demonstrate (Birnbaum & Weinberger, 2017; Gandal et al., 2018). Knowledge of the many mechanisms by which common DNA variants of small effect specifically map on to educationally relevant behaviors and academic outcomes will be essential for effective intervention strategies based on polygenic (and environmental) risk, and for understanding the molecular and neural basis of individual differences in learning.

Genetically Informed Environmental Research

Polygenic scores will also be of use to researchers interested in exploring the interplay between genes and environment during development and controlling for genetic confounding in environmental educational research. One obvious application is in the field of **gene-environment interaction** (GxE) research, which aims to test whether an individual's response to an environmental experience (or exposure) is mediated by their genotype (Rutter, 2006). GxE studies in psychiatry and psychology have historically suffered from poor replication, most probably because they were limited to examining single genetic variants in candidate genes that were not robustly associated with the trait in question to start with (Border et al., 2019). Now that polygenic scores are available that explain meaningful amounts of variance in educational attainment and intelligence, it becomes possible to perform well-powered GxE studies that focus on quantifiable genetic risk and resilience (Assary, Vincent, Keers, & Pluess, 2018). As yet, no GxE studies using the Edu-Years polygenic score have been published, but the approach has been used with some success in GxE studies of psychiatric disease and exposure to environmental risk factors (Mullins et al., 2016) and smoking behavior (Meyers et al., 2013). An area ripe for exploration will be identification of specific environments (for example, parenting behaviors, peer group characteristics or classroom features) that seem to moderate or mitigate outcomes in individuals considered at high polygenic 'risk'.

Polygenic scores can also be used as an individual-specific control to remove the possible confounding influence of genetic influences in observational studies. For example, Smith-Woolley et al. found that when looking at differences in educational achievement and well-being between state and private schools, the educational 'boost' provided by private education was markedly reduced when polygenic scores were used to control for genetic differences between the children (Smith-Woolley, Pingault et al., 2018). What this study demonstrated was that—at least in terms of scholastic achievement—private schools are selecting for heritable characteristics of children during the admissions process.

Conclusion

What Has Behavior Genetics Added to Our Understanding Over and Above Psychology?

The focus of this chapter has been to consider what modern behavioral genetic research has told us about the origins of individual differences in higher-level cognitive traits and behaviors related to education. The leading message is that a student's educational journey, experiences, and academic performance are influenced by the sequence of 3 billion As, Cs, Gs and Ts that they are born with. The question is no longer *whether* genes influence educational outcomes but *how*, and in what environmental contexts are genetic effects most salient. Advances in molecular genetic technologies coupled with careful study design and very large sample sizes have shown that the combined action of *thousands* of alleles that are common in the population collectively contribute to variability in educational and learning outcomes. However, at present we lack a comprehensive understanding of the precise mechanistic links between polygenic load, genome function and regulation, brain development, and cognitive outcomes. Emerging studies indicate polygenic effects converge on general neurobiological functions, such as neuronal development, synaptic transmission, and plasticity. This generality has highlighted the pleiotropic nature of genes and demonstrated that shared biology partly underpins the observed relationships between educational performance and a diverse array of social, economic, and physical and mental health outcomes. Future work will undoubtedly be focused on unpicking the causal nature of these relationships across the lifespan, aided by the availability of genetic datasets and innovative statistical methods that utilize polygenic scores (e.g., see **Mendelian randomisation**; (Pingault et al., 2018).

Concrete Implications of Research and Opportunities for Translation

Identification of the top 'hits' from genome-wide association studies have started to shed some light on mechanisms, which is the first step required for understanding the biological basis of learning and enabling informed decision making about what might be the most effective pedagogical approaches, learning environments, and interventions. Figuring out exactly how specific DNA variants alter molecular and biological processes to result in cognitive and behavioral differences between people remains a significant challenge for researchers, not least because the phenotypes currently used (such as educational attainment) capture many things and are typically measured in adulthood. For translational opportunity, we will need to be clear on the precise phenotypes that we are interested in and measure them appropriately and at the correct developmental stage, and examine the specificity of identified associations at multiple levels of analysis, including at the neurocognitive, behavioral, and structural level (Dick et al., 2018).

Finally, there is great interest—although not without debate—about the use of polygenic scores for prediction of educationally relevant outcomes. It is important to emphasize that polygenic scores are not a crystal ball, nor will they ever be, but their predictive accuracy will grow as we gain more comprehensive insights into the full spectrum of genetic contributions to differences in educational phenotypes, include additional non-genetic predictors in the model, and are better able to account for the developmental interplay between genes and the environment (Aschard et al., 2012); Figure 3.1). Some of the enthusiasm for genetic prediction has undoubtedly been motivated by the recent inroads made with polygenic prediction of chronic diseases and the viability of 'precision medicine' (e.g., see (Chatterjee, Shi, & García-Closas, 2016; Mavaddat et al., 2019). However, the classroom is very different from the clinic and we posit that the same approaches and concerns associated with polygenic risk prediction for chronic disease cannot be cut and pasted to education. There needs to be a demonstrated desire by both parents and educators for genetically informed classrooms, and open and informed discussion about the ethical, social, and policy issues it raises. For example, how polygenic scores are employed will depend on what we want from our educational system. Do we want to use genetic information to maximize every student's educational potential (that will potentially increase individual differences in the classroom), to flatten out and fight genetic inequalities in an effort to narrow the gaps in achievement between students, or focus resources on identifying those students most likely to struggle so that we can intervene early on? These are difficult—but important—questions to answer, and will require open, informed and continued discussions between scientists, policy makers and the general public.

Notes

1. https://wir2018.wid.world/
2. Readers interested in a more detailed overview of the scientific and technical developments that paved the way for genome-wide association studies, the advantages and limitations of the approach, and key sights gleaned from the past 10 years of GWAS are referred to these reviews: Pearson & Manolio (2008); Tam et al. (2019); and Visscher et al. (2017).
3. www.thessgac.org/
4. Readers interested in more in-depth discussion of molecular genetic investigations of cognitive function and educational attainment are referred to recent reviews (Plomin & Deary, 2014; Plomin & von Stumm, 2018).
5. For the interested reader, a number of reviews of the technical considerations of polygenic score construction, their interpretation, and usefulness for research purposes and prediction have been written. See: Bogdan, Baranger, & Agrawal (2018); Chatterjee et al. (2016); Choi, Mak, & O'Reilly (2018); Dudbridge (2016); and Wray et al. (2014).

Suggested Further Reading

Cesarini, D., & Visscher, P. M. (2017). Genetics and educational attainment. *npj Science of Learning, 2*, Article number 4.

Plomin, R., DeFries, J. C., Knopik, V. S., & Neiderhiser, J. M. (2016, January 11). Top 10 replicated findings from behavioral genetics. *Perspectives on Psychological Science, 11*(1), 3–23.

Turkheimer, E. (2000). Three laws of behavior genetics and what they mean. *Current Directions in Psychological Science, 9*(5), 160–164.

Turkheimer, E. (2016). Weak genetic explanation 20 years later: Reply to Plomin et al. *Perspectives on Psychological Science, 11*(1), 24–28.

References

Anderson, J. S., Shade, J., DiBlasi, E., Shabalin, A. A., & Docherty, A. R. (2019). Polygenic risk scoring and prediction of mental health outcomes. *Current Opinion in Psychology, 27*, 77–81. https://doi.org/10.1016/j.copsyc.2018.09.002

Asbury, K., & Plomin, R. (2014). *G is for genes: The impact of genetics on education and achievement*. Wiley-Blackwell. ISBN:978-1-118-48281-0.

Aschard, H., Lutz, S., Maus, B., Duell, E. J., Fingerlin, T. E., Chatterjee, N., . . . Van Steen, K. (2012). Challenges and opportunities in genome-wide environmental interaction (GWEI) studies. *Human Genetics, 131*(10), 1591–1613. https://doi.org/10.1007/s00439-012-1192-0

Assary, E., Vincent, J. P., Keers, R., & Pluess, M. (2018). Gene-environment interaction and psychiatric disorders: Review and future directions. *Seminars in Cell & Developmental Biology, 77*, 133–143. https://doi.org/10.1016/j.semcdb.2017.10.016

Auton, A., Abecasis, G. R., Altshuler, D. M., Durbin, R. M., Bentley, D. R., Chakravarti, A., . . . Schloss, J. A. (2015, October 30). A global reference for human genetic variation. *Nature, 526*, 68–74. https://doi.org/10.1038/nature15393

Balding, D. J. (2006). A tutorial on statistical methods for population association studies. *Nature Reviews: Genetics, 7*(10), 781–791. https://doi.org/10.1038/nrg1916

Bartels, M. (2015). Genetics of wellbeing and its components satisfaction with life, happiness, and quality of life: A review and meta-analysis of heritability studies. *Behavior Genetics, 45*(2), 137–156. https://doi.org/10.1007/s10519-015-9713-y

Belsky, D. W., Moffitt, T. E., Corcoran, D. L., Domingue, B., Harrington, H., Hogan, S., . . . Caspi, A. (2016). The genetics of success: How single-nucleotide polymorphisms associated with educational attainment relate to life-course development. *Psychological Science, 27*(7), 957–972. https://doi.org/10.1177/0956797616643070

Benyamin, B., Pourcain, B., Davis, O. S., Davies, G., Hansell, N. K., Brion, M.-J., . . . Visscher, P. M. (2014). Childhood intelligence is heritable, highly polygenic and associated with FNBP1L. *Molecular Psychiatry, 19*(2), 253–258. https://doi.org/10.1038/mp.2012.184

Birnbaum, R., & Weinberger, D. R. (2017). Genetic insights into the neurodevelopmental origins of schizophrenia. *Nature Reviews Neuroscience, 18*(12), 727–740. https://doi.org/10.1038/nrn.2017.125

Bishop, D. V. M. (2015). The interface between genetics and psychology: Lessons from developmental dyslexia. *Proceedings of the Royal Society B: Biological Sciences*. https://doi.org/10.1098/rspb.2014.3139

Bogdan, R., Baranger, D. A. A., & Agrawal, A. (2018). Polygenic risk scores in clinical psychology: Bridging genomic risk to individual differences. *Annual Review of Clinical Psychology, 14*(1), 119–157. https://doi.org/10.1146/annurev-clinpsy-050817-084847

Border, R., Johnson, E. C., Evans, L. M., Smolen, A., Berley, N., Sullivan, P. F., & Keller, M. C. (2019). No support for historical candidate gene or candidate gene-by-interaction hypotheses for major depression across multiple large samples. *American Journal of Psychiatry, 176*(5), 376–387. https://doi.org/10.1176/appi.ajp.2018.18070881

Boyle, E. A., Li, Y. I., & Pritchard, J. K. (2017). An expanded view of complex traits: From polygenic to omnigenic. *Cell, 169*(7), 1177–1186. https://doi.org/10.1016/j.cell.2017.05.038

Bulik-Sullivan, B. K., Loh, P.-R., Finucane, H. K., Ripke, S., Yang, J., Patterson, N., . . . Neale, B. M. (2015). LD score regression distinguishes confounding from polygenicity in genome-wide association studies. *Nature Genetics, 47*(3), 291–295. https://doi.org/10.1038/ng.3211

Carroll, J. B. (1993). *Human cognitive abilities.* https://doi.org/10.1017/CBO9780511571312

Chabris, C. F., Hebert, B. M., Benjamin, D. J., Beauchamp, J., Cesarini, D., van der Loos, M., . . . Laibson, D. (2012). Most reported genetic associations with general intelligence are probably false positives. *Psychological Science, 23*(11), 1314–1323. https://doi.org/10.1177/0956797611435528

Chatterjee, N., Shi, J., & García-Closas, M. (2016). Developing and evaluating polygenic risk prediction models for stratified disease prevention. *Nature Reviews Genetics, 17*(7), 392–406. https://doi.org/10.1038/nrg.2016.27

Cheesman, R., Selzam, S., Ronald, A., Dale, P. S., McAdams, T. A., Eley, T. C., & Plomin, R. (2017). Childhood behaviour problems show the greatest gap between DNA-based and twin heritability. *Translational Psychiatry, 7*(12), 1284. https://doi.org/10.1038/s41398-017-0046-x

Chiurazzi, P., & Pirozzi, F. (2016). Advances in understanding—genetic basis of intellectual disability. *F1000Research, 5,* 599. https://doi.org/10.12688/f1000research.7134.1

Choi, S. W., Mak, T. S. H., & O'Reilly, P. F. (2018). *A guide to performing polygenic risk score analyses.* bioRxiv Server. https://doi.org/10.1101/416545

Crosswaite, M., & Asbury, K. (2019). Teacher beliefs about the aetiology of individual differences in cognitive ability, and the relevance of behavioural genetics to education. *British Journal of Educational Psychology, 89*(1), 95–110. https://doi.org/10.1111/bjep.12224

Cullen, H., Krishnan, M. L., Selzam, S., Ball, G., Visconti, A., Saxena, A., . . . Edwards, A. D. (2018). *Genes associated with neuropsychiatric disease increase vulnerability to abnormal deep grey matter development.* bioRxiv Server. https://doi.org/10.1101/342394

Cutler, D., Lleras-Muney, A., & Vogl, T. (2008). *Socioeconomic status and health: Dimensions and mechanisms.* https://doi.org/10.3386/w14333

Davies, G., Tenesa, A., Payton, A., Yang, J., Harris, S. E., Liewald, D., . . . Deary, I. J. (2011). Genome-wide association studies establish that human intelligence is highly heritable and polygenic. *Molecular Psychiatry, 16*(10), 996–1005. https://doi.org/10.1038/mp.2011.85

Davis, O. S. P., Butcher, L. M., Docherty, S. J., Meaburn, E. L., Curtis, C. J. C., Simpson, M. A., . . . Plomin, R. (2010). A three-stage genome-wide association study of general cognitive ability: Hunting the small effects. *Behavior Genetics, 40*(6), 759–767. https://doi.org/10.1007/s10519-010-9350-4

Davis, O. S. P., Haworth, C. M. A., Lewis, C. M., & Plomin, R. (2012). Visual analysis of geocoded twin data puts nature and nurture on the map. *Molecular Psychiatry*, 17(9), 867–874. https://doi.org/10.1038/mp.2012.68

de Zeeuw, E. L., de Geus, E. J. C., & Boomsma, D. I. (2015). Meta-analysis of twin studies highlights the importance of genetic variation in primary school educational achievement. *Trends in Neuroscience and Education*, 4(3), 69–76. https://doi.org/10.1016/J.TINE.2015.06.001

de Zeeuw, E. L., van Beijsterveldt, C. E. M., Glasner, T. J., Bartels, M., Ehli, E. A., Davies, G. E., . . . Boomsma, D. I. (2014). Polygenic scores associated with educational attainment in adults predict educational achievement and ADHD symptoms in children. *American Journal of Medical Genetics Part B: Neuropsychiatric Genetics*, 165(6), 510–520. https://doi.org/10.1002/ajmg.b.32254

Deary, I. J. (2012). Intelligence. *Annual Review of Psychology*, 63(1), 453–482. https://doi.org/10.1146/annurev-psych-120710-100353

Deary, I. J., Strand, S., Smith, P., & Fernandes, C. (2007). Intelligence and educational achievement. *Intelligence*, 35(1), 13–21. https://doi.org/10.1016/J.INTELL.2006.02.001

Department for Education. (2015). *The purpose of education—GOV.UK*. Schools Minister Nick Gibb addresses the Education Reform Summit. Retrieved May 29, 2019, from www.gov.uk/government/speeches/the-purpose-of-education

Dick, D. M., Barr, P. B., Cho, S. B., Cooke, M. E., Kuo, S. I.-C., Lewis, T. J., . . . Su, J. (2018). Post-GWAS in psychiatric genetics: A developmental perspective on the "other" next steps. *Genes, Brain and Behavior*, 17(3), e12447. https://doi.org/10.1111/gbb.12447

Docherty, A. R., Moscati, A., Peterson, R., Edwards, A. C., Adkins, D. E., Bacanu, S. A., . . . Kendler, K. S. (2016). SNP-based heritability estimates of the personality dimensions and polygenic prediction of both neuroticism and major depression: Findings from CONVERGE. *Translational Psychiatry*, 6(10), e926–e926. https://doi.org/10.1038/tp.2016.177

Docherty, S. J., Davis, O. S. P., Kovas, Y., Meaburn, E. L., Dale, P. S., Petrill, S. A., . . . Plomin, R. (2010). A genome-wide association study identifies multiple loci associated with mathematics ability and disability. *Genes, Brain and Behavior*, 9(2), 234–247. https://doi.org/10.1111/j.1601-183X.2009.00553.x

Domingue, B. W., Belsky, D. W., Conley, D., Harris, K. M., & Boardman, J. D. (2015). Polygenic influence on educational attainment. *AERA Open*, 1(3). https://doi.org/10.1177/2332858415599972

Dudbridge, F. (2016). Polygenic epidemiology. *Genetic Epidemiology*, 40(4), 268–272. https://doi.org/10.1002/gepi.21966

Dudbridge, F., & Gusnanto, A. (2008). Estimation of significance thresholds for genomewide association scans. *Genetic Epidemiology*, 32(3), 227–234. https://doi.org/10.1002/gepi.20297

Duncan, L., Shen, H., Gelaye, B., Ressler, K., Feldman, M., Peterson, R., & Domingue, B. (2018). *Analysis of polygenic score usage and performance in diverse human populations*. bioRxiv Server. https://doi.org/10.1101/398396

Elliott, M. L., Belsky, D. W., Anderson, K., Corcoran, D. L., Ge, T., Knodt, A., . . . Hariri, A. R. (2018). *A polygenic score for higher educational attainment is associated with larger brains*. bioRxiv Server. https://doi.org/10.1101/287490

Gandal, M. J., Haney, J. R., Parikshak, N. N., Leppa, V., Ramaswami, G., Hartl, C., . . . Geschwind, D. H. (2018). Shared molecular neuropathology across major psychiatric

disorders parallels polygenic overlap. *Science, 359*(6376), 693–697. https://doi.org/
10.1126/science.aad6469

Gilissen, C., Hoischen, A., Brunner, H. G., & Veltman, J. A. (2011). Unlocking mendelian disease using exome sequencing. *Genome Biology, 12*(9), 228. https://doi.org/
10.1186/gb-2011-12-9-228

Hagenaars, S. P., Harris, S. E., Davies, G., Hill, W. D., Liewald, D. C. M., Ritchie,
S. J., . . . Deary, I. J. (2016). Shared genetic aetiology between cognitive functions and physical and mental health in UK biobank (N=112 151) and 24 GWAS
consortia. *Molecular Psychiatry, 21*(11), 1624–1632. https://doi.org/10.1038/
mp.2015.225

Hardy, J., & Singleton, A. (2009). Genomewide association studies and human disease. *New England Journal of Medicine, 360*(17), 1759–1768. https://doi.org/10.1056/
NEJMra0808700

Harlaar, N., Meaburn, E. L., Hayiou-Thomas, M. E., Davis, O. S. P., Docherty, S., Hanscombe, K. B., . . . Plomin, R. (2014). Genome-wide association study of receptive
language ability of 12-year-olds. *Journal of Speech, Language, and Hearing Research,
57*(1), 96–105. https://doi.org/10.1044/1092-4388(2013/12-0303)

Haworth, C. M. A., & Davis, O. S. P. (2014). From observational to dynamic genetics.
Frontiers in Genetics, 5, 6. https://doi.org/10.3389/fgene.2014.00006

Haworth, C. M. A., Davis, O. S. P., & Plomin, R. (2013). Twins early development
study (TEDS): A genetically sensitive investigation of cognitive and behavioral
development from childhood to young adulthood. *Twin Research and Human Genetics: The Official Journal of the International Society for Twin Studies, 16*(1), 117–125.
https://doi.org/10.1017/thg.2012.91

Haworth, C. M. A., Wright, M. J., Luciano, M., Martin, N. G., de Geus, E. J. C., van
Beijsterveldt, C. E. M., . . . Plomin, R. (2010). The heritability of general cognitive
ability increases linearly from childhood to young adulthood. *Molecular Psychiatry,
15*(11), 1112–1120. https://doi.org/10.1038/mp.2009.55

Hill, W. D., Hagenaars, S. P., Marioni, R. E., Harris, S. E., Liewald, D. C. M., Davies,
G., . . . Deary, I. J. (2016). Molecular genetic contributions to social deprivation and
household income in UK biobank. *Current Biology, 26*(22), 3083–3089. https://doi.
org/10.1016/J.CUB.2016.09.035

Hill, W. D., Harris, S. E., & Deary, I. J. (2019). What genome-wide association studies
reveal about the association between intelligence and mental health. *Current Opinion in Psychology, 27*, 25–30. https://doi.org/10.1016/J.COPSYC.2018.07.007

Jelenkovic, A., Sund, R., Hur, Y.-M., Yokoyama, Y., Hjelmborg, J. V. B., Möller, S., . . .
Silventoinen, K. (2016). Genetic and environmental influences on height from
infancy to early adulthood: An individual-based pooled analysis of 45 twin cohorts.
Scientific Reports, 6(1). https://doi.org/10.1038/srep28496

Johnson, W., Deary, I. J., & Iacono, W. G. (2009). Genetic and environmental transactions underlying educational attainment. *Intelligence, 37*(5), 466–478. https://doi.
org/10.1016/J.INTELL.2009.05.006

Kendler, K. S., Neale, M. C., Kessler, R. C., Heath, A. C., & Eaves, L. J. (1993).
A test of the equal-environment assumption in twin studies of psychiatric illness.
Behavior Genetics, 23(1), 21–27. Retrieved from www.ncbi.nlm.nih.gov/pubmed/
8476388

Knopik, V. S., Neiderhiser, J. M., DeFries, J. C., & Plomin, R. (2016). *Behavioral genetics* (7th ed.). New York: Worth Publishers. Retrieved from www.macmillanihe.com/
page/detail/behavioral-genetics/?k=9781464176050&loc=uk

Kong, A., Thorleifsson, G., Frigge, M. L., Vilhjalmsson, B. J., Young, A. I., Thorgeirsson, T. E., . . . Stefansson, K. (2018). The nature of nurture: Effects of parental genotypes. *Science, 359*(6374), 424–428. https://doi.org/10.1126/science.aan6877

Kovas, Y., Harlaar, N., Petrill, S. A., & Plomin, R. (2005). "Generalist genes" and mathematics in 7-year-old twins. *Intelligence, 33*(5), 473–489. https://doi.org/10.1016/j.intell.2005.05.002

Kovas, Y., Voronin, I., Kaydalov, A., Malykh, S. B., Dale, P. S., & Plomin, R. (2013). Literacy and numeracy are more heritable than intelligence in primary school. *Psychological Science, 24*(10), 2048–2056. https://doi.org/10.1177/0956797613486982

Krapohl, E., Euesden, J., Zabaneh, D., Pingault, J.-B., Rimfeld, K., von Stumm, S., . . . Plomin, R. (2016). Phenome-wide analysis of genome-wide polygenic scores. *Molecular Psychiatry, 21*(9), 1188–1193. https://doi.org/10.1038/mp.2015.126

Krapohl, E., & Plomin, R. (2016). Genetic link between family socioeconomic status and children's educational achievement estimated from genome-wide SNPs. *Molecular Psychiatry, 21*(3), 437–443. https://doi.org/10.1038/mp.2015.2

Krapohl, E., Rimfeld, K., Shakeshaft, N. G., Trzaskowski, M., McMillan, A., Pingault, J.-B., . . . Plomin, R. (2014). The high heritability of educational achievement reflects many genetically influenced traits, not just intelligence. *Proceedings of the National Academy of Sciences of the United States of America, 111*(42), 15273–15278. https://doi.org/10.1073/pnas.1408777111

Kruglyak, L. (2008). The road to genome-wide association studies. *Nature Reviews Genetics, 9*(4), 314–318. https://doi.org/10.1038/nrg2316

Lee, J. J., Wedow, R., Okbay, A., Kong, E., Maghzian, O., Zacher, M., . . . Cesarini, D. (2018). Gene discovery and polygenic prediction from a genome-wide association study of educational attainment in 1.1 million individuals. *Nature Genetics, 50*(8), 1112–1121. https://doi.org/10.1038/s41588-018-0147-3

Maier, R. M., Visscher, P. M., Robinson, M. R., & Wray, N. R. (2018). Embracing polygenicity: A review of methods and tools for psychiatric genetics research. *Psychological Medicine, 48*(7), 1055–1067. https://doi.org/10.1017/S0033291717002318

Martin, A. R., Kanai, M., Kamatani, Y., Okada, Y., Neale, B. M., & Daly, M. J. (2019). *Current clinical use of polygenic scores will risk exacerbating health disparities.* bioRxiv Server. https://doi.org/10.1101/441261

Mavaddat, N., Michailidou, K., Dennis, J., Lush, M., Fachal, L., Lee, A., . . . Easton, D. F. (2019). Polygenic risk scores for prediction of breast cancer and breast cancer subtypes. *The American Journal of Human Genetics, 104*(1), 21–34. https://doi.org/10.1016/j.ajhg.2018.11.002

Mayhew, A. J., & Meyre, D. (2017). Assessing the heritability of complex traits in humans: Methodological challenges and opportunities. *Current Genomics, 18*(4), 332. https://doi.org/10.2174/1389202918666170307161450

Meaburn, E. L., Harlaar, N., Craig, I. W., Schalkwyk, L. C., & Plomin, R. (2008). Quantitative trait locus association scan of early reading disability and ability using pooled DNA and 100K SNP microarrays in a sample of 5760 children. *Molecular Psychiatry, 13*(7), 729–740. https://doi.org/10.1038/sj.mp.4002063

Meyers, J. L., Cerdá, M., Galea, S., Keyes, K. M., Aiello, A. E., Uddin, M., . . . Koenen, K. C. (2013). Interaction between polygenic risk for cigarette use and environmental exposures in the Detroit neighborhood health study. *Translational Psychiatry, 3*(8), e290–e290. https://doi.org/10.1038/tp.2013.63

Morris, T. T., Davies, N. M., Dorling, D., Richmond, R. C., & Smith, G. D. (2018). *Examining the genetic influences of educational attainment and the validity of value-added measures of progress.* bioRxiv Server. https://doi.org/10.1101/233635

Mullins, N., Power, R. A., Fisher, H. L., Hanscombe, K. B., Euesden, J., Iniesta, R., . . . Lewis, C. M. (2016). Polygenic interactions with environmental adversity in the aetiology of major depressive disorder. *Psychological Medicine, 46*(4), 759–770. https://doi. org/10.1017/S0033291715002172

Neale, M. C., & Cardon, L. R. (1992). *Methodology for genetic studies of twins and families.* https://doi.org/10.1007/978-94-015-8018-2

Okbay, A., Beauchamp, J. P., Fontana, M. A., Lee, J. J., Pers, T. H., Rietveld, C. A., . . . Benjamin, D. J. (2016). Genome-wide association study identifies 74 loci associated with educational attainment. *Nature, 533*(7604), 539–542. https://doi.org/10.1038/ nature17671

Open Science Collaboration. (2015). Estimating the reproducibility of psychological science. *Science, 349*(6251), aac4716–aac4716. https://doi.org/10.1126/science.aac4716

Palk, A. C., Dalvie, S., de Vries, J., Martin, A. R., & Stein, D. J. (2019). Potential use of clinical polygenic risk scores in psychiatry—ethical implications and communicating high polygenic risk. *Philosophy, Ethics, and Humanities in Medicine, 14*(1), 4. https://doi.org/10.1186/s13010-019-0073-8

Pearson, T. A., & Manolio, T. A. (2008). How to interpret a genome-wide association study. *JAMA, 299*(11). https://doi.org/10.1001/jama.299.11.1335

Pickrell, J. K., Berisa, T., Liu, J. Z., Ségurel, L., Tung, J. Y., & Hinds, D. A. (2016). Detection and interpretation of shared genetic influences on 42 human traits. *Nature Genetics, 48*(7), 709–717. https://doi.org/10.1038/ng.3570

Pingault, J.-B., O'Reilly, P. F., Schoeler, T., Ploubidis, G. B., Rijsdijk, F., & Dudbridge, F. (2018). Using genetic data to strengthen causal inference in observational research. *Nature Reviews Genetics, 19*(9), 566–580. https://doi.org/10.1038/s41576-018-0020-3

Plomin, R. (2011). Commentary: Why are children in the same family so different? Non-shared environment three decades later. *International Journal of Epidemiology, 40*(3), 582–592. https://doi.org/10.1093/ije/dyq144

Plomin, R. (n.d.). *The future of your health could soon be in the NHS's hands | the spectator.* Retrieved from www.spectator.co.uk/2019/02/the-future-of-your-health-could-soon-be-in-the-nhss-hands/

Plomin, R., & Deary, I. J. (2015). Genetics and intelligence differences: Five special findings. *Molecular Psychiatry, 20*(1), 98–108. https://doi.org/10.1038/mp.2014.105

Plomin, R., & von Stumm, S. (2018). The new genetics of intelligence. *Nature Reviews: Genetics, 19*(3), 148–159. https://doi.org/10.1038/nrg.2017.104

Polderman, T. J. C., Benyamin, B., de Leeuw, C. A., Sullivan, P. F., van Bochoven, A., Visscher, P. M., & Posthuma, D. (2015). Meta-analysis of the heritability of human traits based on fifty years of twin studies. *Nature Genetics, 47*(7), 702–709. https:// doi.org/10.1038/ng.3285

Power, R. A., & Pluess, M. (2015). Heritability estimates of the big five personality traits based on common genetic variants. *Translational Psychiatry, 5*(7), e604–e604. https://doi.org/10.1038/tp.2015.96

Reader, R. H., Covill, L. E., Nudel, R., & Newbury, D. F. (2014). Genome-wide studies of specific language impairment. *Current Behavioral Neuroscience Reports, 1*(4), 242–250. https://doi.org/10.1007/s40473-014-0024-z

Rietveld, C. A., Conley, D., Eriksson, N., Esko, T., Medland, S. E., Vinkhuyzen, A. A., . . . Social Science Genetics Association Consortium (2014a). Replicability and robustness of genome-wide-association studies for behavioral traits. *Psychological Science, 25*(11), 1975–1986. doi:10.1177/0956797614545132

Rietveld, C. A., Esko, T., Davies, G., Pers, T. H., Turley, P., Benyamin, B., . . . Koellinger, P. D. (2014b). Common genetic variants associated with cognitive performance identified using the proxy-phenotype method. *Proceedings of the National Academy of Sciences of the United States of America*, *111*(38), 13790–13794. https://doi.org/10.1073/pnas.1404623111

Rietveld, C. A., Medland, S. E., Derringer, J., Yang, J., Esko, T., Martin, N. W., . . . Koellinger, P. D. (2013). GWAS of 126,559 individuals identifies genetic variants associated with educational attainment. *Science (New York, N.Y.)*, *340*(6139), 1467–1471. https://doi.org/10.1126/science.1235488

Rimfeld, K., Ayorech, Z., Dale, P. S., Kovas, Y., & Plomin, R. (2016). Genetics affects choice of academic subjects as well as achievement. *Scientific Reports*, *6*(1), 26373. https://doi.org/10.1038/srep26373

Rimfeld, K., Kovas, Y., Dale, P. S., & Plomin, R. (2016). True grit and genetics: Predicting academic achievement from personality. *Journal of Personality and Social Psychology*, *111*(5), 780–789. https://doi.org/10.1037/pspp0000089

Rimfeld, K., Malanchini, M., Krapohl, E., Hannigan, L. J., Dale, P. S., & Plomin, R. (2018). The stability of educational achievement across school years is largely explained by genetic factors. *npj Science of Learning*, *3*(1), 16. https://doi.org/10.1038/s41539-018-0030-0

Ritchie, S. J., & Tucker-Drob, E. M. (2018). How much does education improve intelligence? A meta-analysis. *Psychological Science*, *29*(8), 1358–1369. https://doi.org/10.1177/0956797618774253

Rodic, M., Cui, J., Malykh, S., Zhou, X., Gynku, E. I., Bogdanova, E. L., . . . Kovas, Y. (2018). Cognition, emotion, and arithmetic in primary school: A cross-cultural investigation. *British Journal of Developmental Psychology*, *36*(2), 255–276. https://doi.org/10.1111/bjdp.12248

Ross, C. E., & Wu, C. (1995). The links between education and health. *American Sociological Review*, *60*(5), 719. https://doi.org/10.2307/2096319

Rutter, M. (2006). *Genes and behavior: Nature-nurture interplay explained*. Oxford: Blackwell Publishing.

Schwabe, I., Janss, L., & van den Berg, S. M. (2017). Can we validate the results of twin studies? A census-based study on the heritability of educational achievement. *Frontiers in Genetics*, *8*, 160. https://doi.org/10.3389/fgene.2017.00160

Selzam, S., Dale, P. S., Wagner, R. K., DeFries, J. C., Cederlöf, M., O'Reilly, P. F., . . . Plomin, R. (2017a). Genome-wide polygenic scores predict reading performance throughout the school years. *Scientific Studies of Reading*, *21*(4), 334–349. https://doi.org/10.1080/10888438.2017.1299152

Selzam, S., Krapohl, E., von Stumm, S., O'Reilly, P. F., Rimfeld, K., Kovas, Y., . . . Plomin, R. (2017b). Predicting educational achievement from DNA. *Molecular Psychiatry*, *22*(2), 267–272. https://doi.org/10.1038/mp.2016.107

Shakeshaft, N. G., Trzaskowski, M., McMillan, A., Rimfeld, K., Krapohl, E., Haworth, C. M. A., . . . Plomin, R. (2013). Strong genetic influence on a UK nationwide test of educational achievement at the end of compulsory education at age 16. *PloS One*, *8*(12), e80341. https://doi.org/10.1371/journal.pone.0080341

Smith-Woolley, E., Ayorech, Z., Dale, P. S., von Stumm, S., & Plomin, R. (2018). The genetics of university success. *Scientific Reports*, *8*(1), 14579. https://doi.org/10.1038/s41598-018-32621-w

Smith-Woolley, E., Pingault, J.-B., Selzam, S., Rimfeld, K., Krapohl, E., von Stumm, S., . . . Plomin, R. (2018). Differences in exam performance between pupils attending selective and non-selective schools mirror the genetic differences between them. *npj Science of Learning*, *3*(1), 3. https://doi.org/10.1038/s41539-018-0019-8

Smith-Woolley, E., Selzam, S., & Plomin, R. (2019). Polygenic score for educational attainment captures DNA variants shared between personality traits and educational achievement. *Journal of Personality and Social Psychology*. https://doi.org/10.1037/pspp0000241

Sniekers, S., Stringer, S., Watanabe, K., Jansen, P. R., Coleman, J. R. I., Krapohl, E., . . . Posthuma, D. (2017). Genome-wide association meta-analysis of 78,308 individuals identifies new loci and genes influencing human intelligence. *Nature Genetics*, 49(7), 1107–1112. https://doi.org/10.1038/ng.3869

Solovieff, N., Cotsapas, C., Lee, P. H., Purcell, S. M., & Smoller, J. W. (2013). Pleiotropy in complex traits: Challenges and strategies. *Nature Reviews Genetics*, 14(7), 483–495. https://doi.org/10.1038/nrg3461

Spain, S. L., & Barrett, J. C. (2015). Strategies for fine-mapping complex traits. *Human Molecular Genetics*, 24(R1), R111–R119. https://doi.org/10.1093/hmg/ddv260

Spearman, C. (1904). General intelligence, objectively determined and measured. *The American Journal of Psychology*, 15(2), 201–292.

Tam, V., Patel, N., Turcotte, M., Bossé, Y., Paré, G., & Meyre, D. (2019). Benefits and limitations of genome-wide association studies. *Nature Reviews Genetics*, 1. https://doi.org/10.1038/s41576-019-0127-1

Taylor, J., Roehrig, A. D., Hensler, B. S., Connor, C. M., & Schatschneider, C. (2010). Teacher quality moderates the genetic effects on early reading. *Science (New York, N.Y.)*, 328(5977), 512. https://doi.org/10.1126/SCIENCE.1186149

Teare, M. D., & Santibanez Koref, M. F. (2014). Linkage analysis and the study of Mendelian disease in the era of whole exome and genome sequencing. *Briefings in Functional Genomics*, 13(5), 378–383. https://doi.org/10.1093/bfgp/elu024

Thomas, M. S. C., Ansari, D., & Knowland, V. C. P. (2019). Annual research review: Educational neuroscience: Progress and prospects. *Journal of Child Psychology and Psychiatry*, 60(4), 477–492. https://doi.org/10.1111/jcpp.12973

Thomas, M. S. C., Kovas, Y., Meaburn, E. L., & Tolmie, A. (2015). What can the study of genetics offer to educators? *Mind, Brain, and Education*, 9(2), 72–80. https://doi.org/10.1111/mbe.12077

Trzaskowski, M., Yang, J., Visscher, P. M., & Plomin, R. (2014). DNA evidence for strong genetic stability and increasing heritability of intelligence from age 7 to 12. *Molecular Psychiatry*, 19(3), 380–384. https://doi.org/10.1038/mp.2012.191

Tucker-Drob, E. M., Briley, D. A., & Harden, K. P. (2013). Genetic and environmental influences on cognition across development and context. *Current Directions in Psychological Science*, 22(5), 349–355. https://doi.org/10.1177/0963721413485087

Turkheimer, E., Haley, A., Waldron, M., D'Onofrio, B., & Gottesman, I. I. (2003). Socioeconomic status modifies heritability of IQ in young children. *Psychological Science*, 14(6), 623–628. https://doi.org/10.1046/j.0956-7976.2003.psci_1475.x

Visscher, P. M., Brown, M. A., McCarthy, M. I., & Yang, J. (2012). Five years of GWAS discovery. *The American Journal of Human Genetics*, 90(1), 7–24. https://doi.org/10.1016/j.ajhg.2011.11.029

Visscher, P. M., Hill, W. G., & Wray, N. R. (2008). Heritability in the genomics era—concepts and misconceptions. *Nature Reviews Genetics*, 9(4), 255–266. https://doi.org/10.1038/nrg2322

Visscher, P. M., Wray, N. R., Zhang, Q., Sklar, P., McCarthy, M. I., Brown, M. A., & Yang, J. (2017). 10 years of GWAS discovery: Biology, function, and translation. *American Journal of Human Genetics*, 101. https://doi.org/10.1016/j.ajhg.2017.06.005

Waaktaar, T., & Torgersen, S. (2013). Self-efficacy is mainly genetic, not learned: A multiple-rater twin study on the causal structure of general self-efficacy in young people. *Twin Research and Human Genetics, 16*(3), 651–660. https://doi.org/10.1017/thg.2013.25

Wang, K., Dickson, S. P., Stolle, C. A., Krantz, I. D., Goldstein, D. B., & Hakonarson, H. (2010). Interpretation of association signals and identification of causal variants from genome-wide association studies. *American Journal of Human Genetics, 86*(5), 730–742. https://doi.org/10.1016/j.ajhg.2010.04.003

Wellcome Trust Case Control Consortium. (2007). Genome-wide association study of 14,000 cases of seven common diseases and 3,000 shared controls. *Nature, 447*(7145), 661–678. https://doi.org/10.1038/nature05911

Wood, A. R., Esko, T., Yang, J., Vedantam, S., Pers, T. H., Gustafsson, S., . . . Frayling, T. M. (2014). Defining the role of common variation in the genomic and biological architecture of adult human height. *Nature Genetics, 46*(11), 1173–1186. https://doi.org/10.1038/ng.3097

Wray, N. R., Lee, S. H., Mehta, D., Vinkhuyzen, A. A. E., Dudbridge, F., & Middeldorp, C. M. (2014). Research review: Polygenic methods and their application to psychiatric traits. *Journal of Child Psychology and Psychiatry, 55*(10), 1068–1087. https://doi.org/10.1111/jcpp.12295

Wray, N. R., Wijmenga, C., Sullivan, P. F., Yang, J., & Visscher, P. M. (2018). Common disease is more complex than implied by the core gene omnigenic model. *Cell, 173*(7), 1573–1580. https://doi.org/10.1016/j.cell.2018.05.051

Yang, J., Benyamin, B., McEvoy, B. P., Gordon, S., Henders, A. K., Nyholt, D. R., . . . Visscher, P. M. (2010). Common SNPs explain a large proportion of the heritability for human height. *Nature Genetics, 42*(7), 565–569. https://doi.org/10.1038/ng.608

Yang, J., Lee, S. H., Goddard, M. E., & Visscher, P. M. (2011). GCTA: A tool for genome-wide complex trait analysis. *The American Journal of Human Genetics, 88*(1), 76–82. https://doi.org/10.1016/j.ajhg.2010.11.011

Zhang, F., & Lupski, J. R. (2015). Non-coding genetic variants in human disease. *Human Molecular Genetics, 24*(1), 102–110. https://doi.org/10.1093/hmg/ddv259

Glossary: definition of terms and behavioural genomic methods

Allele   An alternate version of a gene or DNA sequence at a specific locus (A or a).

Chromosome   A chromosome is a single long molecule of DNA. In diploid cells the human genome is organised into 46 chromosomes; 23 pairs of autosomes (1–22) and one pair of sex chromosomes (XX = female; XY = males).

DNA (Deoxyribonucleic Acid)   The molecule that contains the genetic instructions for all living things. The DNA molecule is comprised of two strands that coil around each other to form a double helix. Each strand contains a sugar-phosphate backbone, attached to which is one of four bases; Adenine (A), Guanine (G), Thymine (T) or Cytosine (C).

DNA variant (also called 'polymorphism')   Variation in the DNA sequence that is common (occurs with a frequency >1%) in a population. The most common type of polymorphisms are SNPs, but many others exist such as rearrangements, copy number variants, and insertions and deletions of DNA sequence.

Effect size   A statistic that quantifies the strength of a relationship between two measures.

Gene   Genes are arranged along chromosomes and consist of a sequence of DNA that is transcribed to produce a protein or an RNA product. These products carry out biological functions inside or outside the cell, or regulate the transcription of other genes. There are approximately ~21,000 protein genes in the human genome.

Gene-environment correlation   The idea that the environment an individual is exposed to is correlated with the genotype they possess. Such correlations may be passive (e.g., children who inherit genes for poor reading ability from their parents will also be raised in a house with fewer books); evocative (e.g., genetically beautiful individuals may be treated differently by other people – their genetic properties evoke a certain response); or active (e.g., children with a genetic talent for soccer may spend more time looking for opportunities to play soccer). Another example of gene-environment correlation is when people perceive their environments differently, in part based on their genetic propensities.

Genotype-environment interaction   This term refers to both the modification of genetic risk factors by environmental factors, and the role of specific genetic risk factors in determining individual differences in vulnerability to environmental risk factors. When GxE interaction is present, a specific environmental change influences the outcome in different ways depending on the genotype.

Genotype   An individual's combination of alleles (or DNA variants); AA, Aa or aa. If an individual has two copies of the same allele for a gene they are homozygous (AA or aa). If an individual has different alleles for the same gene they are said to be heterozygous (Aa).

Environment   In Behavior Genetic research, the environment is taken to mean anything other than DNA sequence. Environmental factors include diet, socioeconomic status, in utero and post-natal environment, and exposure to toxins and viruses.

Heritability   A population statistic that measures the proportion of phenotypic variability (individual differences) in a trait or behaviour that can be accounted for by genetic variation. When heritability is estimated from twin studies, it is called '*twin heritability*', and the remaining variation is assumed to be of environmental origin and classified as shared or non-shared. We are now able to measure genetic variation across the genome directly, and variance explained by observed DNA sequence differences in a population is called '*SNP heritability*' or '*DNA-based heritability*'.

Locus   The physical location of a gene or DNA sequence on a chromosome.

Human Genome   The full DNA sequence for an individual consisting of 3.1×10^8 bases. Diploid cells contain two copies of the genome, one inherited from each parent (to total 6.2×10^8 bases).

Mendelian (or single-gene) phenotype   A condition or disorder that arises due to a change in DNA sequence in a single gene. The altered gene is both necessary and sufficient for the phenotype to occur and results in characteristic familial inheritance patterns. This is in contrast to complex polygenic diseases and traits that arise due to the aggregate effects of many DNA sequence variants and the environment and lack a one-to-one mapping between genotype and phenotype.

Omnigenic hypothesis   GWAS studies have shown that individual effect sizes for trait-associated variants are vanishingly small and seem to be evenly distributed throughout the genome. This new hypothesis predicts that most of the genetic effects we currently detect do not act on trait-relevant pathways and functions directly, but rather have very weak and distal regulatory effects on a smaller sub-set of 'core' genes. If true, this has implications for how we design molecular genetic studies that aim to identify core genes (of potentially larger effect) and pathways.

Phenotype   Any observable characteristic or trait of an individual. For example, a physical trait such as weight or height, brain processes or quantifiable behaviour.

Pleiotropy   The potential for a single gene (or DNA variant) to affect multiple phenotypes. Broadly speaking, two main types of pleiotropy exist: a) biological (or horizontal) pleiotropy where the gene independently affects two traits and b) mediated (or vertical) pleiotropy where the gene affects one trait, which in turn affects the second trait. When pleiotropy is observed it is often very difficult to figure out which scenario is the most likely.

Polygenic   The contribution of many DNA variants (100s or 1,000s) to the variation in a phenotype.

Polygenic score   A cumulative measure of genetic risk for an individual based on the summed effects of many thousands of risk alleles distributed throughout the genome. Also referred to interchangeably in the literature as polygenic risk scores (PRS), genetic risk scores (GRS), polygenic susceptibility scores, SNP-sets, aggregate risk scores or genome-wide polygenic scores (GPS).

Single Nucleotide Polymorphism   (SNP; pronounced 'SNiP'): A single nucleotide variation in the DNA sequence. SNPs are the most common type of genetic variation in human populations and usually consist of two alleles. Not all SNPs impact gene function, and a high proportion are located in the spaces *between* genes.

Approaches and methods

Behaviour Genetics A field within psychology that uses genetic methods to study the origins of individual differences in human behaviour. It uses statistical approaches that infer or directly measure the contribution of genetic variation to individual differences in behaviour in a population; it may infer the genetic contribution using quantitative genetic methods, e.g., by comparing the behavioural similarity of pairs of individuals with different degrees of genetic relatedness (e.g., identical twins versus non-identical twins) while making assumptions about the respectively similarity of their environments (e.g., assuming identical and non-identical twins have equally similar family environments; thus if identical twins behave more similarly, this can only be due to their greater genetic similarity) or directly measure the genetic contribution by using molecular genetic methods to correlate DNA variation to behavioural variation.

Genome wide association study (GWAS) A method in molecular genetics in which common DNA variations (typically SNPs, but it can be other types of variation) are correlated to variations in some trait or behaviour in a population to see if any variant is associated with the trait. GWASes do not directly show which gene or allele is causally responsible for variation in the trait; rather they indicate locations on the genome from where the signal is originating. These regions are then typically followed up in further experiments designed to assess the likely casual allele(s), pathways on which they act, and their impact on gene function and regulation.

Molecular genetics The study of genes and DNA sequence.

SNP Genotyping arrays A technology that is able to genotype hundreds of thousands of SNPs across the genome per individual in a single reaction. The availability of SNP genotyping arrays enabled genome-wide association studies of large numbers of individuals.

Mendelian Randomisation An analytical method that uses observational data and measures genetic variation to assess causal relationships between modifiable environmental risk factors and phenotypic (e.g., behavioural or health) outcomes. The approach depends on several important assumptions but can overcome issues of confounding and reverse causation that blight observational epidemiological studies.

Useful web resources:

http://www.dorak.info/epi/glosge.html
https://www.genome.gov/glossary/
https://www.ashg.org/education/everyone_1.shtml
https://ghr.nlm.nih.gov/primer

4 Socioeconomic Disparities in Achievement

Insights on Neurocognitive Development and Educational Interventions

Daniel A. Hackman and David J. M. Kraemer

Introduction

How does a child's environment shape neurocognitive development and thereby influence academic achievement? A growing body of research has examined the associations among socioeconomic status (SES), neurocognitive performance, and brain development, as well as educational outcomes related to these factors, highlighting the role of both stressful and nurturing factors in one's environment. SES differences have been found in brain regions and cognitive tasks related to executive function, language, memory, and socioemotional regulation, including the prefrontal cortex and the limbic system. In this chapter, we consider the evidence that SES differences in brain and cognition may be involved in academic achievement or educational success, which exhibit marked socioeconomic disparities. In doing so, we focus on both the evidence for mediation (i.e., differences that may account for SES disparities in achievement) and moderation (i.e., outcomes for which SES changes the relationship between brain and behavior). In this context, we discuss the opportunities afforded by neuroscience research for supporting interventions aimed at improving educational outcomes and facilitating healthy neurocognitive development, as well as the theoretical and empirical limitations of this line of work. Critically, this work has the potential both to inform our understanding of SES-related disparities in achievement, and educational strategies to address them, while at the same time illustrating that neuroscience, and such individual-level factors, is only one part of a complex puzzle and that social factors and systems remain central for researchers and educators to understanding disparities in academic trajectories.

This literature, in an early stage of development, has more specific implications for further research than for educators who are implementing curricula in the schools, as much still remains to be understood. Nevertheless, current findings indicate that it is important for educators to consider their students' social and emotional development in addition to learning, and to note the importance of the multifaceted school, family, neighborhood, and policy contexts that are important for their students' development and success. Future research, including that informed by neuroscience, will be needed to help specify how such school-based curricula, interventions, and policy approaches can most effectively narrow achievement gaps and support improved outcomes for all.

SES: A Multifaceted Predictor of Developmental Outcomes

Socioeconomic status (SES) is a multidimensional construct that reflects many components of a child's environment, including material and financial resources, education, power, and social prestige (Braveman et al., 2005; Evans, 2004; Krieger, Williams, & Moss, 1997). For children and adolescents, this is typically thought of in terms of the family's SES or the parents' SES, often measured with family income, parental education, and/or parental occupation. Although SES is often thought of as a single latent construct, different measures of SES also reflect different aspects of experience and predict health in different ways (Braveman et al., 2005). Moreover, SES is not limited to the individual and family environment—it characterizes larger community units, such as neighborhood environments and school contexts as well (Krieger et al., 1997; Leventhal & Brooks-Gunn, 2000). The SES of such higher-level units is often measured based on an aggregate of individual characteristics, such as the percentage of residents of a United States (U.S.) census tract living in poverty (for neighborhoods) or, for schools, the percentage of students in a U.S. school who receive free and reduced price lunches. Given the early stage of the literature reviewed in this chapter, we will often utilize the term SES to refer to any index or measure of SES, although at times we will note specific associations. As the literature develops, establishing the specificity of relations across SES measures will become important.

SES is also an important predictor of a wide set of psychosocial, environmental, and community exposures, outcomes, and opportunities. In particular, SES is one of the most robust predictors of developmental outcomes for children and adolescents, including child health, socioemotional development, mental health, and school success, and even health in adulthood (Bradley & Corwyn, 2002; Leventhal & Brooks-Gunn, 2000; McLoyd, 1998; Miller & Chen, 2013). With respect to developmental experiences, SES predicts a range of different experiences (for reviews see Conger & Donnellan, 2007; Evans, 2004). Family SES can influence the types of resources and time that parents are able to invest in their children's development, whether it be the provision of books, educational and enrichment programs, or time spent reading together. The stresses associated with poverty can also make it more challenging for parents to be as involved in activities, and as warm and responsive in their role as caregivers as they might intend to be (Conger & Donnellan, 2007). SES is also associated with toxin and pollution exposures, the exposure to dangerous or unpredictable contexts, as well as the quality of schools and early caregiving institutions. Consequently, SES is a predictor of a broad set of experiences and exposures that influence child development.

Disparities in Educational Outcomes as a Function of SES

Children and adolescents from families with lower SES are less likely to suc-ceed in school than their higher SES peers (Reardon, 2011; Sirin, 2005). Such educational disparities are widely observed in performance on standardized achievement tests and differences in educational attainment (Brooks-Gunn & Duncan, 1997; Duncan, Morris, & Rodrigues, 2011; Ferguson, Bovarid, & Mueller, 2007; Magnuson, 2007; Reardon, 2011; Sirin, 2005). Although lower quality schools may be one important factor, it is unlikely to explain all of these disparities, as there are disparities in school readiness skills even at school entry (Magnuson, Meyers, Ruhm, & Waldfogel, 2004; Ryan, Fauth, & Brooks-Gunn, 2006; Wolf, Magnuson, & Kimbro, 2017). Neighborhood SES is also a predictor of academic achievement (Chetty, Hendren, & Katz, 2016; Wolf et al., 2017), and there is some evidence that earlier exposure to poverty is more influential than exposure in adolescence (Chetty et al., 2016; Duncan, Yeung, Brooks-Gunn, & Smith, 1998; Magnuson, 2007).

Experimental and quasi-experimental analyses have found that changes to SES can improve student achievement and educational attainment (Dun-can et al., 2011; Duncan, Ziol-Guest, & Kalil, 2010). For example, income supplements, in the form of policy changes or natural experiments, are asso-ciated with higher child achievement and increased school attendance, high school graduation rates, and total years of schooling (Akee, Copeland, Keeler, Angold, & Costello, 2010; Dahl & Lochner, 2012). Moreover, in the Moving to Opportunities randomized experimental study, moving to a higher-SES neighborhood earlier in childhood results in greater likelihood of college attendance (Chetty et al., 2016). These findings indicate that both family-level SES and neighborhood-level SES can have a causal effect on educational outcomes, and that policies that improve socioeconomic circumstances can improve academic achievement and reduce SES-related disparities.

In the U.S., the role of SES in children's developmental outcomes is par-ticularly salient, as increasing inequality over the past decades has become a more pressing issue (Odgers & Adler, 2017). In fact, disparities in school achievement are increasing. Reardon (2011) found that income-related achievement gaps in large national samples has been increasing over the past decades for both math and for reading, consistent with other studies that have found widening achievement gaps (Wolf et al., 2017).

For educators, researchers, and policy makers, understanding and addressing these disparities is essential in order to determine how best to serve all stu-dents to help them learn, grow, and meet their potential. *Therefore, identifying the complex, multilevel mechanisms at the student, family, school, and community/ societal levels that account for disparities is a central task for addressing and prevent-ing disparities, and promoting equity and healthy development for all children.* More-over, this research suggests that educators and policymakers should consider not only curriculum, classroom, and school-based approaches to supporting health, learning, and development, but also consider the wider context in which students and schools are nested.

SES and Neurocognitive Development

As part of the investigation into the multilevel mechanisms that may account for such disparities, there has been recent interest in the role of the brain as a student-level factor of importance that develops dynamically and interactively in social context. Therefore, the association between SES, brain development, and neurocognitive task performance has been theorized to contribute to an understanding of the mechanisms and processes by which socioeconomic disparities emerge (Amso & Lynn, 2017; Brito & Noble, 2014; Farah, 2018; Hackman & Farah, 2009; Sheridan & McLaughlin, 2016). In the past 15 years, the literature on the association between brain development and SES has grown significantly (Farah, 2018) and comprehensive reviews of this literature are available elsewhere (Brito & Noble, 2014; Farah, 2017; Hackman & Farah, 2009; Johnson, Riis, & Noble, 2016; Lipina & Evers, 2017; Ursache & Noble, 2016a).

To consider the potential relevance of this work for educational success and the achievement gap we first highlight some its major themes and findings. In summarizing the themes and findings of this literature, it is important to consider these associations as differences, or correlations, rather than necessarily interpreting differences as SES-related deficits, for multiple reasons. First, it is possible that many differences may actually reflect adaptations to circumstances that can have both positive or negative consequences, depending on the context, task, and outcome of interest. Second, it is also possible that such differences may simply reflect variability that has no particular consequences for differences in achievement. Finally, as will be discussed in the following, it may also be that what is most important for achievement is not the association between SES and neurocognitive development, but the interaction between these factors.

SES and Neurocognitive Performance

Performance on neurocognitive tasks, such as on tasks of executive function, memory, and language, varies by SES level (Blair et al., 2011; Hackman et al., 2014; Hackman, Gallop, Evans, & Farah, 2015; Lawson, Hook, & Farah, 2018; Noble, McCandliss, & Farah, 2007; Raver, Blair, & Willoughby, 2013; Sarsour et al., 2011; Ursache & Noble, 2016a). SES differences in language development have been found for vocabulary and other components of language performance, even in toddlers and in early childhood (Fernald, Marchman, & Weisleder, 2013; Huang, Leech, & Rowe, 2017; Noble et al., 2007; Noble, Norman, & Farah, 2005; Ursache & Noble, 2016a). Language differences have also been found for concentrated neighborhood disadvantage as well local stressors, such as recent community violence (Sampson, Sharkey, & Raudenbush,

2008; Sharkey, 2010), indicative of acute as well as persistent effects. Never-theless, this literature has been the subject of important critiques noting that some of these findings may not indicate differences in language ability per se, nor deficits, but may be related to issues in measurement, bilingualism or other diverse and valuable language experiences not captured in standardized tasks (Ellwood-Lowe, Sacchet, & Gotlib, 2016; Farah, 2018).

The largest evidence base has developed in the area of executive function. Cross-sectional associations, often small to moderate in size, have been found at multiple developmental stages between SES and broader executive func-tion factors as well as working memory, inhibitory control, flexibility, or atten-tion (Blair et al., 2011; Farah et al., 2006; Hackman et al., 2014, 2015; Lawson et al., 2018; Lipina, Martelli, Vuelta, & Colombo, 2005; Lipina, Martelli, Vuelta, Injoque-Ricle, & Colombo, 2004; Mezzacappa, 2004; Noble et al., 2007; Raver et al., 2013; Sarsour et al., 2011; Wiebe et al., 2011), though the literature on neighborhood effects is mixed (Hackman et al., 2014; McCoy, Roy, & Raver, 2016; Raver et al., 2013). There is some evidence that early childhood SES prospectively predicts working memory and planning in later childhood (Hackman et al., 2015), and that childhood SES predicts work-ing memory in late adolescence and early adulthood (Evans, 2016; Evans & Schamberg, 2009; Hackman et al., 2014). Nevertheless, there are no asso-ciations between SES and the rate of development after early childhood, suggesting that early executive function differences may be persistent across time (Hackman et al., 2014, 2015). This does not necessarily imply, how-ever, that interventions that produce meaningful changes in SES, or in sup-portive environments and resources, cannot also influence executive function development.

Consistent with this proposition, there is evidence that these effects are potentially reversible, as acute changes in socioeconomic conditions, scarcity, and contextual stressors are associated with changes in executive function. Time-limited community stressors, such as recent local violence, have been associated with decreases in children's attention and impulse control, though not necessarily EF (McCoy & Raver, 2014; McCoy, Raver, & Sharkey, 2015; Sharkey, Tirado-Strayer, Papachristos, & Raver, 2012). Moreover, there is evi-dence that acute income shocks, and real-world and lab-based manipulations that increase a sense of scarcity, result in lower performance on tasks of EF and more evidence of impulsivity (Haushofer & Fehr, 2014; Mani, Mullaina-than, Shafir, & Zhao, 2013; Shah, Mullainathan, & Shafir, 2012). Such work, indicative of plasticity, is consistent with studies that find that improving fam-ily or neighborhood SES has positive influences on achievement (Akee et al., 2010; Chetty et al., 2016; Dahl & Lochner, 2012; Duncan et al., 2011, 2010).

SES and Brain Structure

SES is associated with differences in the structure of multiple brain regions, dependent on the measure of SES (Brito & Noble, 2014; Johnson et al., 2016).

Indices of SES have been positively correlated with hippocampal volume, such that lower SES is associated with smaller hippocampi (Ellwood-Lowe et al., 2018; Hanson, Chandra, Wolfe, & Pollak, 2011; Hanson, Nacewicz et al., 2015; Noble, Houston, Kan, & Sowell, 2012). Similarly, SES has been demonstrated to be positively correlated with both the volume and thickness of prefrontal and temporal cortices (Hanson, Hair et al., 2015; Holz et al., 2014; Lawson, Duda, Avants, Wu, & Farah, 2013, p. 20; Mackey et al., 2015). Nevertheless, for the amygdala there have been mixed findings, with reports of null (Hanson et al., 2011; Merz, Tottenham, & Noble, 2018), negative (Noble et al., 2012), and positive (Hanson, Nacewicz et al., 2015) associations. Although there is some early evidence of associations between SES and developmental change in the hippocampus and in lobar volumes (Ellwood-Lowe et al., 2018; Hanson, Hair et al., 2015) most studies are cross-sectional and provide limited insight into issues of developmental timing or trajectories.

One challenge for SES and neuroscience research is related to sampling, both in terms of recruiting diverse samples and in conducting studies with sufficient sample size and power to increase confidence in the pattern of results observed. Due to this issue, the Pediatric Imaging, Neurocognition and Genetics (PING) study has been important, as it is a multi-site neuroimaging study of more than 1,000 children between the ages of 3 and 20 (Noble et al., 2015; Ursache & Noble, 2016b). In this study, indices of SES were positively associated with brain structure in many regions including the volume of the hippocampus, and cortical surface area in prefrontal cortex and temporal lobe regions, as well as others. Additionally, higher parental education was uniquely associated with larger hippocampal volumes. However, no associations were found between SES and amygdala volume.

With regard to structural connectivity, there are also some mixed findings from studies with smaller sample sizes. In one study, lower family income was associated with lower fractional anisotropy (FA) across a number of tracts, an index of structural integrity and connectivity (Dufford & Kim, 2017). However, with respect to white matter volume, one study found positive associations (Luby et al., 2013) while two studies found no associations with SES (Hanson, Hair et al., 2015; Mackey et al., 2015). In the PING study, indices of higher SES were associated with higher FA in right parahippocampal cingulum, and the left superior cortiostriate tract in parietal cortex, though there were different effects for family income and parental education and many tracts did not show associations with SES (Ursache & Noble, 2016b). Altogether, this suggests that there may be some positive associations between SES and structural connectivity in a subset of tracts, with more equivocal evidence for white matter volume.

SES and Brain Function

SES has been associated with differences in brain function across a variety of tasks. For example, there are SES differences in activation during various executive function tasks, such as working memory and inhibition tasks, with differences not only in the degree of prefrontal activation but also in the patterns of correlation with task success (Finn et al., 2017; Sheridan, Peverill, Finn, & McLaughlin, 2017; Spielberg et al., 2015). Some authors have even argued that the patterns of activation associated with lower-SES are inefficient, as they tend to result in lower performance levels (Sheridan et al., 2017; Spielberg et al., 2015). In contrast, lower SES has been associated with increased amygdala activity in response to emotional faces (Javanbakht et al., 2015; Muscatell et al., 2012) and heightened activity in the anticipation of rewards in mesolimbic regions (Gonzalez, Allen, & Coan, 2016) and medial prefrontal cortex (Romens et al., 2015). Moreover, lower SES has been associated prospectively with decreased recruitment of prefrontal cortex during emotion regulation, in particular reappraisal (Kim et al., 2013). These effects suggest SES-related differences in neural processing during tasks that are central to navigating both the curricular and complex social and emotional demands of schools, which often require self-regulation to meet academic goals.

There is also emerging evidence of SES-related differences in functional connectivity at rest, with lower SES largely associated with reduced connectivity. For example, in one longitudinal study lower early childhood income-to-needs was associated with reduced connectivity between both the hippocampus and amygdala with multiple regions, such as the superior frontal gyrus and posterior cingulate, which accounted for differences in negative mood symptoms (Barch et al., 2016). In addition, two longitudinal studies have also found associations with default mode connectivity. This fMRI measure is collected during periods of time that are not task related (i.e., rest) and therefore reflects the endogenous functional connectivity in an individual's brain independent of task demands (Greicius, Supekar, Menon, & Dougherty, 2009; Raichle et al., 2001). One study found that lower family income predicted reduced connectivity between posterior cingulate cortex, hippocampus, and prefrontal cortex (Sripada, Swain, Evans, Welsh, & Liberzon, 2014), and another found that income increases for low-income families were associated with increased connectivity across multiple prefrontal and parietal regions (Weissman, Conger, Robins, Hastings, & Guyer, 2018). These results suggest that either low income in general, or consistent, stable low income for families is associated with lower levels of functional connectivity at rest, indicating there are differences in neural activity that extend beyond particular laboratory-based tasks.

Possible Mechanisms

There are multiple plausible mechanisms that may link SES to neural and neurocognitive development, beyond the scope of this review, that can be drawn from an integration of neuroscientific, psychological, sociological, educational, and social work research traditions (Bradley & Corwyn, 2002; Conger & Donnellan, 2007; Duncan & Murnane, 2011; Evans, 2004; Hackman, Farah, & Meaney, 2010; Luby et al., 2013; McEwen & Gianaros, 2010;

McLoyd, 1998; Sheridan & McLaughlin, 2016; Ursache & Noble, 2016a). Although there remains to be consensus on the best way to examine individual exposures versus cumulative or aggregate factors or themes in the experience of adversity (Evans, Li, & Whipple, 2013; Sheridan & McLaughlin, 2016), there are a number of commonly proposed mechanisms. First are different *factors that comprise the formal or informal learning environment*, and the resources, investments, and opportunities that allow for an enriched environment that support development. These factors can include books in the home, preschools, music lessons, language classes, or other enrichment activities. A related construct, capturing more extreme variation, is the notion of deprivation of cognitive stimulation. Second is the *general experience of stress*, which may influence behavioral, or coping responses, as well as elicit biological stress responses that may have a cumulative toll over time. Third, the *stressors related to SES influence parents* as well as children, and make it more challenging for parents to be as supportive, responsive, and warm as often as they might otherwise intend. Fourth, *prenatal factors*, such as maternal stress and toxin exposure, may be important influences. Fifth, *experiences of threat and potential harm*, such as exposure to community violence, and certain types of abuse or maltreatment, may also be central components of how SES may influence psychological and neurobiological development. Future research establishing the mechanisms underlying these differences is important, as well as understanding the role of adaptations to environmental constraints and conditions that may be context-dependent and reversible.

Advancing Academic Achievement and Reducing Disparities: What Role Can Cognitive Neuroscience Play?

At this stage, it is important to consider the ways in which cognitive neuroscience research may contribute to efforts aimed at mitigating the impact of SES disparity. The consideration of disparities in educational success is of necessity a multilevel endeavor, as noted previously, considering mechanisms from the societal, school, family, and individual levels, as well as their interplay. Consequently, the economic pressures felt by families and the strategies and time needed to cope with them, and many other environmental factors, all are likely to be important mechanisms that contribute to disparities in school readiness, academic achievement, and educational attainment. Although many such mechanisms may not include any relation to brain development, neuroscience may also contribute to understanding this complexity, especially in terms of development on the level of the individual child.

Farah (2018) outlined three potential ways in which a neuroscience approach may help elucidate the etiology of disparities and potentially inform policy. First, neurobiological differences themselves may play a role in disparities, both uniquely and in terms of their relation to important patterns of emotional, cognitive, or social and psychological functioning (see Figure 4.1). Academic success relies on a combination of cognitive and socioemotional

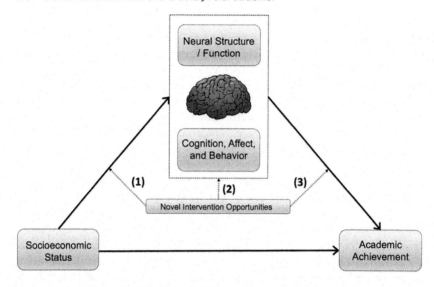

Figure 4.1 Mediation: A schematic of how neural and neurocognitve factors may be part of the mechanism that relates socioeconomic status to academic achievement.

Illustration of mediation, a causal model in which cognition, affect, and behavior, and/ or neural factors, are part of the pathway by which SES influences academic achievement. The direct arrow between SES and achievement represents the degree to which such mechanisms do not explain the achievement gap.

There are three novel intervention (or prevention) targets based upon this model, indicated by the numerals:

(1) Reduce social-contextual risk factors, or increase social-contextual protective or promotive factors, in order to reduce the association between SES and neural or cognitive factors.

(2) Intervene to directly influence the development of neural or cognitive factors, such as increasing executive function or emotion regulation abilities.

(3) Decrease the degree to which such neural or cognitive factors are predictive of academic achievement. An example might be designing classroom environments that reduce demand on executive function for school.

Note of caution: To the degree that neural, cognitive, affective or behavioral differences are adaptive, such interventions might have unanticipated effects on child development in contexts outside of school, and thus should be pursued with caution.

skills, and neuroscience research, convergent with other data sources, has focused on the ways in which these cognitive and emotional skills are rooted in brain structure and brain function. Second, and related to the first point, neuroscience measures may simply be sensitive to differences that are not as easily detectable using other methods. In addition to providing convergent evidence to other approaches, neuroscience research therefore has the potential to generate new hypotheses as well, based on our current understanding of neural systems underlying brain function and brain structure. Even surprising findings from neuroscience studies may help to point classroom-based research in new and useful directions.

A third possibility is that neuroscience measures, as with other levels of measurement, may provide insight into qualitative differences in the mechanisms predicting educational success at different SES levels (Farah, 2018). In other words, there may be systematic differences in brain-behavior relationships associated with SES, in which SES acts as a *moderator* (see Figure 4.2), rather than neural differences providing insight into *mediation* (see Figure 4.1). Put another way, differential relationships between neurocognitive development and educational outcomes may be found for different levels of SES, and aspects of brain structure or function may have more or less relevance at different levels of SES. This would suggest that different interventions are optimal for different individuals or groups depending on the context, though there would likely be significant variability such that broad, multifaceted approaches would still be necessary. This approach would be consistent with an adaptation perspective, in which observed SES-related effects are not necessarily indicative of a deficit but instead adaptations to environmental conditions, and thus differences in how tasks important to academic success are completed, either at the neural or psychological levels. Consequently, use of a neuroscience approach does not need to be focused on, or interpreted as, a deficit-based approach but instead can elucidate adaptation and variation.

Although the framework of neuroscience has already been utilized within the context of policy debates (Farah, 2018), empirical work to address these implications for education are still in a relatively early stage of development (Ansari & Coch, 2006; Howard-Jones, 2014; Sigman, Peña, Goldin, & Ribeiro, 2014; Willingham & Lloyd, 2007). Therefore, additional research is needed to determine the extent of the unique contributions of a neuroscience approach to educational interventions, curriculum, or policy, and to determine the extent of any unique insights into the effects of the larger scale social forces that account for educational disparities and how to refine policy and practice to promote educational success and reduce disparities.

Rationale for Implications of Neurocognitive Measures

The aforementioned SES-related differences in neurocognitive measures may plausibly contribute to disparities in educational outcomes, either via mediation or moderation. Review of the importance of these neural systems is beyond the scope of this paper. However, it is worthwhile to highlight how executive function and emotion regulation, in particular, are important predictors of academic achievement and are essential for navigating the social and emotional complexities of the school environment (Alloway & Alloway, 2010; Graziano, Reavis, Keane, & Calkins, 2007; St. Clair-Thompson & Gathercole, 2006). Executive function refers to a set of cognitive skills including

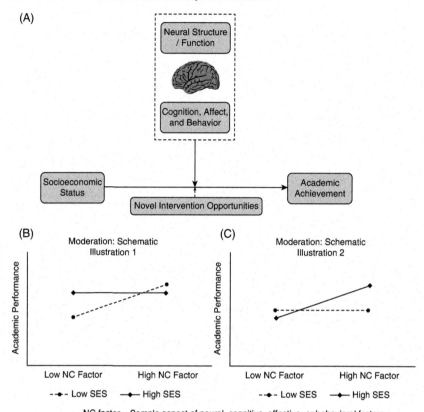

Figure 4.2 Moderation: A Schematic of Associations Between Socioeconomic Status, Neural, and Neurocognitve Factors, and Academic Achievement.

(A) Conceptual illustrations of moderation, in which a neural, cognitive, affective, or behavioral factor (NC) moderates the association between SES and academic achievement. In this model, it is the intersection or interaction between SES and NC factors that matter for achievement. Consequently, novel interventions based on this approach must be informed by research focused on the ways in which these factors are found to interact, rather than their associations. Critically, intervention implications would be dependent on the nature of this moderation, which can follow multiple patterns.

In Sections (B) and (C), two of many different potential moderation patterns are presented in schematic fashion to illustrate possible patterns of moderation, as a heuristic (not using real data). In both examples, there is both a main effect of SES and a main effect of NC factor.

(B) Here the combination of low-SES and low NC factor is associated with lower achievement, as SES is only associated with achievement in the context of low NC. Conversely, there is only a relationship between NC and achievement at low SES levels. This pattern suggests that lifting performance and closing the achievement gap can be achieved either by improving NC performance or by improving family SES. This may also suggest a targeted approach supporting those at greatest risk may also be effective.

(C) The association between NC and achievement is only present at high SES levels, and high NC only promotes achievement at higher SES levels. In this model, there is no association between SES and achievement at low NC levels, but there is an association between SES and achievement at higher NC levels. This model suggests that lifting performance and closing the achievement gap requires a more universal and broad approach that focuses on both improving NC performance and family SES.

Figures 4.2 (Continued)

attention, working memory, and inhibition that function together to facilitate goal-oriented behavior, which is required for staying focused on tasks in the lab (e.g., Stroop color-word responses) and while attending to lectures in the classroom (Fan, McCandliss, Sommer, Raz, & Posner, 2002; Welsh, Pennington, & Groisser, 1991; Zelazo & Müller, 2002). In particular, although various tasks have been developed to tap different aspects of executive functions, they all seem to share common variance related to the cognitive skill of inhibition (McCabe, Roediger III, McDaniel, Balota, & Hambrick, 2010; Miyake & Friedman, 2012). Moreover, this same inhibition skill is not only associated with "cold cognitive" tasks that tap executive function directly, but also with inhibition of emotion-related behaviors, such that a lack of inhibitory capacity is linked to externalizing behaviors in the classroom (Young et al., 2009). Indeed, cognitive skills related to inhibition, including delay of gratification, grit, and self-control, have all been associated with educational achievement and other long-term positive life outcomes (Casey et al., 2011; Duckworth, Peterson, Matthews, & Kelly, 2007; Duckworth & Seligman, 2005; Mischel et al., 2011) and early measures of executive functions are correlated with concurrent and later language and math skills (Allan, Hume, Allan, Farrington, & Lonigan, 2014; McClelland et al., 2007, 2014; Ponitz, McClelland, Matthews, & Morrison, 2009; St. Clair-Thompson & Gathercole, 2006). On a neural systems level, this inhibition system is associated with prefrontal cortex, including the anterior cingulate and inferior frontal gyrus, for cognitive tasks (Fan et al., 2002) as well as for emotion regulation (Casey et al., 2011). Consequently, many of the same aspects of neurocognitive performance and brain development that are associated with SES are also predictive of educational outcomes. However, documenting these correlations are only the first step in establishing the relevance of this approach, as it is critical to understand the relationships between these factors on multiple levels. Therefore, in the remainder of this chapter, we consider early evidence for how they are all related.

How Are SES, Neurocognitive Development, and Academic Achievement Interrelated?

In general, there are two broad ways in which SES, neurocognitive development, and academic achievement might be interrelated: *mediation* and moderation. Understanding the conditions under which either might operate is essential to understanding both etiology as well as how neuroscience research might help guide intervention targets or measures of intervention success.

In this context, mediation refers to the notion that SES-related differences in brain and neurocognitive development may play a mechanistic role in accounting for educational disparities (see Figure 4.1). In other words, factors related to SES may cause the changes in neurodevelopment that lead to certain educational outcomes. Relatedly, moderation refers to the idea that differences associated with SES may change the relationship between specific neurocognitive factors and specific educational outcomes for different individuals or groups (see Figure 4.2a). As illustrated in Figures 4.2b and 4.2c, for moderation it is the intersection between SES and neurocognitive factors that may matter for achievement, and such moderation can take many distinct patterns that have different implications. Among the reasons this might occur is if at different SES levels non-neural environmental factors are more prominent predictors of achievement or the challenge of differing social conditions highlight the importance of different social, cognitive, and affective tasks necessary to succeed. In both circumstances, the central issue is context dependence, and no SES differences are deficits, per se. Here we consider evidence for both mediation and moderation with respect to the relation of neurocognitive performance and brain development with SES and academic achievement.

The Role of Neurocognitive Performance

In terms of mediation, evidence is beginning to accumulate that differences in executive function may partially account for the association between SES and school readiness as well as early performance on standardized achievement tests. Multiple cross-sectional studies have provided evidence that EF may account for a significant portion of the SES-related differences in school readiness and achievement, especially for math (Dilworth-Bart, 2012; Fitzpatrick, McKinnon, Blair, & Willoughby, 2014; Korzeniowski, Cupani, Ison, & Difabio, 2016), though they do not establish the temporal order necessary for mediation.

Three studies have been longitudinal in nature, providing stronger evidence of mediation. The association between early childhood income-to-needs and first grade achievement was mediated by executive function in kindergarten in one study, with stronger effects for completing math problems than literacy or reading skills (Nesbitt, Baker-Ward, & Willoughby, 2013). In a large, national sample of children followed from birth, it was found that planning performance in 3rd grade was a mediator of the association between early childhood income-to-needs ratio and achievement scores in 5th grade, though this effect was also stronger in mathematics than in reading performance (Crook & Evans, 2014). Similarly, in a different national sample of children aged 6–15 years, a composite of executive function measures mediated the association between SES and the change in mathematics performance, but not reading comprehension (Lawson & Farah, 2017). Across all studies, the evidence supports a role for executive function in performance of mathematics achievement tests, though this role does not preclude other important mediators as well. This highlights the potential utility of incorporating a neuroscience pathway to identify specificity in SES differences in academic achievement, as it suggests that different outcomes (e.g., mathematics versus language-based skills) may have different mediators.

Few studies have tested the hypothesis that the relation between executive function and school achievement will differ based on SES. One study examined this question in a sample of 100 preschool children of lower SES in the Head Start preschool program and a comparison group (Duncan, McClelland, & Acock, 2017). Results showed two significant interactions (of nine examined) in which performance on the EF task had a smaller association with achievement in the low-SES group, suggesting that factors other than EF may be more influential for low-income preschoolers.

The Role of Brain Structure

Three studies focus on either explicitly examining if brain structure may account for, or mediate, the association between SES and academic achievement. One cross-sectional study of 58 adolescents found that higher family income was associated with increased cortical thickness and grey matter volume in the prefrontal cortex and occipital and temporal lobes (Mackey et al., 2015). Morphometry of some of these regions correlated, in a manner consistent with mediation, with achievement scores on standardized statewide assessment for mathematics and language arts in the 7th and 8th grades (though not prefrontal cortex). A separate investigation utilized three waves of data for 4–22-year-olds from National Institutes of Health Magnetic Resonance Imaging Study of Normal Brain Development (Hair, Hanson, Wolfe, & Pollak, 2015). They found that gray matter volume in the frontal and temporal lobes, as well as the hippocampus, mediated the association between family income and both math and reading achievement measures, accounting for between about 8 and 15% of the association.

Finally, Whittle et al. (2017) followed 166 Australian youth to determine if interactions between parenting and socioeconomic disadvantage might account for differences in school completion via structural brain development. They found an interaction between parenting and both neighborhood disadvantage and family-level-SES, primarily in boys. In particular for boys who grow up in disadvantaged neighborhoods but without the benefit of very positive, supportive parenting, development in the dorsal frontal cortex accounted for rates of school non-completion. However, although across all these studies there is some conceptual support for mediation, there remain a number of key issues and limitations in the literature. First, mediation analyses regarding brain structure invite the question of whether such effects are driven by aspects of cognition and behavior related to the structure of these brain regions. Second, such mediation analyses actually leave the majority of SES effects on achievement unexplained, which suggests that social factors or other individual-level factors account for a larger part of the SES-achievement relationship. Finally, these studies exhibit inconsistent findings regarding which regions are mediators, which suggests that thus far the literature does not strongly support a consensus, with replication, regarding which brain regions play a mediational role.

In terms of moderation effects, only a few studies have focused on whether or not there is evidence of different relationships between brain structure and behavior by SES level. In a small sample spanning middle childhood and early adolescence, Gullick, Demir-Lira, and Booth (2016) examined if the association between white matter integrity and reading skill was moderated by parental education level. Results largely suggested that tracts in the right hemisphere were positively correlated with reading in the low parental education group, while those in the left hemisphere were associated with reading in children whose parents had higher education levels. The authors speculate that this might be due to an increased recruitment of visuospatial processing for reading in lower-SES children and thus suggestion of different neural and cognitive strategies used to complete the same academic tasks.

Separately, Brito, Piccolo, and Noble (2017) focused on the role of cortical thickness in the larger PING dataset, a sample that ranged from 3 to 20 years of age. In this case, they found that for both language and EF, there was a stronger link between cortical thickness and performance in low-income children and adolescents. Similarly, in the PING dataset, higher FA was only associated with better performance on tasks of cognitive flexibility in the low-income group (Ursache & Noble, 2016b). This pattern of results may arise because environmental stressors may accentuate the role of neural processes in the context of adversity and disadvantage, whereas resources associated with higher income may lead to better reading performance, even when neural differences are present. Such moderation effects might suggest that a focus on neural processes to reduce the achievement gap may not be the most effective strategy, and that instead focusing on more structural and systematic resources available to families to reduce stress and support learning may be most effective.

The Role of Brain Function

In terms of brain activity, one study has examined whether differences in brain function during a working memory task mediate SES-related differences in achievement (Finn et al., 2017). In this study, middle-school children completed an N-back working memory task, in which working memory load was varied parametrically. As working memory load increased, the higher income group showed patterns of increased recruitment of multiple brain regions, including regions such as bilateral middle and inferior frontal gyri (MFG and IFG) in the prefrontal cortex, the intraparietal sulcus, as well as regions in the basal ganglia. The authors found that this set of neural differences, as well as working-memory task performance, both mediated the effect of income group on performance on a statewide standardized achievement test for mathematics.

Two recent studies provide excellent examples of work examining whether SES may moderate how the patterns or strengths of neural activation during tasks relate to differences in academic performance (Demir-Lira, Prado, & Booth, 2015, 2016). In overlapping samples between the ages of 8 and 13, the authors focused on whether the neural activity during an arithmetic task had differential associations, based on parental educational level, with both mathematics achievement measured concurrently (Demir-Lira et al., 2015) as well as with the growth in math achievement over the next 1.5 years, on average (Demir-Lira et al., 2016). They found that, cross-sectionally, different regions were associated with math performance based on parental education: at high levels of parental education, activity in the left middle temporal gryus predicted math achievement, while at lower levels activity in the right intraparietal sulcus predicted achievement. For gains, they found that two regions had inverse relationships with achievement based on SES level. In the left inferior frontal gyrus, there was a positive correlation with math gains at higher parental education levels and a negative correlation at lower parental education levels, while the inverse pattern was observed for the superior parietal sulcus. As with moderation for structural differences (Gullick et al., 2016), the authors speculate that this may mean that higher-SES children and adolescents with greater levels of math achievement may generally rely on more verbal processing, while the lower-SES children with higher achievement rely more on visuospatial processing (Demir-Lira et al., 2015, 2016). Interactions have also been found for reading (Noble, Wolmetz, Ochs, Farah, & McCandliss, 2006) as well as for accuracy in a visuospatial memory task (Duval et al., 2017), suggesting that such moderation effects may not be limited to math achievement.

Therefore, while this line of research is still in its early days, there are some indications that SES-related differences in functional brain activity may be useful in understanding the relation between SES and achievement, especially in terms of moderation or adaptation.

Effects of SES on Multivariate Outcome Measures

One of the limitations of the prior analyses is that few studies simultaneously test mediation by multiple neural and behavioral processes to contrast possible causal pathways. To our knowledge only one study has examined multiple mediators simultaneously, in a small sample of youth from middle childhood through the end of adolescence (Rosen, Sheridan, Sambrook, Meltzoff, & McLaughlin, 2018). Participants underwent a battery that included an executive function task during functional imaging, diffusion tensor imaging for measuring structural integrity, and a structural image to measure cortical thickness. Working memory performance, as well as functional activity and structural integrity in regions and tracts of interest were associated with family income, and they jointly mediated the association between family income and parent reports of achievement. Cortical thickness, however, did not mediate this association, and they did not examine whether SES moderated the brain-achievement relationships. In addition, cognitive stimulation in the household was found to be a reliable mediator, and therefore the authors concluded that additional environmental exposures continued to remain important.

Influence of Supportive School and Family Environments: The Role of Neuroscience in Potential Intervention Design

Altogether, the early literature provides some evidence for a link between SES and neural and cognitive development both in terms of mediation and moderation. However, these pathways do not explain all of the variance. This raises the question, though, of what the mediation or moderation means for intervention and prevention strategies. Although incorporating a neuroscience perspective might suggest that the function of neural, cognitive, and affective systems be a novel target of interventions, the implications of this research are actually far broader and suggest that a focus on multilevel social factors are potentially important as well. In part, this is due to the fact that such factors, at best, seem to explain only part of the SES-achievement relationship.

In addition, a basic consideration of mediation and moderation suggest the potential importance of a broader approach. With respect to moderation, achievement may be more related to the intersection of SES and neural, cognitive, and affective factors, suggesting that an integrated, multilevel approach might be warranted (see Figure 4.2). Even with respect to mediation, however, there are three possible approaches to refining intervention or prevention approaches that are suggested by incorporating neuroscience research (see Figure 4.1). First, intervening to influence the development of neural, cognitive or affective factors, such as increasing executive function, may be promising. Second, it may still be most effective to intervene by reducing social-contextual risk factors, or by increasing promotive or protective factors at the social or system level, in order to reduce the association between SES and mediating neural or cognitive systems. From this perspective, a neuroscience approach may help refine our understanding of which contextual risk or promotive factors to target. Finally, it is also potentially promising to intervene to create conditions, such as in schools, that decrease the degree to which such neural, cognitive, or affective factors predict academic achievement. For example, it may be promising to focus on creating classroom environments that are less stressful and reduce demands on executive function to succeed when it is not necessary. Having multiple strategies to promote student success and reduce disparities is important, because caution should be exercised in targeting interventions at the individual level to uniformly influence cognitive or affect function. As noted earlier, one hypothesis is that such differences may be adaptive (Belsky & Pluess, 2009; Del Giudice, Ellis, & Shirtcliff, 2011; Ellis & Boyce, 2008), and if this is the case then intervention focused on such neural, cognitive, and affective systems may have unintended consequences. Together, this suggests that careful and rigorous research is warranted to identify the best set of approaches to programs and policies designed to support achievement and reduce disparities.

Consequently, utilizing interventions at the societal or systemic level to create supportive environments is a promising strategy. Importantly, an emerging literature suggests that *the associations between SES and neurocognitive development are not fixed, nor only sensitive to early influences, but may be mutable over time* if a child's later environment is highly supportive.

To highlight one recurring example, positive parenting and warmth during late childhood and early adolescence have been found to moderate, and at times eliminate, the association between disadvantage and brain volume. For instance, in one longitudinal observation study of Australian adolescents (Whittle et al., 2017), positive parenting appeared to buffer the effect of disadvantage. Especially for males from families living in areas of high disadvantage, positive and supportive parenting was associated with patterns in prefrontal cortex more similar to youth from less disadvantaged neighborhoods. A further study moved beyond longitudinal observations and examined whether an ecologically relevant intervention designed to increase positive parenting also reduced the association between SES and brain structure (Brody et al., 2017). This randomized controlled study of the Strong African-American Families prevention program for low-income, rural African Americans, followed children from age 11, when they received the intervention, until age 25, when they underwent structural MRI scans. There was no association between poverty and brain volume in the intervention group, while in the control group, greater exposure to poverty across adolescence was associated with reduced volume in the left amygdala as well as in hippocampal subfields. While these studies did not measure academic achievement outcomes directly, these results suggest that positive parenting may buffer adolescents from the effects of both neighborhood and family SES on brain development, and that the effects of SES may be malleable through adolescence.

In addition, two studies have examined the influence of school environments on executive function and brain function, using quasi-experimental designs. One study compared students born within 4 months of each other but on either side of the school entry cutoff, in order to study the effect of one year of structured kindergarten schooling compared to one year of less-structured preschool for two nearly-matched groups (Burrage et al., 2008). The authors found evidence for schooling effects on executive function as well as word decoding, conveying a benefit in these skills from the more structured school environment. Using a similar design, Brod, Bunge, and Shing (2017) found similar benefits of one year of first-grade classes compared to students who stayed in kindergarten for a second year. Moreover, fMRI results implicated increased activity in posterior parietal cortex and dorsolateral prefrontal cortex for the first graders. Although not related to SES directly, these findings confirm that school-related experiences influence brain development and cognition in a manner that is potentially relevant to interventions addressing disparities.

Consequently, these studies raise the possibility that SES differences in brain and behavior are malleable and can be reduced or eliminated by interventions later in development that increase supportive environments. Moreover, given the potential influence of both early school environments and family environments in adolescence, the implication is that whereas *developmental timing is important, it is not deterministic—both earlier and later interventions may serve to reduce disparities* in neurocognitive development and academic success.

Summary, Critique, and Future Directions

Across all studies, not only is SES associated with differences in neurocognitive performance and brain development, but there is some evidence suggesting these differences partially mediate the relationship between SES and educational outcomes. The largest and strongest body of evidence is in the domain of executive function, which accounts in part for SES-related disparities in achievement scores, particularly for mathematics. Therefore, programs that support executive function development may play a role in narrowing the achievement gap, as there is some evidence that executive function may be influenced by formal schooling (Brod et al., 2017; Burrage et al., 2008) and additional training activities, though the strength, breadth, and durability of such effects remain to be determined (Diamond & Ling, 2016; Melby-Lervåg & Hulme, 2013; Shipstead, Redick, & Engle, 2012). However, to date there is no evidence to support this speculation, and such mediation effects may instead suggest a more targeted focus on social context and school environments. In terms of moderating effects, the early literature provides proof of concept for the notion that SES may, under certain conditions, moderate the relationship between the brain and behavior or achievement. Some findings from this research highlight how access to resources associated with higher SES lessen the influence of neural variation on educational outcomes and executive function (Brito et al., 2017; Ursache & Noble, 2016b), possibly by increasing the availability of beneficial environmental influences (Brod et al., 2017; Brody et al., 2017; Burrage et al., 2008; Whittle et al., 2017). These findings, therefore, place increased emphasis on efforts to increase access to such resources. Nevertheless, the possibility that mediation or moderation results might inform curricular or policy approaches remains highly speculative and should mainly be used to inform hypotheses for future research.

There are a number of important methodological considerations and conceptual challenges that must inform cautious interpretation and application of this literature. With respect to methodology, first, additional studies with larger sample sizes and diverse, representative samples are needed. Under-powered studies may hamper the literature, particularly for mediation analyses (Fritz & MacKinnon, 2007), while early findings suggest that conclusions regarding neural data may differ with representative samples or with use of population weights (LeWinn, Sheridan, Keyes, Hamilton, & McLaughlin, 2017). Second, longitudinal studies are needed to establish the time course necessary for mediation. Third, observational associations and mediation or moderation analyses do not establish causality. In terms of education, this is particularly important for how such findings at the neural or neurocognitive level inform hypotheses for intervention studies. Consequently, intervention studies targeting these neural systems will be needed to determine if these pathways are potentially causal and are effective intervention targets to increase achievement and reduce educational disparities. Finally, there is no evidence yet that neural measures mediate or moderate the associations of SES with educational attainment rather than performance on achievement tests. Given that attainment may be plausibly influenced by additional challenges, constraints, and opportunities at the societal level, it is important for future work to consider attainment as well.

With respect to conceptual limitations and cautions, the first to consider is variability. Despite the associations described here SES is neither a sensitive nor specific predictor of any particular patterns of neurocognitive performance or brain development, nor do the mediation/moderation pathways apply for everyone. Consequently, one cannot infer any particular pattern of performance or brain development from someone's SES level, and in fact this variance should be a focus of future research, especially in terms of resilience processes. In addition, this suggests that a one-size-fits-all approach to tailoring interventions, based on moderation or mediation analyses, is unlikely to be successful. Instead, these results might better inform hypotheses about a multiplicity of strategies to support children's academic development.

Second, and relatedly, none of the reported associations can be interpreted as reflecting inherent or, more importantly, irreversible differences that are deterministic in nature (Farah, 2018; Hackman & Farah, 2009). Indeed, the literature on genetic contributions to educational attainment (Lee et al., 2018), socioeconomic mobility (Belsky et al., 2018), and the link between SES and academic achievement (Krapohl & Plomin, 2016), which include large and diverse samples, indicates that the vast majority of the variance in each of these factors is not explained by genetic variation alone. Moreover, heritability estimates from such studies can not necessarily be interpreted as causal (Krapohl & Plomin, 2016), and there is even some evidence that environmental factors may mediate, or account for, some genetic associations (Belsky et al., 2018). Therefore, environmental and developmental factors such as those described here and many others, as well as interactions between these factors and genetic predispositions, likely contribute to achievement. The degree of plasticity in response to environmental factors or interventions, the mechanisms underlying such differences, and the nature of plasticity based on the timing of both exposures as well as interventions or social and contextual changes are open, empirical questions. In fact, the reduction of academic disparities by policies that influence SES, and research on the main or buffering effects of other social contextual factors, such as supportive parenting and school environments, suggests both malleability and the promise of interventions at multiple developmental stages.

Third, and as noted in this chapter, SES-related differences in brain or neurocognitive development should not be reflexively interpreted as deficits. On the one hand, many differences may instead represent adaptations that can have both positive or negative consequences, depending on the context or the developmental task. However, even when studies exhibit evidence of mediation, it is not observed for all regions or tasks that show SES-related differences, even within the same study. This issue is also seen in moderation analyses, as many neural or neurocognitive measures do not exhibit moderation. This pattern suggests that many SES-related differences in brain development may not necessarily contribute to differences in achievement all. Although it is possible they may be of importance for mental and physical health (Chan et al., 2018; Hackman, Kuan, Manuck, & Gianaros, 2018; Merz et al., 2018), they may also simply represent variability without a functional consequence. Moreover, the typically small size of mediation effects, as well as moderation effects suggesting that neural measures are less correlated with behavior at higher SES levels, indicates that while currently available neural and behavioral measures may be important, other child-based, social, systemic, and environmental mechanisms remain critical as well (in addition to neural measures not yet developed). In this way, the neuroscience approach both provides an additional perspective on child-level factors and also refocuses attention on the importance of population-level, social and systemic factors that are important for child development and educational success.

What Has Cognitive, Affective, and Educational Neuroscience Added to Our Understanding Over and Above Psychology?

The promise of a neuroscience approach to understanding SES-related disparities, as previously articulated, lies in providing another level of analysis with additional measurement approaches that may help identify the processes linking children's experience of social and economic contexts with achievement. Thus far, SES has been associated with executive function, language, memory, and emotion regulation, and there is some evidence of SES association with the neural underpinnings of these cognitive functions. For educators and policymakers, though, the real promise lies in understanding how these factors relate to academic achievement. This work has thus far suggested that aspects of executive function may account for some SES differences in achievement, and that there is evidence of qualitative differences in brain-behavior relationships that highlight the potential importance of multiple curricular and societal strategies to support child development. However, this literature is in its early stages, and the clearest implication is the need for further research, as additional empirical work to fulfill this promise is needed to determine the extent and nature of unique contributions from a neuroscience approach.

What Are Some Concrete Implications of This Research and Opportunities for Translation?

Research on SES-related disparities, adopting a neuroscience approach, has important conceptual implications and concrete implications for future research. Even though this work cannot yet point to any specific curricula, policy changes, or classroom-based practices, the implications are important for educators to consider.

First, consideration of the broad range of children's cognitive and socioemotional competencies is warranted, in addition to a focus on learning. SES is associated with a range of neurocognitive systems that are important for all the academic, social, and developmental tasks necessary for school success. Although it is not clear yet how these factors are all interrelated with academic performance, let alone which approaches are successful for all students and for narrowing achievement gaps, it can be hypothesized that many of these domains are important. Moderation analyses, though, suggest that there may be variation in what predicts academic success both within and across SES levels, and thus a *multiplicity of strategies, rather than specific tailored approaches, may be most effective*. These are important areas for future research.

Second, to support students and families most effectively, it is important for educators and policymakers to consider the wider societal context in which students and schools are nested, in addition to considering the curricula and practice within the classroom. In fact, an over-emphasis on neural processes and systems in isolation may be less effective than changing the resources, systems, supports, and contexts that influence families and students. Neuroscience may thus be most useful when it helps guide more refined interventions that focus on social systems and processes rather than on curricula or on individuals. Consequently, a comprehensive approach is warranted, considering neurocognitive measures within the broader context.

Third, the tools of neuroscience provide an important means of tracking the effectiveness of specific interventions over time, at least in the context of research to identify best practices. In addition to the important dependent measures of such interventions that can be measured from school records (e.g., class grades and test scores), analyzing neurocognitive batteries that tap executive function and emotion regulation, as well as the brain structures and functions that correspond to these cognitive characteristics, may be important for collaborative translational research.

Consequently, as children develop in multilevel systems, a multilevel approach to research to eventually refine and enhance policy and interventions is promising. Neuroscience may thus have an important role to play, in addition to continued focus on societal and school contexts, to identify ways to effectively narrow achievement gaps and support healthy development for all children.

Further Resources for the Reader

Here we make suggestions for additional literature and reviews of particular relevance to the following areas, to learn more about this topic:

- SES, its operationalization and meaning for child development: Bradley & Corwyn, 2002; Conger & Donnellan, 2007; Duncan & Murnane, 2011; Evans, 2004; Krieger et al., 1997; Leventhal & Brooks-Gunn, 2000; McLoyd, 1998; Reardon, 2011.
- SES and differences in brain development and neurocognitive performance: Brito & Noble, 2014; Farah, 2017; Hackman & Farah, 2009; Hackman et al., 2010; Johnson et al., 2016; Noble et al., 2015.
- Discussion of the role of neuroscience for SES-related research and policy, including critiques and cautions: Ellwood-Lowe et al., 2016; Farah, 2018; Lipina & Evers, 2017.

References

Akee, R. K. Q., Copeland, W. E., Keeler, G., Angold, A., & Costello, E. J. (2010). Parents' incomes and children's outcomes: A quasi-experiment. *American Economic Journal: Applied Economics, 2*(1), 86–115.

Allan, N. P., Hume, L. E., Allan, D. M., Farrington, A. L., & Lonigan, C. J. (2014). Relations between inhibitory control and the development of academic skills in preschool and kindergarten: A meta-analysis. *Developmental Psychology, 50*(10), 2368–2379. https://doi.org/10.1037/a0037493

Alloway, T. P., & Alloway, R. G. (2010). Investigating the predictive roles of working memory and IQ in academic attainment. *Journal of Experimental Child Psychology, 106*(1), 20–29.

Amso, D., & Lynn, A. (2017). Distinctive mechanisms of adversity and socioeconomic inequality in child development: A review and recommendations for evidence-based policy. *Policy Insights from the Behavioral and Brain Sciences, 4*(2), 139–146. https://doi.org/10.1177/2372732217721933

Ansari, D., & Coch, D. (2006). Bridges over troubled waters: Education and cognitive neuroscience. *Trends in Cognitive Sciences, 10*(4), 146–151. https://doi.org/10.1016/j.tics.2006.02.007

Barch, D. M., Pagliaccio, D., Belden, A., Harms, M. P., Gaffrey, M., Sylvester, C. M., ... Luby, J. (2016). Effect of hippocampal and amygdala connectivity on the relationship between preschool poverty and school-age depression. *American Journal of Psychiatry, 173*, 625–634.

Belsky, D. W., Domingue, B. W., Wedow, R., Arseneault, L., Boardman, J. D., Caspi, A., ... Harris, K. M. (2018). Genetic analysis of social-class mobility in five longitudinal studies. *Proceedings of the National Academy of Sciences, 115*(31), e7275. https://doi.org/10.1073/pnas.1801238115

Belsky, J., & Pluess, M. (2009). Beyond diathesis stress: Differential susceptibility to environmental influences. *Psychological Bulletin, 135*(6), 885–908.

Blair, C., Granger, D. A., Willoughby, M., Mills-Koonce, R., Cox, M., Greenberg, M. T., ... Family Life Project Investigators. (2011). Salivary cortisol mediates effects of poverty and parenting on executive functions in early childhood. *Child Development, 82*(6), 1970–1984.

Bradley, R. H., & Corwyn, R. F. (2002). Socioeconomic status and child development. *Annual Review of Psychology, 53*(1), 371–399.

Braveman, P. A., Cubbin, C., Egerter, S., Chideya, S., Marchi, K. S., Metzler, M., & Posner, S. (2005). Socioeconomic status in health research: One size does not fit all. *Journal of the American Medical Association, 294*(22), 2879–2888. https://doi.org/10.1001/jama.294.22.2879

Brito, N. H., & Noble, K. G. (2014). Socioeconomic status and structural brain development. *Frontiers in Neuroscience, 8*, 276. https://doi.org/10.3389/fnins.2014.00276

Brito, N. H., Piccolo, L. R., & Noble, K. G. (2017). Associations between cortical thickness and neurocognitive skills during childhood vary by family socioeconomic factors. *Brain and Cognition, 116*, 54–62. https://doi.org/10.1016/j.bandc.2017.03.007

Brod, G., Bunge, S. A., & Shing, Y. L. (2017). Does one year of schooling improve children's cognitive control and alter associated brain activation? *Psychological Science, 28*(7), 967–978. https://doi.org/10.1177/0956797617699838

Brody, G. H., Gray, J. C., Yu, T., Barton, A. W., Beach, S. R. H., Galvan, A., . . . Sweet, L. H. (2017). Protective prevention effects on the association of poverty with brain development. *JAMA Pediatrics, 171*(1), 46–52.

Brooks-Gunn, J., & Duncan, G. J. (1997). The effects of poverty on children. *The Future of Children, 7*(2), 55–71.

Burrage, M. S., Ponitz, C. C., McCready, E. A., Shah, P., Sims, B. C., Jewkes, A. M., & Morrison, F. J. (2008). Age- and schooling-related effects on executive functions in young children: A natural experiment. *Child Neuropsychology, 14*(6), 510–524.

Casey, B. J., Somerville, L. H., Gotlib, I. H., Ayduk, O., Franklin, N. T., Askren, M. K., . . . Shoda, Y. (2011). Behavioral and neural correlates of delay of gratification 40 years later. *Proceedings of the National Academy of Sciences, 108*(36), 14998. https://doi.org/10.1073/pnas.1108561108

Chan, M. Y., Na, J., Agres, P. F., Savalia, N. K., Park, D. C., & Wig, G. S. (2018). Socioeconomic status moderates age-related differences in the brain's functional network organization and anatomy across the adult lifespan. *Proceedings of the National Academy of Sciences.* https://doi.org/10.1073/pnas.1714021115

Chetty, R., Hendren, N., & Katz, L. F. (2016). The effects of exposure to better neighborhoods on children: New evidence from the moving to opportunity experiment. *American Economic Review, 106*(4), 855–902.

Conger, R. D., & Donnellan, M. B. (2007). An interactionist perspective on the socioeconomic context of human development. *Annual Review of Psychology, 58*, 175–199.

Crook, S. R., & Evans, G. W. (2014). The role of planning skills in the income—achievement gap. *Child Development, 85*(2), 405–411.

Dahl, G. B., & Lochner, L. (2012). The impact of family income on child achievement: Evidence from the earned income tax credit. *American Economic Review, 102*(5), 1927–1956.

Del Giudice, M., Ellis, B. J., & Shirtcliff, E. A. (2011). The adaptive calibration model of stress responsivity. *Neuroscience & Biobehavioral Reviews, 35*(7), 1562–1592.

Demir-Lira, Ö. E., Prado, J., & Booth, J. R. (2015). Parental socioeconomic status and the neural basis of arithmetic: Differential relations to verbal and visuo-spatial representations. *Developmental Science, 18*(5), 799–814. https://doi.org/10.1111/desc.12268

Demir-Lira, Ö. E., Prado, J., & Booth, J. R. (2016). Neural correlates of math gains vary depending on parental socioeconomic status (SES). *Frontiers in Psychology, 7*, 892. https://doi.org/10.3389/fpsyg.2016.00892

Diamond, A., & Ling, D. S. (2016). Conclusions about interventions, programs, and approaches for improving executive functions that appear justified and those that, despite much hype, do not. *Flux Congress 2014, 18,* 34–48. https://doi.org/10.1016/j. dcn.2015.11.005

Dilworth-Bart, J. E. (2012). Does executive function mediate SES and home quality associations with academic readiness? *Early Childhood Research Quarterly, 27*(3), 416–425. https://doi.org/10.1016/j.ecresq.2012.02.002

Duckworth, A. L., Peterson, C., Matthews, M. D., & Kelly, D. R. (2007). Grit: Perseverance and passion for long-term goals. *Journal of Personality and Social Psychology, 92*(6), 1087–1101.

Duckworth, A. L., & Seligman, M. E. P. (2005). Self-discipline outdoes IQ in predicting academic performance of adolescents. *Psychological Science, 16*(12), 939–944.

Dufford, A. J., & Kim, P. (2017). Family income, cumulative risk exposure, and white matter structure in middle childhood. *Frontiers in Human Neuroscience, 11,* 547. https://doi.org/10.3389/fnhum.2017.00547

Duncan, G. J., Morris, P. A., & Rodrigues, C. (2011). Does money really matter? Estimating impacts of family income on young children's achievement with data from random-assignment experiments. *Developmental Psychology, 47*(5), 1263–1279.

Duncan, G. J., & Murnane, R. J. (2011). *Whither opportunity? Rising inequality, schools, and children's life chances.* New York: Russell Sage Foundation Press.

Duncan, G. J., Yeung, W. J., Brooks-Gunn, J., & Smith, J. R. (1998). How much does childhood poverty affect the life chances of children? *American Sociological Review, 63*(3), 406–423.

Duncan, G. J., Ziol-Guest, K. M., & Kalil, A. (2010). Early-childhood poverty and adult attainment, behavior, and health. *Child Development, 81*(1), 306–325. https://doi.org/10.1111/j.1467-8624.2009.01396.x

Duncan, R. J., McClelland, M. M., & Acock, A. C. (2017). Relations between executive function, behavioral regulation, and achievement: Moderation by family income. *Journal of Applied Developmental Psychology, 49,* 21–30. https://doi.org/10.1016/j.appdev.2017.01.004

Duval, E. R., Garfinkel, S. N., Swain, J. E., Evans, G. W., Blackburn, E. K., Angstadt, M., . . . Liberzon, I. (2017). Childhood poverty is associated with altered hippocampal function and visuospatial memory in adulthood. *Developmental Cognitive Neuroscience, 23,* 39–44. https://doi.org/10.1016/j.dcn.2016.11.006

Ellis, B. J., & Boyce, W. T. (2008). Biological sensitivity to context. *Current Directions in Psychological Science, 17*(3), 183–187.

Ellwood-Lowe, M. E., Humphreys, K. L., Ordaz, S. J., Camacho, M. C., Sacchet, M. D., & Gotlib, I. H. (2018). Time-varying effects of income on hippocampal volume trajectories in adolescent girls. *Developmental Cognitive Neuroscience, 30,* 41–50. https://doi.org/10.1016/j.dcn.2017.12.005

Ellwood-Lowe, M. E., Sacchet, M. D., & Gotlib, I. H. (2016). The application of neuroimaging to social inequity and language disparity: A cautionary examination. *Developmental Cognitive Neuroscience, 22,* 1–8. https://doi.org/10.1016/j.dcn.2016.10.001

Evans, G. W. (2004). The environment of childhood poverty. *American Psychologist, 59*(2), 77–92.

Evans, G. W. (2016). Childhood poverty and adult psychological well-being. *Proceedings of the National Academy of Sciences, 113*(52), 14949–14952.

Evans, G. W., Li, D., & Whipple, S. S. (2013). Cumulative risk and child development. *Psychological Bulletin, 139*(6), 1342–1396. https://doi.org/10.1037/a0031808

Evans, G. W., & Schamberg, M. A. (2009). Childhood poverty, chronic stress, and adult working memory. *Proceedings of the National Academy of Sciences, 106*(16), 6545–6549. https://doi.org/10.1073/pnas.0811910106

Fan, J., McCandliss, B. D., Sommer, T., Raz, A., & Posner, M. I. (2002). Testing the efficiency and independence of attentional networks. *Journal of Cognitive Neuroscience, 14*(3), 340–347. https://doi.org/10.1162/089892902317361886

Farah, M. J. (2017). The neuroscience of socioeconomic status: Correlates, causes, and consequences. *Neuron, 96*(1), 56–71. https://doi.org/10.1016/j.neuron.2017.08.034

Farah, M. J. (2018). Socioeconomic status and the brain: Prospects for neuroscience-informed policy. *Nature Reviews Neuroscience.* https://doi.org/10.1038/s41583-018-0023-2

Farah, M. J., Shera, D. M., Savage, J. H., Betancourt, L., Giannetta, J. M., Brodsky, N. L., . . . Hurt, H. (2006). Childhood poverty: Specific associations with neurocognitive development. *Brain Research, 1110*(1), 166–174.

Ferguson, H. B., Bovarid, S., & Mueller, M. P. (2007). The impact of poverty on educational outcomes for children. *Paedtric Child Health, 12*(8), 701–706.

Fernald, A., Marchman, V. A., & Weisleder, A. (2013). SES differences in language processing skill and vocabulary are evident at 18 months. *Developmental Science, 16*(2), 234–248. https://doi.org/10.1111/desc.12019

Finn, A. S., Minas, J. E., Leonard, J. A., Mackey, A. P., Salvatore, J., Goetz, C., . . . Gabrieli, J. D. E. (2017). Functional brain organization of working memory in adolescents varies in relation to family income and academic achievement. *Developmental Science, 20*(5), 1–15. https://doi.org/10.1111/desc.12450

Fitzpatrick, C., McKinnon, R. D., Blair, C. B., & Willoughby, M. T. (2014). Do preschool executive function skills explain the school readiness gap between advantaged and disadvantaged children? *Learning and Instruction, 30*, 25–31. https://doi.org/10.1016/j.learninstruc.2013.11.003

Fritz, M. S., & MacKinnon, D. P. (2007). Required sample size to detect the mediated effect. *Psychological Science, 18*(3), 233–239.

Gonzalez, M. Z., Allen, J. P., & Coan, J. A. (2016). Lower neighborhood quality in adolescence predicts higher mesolimbic sensitivity to reward anticipation in adulthood. *Developmental Cognitive Neuroscience, 22*, 48–57. https://doi.org/10.1016/j.dcn.2016.10.003

Graziano, P. A., Reavis, R. D., Keane, S. P., & Calkins, S. D. (2007). The role of emotion regulation in children's early academic success. *Journal of School Psychology, 45*(1), 3–19.

Greicius, M. D., Supekar, K., Menon, V., & Dougherty, R. F. (2009). Resting-state functional connectivity reflects structural connectivity in the default mode network. *Cerebral Cortex, 19*(1), 72–78. https://doi.org/10.1093/cercor/bhn059

Gullick, M. M., Demir-Lira, Ö. E., & Booth, J. R. (2016). Reading skill—fractional anisotropy relationships in visuospatial tracts diverge depending on socioeconomic status. *Developmental Science, 19*(4), 673–685. https://doi.org/10.1111/desc.12428

Hackman, D. A., Betancourt, L. M., Gallop, R., Romer, D., Brodsky, N. L., Hurt, H., & Farah, M. J. (2014). Mapping the trajectory of socioeconomic disparity in working memory: Parental and neighborhood factors. *Child Development, 85*(4), 1433–1445. https://doi.org/10.1111/cdev.12242

Hackman, D. A., & Farah, M. J. (2009). Socioeconomic status and the developing brain. *Trends in Cognitive Sciences, 13*(2), 65–73.

Hackman, D. A., Farah, M. J., & Meaney, M. J. (2010). Socioeconomic status and the brain: Mechanistic insights from human and animal research. *Nature Reviews Neuroscience, 11*, 651–659.

Hackman, D. A., Gallop, R., Evans, G. W., & Farah, M. J. (2015). Socioeconomic status and executive function: Developmental trajectories and mediation. *Developmental Science, 18*(5), 686–702.

Hackman, D. A., Kuan, D. C.-H., Manuck, S. B., & Gianaros, P. J. (2018). Socio-economic position and age-related disparities in regional cerebral blood flow within the prefrontal cortex. *Psychosomatic Medicine, 80*(4). Retrieved from https://journals.lww.com/psychosomaticmedicine/Fulltext/2018/05000/Socioeconomic_Position_and_Age_Related_Disparities.2.aspx

Hair, N. L., Hanson, J. L., Wolfe, B. L., & Pollak, S. D. (2015). Association of child poverty, brain development, and academic achievement. *JAMA Pediatrics, 169*(9), 822–829. https://doi.org/10.1001/jamapediatrics.2015.1475

Hanson, J. L., Chandra, A., Wolfe, B. L., & Pollak, S. D. (2011). Association between income and the hippocampus. *PLoS One, 6*(5), e18712. https://doi.org/10.1371/journal.pone.0018712

Hanson, J. L., Hair, N. L., Shen, D. G., Shi, F., Gilmore, J. H., Wolfe, B. L., & Pollak, S. D. (2015). Family poverty affects the rate of human infant brain growth. *PLoS One, 10*(12), e0146434.

Hanson, J. L., Nacewicz, B. M., Sutterer, M. J., Cayo, A. A., Schaefer, S. M., Rudolph, K. D., . . . Davidson, R. J. (2015). Behavioral problems after early life stress: Contributions of the hippocampus and amygdala. *Early Life Stress, Epigenetics, and Resilence, 77*(4), 314–323. https://doi.org/10.1016/j.biopsych.2014.04.020

Haushofer, J., & Fehr, E. (2014). On the psychology of poverty. *Science, 344*(6186), 862–867.

Holz, N. E., Boecker, R., Hohm, E., Zohsel, K., Buchmann, A. F., Blomeyer, D., . . . Laucht, M. (2014). The long-term impact of early life poverty on orbitofrontal cortex volume in adulthood: Results from a prospective study over 25 years. *Neuropsychopharmacology, 40*, 996.

Howard-Jones, P. A. (2014). Neuroscience and education: Myths and messages. *Nature Reviews Neuroscience, 15*, 817.

Huang, Y. T., Leech, K., & Rowe, M. L. (2017). Exploring socioeconomic differences in syntactic development through the lens of real-time processing. *Cognition, 159*, 61–75. https://doi.org/10.1016/j.cognition.2016.11.004

Javanbakht, A., King, A. P., Evans, G. W., Swain, J. E., Angstadt, M., Phan, K. L., & Liberzon, I. (2015). Childhood poverty predicts adult amygdala and frontal activity and connectivity in response to emotional faces. *Frontiers in Behavioral Neuroscience, 9*, 154. https://doi.org/10.3389/fnbeh.2015.00154

Johnson, S. B., Riis, J. L., & Noble, K. G. (2016). State of the art review: Poverty and the developing brain. *Pediatrics.* https://doi.org/10.1542/peds.2015-3075

Kim, P., Evans, G. W., Angstadt, M., Ho, S. S., Sripada, C. S., Swain, J. E., . . . Phan, K. L. (2013). Effects of childhood poverty and chronic stress on emotion regulatory brain function in adulthood. *Proceedings of the National Academy of Sciences, 110*(46), 18442–18447.

Korzeniowski, C., Cupani, M., Ison, M., & Difabio, H. (2016). School performance and poverty: The mediating role of executive functions. *Electronic Journal of Research in Educational Psychology, 14*(3), 474–494.

Krapohl, E., & Plomin, R. (2016). Genetic link between family socioeconomic status and children's educational achievement estimated from genome-wide SNPs. *Molecular Psychiatry, 21*, 437.

Krieger, N., Williams, D. R., & Moss, N. E. (1997). Measuring social class in U.S. public health research: Concepts, methodologies, and guidelines. *Annual Review of Public Health, 18*(1), 341–378. https://doi.org/doi:10.1146/annurev.publhealth.18.1.341

Lawson, G. M., Duda, J. T., Avants, B. B., Wu, J., & Farah, M. J. (2013). Associations between children's socioeconomic status and prefrontal cortical thickness. *Developmental Science, 16*(5), 641–652. https://doi.org/10.1111/desc.12096

Lawson, G. M., & Farah, M. J. (2017). Executive function as a mediator between SES and academic achievement throughout childhood. *International Journal of Behavioral Development, 41*(1), 94–104.

Lawson, G. M., Hook, C. J., & Farah, M. J. (2018). A meta-analysis of the relationship between socioeconomic status and executive function performance among children. *Developmental Science, 21*(2). https://doi.org/10.1111/desc.12529

Lee, J. J., Wedow, R., Okbay, A., Kong, E., Maghzian, O., Zacher, M., . . . Social Science Genetic Association Consortium. (2018). Gene discovery and polygenic prediction from a genome-wide association study of educational attainment in 1.1 million individuals. *Nature Genetics, 50*(8), 1112–1121. https://doi.org/10.1038/s41588-018-0147-3

Leventhal, T., & Brooks-Gunn, J. (2000). The neighborhoods they live in: The effects of neighborhood residence on child and adolescent outcomes. *Psychological Bulletin, 126*(2), 309–337.

LeWinn, K. Z., Sheridan, M. A., Keyes, K. M., Hamilton, A., & McLaughlin, K. A. (2017). Sample composition alters associations between age and brain structure. *Nature Communications, 8*(1), 874. https://doi.org/10.1038/s41467-017-00908-7

Lipina, S. J., & Evers, K. (2017). Neuroscience of childhood poverty: Evidence of impacts and mechanisms as vehicles of dialog with ethics. *Frontiers in Psychology, 8*, 61. https://doi.org/10.3389/fpsyg.2017.00061

Lipina, S. J., Martelli, M. I., Vuelta, B., & Colombo, J. A. (2005). Performance on the A-not-B task of Argentinean infants from unsatisfied and satisfied basic needs homes. *Interamerican Journal of Psychology, 39*(1), 49–60.

Lipina, S. J., Martelli, M. I., Vuelta, B. L., Injoque-Ricle, I., & Colombo, J. A. (2004). Pobreza y desempeno ejecutivo en alumnos preescolares de la ciudad de Buenos Aires (Republica Argentina). Poverty and executive performance in preschool pupils from Buenos Aires city (Republica Argentina). *Interdisciplinaria, 21*(2), 153–193.

Luby, J., Belden, A., Botteron, K., Marrus, N., Harms, M. P., Babb, C., . . . Barch, D. M. (2013). The effects of poverty on childhood brain development: The mediating effect of caregiving and stressful life events. *JAMA Pediatrics, 167*(12), 1135–1142.

Mackey, A. P., Finn, A. S., Leonard, J. A., Jacoby Senghor, D. S., West, M. R., Gabrieli, C. F. O., & Gabrieli, J. D. E. (2015). Neuroanatomical correlates of the income achievement gap. *Psychological Science, 26*(6), 925–933. https://doi.org/10.1177/0956797615572233

Magnuson, K. A. (2007). Maternal education and children's academic achievement during middle childhood. *Developmental Psychology, 43*(6), 1497–1512.

Magnuson, K. A., Meyers, M. K., Ruhm, C., & Waldfogel, J. (2004). Inequality in preschool education and school readiness. *American Educational Research Journal, 41*(1), 115–157.

Mani, A., Mullainathan, S., Shafir, E., & Zhao, J. (2013). Poverty impedes cognitive function. *Science, 341*, 976–980.

McCabe, D. P., Roediger III, H. L., McDaniel, M. A., Balota, D. A., & Hambrick, D. Z. (2010). The relationship between working memory capacity and executive functioning: Evidence for a common executive attention construct. *Neuropsychology, 24*(2), 222–243. https://doi.org/10.1037/a0017619

McClelland, M. M., Cameron, C. E., Connor, C. M., Farris, C. L., Jewkes, A. M., & Morrison, F. J. (2007). Links between behavioral regulation and preschoolers' literacy, vocabulary, and math skills. *Developmental Psychology, 43*(4), 947–959. https://doi.org/10.1037/0012-1649.43.4.947

McClelland, M. M., Cameron, C. E., Duncan, R., Bowles, R. P., Acock, A. C., Miao, A., & Pratt, M. E. (2014). Predictors of early growth in academic achievement: The head-toes-knees-shoulders task. *Frontiers in Psychology, 5,* 599. https://doi.org/10.3389/fpsyg.2014.00599

McCoy, D. C., & Raver, C. C. (2014). Household instability and self-regulation among poor children. *Journal of Child Poverty, 20*(2), 131–152.

McCoy, D. C., Raver, C. C., & Sharkey, P. (2015). Children's cognitive performance and selective attention following recent community violence. *Journal of Health and Social Behavior, 56*(1), 19–36.

McCoy, D. C., Roy, A. L., & Raver, C. C. (2016). Neighborhood crime as a predictor of individual differences in emotional processing and regulation. *Developmental Science, 19*(1), 164–174.

McEwen, B. S., & Gianaros, P. J. (2010). Central role of the brain in stress and adaptation: Links to socioeconomic status, health, and disease. *Annals of the New York Academy of Sciences, 1186,* 190–222.

McLoyd, V. C. (1998). Socioeconomic disadvantage and child development. *American Psychologist, 53*(2), 185–204.

Melby-Lervåg, M., & Hulme, C. (2013). Is working memory training effective? A meta-analytic review. *Developmental Psychology, 49*(2), 270–291. https://doi.org/10.1037/a0028228

Merz, E. C., Tottenham, N., & Noble, K. G. (2018). Socioeconomic status, amygdala volume, and internalizing symptoms in children and adolescents. *Journal of Clinical Child & Adolescent Psychology, 47*(2), 312–323. https://doi.org/10.1080/15374416.2017.1326122

Mezzacappa, E. (2004). Alerting, orienting, and executive attention: Developmental properties and sociodemographic correlates in an epidemiological sample of young, urban children. *Child Development, 75*(5), 1373–1386.

Miller, G. E., & Chen, E. (2013). The biological residue of childhood poverty. *Child Development Perspectives, 7*(2), 67–73.

Mischel, W., Ayduk, O., Berman, M. G., Casey, B. J., Gotlib, I. H., Jonides, J., . . . Shoda, Y. (2011). "Willpower" over the life span: Decomposing self-regulation. *Social Cognitive and Affective Neuroscience, 6*(2), 252–256. https://doi.org/10.1093/scan/nsq081

Miyake, A., & Friedman, N. P. (2012). The nature and organization of individual differences in executive functions: Four general conclusions. *Current Directions in Psychological Science, 21*(1), 8–14. https://doi.org/10.1177/0963721411429458

Muscatell, K. A., Morelli, S. A., Falk, E. B., Way, B. M., Pfeifer, J. H., Galinsky, A. D., . . . Eisenberger, N. I. (2012). Social status modulates neural activity in the mentalizing network. *NeuroImage, 60*(3), 1771–1777. https://doi.org/10.1016/j.neuroimage.2012.01.080

Nesbitt, K. T., Baker-Ward, L., & Willoughby, M. T. (2013). Executive function mediates socio-economic and racial differences in early academic achievement. *Early Childhood Research Quarterly, 28,* 774–783.

Noble, K. G., Houston, S. M., Brito, N. H., Bartsch, H., Kan, E., Kuperman, J. M., . . . Sowell, E. R. (2015). Family income, parental education and brain structure in children and adolescents. *Nature Neuroscience, 18,* 773–778.

Noble, K. G., Houston, S. M., Kan, E., & Sowell, E. R. (2012). Neural correlates of socioeconomic status in the developing human brain. *Developmental Science, 15*(4), 516–527.

Noble, K. G., McCandliss, B. D., & Farah, M. J. (2007). Socioeconomic gradients predict individual differences in neurocognitive abilities. *Developmental Science, 10*(4), 464–480.

Noble, K. G., Norman, M. F., & Farah, M. J. (2005). Neurocognitive correlates of socioeconomic status in kindergarten children. *Developmental Science, 8*(1), 74–87.

Noble, K. G., Wolmetz, M. E., Ochs, L. G., Farah, M. J., & McCandliss, B. D. (2006). Brain-behavior relationships in reading acquisition are modulated by socioeconomic factors. *Developmental Science, 9*(6), 642–654.

Odgers, C. L., & Adler, N. E. (2017). Challenges for low-income children in an era of increasing income inequality. *Child Development Perspectives.* https://doi.org/10.1111/cdep.12273

Ponitz, C. C., McClelland, M. M., Matthews, J. S., & Morrison, F. J. (2009). A structured observation of behavioral self-regulation and its contribution to kindergarten outcomes. *Developmental Psychology, 45*(3), 605–619. https://doi.org/10.1037/a0015365

Raichle, M. E., MacLeod, A. M., Snyder, A. Z., Powers, W. J., Gusnard, D. A., & Shulman, G. L. (2001). A default mode of brain function. *Proceedings of the National Academy of Sciences, 98*(2), 676. https://doi.org/10.1073/pnas.98.2.676

Raver, C. C., Blair, C., & Willoughby, M. (2013). Poverty as a predictor of 4-year-olds' executive function: New perspectives on models of differential susceptibility. *Developmental Psychology, 49*(2), 292–304.

Reardon, S. F. (2011). The widening academic achievement gap between the rich and the poor: New evidence and possible explanations. In R. J. Murnane & G. J. Duncan (Eds.), *Whither opportunity? Rising inequality and the uncertain life chances of low-income children* (pp. 91–115). New York: Russell Sage Foundation Press.

Romens, S. E., Casement, M. D., McAloon, R., Keenan, K., Hipwell, A. E., Guyer, A. E., & Forbes, E. E. (2015). Adolescent girls' neural response to reward mediates the relation between childhood financial disadvantage and depression. *Journal of Child Psychology and Psychiatry, 56*(11), 1177–1184.

Rosen, M. L., Sheridan, M. A., Sambrook, K. A., Meltzoff, A. N., & McLaughlin, K. A. (2018). Socioeconomic disparities in academic achievement: A multi-modal investigation of neural mechanisms in children and adolescents. *NeuroImage, 173*, 298–310. https://doi.org/10.1016/j.neuroimage.2018.02.043

Ryan, R., Fauth, R., & Brooks-Gunn, J. (2006). Childhood poverty: Implications for school readiness and early childhood education. In O. Saracho & B. Spodek (Eds.), *Handbook of research on the education of young children* (2nd ed., pp. 323–346). Mahwah, NJ: Lawrence Erlbaum Associates.

Sampson, R. J., Sharkey, P., & Raudenbush, S. W. (2008). Durable effects of concentrated disadvantage on verbal ability among African-American children. *Proceedings of the National Academy of Sciences, 105*(3), 845–852. https://doi.org/10.1073/pnas.0710189104

Sarsour, K., Sheridan, M., Jutte, D., Nuru-Jeter, A., Hinsh, S., & Boyce, W. T. (2011). Family socioeconomic status and child executive functions: The roles of language, home environment, and single parenthood. *Journal of the International Neuropsychological Society, 17*(1), 120–132.

Shah, A. K., Mullainathan, S., & Shafir, E. (2012). Some consequences of having too little. *Science, 338*(6107), 682–685.

Sharkey, P. (2010). The acute effect of local homicides on children's cognitive performance. *Proceedings of the National Academy of Sciences*, 107(26), 11733–11738.

Sharkey, P., Tirado-Strayer, N., Papachristos, A. V., & Raver, C. C. (2012). The effect of local violence on children's attention and impulse control. *American Journal of Public Health*, 102(12), 2287–2293.

Sheridan, M. A., & McLaughlin, K. A. (2016). Neurobiological models of the impact of adversity on education. *Neuroscience of Education*, 10, 108–113. https://doi.org/10.1016/j.cobeha.2016.05.013

Sheridan, M. A., Peverill, M., Finn, A. S., & McLaughlin, K. A. (2017). Dimensions of childhood adversity have distinct associations with neural systems underlying executive functioning. *Development and Psychopathology*, 29(5), 1777–1794. https://doi.org/10.1017/S0954579417001390

Shipstead, Z., Redick, T. S., & Engle, R. W. (2012). Is working memory training effective? *Psychological Bulletin*, 138(4), 628–654. https://doi.org/10.1037/a0027473

Sigman, M., Peña, M., Goldin, A. P., & Ribeiro, S. (2014). Neuroscience and education: Prime time to build the bridge. *Nature Neuroscience*, 17, 497.

Sirin, S. R. (2005). Socioeconomic status and academic achievement: A meta-analytic review of research. *Review of Educational Research*, 75(3), 417–453.

Spielberg, J. M., Galarce, E. M., Ladouceur, C. D., McMakin, D. L., Olino, T. M., Forbes, E. E., . . . Dahl, R. E. (2015). Adolescent development of inhibition as a function of SES and gender: Converging evidence from behavior and fMRI. *Human Brain Mapping*, 36(8), 3194–3203. https://doi.org/10.1002/hbm.22838

Sripada, R. K., Swain, J. E., Evans, G. W., Welsh, R. C., & Liberzon, I. (2014). Childhood poverty and stress reactivity are associated with aberrant functional connectivity in default mode network. *Neuropsychopharmacology*, 39, 2244–2251.

St. Clair-Thompson, H. L., & Gathercole, S. E. (2006). Executive functions and achievements in school: Shifting, updating, inhibition, and working memory. *The Quarterly Journal of Experimental Psychology*, 59(4), 745–759.

Ursache, A., & Noble, K. G. (2016a). Neurocognitive development in socioeconomic context: Multiple mechanisms and implications for measuring socioeconomic status. *Psychophysiology*, 53(1), 71–82. https://doi.org/10.1111/psyp.12547

Ursache, A., & Noble, K. G. (2016b). Socioeconomic status, white matter, and executive function in children. *Brain and Behavior*, 6(10), e00531. https://doi.org/10.1002/brb3.531

Weissman, D. G., Conger, R. D., Robins, R. W., Hastings, P. D., & Guyer, A. E. (2018). Income change alters default mode network connectivity for adolescents in poverty. *Developmental Cognitive Neuroscience*, 30, 93–99. https://doi.org/10.1016/j.dcn.2018.01.008

Welsh, M. C., Pennington, B. F., & Groisser, D. B. (1991). A normative-developmental study of executive function: A window on prefrontal function in children. *Developmental Neuropsychology*, 7(2), 131–149. https://doi.org/10.1080/87565649109540483

Whittle, S., Vijayakumar, N., Simmons, J. G., Dennison, M., Schwartz, O., Pantelis, C., . . . Allen, N. B. (2017). Role of positive parenting in the association between neighborhood social disadvantage and brain development across adolescence. *JAMA Psychiatry*, 74(8), 824–832.

Wiebe, S. A., Sheffield, T., Nelson, J. M., Clark, C. A. C., Chevalier, N., & Espy, K. A. (2011). The structure of executive function in 3-year-olds. *Journal of Experimental Child Psychology*, 108(3), 436–452.

Willingham, D. T., & Lloyd, J. W. (2007). How educational theories can use neuro-scientific data. *Mind, Brain, and Education*, *1*(3), 140–149. https://doi.org/10.1111/j.1751-228X.2007.00014.x

Wolf, S., Magnuson, K. A., & Kimbro, R. T. (2017). Family poverty and neighborhood poverty: Links with children's school readiness before and after the great recession. *Children and Youth Services Review*, *79*, 368–384.

Young, S. E., Friedman, N. P., Miyake, A., Willcutt, E. G., Corley, R. P., Haberstick, B. C., & Hewitt, J. K. (2009). Behavioral disinhibition: Liability for externalizing spectrum disorders and its genetic and environmental relation to response inhibition across adolescence. *Journal of Abnormal Psychology*, *118*(1), 117–130. https://doi.org/10.1037/a0014657

Zelazo, P. D., & Müller, U. (2002). Executive function in typical and atypical development. In *Blackwell handbook of childhood cognitive development* (pp. 445–469). Malden: Blackwell Publishing. https://doi.org/10.1002/9780470996652.ch20

Section 2

Discipline-Specific Abilities

Literacy, Numeracy, and Science

5 Neuroscience in Reading and Reading Difficulties

Xiuhong Tong and Catherine McBride

Neuroscience in Reading and Reading Difficulties

Reading is a complex and multifaceted skill, which has to be acquired through years of extensive and explicit teaching and practice (Herbster, Mintun, Nebes, & Becker, 1997). More than 10% of children have been found to have relatively severe impairments in reading despite adequate intelligence; those children are defined as having developmental dyslexia (Catts, Adlof, Hogan, & Weismer, 2005). With the development of research methods and technology, our understanding of reading and reading difficulties has advanced over the decades. In particular, advances in neuroscience methods have provided important insights on some critical issues related to reading. The most widely used neuroscience methods applied to investigate reading and reading difficulty thus far are the event-related potential (ERP) and functional magnetic resonance imaging (fMRI) techniques. Both ERP and fMRI techniques are noninvasive approaches that can be used in both typically developing child and adult readers and in readers with reading difficulties. To provide a better understanding of neuroscience in reading and reading difficulty, this review will overview important neuropsychological (i.e., ERP and fMRI) evidence that favors temporal brain wave patterns and abnormalities of ERP studies as well as brain activation patterns and weaknesses as shown in fMRI studies on reading and reading difficulty. Moreover, we will highlight some noncognitive factors such as socio-economic status (SES) that modulate the brain regions that we use when we read. Finally, issues of neuroscience research to reading practice and reading difficulty diagnosis and remediation will be discussed.

What Has Neuroscience Added to Our Understanding Over and Above Psychology on Reading and Reading Difficulties?

Visual word reading/recognition starts with the analysis of visual features of a word and then maps the orthographic/graphic units, referring to written letters, strings of letters, or other graphemes, onto phonological units such as phonemes or syllables; meaning is, thus, accessed. In this chapter, phonology refers to the speech sounds comprising words. The meanings of these words are referred to as semantics. Finally, the ways in which these words appear in print constitute the orthographic aspects of word reading. Ways to study our understanding of phonology, semantics, and orthographic aspects of word reading depend largely upon behavioral experiments that make use of different paradigms. For example, in the lexical decision paradigm, readers are required to make a decision as to whether what they see in print is a word or not. Similarly, in a priming task, children are asked to make decisions about words that they see. These decisions are sometimes "primed" with a word that come before the target word. This "prime" may or may not influence the decision that is made about the following word.

Thus, many experimental methods have facilitated the investigation of how orthographic, phonological, and semantic information is accessed during visual word recognition. However, traditional behavioral research methods that make use of reaction time or response accuracy as indices of cognitive information processing are often very indirect and rarely straightforward. This is especially the case in reading, a skill that involves multiple cognitive and linguistic information processing. The result of a given behavioral test is a compound function of perception, cognition, attention, and motor control such as naming a word or pressing a button. Therefore, variations in reaction time and accuracy may be difficult to attribute to variations in a specific cognitive process (Landi & Perfetti, 2007). In contrast, the ERP measure is well known for its excellent temporal resolution and provides a powerful tool to probe word recognition and broader language comprehension more directly. An ERP measure is defined as changes in voltage potential collected by electrodes placed on the scalp; the changes in voltage are produced by the collective action of underlying neural activity induced by stimulus presentation. In comparison to traditional behavioral measures used in language and reading research (e.g., reaction time and response accuracy), the ERP approach has at least three advantages. First, ERP provides a continuous record of brain activity with millisecond temporal resolution (Molfese, Molfese, & Espy, 1999). Second, ERPs are time-locked to the onset of stimuli. The ERP can thus be used effectively to determine which stage or stages of word recognition are affected by specific linguistic information. Third, ERPs can be obtained in passive or active tasks and are relatively noninvasive. Therefore, the ERP is particularly valuable in studying reading/language comprehension in children of all ages, even infants, and in readers with reading difficulty (Molfese, Freeman, & Palermo, 1975). Indeed, the ERP technique has been widely used in both infant and young children's language and reading research studies, which provide converging lines of evidence for a better understanding of the processes involved in visual word reading.

ERPs reflect neural activity from large populations of neurons linked to specific cognitive processing (Taylor & Baldeweg, 2002). Within ERPs, the brain changes in relation to cognitive processes are typically measured via fluctuations in the amplitude or latency of various positive or negative components that occur at different time points throughout their time course (Callaway,

Tueting, & Koslow, 1978). Over time, ERP studies have noted signatures that can be used as predictors of language and reading abilities; several ERP components, including early components (e.g., N1/N170, P200) and later components (e.g., N400), have been reported to relate to different aspects of language information processing (Friederici, Hahne, & Mecklinger, 1996; Penke et al., 1997). The names of these components of electrical activity are usually determined by whether they are Positive (P) or Negative (N) and approximately how many milliseconds they occur following the stimulus presentation. Using the ERP technique, Molfese and colleagues conducted a series of studies to examine whether and how children's abilities in neural discrimination of speech information (e.g., voice onset time, and place of articulation) predicted their later language and reading performance from infancy into childhood and adulthood (Molfese & Betz, 1988). The authors found that newborn infants who could discriminate between consonant sounds alone and consonant sounds in combination with different vowel sounds as reflected by an ERP component peaked between 88–240 ms, and a later peak latency of 664 ms, showed better performance on language tasks at age 5 years; this peak could also predict their verbal skills and reading skills through 8 years of age (Molfese & Molfese, 1997).

Studies on children's neural sensitivity to print using ERP techniques demonstrate that the N1 component is a neural indicator of children's ability to distinguish words from objects (e.g., circles) and word-like stimuli (e.g., consonant strings). The N1/N170, a negative-going ERP component of the ERP, has been suggested to reflect visual-orthographic processing in visual word recognition peaking at around 200 ms after stimulus onset with localization over the left occipital-temporal cortex (Maurer & McCandliss, 2008; Michel et al., 2004; Rossion, Gauthier, Goffaux, Tarr, & Crommelinck, 2002; Tarkiainen, Helenius, Hansen, Cornelissen, & Salmelin, 1999). This component has been found to relate highly with children's experience in formal literacy training. For example, the N1 was absent in German-speaking kindergarteners with a mean age of 6.47 years old, but a larger N1 for German words than symbol strings was shown in the same children only after they had received 1.5 years of schooling at the age of 8.26 years old (Maurer et al., 2006). A recent study conducted in our lab revealed that the change of N1 amplitude was moderately and negatively correlated with children's reading fluency and accuracy. That is, children with high reading ability showed better performance in distinguishing words from symbols (Tong et al., 2016).

Two other important ERP components that are worth introducing in this chapter are the N400 and MMN components. The N400 is a scalp negative deflection peaking around 400 ms post stimulus. It is taken as a measure for the semantic evaluation of words generally observed in lexical decision/priming tasks or sentence acceptance tasks (Deacon, Hewitt, Yang, & Nagata, 2000; Gomes, Ritter, Tartter, Vaughan, & Rosen, 1997; Holcomb, 1988; Kutas & Hillyard, 1984). In addition, the N400 component has been found to be sensitive to morphological structure processing (Gross, Say, Kleingers,

Clahsen, & Münte, 1998; Huang, Lee, Tsai, & Tzeng, 2011; Münte, Say, Clahsen, Schiltz, & Kutas, 1999). For example, one of our studies has shown that typically developing Chinese children had most difficulty in processing the nonwords composed of real word morphemes that were reversed relative to nonwords composed of two random single morphemes as reflected by a strong N400 effect found in the reversed condition (Tong, Chung, & McBride, 2014). The mismatch negativity (MMN) component, characterized by a negative deflection with a frontocentral distribution, is another important component. Using MMN, we can determine whether the auditory system is able to distinguish the deviation between two stimuli with very small acoustic changes (Näätänen, Paavilainen, Rinne, & Alho, 2007). The N1, N400, and MMN components, thus, can be used as neural indicators of phonological, visual-orthographic processing and morphological /semantic information processing.

The aforementioned ERP research has contributed to our knowledge of the temporal course of reading. We cannot, however, accurately infer the brain regions that engage in reading by using ERP alone. Fortunately, the functional magnetic resonance imaging (fMRI) technique, which is a sensitive measure of brain structure, and spatial location of function, has facilitated tremendous methodological advances in terms of spatial resolution compared to traditional research methods and the ERP technique. The fMRI measures blood flow, and is sensitive to the level of oxygen in the blood. It measures the BOLD signal, standing for the blood oxygen level dependent signal. Oxygenated blood flow increases to regions of neural activity over the time course of a few seconds, and therefore the BOLD signal can serve as an indirect measure of neural activity associated with the performance of a cognitive task. Compared to the traditional research approaches and other neural imaging methods such as PET, fMRI has relatively high spatial resolution and is easy to use. Moreover, fMRI is noninvasive, and it can thus examine brain functioning safely and effectively. fMRI is also potentially more objective than traditional psychological research methods. As mentioned earlier, the result of a given behavioral test such as reaction time is a compound of multiple cognitive activities (e.g., perception, attention, and motor control). Moreover, most traditional psychological research methods require children to be involved in explicit tasks. In contrast, the fMRI method, with its implicit tasks, can provide direct evidence on the neural activities associated with certain cognitive processing as well as the untypical activities related to certain deficits in reading or language processing. Given the preceding advantages, fMRI has been widely employed to examine cognitive processes, including reading, in both typical readers and readers with learning difficulties such as dyslexia (Hoeft et al., 2007).

fMRI has been widely used to examine some issues that could not be answered using traditional behavioral methods in reading and language research in both young and adult readers, such as the following: (1) Are there specific brain areas for reading and what are those areas? (2) Do children use the same neural networks as adults? (3) What are the developmental connections from brain functions to children's reading/language development and education? (4) How might two different writing systems shape the reading areas in the brain in bilingual learners?

To date, fMRI studies have yielded important insights into the preceding issues. For example, neuroimaging studies of reading in skilled readers suggest that reading engages a large-scale network of left frontal, temporoparietal, and occipitotemporal regions (Turkeltaub, Gareau, Flowers, Zeffiro, & Eden, 2003). More specifically, the brain areas of the inferior frontal gyrus and the precentral gyrus are active in processing phonological elements within words. The inferior, middle, and superior temporal gyri, and the inferior parietal gyrus have been found to be responsible for mapping orthographic information onto phonological and semantic representations (Turkeltaub et al., 2003). In particular, the left occipitotemporal cortex, labelled the 'visual word form area' (VWFA) is consistently activated by visual word reading across writing systems (Houdé, Rossi, Lubin, & Joliot, 2010) although there is still a debate as to whether the VWFA is a brain area of abstract representations of visual words (Nakamura, Dehaene, Jobert, Le, & Kouider, 2005); some researchers argue that the VWFA is a brain region that is involved in more general sensorimotor integration (Price & Devlin, 2003). A recent fMRI meta-analysis has revealed that children use similar brain areas during reading: The frontal, temporoparietal, and occipitotemporal regions are the main brain areas for reading (Houdé et al., 2010).

A majority of neuroimaging studies in bilinguals suggest that two languages spoken by bilinguals activate common brain regions, irrespective of the age at which learners begin to acquire the L2 (Briellmann et al., 2004; Frenck-Mestre, Anton, Roth, Vaid, & Viallet, 2005; Gandour et al., 2007; Halsband, Krause, Sipila, Teras, & Laihinen, 2002; Hasegawa, Carpenter, & Just, 2002; Hernandez, Martinez, & Kohnert, 2000; Illes et al., 1999; Klein, Milner, Zatorre, Meyer, & Evans, 1995; Klein, Milner, Zatorre, Zhao, & Nikelski, 1999; Klein, Watkins, Zatorre, & Milner, 2006; Klein, Zatorre, Milner, Meyer, & Evans, 1994; Mahendra, Plante, Magloire, Milman, & Trouard, 2003; Perani et al., 1998; Yokoyama et al., 2006). For example, in one fMRI study, Illes et al. (1999) reported an overlapping activation in the frontal lobe region for L1 and L2 in Spanish-English bilinguals completing a semantic task (here, participants were required to decide whether words were concrete or abstract in meaning) vs. a non-semantic decision task (here, participants were asked to judge whether words were printed in uppercase or lowercase). Studies of Chinese-English bilinguals also found similar patterns of cortical activation for L1 and L2, in spite of the remarkably different orthography, phonology, and syntax of the two languages (Chee, Soon, & Lee, 2003; Chee, Tan, & Thiel, 1999; Chee et al., 2000; Pu et al., 2001; Xue, Dong, Jin, Zhang, & Wang, 2004). Using an fMRI measure, Chee et al. (1999) examined the cortical organization of language of both early and late Mandarin-English bilinguals using a word stem completion task. They found that in both languages, activations were observed in the prefrontal, temporal, and parietal regions, as well as the supplementary motor area of the brain.

Concrete Implications of Research and Opportunities for Translation

The ERP and fMRI approaches are particularly useful in identifying infants and young children who are at risk for dyslexia. Dyslexia involves difficulties in reading and spelling despite normal schooling, adequate intelligence, and equal social economic opportunities, as well as a lack of sensory acuity deficits, and neurological and psychiatric diseases (Critchley, 1970; WHO, 1994).

As mentioned previously, reading is a complex cognitive skill, entailing several levels of brain organization, which are difficult to differentiate with traditional psychological measures. However, ERPs are time-locked and have very high temporal resolution, and thus are well suited for examinations of the time course of cognitive processing required for reading, in particular in children with reading difficulties (Hillyard & Kutas, 1983). ERP studies accumulating to date demonstrate that certain abnormalities of both early events (e.g., MMN, N1, P2, or N2) and late events (e.g., P300, N400) in both cognitive and linguistic task processing are implicated in dyslexia (Bentin, Mouchetant-Rostaing, Giard, Echallier, & Pernier, 1999; Bonte, Poelmans, & Blomert, 2007; Breznitz & Meyler, 2003; Caylak, 2009; Guttorm, Leppanen, Richardson, & Lyytinen, 2001).

Using an MMN paradigm, a number of studies have consistently found that those with dyslexia have deficits in processing both general acoustic (Baldeweg, Richardson, Watkins, Foale, & Gruzelier, 1999) and speech information (Schulte-Körne, Deimel, Bartling, & Remschmidt, 1998, 2001). In terms of acoustic processing deficits, MMN studies show that those with dyslexia show an untypical MMN in frequency discrimination and modulation (Baldeweg et al., 1999). For example, Baldeweg et al. (1999) conducted a study examining frequency discrimination deficits in dyslexic adults using an MMN paradigm. The authors found that dyslexic adults showed delayed and reduced MMN responses for tone frequency deviants of 1015, 1030, and 1060 Hz, but not for 1090 Hz to a standard stimulus of 1000Hz. At the same time, the dyslexics showed a similar N1 pattern as the controls, suggesting that adults with dyslexia might have difficulties in tone perception. Moreover, they found significant correlations between MMN latencies and errors in both word and nonword reading (r = .52 and .71, respectively). Adult dyslexics were also found to have deficits in pitch discrimination as reflected by an attenuated MMN for pitch contrasts (e.g., Maurer Bucher, Brem, & Brandeis, 2003). Maurer and colleagues (2003) reported a study showing that children at familial risk for dyslexia had similar deficits as dyslexic adults in pitch differences of 30 and 60 Hz. For speech information perception, the MMN studies mainly focus on discrimination between formant transitions (spectral changes) and voice onset timing transitions (temporal changes). Both adults and children with dyslexia show untypical MMNs in speech information perception at both the spectral and temporal level. For example, Schulte-Körne et al. (1998) reported an attenuated MMN that peaked between 176–302 ms to /da/-/ba/ contrasts in dyslexic children with a mean age of 12.5 years. The spectral discrimination deficit was also found in Chinese children with developmental dyslexia in a study conducted by Meng et al. (2005) with a smaller MMN shown in the dyslexic group to /da/-/ga/ contrasts in the time window of 0–100 ms. Collectively, the MMN can serve as a neural discrimination marker of acoustic and speech information perception deficits for dyslexia (e.g., Huttunen-Scott, Kaartinen, Tolvanen, & Lyytinen, 2008).

Deficits in visual word processing were reported in a number of ERP studies in dyslexia. Three ERP components, i.e., N1/N170, P200, and N400, have been linked to visual word processing (Sereno & Rayner, 2003). The N1/N170 and P200 components are sensitive to early orthographic processing during word recognition (Meng, Tian, Jian, & Zhou, 2007; Pratarelli, 1995); the N400 is a component taken as a measure for semantic evaluation of words, and it is generally observed in lexical decision/priming tasks or sentence acceptance tasks (Deacon et al., 2000; Gomes et al., 1997; Holcomb, 1988; Kutas & Hillyard, 1980, 1984, 1989; Lovrich, Cheng, & Velting, 2003; Lovrich, Cheng, Velting, & Kazmerski, 1997; Meng et al., 2007). Empirical evidence has demonstrated that dyslexics tend to have reduced reading-related N170 specialization (e.g., Maurer et al., 2007) and smaller or no P200 and N400 effects in some visual word processing tasks (e.g., Chung, Tong, & McBride-Chang, 2012).

For example, Maurer et al. (2007) conducted a study investigating how N1 tuning for print developed in children in kindergarten and second grade from families with and without familial risk for dyslexia using a repetition detection task. This task consisted of four experimental conditions, including words, symbol strings, pseudowords, and pictures. The ERP results revealed that the increase in N1 specialization was increasingly specific to written words only. That is, there was no specialization for other visual input such as nonsense symbols or pictures of objects. Results likely reflect the increasing specialization of the underlying cortex to recognizing visual word forms. Importantly, reading training was not significant for children with dyslexia from kindergarten to second grade, but the children with normal reading ability showed a significant increase in the N1 specialization with an increase of formal reading training, and the N1 specialization was smaller in second grade children with dyslexia compared to those typically developing children in second grade. The researchers also found that the N1 specialization effect in second grade was significantly correlated with reading speed across the whole sample. These findings suggest that the N1 specialization is a neural marker of emerging literacy.

In a study in Chinese developmental dyslexia, Meng and colleagues (2007) investigated orthographic and phonological processing conveyed by characters during sentence reading in Chinese children with dyslexia and typically developing children. Two ERP components, P200 and N400, were found in their study. The results from the study by Meng et al. (2007) revealed that for the control children, more negative ERP responses in both P200 and N400 time windows were found in the orthographic and phonological mismatches conditions compared with the baseline condition at the central—posterior scalp regions, but dyslexic children did not differ across experimental conditions in either of the P200 or the N400 components. They also found that dyslexic children exhibited a less negative response in the mean amplitude of the N400 component compared with control children. Meng et al. suggested that Chinese dyslexic children might have a deficiency in processing orthographic and phonological information during sentence comprehension. Their findings also indicated that compared with typically developing children, dyslexic children relied more on phonological information to access word meanings.

However, in our own study (Chung, Tong, & McBride-Chang, 2012), we did not find a difference in the P200 component between our dyslexic children and the control group in processing orthographic information. The particular focus was radical positional information. A radical is a graphical component of a Chinese character, often a semantic indicator or a phonetic component, and radicals are often used to list characters in Chinese dictionaries. However, the two groups did show differences in the mean amplitude of the N400 component. In this case, control children exhibited differences across experimental conditions, but dyslexic children did not show any effects of the N400 component. One possible interpretation is that the positional information of radicals within a Chinese compound character may influence the recognition of the Chinese character at a late stage as reflected in the N400 component. The different result in the P200 component between our study and the study by Meng et al. may be attributable to the following: first, the manipulation of orthography in the study by Meng et al. (2007) was based on the whole character, rather than on radical positioning (at the sub-character level). Second, the mean frequencies of the base words, from which the critical compound nonwords were derived, were different between the homophonic condition (43 per million) and the baseline condition (115 per million) in the study by Meng and colleagues. Finally, the operation of orthography in that study was embedded within sentences. Indeed, their task required children to make sentence acceptance judgments. Therefore, their study may have tapped into different levels of lexical processing, which may have resulted in different ERP effects, such as the P200 effect.

In another ERP study (Tong et al., 2014), we examined morphological processing in Chinese dyslexics. Morphemes are the smallest meaning-carrying components of characters. We manipulated the position of morphemes within a Chinese two-character compound word. Three experimental conditions were created: (1) real word condition (e.g., 天氣 (weather)); (2) reversed condition, where a nonword was generated by reversing the order of morphemes in a real compound words (e.g., 期假 came from the character 假期 (holiday)), and (3) random condition, in which two free morphemes were randomly combined (e.g., 架旅). Children with dyslexia showed different ERP patterns in processing morphological information as reflected by the N400 component. That is, there was no difference across the three experimental conditions for the dyslexic group, but for the control group, there were significant differences across experimental conditions, with the most negative mean amplitude occurring in the reversed condition, followed by the random condition and the real condition. Even though we cannot provide conclusive evidence that Chinese dyslexic children have a deficit in processing of positional information of the morpheme within a Chinese compound word based on this single study, we believe that those with and without dyslexia tend to perform somewhat differently in processing of morpheme position information. Collectively, the ERP studies have developed some neural signatures for dyslexia at different levels of information processing during visual word processing.

The fMRI studies accumulating to date have identified some important neural correlates of visual word processing focused on both brain structure and functional levels in dyslexia as well (e.g., Eckert, 2004; Richlan, Kronbichler, & Wimmer, 2009). At the structural level, brain-imaging studies have revealed that children with dyslexia differ from those without dyslexia in some subtle anatomical structures in the brain (Galaburda, Sherman, Rosen, Aboitiz, & Geschwind, 1985; Geschwind & Levitsky, 1968; Jenner, Rosen, & Galaburda, 1999; Livingstone, Rosen, Drislane, & Galaburda, 1991). For example, several studies have found that, compared to typically developing readers, individuals with dyslexia exhibit either a rightward asymmetry or symmetrical planum temporale, a brain region often referred to as Wernicke's area, and one of the most important functional areas for language processing; normal readers tend to demonstrate a leftward asymmetry of the planum temporale (Galaburda et al., 1985; Geschwind & Levitsky, 1968; Jenner et al., 1999; Livingstone et al., 1991). Researchers have suggested that those with non-leftward planum temporale asymmetry might show deficits in verbal comprehension, phonological decoding, and expressive language (for a review, see Caylak, 2009). In addition, a line of MRI studies has indicated that dyslexic children show an increase in the size of the corpus callosum (Duara et al., 1991; Rumsey et al., 1996), and some other studies on the morphology of the cerebellum have found that individuals with dyslexia exhibit a significantly smaller right anterior lobe of the cerebellum as well as a smaller total cerebral volume compared to the typically developing readers (Middleton & Strick, 1997; Schmahmann & Pandya, 1997).

Studies using voxel-based morphometry (VBM), a technique allowing examination of focal differences in brain anatomy, have also demonstrated that individuals with dyslexia sometimes have reduced gray matter density and/or smaller gray matter volume in some regions of the brain (e.g., left posterior temporal region, the left posterior middle temporal gyrus, and left inferior occipitotemporal cortex) (e.g., Brambati et al., 2004; Brown et al., 2001; Eckert, 2004; Hoeft et al., 2007; Jednorog et al., 2015; Kronbichler, Wimmer, Staffen, Hutzler, Mair, & Ladurner, 2008; Ramus, Altarelli, Jednoróg, Zhao, & di Covella, 2017; Silani et al., 2005). It has been suggested that the reductions of gray matter might reflect a regional decrease in neuronal number or neuropil, which in turn might result in reading disabilities (Caylak, 2009).

In most previous anatomical structure studies, the functional significance of the brain structural differences between those with and without dyslexia has not been clear. We often do not even know which of those differences are specifically relevant to dyslexia considering the well-known comorbidity between dyslexia and many other developmental disorders (Middleton & Strick, 1997; Schmahmann & Pandya, 1997). For example, among readers with dyslexia, around 18–42% of them tend to meet criteria for attention deficit hyperactivity disorder (Mayes, Calhoun, & Crowell, 2000) given the fact reading is highly associated with attention. Functional neuroimaging techniques have been widely used in reading development, reading disability, and intervention (Pugh et al., 2000; Sarkari et al., 2002); in these studies, the functional significance of brain abnormalities has been studied in detail. Numerous studies have revealed that developmental dyslexics showed atypical activation in the occipitotemporal, temporoparietal, and anterior areas related to specific reading or language processes (Hoeft et al., 2007; Kronbichler et al., 2006; Meyler et al., 2007; Shaywitz et al., 2002). For example, in phonological tasks (e.g., a rhyme judgment task in which the participant had to indicate whether two words rhymed or not), there was evidence of reduced activation in the left temporoparietal region in dyslexic children compared with typically developing children who were three years younger but reading at the same level as the dyslexic children (Hoeft et al., 2007). There is substantially converging evidence that dyslexics of alphabetic languages commonly exhibit abnormal activation in the left posterior temporoparietal region ((Kronbichler et al., 2006; Meyler et al., 2007; Paulesu et al., 2001; B. A. Shaywitz et al., 2002; S. E. Shaywitz et al., 2003). This region is proposed to play "a plausible role in mediating the visual entry into the linguistic system, combining orthographic, lexical and phonological information about words" (see a review, Habib, 2000, p. 2390). In contrast, Siok and colleagues (2004, 2008) have found significantly reduced activation in the left middle frontal gyrus (LMFG) in Chinese dyslexic children as compared to typically developing Chinese children. This finding suggests that Chinese developmental dyslexia differs somewhat in its neural basis from those of alphabetic languages. The difference in brain regions between Chinese and alphabetic dyslexia is likely attributable to the difference in the orthographies used. The complex visual-spatial structure of Chinese characters demands detailed visuospatial computation, and the LMFG is proposed to be associated with the processing of visuospatial and verbal information as well as to coordinate cognitive resources (Tan, Laird, Li, & Fox, 2005; Tan et al., 2003). Siok and colleagues, therefore, suggested that LMFG might be a neuroanatomical marker of Chinese reading disability.

However, researchers have hotly debated the extent to which there may be Chinese-specific regions involved in dyslexia as argued by Siok et al. (2004, 2008). In another study (Hu et al., 2010), Hu and colleagues found that developmental dyslexics in Chinese exhibited very similar brain patterns to their English counterparts, with a direct comparison of Chinese and English monolingual reading. Hu et al. reported that compared with culturally matched normal readers, both Chinese and English dyslexics showed reduced activation in the left middle frontal gyrus, left posterior middle temporal gyrus, left occipitotemporal cortex, and left angular gyrus. The authors concluded that "this pattern of similarities and differences strongly suggests a common neural basis for dyslexia regardless of the language spoken and its orthography" (p. 1705). However, across these studies, different tasks were employed. In the study by Siok et al. (2004), they used homophone judgment and lexical decision tasks, which required the mapping from orthography to phonology. In contrast, a semantic decision task, which requires explicit semantic processing, was applied in the study by Hu et al. (2010). The differences between tasks may account for the differences in brain regions. However, there are really few conclusive neuroimaging studies in Chinese dyslexia. We can expect important news in the near future if the very recent representations can be used as a basis for prognosis. The ERP and fMRI methodologies can also help to diagnose language/reading impairments potentially earlier than would be conceivable via behavioral or psychological inspection alone. Additionally, the ERP and fMRI studies help to predict the degree to which children with dyslexia benefit from a subsequent intervention (Raizada & Kishiyama, 2010). There have been some valuable longitudinal ERP and fMRI data in predicting risk for language and reading difficulty at early ages (e.g., Hoeft et al., 2011; Lyytinen, Eklund, & Lyytinen, 2005; Molfese, 2000). For example, Molfese (2000) used the ERP measure to record 186 infants within 36 hours of birth with a passive listening experiment in which the infants were required to listen to synthetic speech stimuli /gi/, /bi/, and /di/ during sleep. The authors then conducted a discriminate analysis at 8 years of age of those children to classify them according to their speech ERPs at birth. The authors found that the ERPs (i.e., N1, P2, and N2 components) at birth could distinguish 76.5% of children with dyslexia, 100% of poor readers (low IQ and reading ability), and 79% of control children at age 8. In another longitudinal study conducted by Lyytinen et al. (2005), ERPs in relation to both synthetic and natural spoken speech were recorded in 100 children with risk for dyslexia and 100 children in a control group. The children with risk for dyslexia had different brain distributions for the standard and deviant responses to the natural speech sound /ka/ compared to the control group at birth. The two groups also showed differences in response to synthetic speech stimuli between 540–630 ms at birth with a larger and more prolonged response between standard and deviant stimuli in the right hemisphere for the children with risk for dyslexia but with the largest difference between the standard and deviant speech sounds in the left hemisphere for the control group. The correlation analysis revealed that the ERP activity in the right hemisphere in children with risk for dyslexia correlated with lower word and nonword reading accuracy in the first grade of school, poorer language skills at 2.5 years, poorer verbal memory and reduced phonological skills at age 5 years, and slower lexical access and less knowledge of letters at 6.5 years (Lyytinen et al., 2005). These two important longitudinal studies demonstrate that neuroscience methods can be used as a tool to predict which children are at risk for reading difficulties.

In a longitudinal study, Hoeft and colleagues (Hoeft et al., 2011) used fMRI and DTI brain measures to examine whether functional and structural brain measures could predict reading improvement in dyslexia over a 2.5-year period. Twenty-five children with dyslexia and 20 typically developing children were administered a series of standardized tests of reading and language, and they also participated in an fMRI experiment in which they were asked to perform a printed-word rhyme judgment task at time 1 (e.g., participants were required to judge whether two visually presented words such as *bait* and *gate* rhymed or not). At follow-up 2.5 years later, the two groups of children were reassessed with those standardized reading tests used in Time 1. Behavioral results showed that none of the standardized behavioral scores from Time 1 significantly predicted improvement of reading scores in the dyslexic group. However, neuroimaging data analyses demonstrated that the increase in the right prefrontal activation during the printed-word rhyme judgment task and the right superior longitudinal fasciculus white matter organization were significantly predictive of reading gains in dyslexia. These findings suggest that right prefrontal brain areas might be important for reading improvement in dyslexia. As mentioned earlier, the main brain regions responsible for language and reading locate in the left hemisphere of the brain. The involvement of the right hemisphere for readers with dyslexia suggests that some regions located at the right hemisphere of the brain might play certain compensatory roles for those with dyslexia vis-a-vis language and reading. These findings are especially notable for demonstrating the power of neuroimaging measurements in predicting reading gains in dyslexia with higher accuracy than available behavioral measures.

The previously reviewed ERP and fMRI findings on the neural basis of reading and reading difficulties are informative for parents, teachers, practitioners, and educators at least from the following aspects: (1) Reading and reading difficulties are not only evident in behavioral results, but also associate with the neural basis for reading at both structural and functional levels. When a child shows specific and significant problems in reading over time, parents and teachers should not attribute this to their studying attitude problem, that is, assuming that they do not work hard. As brain imaging studies have shown, the brain's activation in those children with dyslexia are atypical, and there are some particular brain regions associated with reading and language dysfunction in dyslexia. (2) Early targeted intervention on language and reading is possible using imaging methods. In particular, children with familial risk for dyslexia should receive early intervention in relation to language and reading ability based on a number of imaging studies' findings that early training in language and reading at early ages can improve children's reading abilities at later ages. (3) With development of technology, some imaging equipment such as portable EEG can be used in classrooms to help teachers monitor students' learning processes and then to understand individual differences in language and reading learning processes.

Further Resources to Learn More About Reading and Reading Difficulties

It is well-established that reading is not only shaped by linguistic and cognitive abilities, but also by social and cultural factors (Aikens & Barbarin, 2008).

According to Bronfenbrenner's (1979) theory, children's development unfolds within multiple settings and in relationships with multiple others. For example, correlational studies have revealed that socioeconomic status (SES), usually measured by parental education level, occupation, and income, is a strong predictor of children's reading development not only in L1 (e.g., Noble, Wolmetz, Ochs, Farah, & Mccandliss, 2006) but also in L2 (e.g., Liu, Chung, & McBride, 2016). For example, Liu and colleagues (2016) found that SES longitudinally explained 3% and 16.7% variance in K3 Chinese word reading and English word reading, respectively, statistically controlling for children's age (Liu et al., 2016). Children from families with higher SES exhibit higher performance in reading and language skills; in contrast, children from families with lower SES are more likely to have troubles in reading and language acquisition and are at risk for reading difficulties (e.g., Aikens, & Barbarin, 2008).

A few neuroscience studies have further contributed to our understanding of how social factors such as SES influence the brain basis of reading and reading difficulties (e.g., Noble et al., 2006). Noble et al. (2006) conducted a fMRI study examining the relations among SES, phonological language skills and reading-related brain activity in children with equivalent phonological skills but diverse socioeconomic backgrounds. They found that in the group with lower SES, children's phonological skill was more strongly associated with left fusiform activation, a brain area supporting rapid visual word recognition, whereas in the group with higher SES, the association between phonological skills and left fusiform was reduced. The findings suggest that SES is a significant factor that modulates the relationship between phonological language skills and reading-related brain activity in the left fusiform and perisylvian regions, which have been found to associate with visual-orthographic processes in reading (e.g., Price & Devlin, 2004). As the authors proposed, among children with fewer resources for literacy support (i.e., lower SES), learning to use the above-listed brain regions during reading tasks may be linked to differences in phonological ability. In contrast, children from families with more literacy resources may reduce the influence of individual differences in phonological abilities. This finding somewhat implies that more literacy support associated with higher SES may influence the development of orthographic processes.

In another fMRI study, Raizada, Richards, Meltzoff, and Kuhl (2008) investigated the relationship between SES, neural activity recorded by fMRI, and a battery of standardized cognitive and linguistic tests in 5-year-old children. Correlational analysis revealed that there was a significant correlation between SES and the degree of hemispheric specialization in the left inferior frontal gyrus (IFG) at the functional level, and at the structural level, marginally significant correlations between SES and grey and whiter matter volumes of the IFG were found. These results highlight the possibility that SES might influence the brain regions of reading and language at both brain anatomical and functional levels. The neuroscience findings on the relationship between social factors and neural activity of reading and language are exciting and promising. On the one hand, these studies further suggest that reading development is also shaped by social factors, to the point that social factors such as SES can modulate the neural basis of reading. On the other hand, neuroscience measurements are effective and direct in uncovering the relation between neural representational competence and performance in behavioral tasks.

Although the preceding reviewed exciting neuroscience findings have advanced our understanding of the neural basis of reading and reading difficulty, there is still a big gap between laboratory research and practice (Seidenberg, 2013). Results of neuroscience research have not been directly and commonly used in practice (Katzir & Pare-Blagoev, 2006), and there has been much resistance to the use of neuroscience approaches in the real world of the classroom (Ansari & Coch, 2006). Teachers, practitioners, and policy makers have not noted the potential influence of neuroscience research on individuals' education (Ansari & Coch, 2006). The public, in particular children's parents, have concerns about safety in using neuroscience methods such as ERP and fMRI on their children despite reassurances that the ERP and fMRI techniques are noninvasive. Moreover, neuroscientists are not necessarily familiar with educational needs in practice.

To bridge the gap between research and practice, conversations between neuroscientists, educators, and teachers are necessary (Ansari & Coch, 2006). First, some training courses with a basic introduction to structural and functional brain development and brain mechanisms subserving reading and reading difficulty should be provided to teachers in order to train teachers to make connections across different sources of evidence and to think about how the neuroscience findings can affect literacy teaching, and then apply empirical findings to their teaching. The existing training programs for teachers are mostly based on behavioral research findings; there are few training courses that are brain evidence based. Second, it is essential for neuroscientists to study classroom teaching environments and educational policies in reality and to integrate teachers' knowledge to understand pedagogical practice. The issues of how cognitive neuroscience informs education and what the best intervention practices are for children with reading difficulties are still unclear thus far. It is a must for neuroscientists to design research paradigms that can meet the requirements of increased compatibility with future applied research. To summarize, collaboration among teachers, educators, and neuroscientists is crucial to build connections between neuroscience research and implementation of research findings.

Acknowledgements

The research leading to these results has received funding from the People Programme (Marie Curie Actions) of the European Union's Seventh Framework Programme (FP7/2007–2013) under REA grant agreement n [609400].

References

Aikens, N. L., & Barbarin, O. (2008). Socioeconomic differences in reading trajectories: The contribution of family, neighborhood, and school contexts. *Journal of Educational Psychology, 100*(2), 235–251.

Ansari, D., & Coch, D. (2006). Bridges over troubled waters: Education and cognitive neuroscience. *Trends in Cognitive Sciences, 10*(4), 146–151.

Baldeweg, T., Richardson, A., Watkins, S., Foale, C., & Gruzelier, J. (1999). Impaired auditory frequency discrimination in dyslexia detected with mismatch evoked potentials. *Annals of Neurology, 45*(4), 495–503.

Bentin, S., Mouchetant-Rostaing, Y., Giard, M. H., Echallier, J. F., & Pernier, J. (1999). ERP manifestations of processing printed words at different psycholinguistic levels: Time course and scalp distribution. *Journal of Cognitive Neuroscience, 11*(3), 235–260.

Bonte, M., Poelmans, H., & Blomert, L. (2007). Deviant neurophysiological responses to phonological regularities in speech in dyslexic children. *Neuropsychologia, 45*(7), 1427–1437.

Brambati, S. M., Termine, C., Ruffino, M., Stella, G., Fazio, F., Cappa, S. F., & Perani, D. (2004). Regional reductions of gray matter volume in familial dyslexia. *Neurology, 63*(4), 742–745.

Breznitz, Z., & Meyler, A. (2003). Speed of lower-level auditory and visual processing as a basic factor in dyslexia: Electrophysiological evidence. *Brain & Language, 85*(2), 166–184.

Briellmann, R. S., Saling, M. M., Connell, A. B., Waites, A. B., Abbott, D. F., & Jackson, G. D. (2004). A high-field functional MRI study of quadri-lingual subjects. *Brain & Language, 89*(3), 531–542.

Bronfenbrenner, U. (1979). *The ecology of human development: Experiments by nature and design.* Cambridge, MA: Harvard University Press.

Brown, W. E., Eliez, S., Menon, V., Rumsey, J. M., White, C. D., & Reiss, A. L. (2001). Preliminary evidence of widespread morphological variations of the brain in dyslexia. *Neurology, 56*(6), 781–783.

Callaway, C., Tueting, P., & Koslow, S. (1978). *Event-related brain potentials and behavior.* New York: Academic.

Catts, H. W., Adlof, S. M., Hogan, T. P., & Weismer, S. E. (2005). Are specific language impairment and dyslexia distinct disorders? *Journal of Speech, Language, and Hearing Research, 48*(6), 1378–1396.

Caylak, E. (2009). Neurobiological approaches on brains of children with dyslexia: Review. *Academic Radiology, 16*(8), 1003–1024. doi:10.1016/j.acra.2009.02.012

Chee, M. W., Soon, C. S., & Lee, H. L. (2003). Common and segregated neuronal networks for different languages revealed using functional magnetic resonance adaptation. *Journal of Cognitive Neuroscience, 15*(1), 85–97.

Chee, M. W., Tan, E. W., & Thiel, T. (1999). Mandarin and English single word processing studied with functional magnetic resonance imaging. *Journal of Neuroscience, 19*(8), 3050–3056.

Chee, M. W., Weekes, B., Lee, K. M., Soon, C. S., Schreiber, A., Hoon, J. J., & Chee, M. (2000). Overlap and dissociation of semantic processing of Chinese characters, English words, and pictures: Evidence from fMRI. *Neuroimage, 12*(4), 392–403.

Chung, K. K., Tong, X., & McBride-Chang, C. (2012). Evidence for a deficit in orthographic structure processing in Chinese developmental dyslexia: An event-related potential study. *Brain Research, 1472*, 20–31.

Critchley, M. (1970). *The dyslexic child.* London: Heinemann Medical.

Deacon, D., Hewitt, S., Yang, C. M., & Nagata, M. (2000). Event-related potential indices of semantic priming using masked and unmasked words: Evidence that the N400 does not reflect a post-lexical process. *Brain Research Cognitive Brain Research, 9*(2), 137–146.

Duara, R., Kushch, A., Grossglenn, K., Barker, W. W., Jallad, B., Pascal, S., & Levin, B. (1991). Neuroanatomic differences between dyslexic and normal readers on magnetic resonance imaging scans. *Archives of Neurology, 48*(4), 410–416.

Eckert, M. (2004). Neuroanatomical markers for dyslexia: A review of dyslexia structural imaging studies. *Neuroscientist, 10*(4), 362–371.

Frenck-Mestre, C., Anton, J. L., Roth, M., Vaid, J., & Viallet, F. (2005). Articulation in early and late bilinguals' two languages: Evidence from functional magnetic resonance imaging. *Neuroreport, 16*(7), 761–765.

Friederici, A. D., Hahne, A., & Mecklinger, A. (1996). Temporal structure of syntactic parsing: Early and late event-related brain potential effects. *J Exp Psychol Learn Mem Cogn, 22*(5), 1219–1248.

Galaburda, A. M., Sherman, G. F., Rosen, G. D., Aboitiz, F., & Geschwind, N. (1985). Developmental dyslexia: Four consecutive patients with cortical anomalies. *Annals of Neurology, 18*(2), 222–233.

Gandour, J., Tong, Y., Talavage, T., Wong, D., Dzemidzic, M., Xu, Y., & Lowe, M. (2007). Neural basis of first and second language processing of sentence-level linguistic prosody. *Hum Brain Mapp, 28*(2), 94–108.

Geschwind, N., & Levitsky, W. (1968). Human brain: Left-right asymmetries in temporal speech region. *Science, 161*(3837), 186–187.

Gomes, H., Ritter, W., Tartter, V. C., Vaughan, H. G., & Rosen, J. J. (1997). Lexical processing of visually and auditorily presented nouns and verbs: Evidence from reaction time and N400 priming data. *Brain Res Cogn Brain Res, 6*(2), 121–134.

Gross, M., Say, T., Kleingers, M., Clahsen, H., & Münte, T. F. (1998). Human brain potentials to violations in morphologically complex Italian words. *Neuroscience Letters, 241*(2–3), 83–86.

Guttorm, T. K., Leppanen, P. H., Richardson, U., & Lyytinen, H. (2001). Event-related potentials and consonant differentiation in newborns with familial risk for dyslexia. *J Learn Disabil, 34*(6), 534–544.

Habib, M. (2000). The neurological basis of developmental dyslexia: An overview and working hypothesis. *Brain, 123*(12), 2373–2399.

Halsband, U., Krause, B. J., Sipila, H., Teras, M., & Laihinen, A. (2002). PET studies on the memory processing of word pairs in bilingual Finnish-English subjects. *Behav Brain Res, 132*(1), 47–57.

Hasegawa, M., Carpenter, P. A., & Just, M. A. (2002). An fMRI study of bilingual sentence comprehension and workload. *Neuroimage, 15*(3), 647–660.

Herbster, A. N., Mintun, M. A., Nebes, R. D., & Becker, J. T. (1997). Regional cerebral blood flow during word and nonword reading. *Human Brain Mapping, 5*(2), 84–92.

Hernandez, A. E., Martinez, A., & Kohnert, K. (2000). In search of the language switch: An fMRI study of picture naming in Spanish-English bilinguals. *Brain & Language, 73*(3), 421–431.

Hillyard, S. A., & Kutas, M. (1983). Electrophysiology of cognitive processing. *Annu Rev Psychol, 34*(1), 33–61.

Hoeft, F., McCandliss, B. D., Black, J. M., Gantman, A., Zakerani, N., Hulme, C., & Gabrieli, J. D. (2011). Neural systems predicting long-term outcome in dyslexia. *Proceedings of the National Academy of Sciences, 108*(1), 361–366.

Hoeft, F., Meyler, A., Hernandez, A., Juel, C., Taylor-Hill, H., Martindale, J. L., & Gabrieli, J. D. E. (2007). Functional and morphometric brain dissociation between dyslexia and reading ability. *Proceedings of the National Academy of Sciences, 104*(10), 4234–4239.

Holcomb, P. J. (1988). Automatic and attentional processing: An event-related brain potential analysis of semantic priming. *Brain & Language, 35*(1), 66–85.

Houdé, O., Rossi, S., Lubin, A., & Joliot, M. (2010). Mapping numerical processing, reading, and executive functions in the developing brain: An fMRI meta-analysis of 52 studies including 842 children. *Developmental Science, 13*(6), 876–885.

Hu, W., Lee, H. L., Zhang, Q., Liu, T., Geng, L. B., Seghier, M. L., . . . Price, C. J. (2010). Developmental dyslexia in Chinese and English populations: Dissociating the effect of dyslexia from language differences. *Brain, 133*(6), 1694–1706.

Huang, H. W., Lee, C. Y., Tsai, J. L., & Tzeng, J. L. (2011). Sublexical ambiguity effect in reading Chinese disyllabic compounds. *Brain & Language, 117*(2), 77–87.

Huttunen-Scott, T., Kaartinen, J., Tolvanen, A., & Lyytinen, H. (2008). Mismatch negativity (MMN) elicited by duration deviations in children with reading disorder, attention deficit or both. *International Journal of Psychophysiology, 69*(1), 69–77.

Illes, J., Francis, W. S., Desmond, J. E., Gabrieli, J. D., Glover, G. H., Poldrack, R., & Wagner, A. D. (1999). Convergent cortical representation of semantic processing in bilinguals. *Brain & Language, 70*(3), 347–363.

Jednorog, K., Marchewka, A., Altarelli, I., Monzalvo Lopez, A. K., van Ermingen-Marbach, M., Grande, M., . . . Ramus, F. (2015). How reliable are gray matter disruptions in specific reading disability across multiple countries and languages? Insights from a large-scale voxel-based morphometry study. *Human Brain Mapping, 36*(5), 1741–1754.

Jenner, A. R., Rosen, G. D., & Galaburda, A. M. (1999). Neuronal asymmetries in primary visual cortex of dyslexic and nondyslexic brains. *Annals of Neurology, 46*(2), 189–196.

Katzir, T., & Pare-Blagoev, J. (2006). Applying cognitive neuroscience research to education: The case of literacy. *Educational Psychologist, 41*(1), 53–74.

Klein, D., Milner, B., Zatorre, R. J., Meyer, E., & Evans, A. C. (1995). The neural substrates underlying word generation: A bilingual functional-imaging study. *Proceedings of the National Academy of Sciences, 92*(7), 2899–2903.

Klein, D., Milner, B., Zatorre, R. J., Zhao, V., & Nikelski, J. (1999). Cerebral organization in bilinguals: A PET study of Chinese-English verb generation. *Neuroreport, 10*(13), 2841–2846.

Klein, D., Watkins, K. E., Zatorre, R. J., & Milner, B. (2006). Word and nonword repetition in bilingual subjects: A PET study. *Human Brain Mapping, 27*(2), 153–161.

Klein, D., Zatorre, R. J., Milner, B., Meyer, E., & Evans, A. C. (1994). Left putaminal activation when speaking a second language: Evidence from PET. *Neuroreport*, 5(17), 2295–2297.

Kronbichler, M., Hutzler, F., Staffen, W., Mair, A., Ladurner, G., & Wimmer, H. (2006). Evidence for a dysfunction of left posterior reading areas in German dyslexic readers. *Neuropsychologia*, 44(10), 1822–1832.

Kronbichler, M., Wimmer, H., Staffen, W., Hutzler, F., Mair, A., & Ladurner, G. (2008). Developmental dyslexia: Gray matter abnormalities in the occipitotemporal cortex. *Human Brain Mapping*, 29(5), 613–625.

Kutas, M., & Hillyard, S. A. (1980). Event-related brain potentials to semantically inappropriate and surprisingly large words. *Biological Psychology*, 11(2), 99–116.

Kutas, M., & Hillyard, S. A. (1984). Event-related brain potentials (ERPs) elicited by novel stimuli during sentence processing. *Ann N Y Acad Sci*, 425(1), 236–241.

Kutas, M., & Hillyard, S. A. (1989). An electrophysiological probe of incidental semantic association. *Journal of Cognitive Neuroscience*, 1(1), 38–49.

Landi, N., & Perfetti, C. A. (2007). An electrophysiological investigation of semantic and phonological processing in skilled and less-skilled comprehenders. *Brain & Language*, 102(1), 30–45.

Liu, D., Chung, K. K., & McBride, C. (2016). The role of SES in Chinese (L1) and English (L2) word reading in Chinese-speaking kindergarteners. *Journal of Research in Reading*, 39(3), 268–291.

Livingstone, M. S., Rosen, G. D., Drislane, F. W., & Galaburda, A. M. (1991). Physiological and anatomical evidence for a magnocellular defect in developmental dyslexia. *Proceedings of the National Academy of Sciences*, 88(18), 7943–7947.

Lovrich, D., Cheng, J. C., & Velting, D. M. (2003). ERP correlates of form and rhyme letter tasks in impaired reading children: A critical evaluation. *Child Neuropsychology: A Journal on Normal & Abnormal Development in Childhood & Adolescence*, 9(3), 159–174.

Lovrich, D., Cheng, J. C., Velting, D. M., & Kazmerski, V. (1997). Auditory ERPs during rhyme and semantic processing: Effects of reading ability in college students. *Journal of Clinical & Experimental Neuropsychology*, 19(3), 313–330.

Lyytinen, P., Eklund, K., & Lyytinen, H. (2005). Language development and literacy skills in late-talking toddlers with and without familial risk for dyslexia. *Annals of Dyslexia*, 55(2), 166–192.

Mahendra, N., Plante, E., Magloire, J., Milman, L., & Trouard, T. P. (2003). fMRI variability and the localization of languages in the bilingual brain. *Neuroreport*, 14(9), 1225–1228.

Maurer, U., Brem, S., Bucher, K., Kranz, F., Benz, R., Steinhausen, H. C., & Brandeis, D. (2007). Impaired tuning of a fast occipito-temporal response for print in dyslexic children learning to read. *Brain: A Journal of Neurology*, 130(12), 3200–3210.

Maurer, U., Brem, S., Kranz, F., Bucher, K., Benz, R., Halder, P., & Brandeis, D. (2006). Coarse neural tuning for print peaks when children learn to read. *Neuroimage*, 33(2), 749–758.

Maurer, U., Bucher, K., Brem, S., & Brandeis, D. (2003). Altered responses to tone and phoneme mismatch in kindergartners at familial dyslexia risk. *Neuroreport*, 14(17), 2245–2250.

Maurer, U., & McCandliss, B. D. (2008). The development of visual expertise for words: The contribution of electrophysiology. In E. L. Grigorenko & A. Naples (Eds.), *Single-word reading: Cognitive, behavioral and biological perspectives*. Mahwah, NJ: Lawrence Erlbaum Associates.

Mayes, S. D., Calhoun, S. L., & Crowell, E. W. (2000). Learning disabilities and ADHD: Overlapping spectrum disorders. *Journal of Learning Disabilities, 33*(5), 417–424.

Meng, X., Sai, X., Wang, C., Wang, J., Sha, S., & Zhou, X. (2005). Auditory and speech processing and reading development in Chinese school children: Behavioural and ERP evidence. *Dyslexia, 11*(4), 292–310.

Meng, X., Tian, X., Jian, J., & Zhou, X. (2007). Orthographic and phonological processing in Chinese dyslexic children: An ERP study on sentence reading. *Brain Research, 1179*(3), 119–130.

Meyler, A., Keller, T. A., Cherkassky, V. L., Lee, D. H., Hoeft, F., Whitfield-Gabrieli, S., & Just, M. A. (2007). Brain activation during sentence comprehension among good and poor readers. *Cerebral Cortex, 17*(12), 2780–2787.

Michel, C. M., Murray, M. M., Lantz, G., Gonzalez, S., Spinelli, L., & Grave, D. P. R. (2004). EEG source imaging. *Clinical Neurophysiology, 115*(10), 2195–2222.

Middleton, F. A., & Strick, P. L. (1997). Cerebellar output channels. *International Review of Neurobiology, 41*, 61–82.

Molfese, D. L. (2000). Predicting dyslexia at 8 years of age using neonatal brain responses. *Brain & Language, 72*(3), 238–245.

Molfese, D. L., & Betz, J. C. (1988). Electrophysiological indices of the early development of lateralization for language and cognition and their implications for predicting later development. In D. L. Molfese & S. J. Segalowitz (Eds.), *The developmental implications of brain lateralization for language and cognitive development* (pp. 171–190). New York: Guilford.

Molfese, D. L., Freeman, R. B., & Palermo, D. S. (1975). The ontogeny of brain lateralization for speech and nonspeech stimuli. *Brain & Language, 2*(3), 356–368.

Molfese, D. L., & Molfese, V. J. (1997). Discrimination of language skills at five years of age using event-related potentials recorded at birth. *Developmental Neuropsychology, 13*(2), 135–156.

Molfese, D. L., Molfese, V. J., & Espy, K. A. (1999). The predictive use of event-related potentials in language development and the treatment of language disorders. *Developmental Neuropsychology, 16*(3), 373–377.

Münte, T. F., Say, T., Clahsen, H., Schiltz, K., & Kutas, M. (1999). Decomposition of morphologically complex words in English: Evidence from event-related brain potentials. *Cognitive Brain Research, 7*(3), 241–253.

Näätänen, R., Paavilainen, P., Rinne, T., & Alho, K. (2007). The mismatch negativity (MMN) in basic research of central auditory processing: A review. *Clinical Neurophysiology Official Journal of the International Federation of Clinical Neurophysiology, 118*(12), 2544–2590.

Nakamura, K., Dehaene, S., Jobert, A., Le, B. D., & Kouider, S. (2005). Subliminal convergence of Kanji and Kana words: Further evidence for functional parcellation of the posterior temporal cortex in visual word perception. *Journal of Cognitive Neuroscience, 17*(6), 954–968.

Noble, K. G., Wolmetz, M. E., Ochs, L. G., Farah, M. J., & McCandliss, B. D. (2006). Brain-behavior relationships in reading acquisition are modulated by socioeconomic factors. *Developmental Science, 9*(6), 642–654.

Paulesu, E., Demonet, J. F., Fazio, F., McCrory, E., Chanoine, V., Brunswick, N., & Frith, U. (2001). Dyslexia: Cultural diversity and biological unity. *Science, 291*(5511), 2165–2167.

Penke, M., Weyerts, H., Gross, M., Zander, E., Münte, T. F., & Clahsen, H. (1997). How the brain processes complex words: An event-related potential study of German verb inflections. *Cognitive Brain Research, 6*(1), 37–52.

Perani, D., Paulesu, E., Galles, N. S., Dupoux, E., Dehaene, S., Bettinardi, V., & Mehler, J. (1998). The bilingual brain: Proficiency and age of acquisition of the second language. *Brain, 121*(10), 1841–1852.

Pratarelli, M. E. (1995). Modulation of semantic processing using word length and complexity: An ERP study. *International Journal of Psychophysiology, 19*(3), 233–246.

Price, C. J., & Devlin, J. T. (2003). The myth of the visual word form area. *Neuroimage, 19*(3), 473–481.

Price, C. J., & Devlin, J. T. (2004). The pro and cons of labelling a left occipitotemporal region: "The visual word form area". *Neuroimage, 22*(1), 477.

Pu, Y., Liu, H. L., Spinks, J. A., Mahankali, S., Xiong, J., Feng, C. M., . . . Gao, J. H. (2001). Cerebral hemodynamic response in Chinese (first) and English (second) language processing revealed by event-related functional MRI. *Magnetic Resonance Imaging, 19*(5), 643–647.

Pugh, K. R., Mencl, W. E., Jenner, A. R., Katz, L., Frost, S. J., Lee, J. R., & Shaywitz, B. A. (2000). Functional neuroimaging studies of reading and reading disability (developmental dyslexia). *Ment Retard Dev Disabil Res Rev, 6*(3), 207–213.

Raizada, R. D., & Kishiyama, M. M. (2010). Effects of socioeconomic status on brain development, and how cognitive neuroscience may contribute to levelling the playing field. *Frontiers in Human Neuroscience, 4*, 3.

Raizada, R. D., Richards, T. L., Meltzoff, A., & Kuhl, P. K. (2008). Socioeconomic status predicts hemispheric specialisation of the left inferior frontal gyrus in young children. *Neuroimage, 40*(3), 1392–1401.

Ramus, F., Altarelli, I., Jednoróg, K., Zhao, J., & di Covella, L. S. (2018). Neuroanatomy of developmental dyslexia: Pitfalls and promise. *Neuroscience & Biobehavioral Reviews, 84*, 434–452.

Richlan, F., Kronbichler, M., & Wimmer, H. (2009). Functional abnormalities in the dyslexic brain: A quantitative meta-analysis of neuroimaging studies. *Human Brain Mapping, 30*(10), 3299–3308.

Rossion, B., Gauthier, I., Goffaux, V., Tarr, M. J., & Crommelinck, M. (2002). Expertise training with novel objects leads to left-lateralized facelike electrophysiological responses. *Psychological Science, 13*(3), 250–257.

Rumsey, J. M., Casanova, M., Mannheim, G. B., Patronas, N., De, V. N., Hamburger, S. D., & Aquino, T. (1996). Corpus callosum morphology, as measured with MRI, in dyslexic men. *Biological Psychiatry, 39*(9), 769–775.

Sarkari, S., Simos, P. G., Fletcher, J. M., Castillo, E. M., Breier, J. I., & Papanicolaou, A. C. (2002). Contributions of magnetic source imaging to the understanding of dyslexia. *Seminars in Pediatric Neurology, 9*(3), 229–238.

Schmahmann, J. D., & Pandya, D. N. (1997). The cerebrocerebellar system. *International Review of Neurobiology, 41*, 31–38.

Schulte-Körne, G., Deimel, W., Bartling, J., & Remschmidt, H. (1998). Auditory processing and dyslexia: Evidence for a specific speech processing deficit. *Neuroreport, 9*(2), 337–340.

Schulte-Körne, G., Deimel, W., Bartling, J., & Remschmidt, H. (2001). Speech perception deficit in dyslexic adults as measured by mismatch negativity (MMN). *International Journal of Psychophysiology Official Journal of the International Organization of Psychophysiology, 40*(1), 77–87.

Seidenberg, M. S. (2013). The science of reading and its educational implications. *Language Learning and Development, 9*(4), 331–360.

Sereno, S. C., & Rayner, K. (2003). Measuring word recognition in reading: Eye movements and event-related potentials. *Trends Cogn Sci, 7*(11), 489–493.

Shaywitz, B. A., Shaywitz, S. E., Pugh, K. R., Mencl, W. E., Fulbright, R. K., Skudlarski, P., . . . Gore, J. C. (2002). Disruption of posterior brain systems for reading in children with developmental dyslexia. *Biological Psychiatry, 52*(2), 101–110.

Shaywitz, S. E., Shaywitz, B. A., Fulbright, R. K., Skudlarski, P., Mencl, W. E., Constable, R. T., . . . Gore, J. C. (2003). Neural systems for compensation and persistence: Young adult outcome of childhood reading disability. *Biological Psychiatry, 54*(1), 25–33.

Silani, G., Frith, U., Demonet, J. F., Fazio, F., Perani, D., Price, C., & Paulesu, E. (2005). Brain abnormalities underlying altered activation in dyslexia: A voxel based morphometry study. *Brain, 128*(10), 2453–2461.

Siok, W. T., Niu, Z., Jin, Z., Perfetti, C. A., & Tan, L. H. (2008). A structural-functional basis for dyslexia in the cortex of Chinese readers. *Proceedings of the National Academy of Sciences, 105*(14), 5561–5565.

Siok, W. T., Perfetti, C. A., Jin, Z., & Tan, L. H. (2004). Biological abnormality of impaired reading is constrained by culture. *Nature, 431*(7004), 71–76.

Tan, L. H., Laird, A. R., Li, K., & Fox, P. T. (2005). Neuroanatomical correlates of phonological processing of Chinese characters and alphabetic words: A meta-analysis. *Human Brain Mapping, 25*(1), 83–91.

Tan, L. H., Spinks, J. A., Feng, C. M., Siok, W. T., Perfetti, C. A., Xiong, J., & Gao, J. H. (2003). Neural systems of second language reading are shaped by native language. *Human Brain Mapping, 18*(3), 158–166.

Tarkiainen, A., Helenius, P., Hansen, P. C., Cornelissen, P. L., & Salmelin, R. (1999). Dynamics of letter string perception in the human occipitotemporal cortex. *Brain, 122*(11), 2119–2132.

Taylor, M. J., & Baldeweg, T. (2002). Application of EEG, ERP and intracranial recordings to the investigation of cognitive functions in children. *Developmental Science, 5*(3), 318–334.

Tong, X., Chung, K. K. H., & McBride, C. (2014). Two-character Chinese compound word processing in Chinese children with and without dyslexia: ERP evidence. *Developmental Neuropsychology, 39*(4), 285–301.

Tong, X., Lo, J. C. M., McBride, C., Ho, C. S. H., Waye, M. M. Y., Chung, K. K. H., . . . Chow, B. W. Y. (2016). Coarse and fine N1 tuning for print in younger and older Chinese children: Orthography, phonology, or semantics driven? *Neuropsychologia, 91*, 109–119.

Turkeltaub, P. E., Gareau, L., Flowers, D. L., Zeffiro, T. A., & Eden, G. F. (2003). Development of neural mechanisms for reading. *Nat Neurosci, 6*(7), 767–773.

WHO. (1994). *The ICD-10 classification of mental and behavioural disorders: Diagnostic criteria for research.* Washington, DC: American Psychiatric Press.

Xue, G., Dong, Q., Jin, Z., Zhang, L., & Wang, Y. (2004). An fMRI study with semantic access in low proficiency second language learners. *Neuroreport, 15*(5), 791–796.

Yokoyama, S., Okamoto, H., Miyamoto, T., Yoshimoto, K., Kim, J., Iwata, K., & Kawashima, R. (2006). Cortical activation in the processing of passive sentences in L1 and L2: An fMRI study. *Neuroimage, 30*(2), 570–579.

6 Reading Acquisition and Developmental Dyslexia

Educational Neuroscience and Phonological Skills

Usha Goswami

Reading acquisition by children is predicted across languages by individual differences in phonological (sound-based) skills. Phonological skills reflect in part children's awareness of the phonological structure of words (Ziegler & Goswami, 2005). Phonological awareness is typically measured using simple oral tasks, such as counting the number of syllables in words. For example, there are two syllables in "wigwam", and three syllables in "radio". Children who show better phonological skills at the syllable level are likely to become better readers (Liberman, Shankweiler, Fischer, & Carter, 1974). Similarly, children can be asked to judge whether words rhyme or not ("cat-hat", *yes*, "cat-cot", *no*). Studies show that children who struggle to make accurate rhyme judgements are more likely to have specific reading difficulties (*developmental dyslexia*; Bradley & Bryant, 1978). The relationship between individual differences in phonological skills as measured by oral tasks like these and literacy acquisition across languages appears to be a causal one. Performance in tasks like syllable counting and rhyme judgement are predictive of reading in both alphabetical languages like English and German (e.g., Frith, Wimmer, & Landerl, 1998), and in non-alphabetical languages like Chinese (e.g., Siok & Fletcher, 2001). Furthermore, children with developmental dyslexia in both alphabetic and non-alphabetic languages show difficulties in phonological tasks.

More recently, phonological awareness of syllable stress patterns has also been shown to play a role in explaining individual differences in reading acquisition (Whalley & Hansen, 2006; Wood & Terrell, 1998). When whole phrases rather than single words are the unit of analysis, some syllables will receive greater emphasis or *stress* than others, as in "JACK and JILL went UP the HILL". Children with dyslexia have very poor awareness of relative stress patterns in oral tasks (also termed awareness of "prosodic structure"; Goswami, Gerson, & Astruc, 2010; Goswami et al., 2013). Recent research in auditory neuroscience is beginning to explain why this may be the case.

The different levels of phonological awareness demonstrated in behavioural studies with children can be conceptualised as a linguistic *hierarchy*, discussed in the following. In the linguistic hierarchy, awareness of larger phonological units, like stressed syllables and syllables, emerges prior to awareness of smaller phonological units, like rhymes. Children with developmental dyslexia show reduced awareness of phonology at all levels in the hierarchy. Recent studies in auditory neuroscience have revealed that the linguistic hierarchy is mirrored by an *oscillatory* hierarchy in the brain. Networks of brain cells send signals in the brain by oscillating or alternating from an excited state, during which electrical potentials are generated, to an inhibited state, during which no electrical potentials are generated. This alternation from excitation to inhibition produces an oscillation in electrical rhythm—a brain rhythm or "brain wave". During speech encoding, different brain electrical rhythms re-calibrate their activity until they are in time or in synchrony with rhythmic energy patterns in the speech signal (sound waves). The accuracy of this neural alignment between brain waves and sound waves (called neural "entrainment") governs speech intelligibility. As will be described in this chapter, new brain research suggests that children with good phonological skills encode speech more accurately via this oscillatory process. Children with developmental dyslexia, on the other hand, show atypical oscillatory entrainment to speech. Their brain response is "out of time".

The structure of this chapter will be as follows. I will first give a flavour of the past three decades of behavioural research that documents the importance of phonological skills for learning to read. I will then discuss the linguistic structure of phonological skills, and explain how to model the speech signal in terms of amplitude (~intensity) patterns. This amplitude-based modelling will then be applied to children's nursery rhymes, to show why this particular way of modelling speech is important for children's phonological development. I will next explain how the brain encodes amplitude patterns in speech by using neuroelectric oscillations, systematic temporal variation in neural firing patterns. This is exciting new work, showing the mechanism whereby human speech becomes intelligible. In the final parts of the chapter, I will explain how the dyslexic brain does poorly in perceiving amplitude information, and how neural oscillatory mechanisms are atypical in dyslexia. I will then consider new avenues for remediation in light of this neural/mechanistic knowledge.

Phonological Skills and Learning to Read

Since Goswami and Bryant (1990) reviewed the evidence regarding the importance of children's phonological skills for learning to read, it has been recognised that a child's phonological system is already structured prior to reading development. This structure reflects knowledge about syllables, onsets and rimes. The onset-rime division of the syllable comes from linguistic terminology, and refers to the fact that any syllable can be divided at the vowel into its "onset" and "rime" constituents (e.g., "f—ate", "tr—ait", "str—aight"). Words with more than one syllable, like "carpet", will have more than one rime, as in "c—ar" "p—et". Phonological skills at these larger-unit or 'large grain' sizes have been found in pre-reading children in every language so far studied (Ziegler & Goswami, 2005).

To become an efficient reader, children learning to read in alphabetic orthographies have to develop a further level of phonological awareness, awareness of the smaller sound elements in words that correspond to alphabetic letters—"phonemes". Phoneme awareness appears to develop largely as a consequence of reading instruction, across languages. Adults who have never learned to read, and pre-reading children, perform very poorly on phonological awareness tasks that measure phoneme knowledge. An example is phoneme isolation tasks ("What is the second sound in the word 'train'?"). Children with developmental dyslexia perform poorly in phonological tasks at all levels—syllable, rhyme or phoneme.

Children with dyslexia also have poor *prosodic* awareness. They find it difficult to reflect on the quasi-rhythmic patterning of stressed and unstressed syllables that characterises every language, and that typically forms the basis for poetry and song. For example, English nursery rhymes are frequently metrically regular poems, with nursery rhymes like "Jack and Jill went up the hill" and "Pussycat, Pussycat, where have you been" providing examples of alternating stress patterns. Indeed, language acquisition by infants is thought to *begin* with an implicit awareness of stress patterning (Mehler et al., 1988). For English, for example, stressed syllables usually denote the beginning of words, as in MUMMy, DADDy or BAby. Accordingly, if infants learn the stress patterning of their language, it can help them to parse the continuous speech stream into words.

The Linguistic Hierarchy

Linguistically, we can think of these different levels of phonology as forming a hierarchy, with larger units at the top of the hierarchy. This is depicted schematically in Figure 6.1. Phonemes, the smallest units of sound in words, could represent the end state of the hierarchy, the "goal" for successful literacy tuition. Note that there is some overlap between onset-rime skills and phoneme-level skills. For the first syllable in "carpet", in Southern British accents the 'vowel r' phoneme means that the onset-rime division of the syllable matches its segmentation into two individual phonemes. Indeed, in languages with predominantly consonant-vowel (CV) syllable structures, onsets and rimes are usually single phonemes. In such languages, like Italian or Spanish, the onset-rime division of the syllable also yields the constituent phonemes (English examples are "s-ea", "z-oo", "t-oe"; these words all contain two phonemes).

Research has suggested that the ability to recognise, identify and manipulate phonological units like onsets, rimes, syllables and phonemes appears to reflect a single continuum of ability in children. In a series of comprehensive studies, Anthony et al. (2002, 2003) measured phonological skills in over 1000 American preschool children aged between 2 and 6 years. In order to equate cognitive difficulty across the different phonological "grain sizes" being assessed, they used blending and deletion tasks to measure phonological awareness at each level. For example, children might be asked to blend the

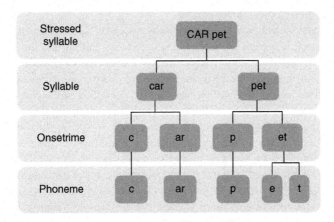

Figure 6.1 The Linguistic Hierarchy Depicted Schematically for the Spoken Word "Carpet".

syllables "sis" and "ter" to make "sister", the onset-rime units "h" and "at" to make "hat", or the phonemes "f"—"ah"—"s"—"t" together to make "fast". Anthony et al. reported that the children generally mastered word-level skills before they mastered syllable-level skills, mastered syllable-level skills before they mastered onset/rime skills, and mastered onset/rime-level skills before they mastered phoneme-level skills. The development of phonological awareness in children thus appeared to follow the hierarchical structure depicted in Figure 6.1, with awareness of larger grain sizes developmentally preceding the awareness of smaller grain sizes. Accordingly, preschool children's phonological skills will depend in part on the richness and variety of their oral language experiences. High-quality oral learning environments at home and preschool will have an enriching effect on the development of phonological skills.

Individual differences in phonological skills do not depend only on enrichment however, as there are intrinsic differences between children in their ability to reflect upon and manipulate phonological units in words. One important source of individual differences lies in children's acoustic processing skills. As pre-literate phonology comprises awareness of syllable stress, syllables and rhymes, the acoustic correlates of these larger-grain phonological units could be an important source of individual differences. Recent research in auditory neuroscience suggests that this is indeed the case.

Amplitude Modulation and the Amplitude Envelope of Speech

In the past decade, work in adult auditory neuroscience has revealed the importance of amplitude modulations (variations in signal intensity) and related "rise times" (times to peak intensity) for the neural processing of speech. This work has turned out to have important consequences for our understanding of children's phonological development.

Amplitude modulation had previously received little attention in the developmental language literature. In simple terms, amplitude modulation is variations in loudness, which have not been expected to govern individual differences in language acquisition. However, as someone is speaking there are variations in loudness *within* the phrases that they are saying, and it is these internal variations in loudness that hold important clues to phonological structure. When someone opens their mouth to speak, they are causing air molecules to move—they are producing a "sound wave". The sound wave of speech can be thought of as energy moving through the air. When there is a lot of energy (loud sound), the signal has greater amplitude than when there is relatively low energy (soft sound). However, as the speaker opens and closes the vocal tract, there are additional naturally varying changes or *modulations* in the energy in the overall signal, however loudly or softly overall that particular signal is being produced. These modulations are caused by simultaneous movements of the vocal folds, the tongue and the vocal tract. These modulations in loudness (amplitude modulations) are broadly experienced as speech rhythm. Even when you are listening to someone speaking in an unknown foreign language, you can hear loudness patterning that sounds quasi-rhythmic. It makes evolutionary sense that the brain has developed to be tuned to encode these variations in amplitude modulation or speech energy as optimally as possible. The simultaneous movements of the vocal folds, tongue and vocal tract together produce quasi-rhythmic variations in amplitude at a number of different temporal rates simultaneously, within the continuous experienced stream of speech. These different patterns of amplitude modulation can be thought of as embedded in an overall "envelope" of sound, which reaches the ear and then excites different parts of the cochlea, the nerve endings in the inner ear. It is the changes or modulations in this overall "amplitude envelope" that is primarily experienced by the listener as speech rhythm (Greenberg, 2006).

Accurate perception of the amplitude envelope turns out to be very important for speech intelligibility. Studies with adults have shown that the brain can recognise speech on the basis of the amplitude and temporal cues in the envelope alone (Shannon et al., 1995). This is also how cochlear implants for deaf people work. The implants reproduce the amplitude envelope in a few of the frequency channels in natural speech, via sophisticated electronics. The energy profile of the amplitude envelope in speech varies relatively slowly in time, and most of the amplitude fluctuations in the envelope reflect the rising and falling "arcs" of energy that coincide with syllable production (Greenberg, 2006). As each syllable is produced by a speaker, peak energy is reached as the vowel is produced, and then falls again. The rising phase of each energy "arc" corresponds to amplitude "rise time", the time taken to reach maximal energy or peak amplitude in a modulation. Sensitivity to these amplitude rise times is important for the neural encoding of speech (discussed further in the following). For child phonology, we can think of the patterns of amplitude modulation that are produced by a speaker as providing important statistical information about language, information potentially relevant to phonological development. The easiest way to think about this is through the amplitude modulation-driven rhythm patterns in children's nursery rhymes.

Children's Nursery Rhymes and the Amplitude Modulation Hierarchy

Nursery rhymes and rhyming games are a ubiquitous part of childhood (Opie & Opie, 1987). As well as being fun, these games and nursery routines play a key role in children's development of phonological awareness (Bryant, Bradley, Maclean, & Crossland, 1989). Recently, a novel acoustic reason for this has been uncovered. Statistical patterns of amplitude modulation in the speech envelope can be used by the brain to compute speech rhythm, and nursery rhymes provide optimal examples of these statistical patterns. In fact, the amplitude modulation structure of children's nursery rhymes holds acoustic statistical clues to phonological units of many different grain sizes. This has been discovered by modelling the amplitude modulation structure of English nursery rhymes (Leong & Goswami, 2015).

Leong and Goswami capitalised on modelling work exploring the amplitude modulation structure of environmental sounds like rain and wind, carried out by Turner (2010). Turner had shown that these natural sounds were characterised by what he termed amplitude modulation "cascades". Rather than being unstructured, a sound like rain has rhythmic patterning because of loudness patterns that are correlated over long time scales and across multiple different temporal rates. The loudness patterns are cascade-like because there are statistical dependencies between different temporal rates. In effect, rain or wind contains *nested hierarchies* of amplitude modulations, with slower rates governing faster rates. Leong and Goswami (2015) applied Turner's approach to the speech signal. As many languages use special rhythmic speech registers with young children, they hypothesised that rhythmic speech may contain particularly strong cascade-like patterning of amplitude modulations.

English nursery rhymes typically have simple metrical structures, with clear rhythmic patterns based on the alternation of stressed (or strong) and unstressed (or weak) syllables, as for example in the English nursery rhyme "DOC-tor FOS-ter WENT to GLOU-cester IN a SHOWer of RAIN". English "tongue twisters" are also rhythmically patterned, for example "PEter PIper PICKED a PECK of PICKled PEPPers". Leong and Goswami (2015) modelled this rhythmic patterning in children's linguistic routines in terms of amplitude modulations. They began by treating the speech signal in the same way as it is filtered by the cochlea in the human ear, and then looked for statistical patterns in the outputs of these filters. The basis for the modelling was 44 English nursery rhymes as spoken by early years teachers at a natural pace. The modelling showed that the speech energy in the nursery rhymes was clustered into three bands of different temporal rates, a very slow band (amplitude modulations centred on 2 Hz, or two modulations per second), a slow band (amplitude modulations centred on 5 Hz, five modulations per second), and a faster band (amplitude modulations centred on 20 Hz). This last band was fairly wide (12–40 Hz). These temporal rates were nested inside each other, so that the timing of the fluctuations at ~2 Hz determined the timing of the fluctuations at ~5 Hz, and the timing of the fluctuations at ~5 Hz in turn determined the timing of the faster fluctuations at ~20 Hz. The output of Leong and Goswami's modelling is depicted in Figure 6.2 for the nursery rhyme sentence "Doctor Foster went to Gloucester".

The dominance of red colour amplitude modulations in Figure 6.2 shows that the rhythmic changes carried by low frequency portions of the speech signal (portions lower in pitch, < ~700 Hz) are particularly salient clues to phonological structure. Interestingly, the modelling also showed that these lower-frequency portions of the speech signal were produced with the largest degree of temporal similarity by the different speakers participating in the study. As can be seen in Figure 6.2, the largest peaks in amplitude modulation are correlated with the occurrence of the *stressed* syllables, like DOC in "doctor" and FOS in "Foster". Smaller peaks are also visible, which approximately correspond to each syllable. When a peak in modulation (energy) at the syllable rate coincides with a peak in modulation at the slower stressed syllable rate, a strong syllable is heard. When a peak in modulation at the syllable rate coincides with a trough in modulation at the slower stressed syllable rate, a weaker syllable is heard. This means that a unique acoustic statistic, the *phase alignment* (rhythmic synchronicity) of the very slow and slow rates of amplitude modulation in speech gives the rhythmic patterning of a phrase like "Doctor Foster went to Gloucester".

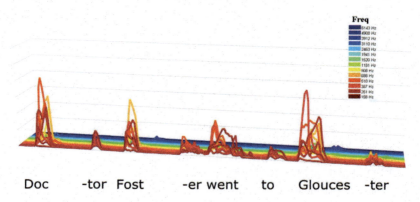

Figure 6.2 Schematic Depiction of the Amplitude Modulations Over Time in the Nursery Rhyme Phrase "Doctor Foster went to Gloucester". The different colours represent the different frequencies in speech and the time frame is about 2 seconds.

Source: Figure by Sheila Flanagan.

The faster amplitude modulations are more difficult to see in Figure 6.2, but they are also statistically important. The faster amplitude modulations turned out to correspond to the occurrence of the onset phonemes in each syllable, such as the "d" in "doc" and the "f" in "Fos". Indeed, all three patterns of amplitude modulation turned out to hold important statistical clues to phonological units. When Leong and Goswami (2015) applied the model to new nursery rhymes, the model was able to detect the stressed syllables, syllables and onset-rime units in the new speech material quite successfully. For nursery rhymes spoken to a metronome beat, hence with perfect rhythmic timing, the model identified 95% of stressed syllables accurately, 98% of syllables accurately, and 91% of the onset-rime units accurately. For nursery rhymes spoken freely, the model identified 72% of stressed syllables accurately, 82% of syllables accurately, and 78% of the onset-rime units accurately. The performance of the model suggests that the acoustic structure of the amplitude envelope of rhythmic child-directed speech carries important statistical information for phonological development. If encoded accurately by the brain, these acoustic statistics would yield the linguistic hierarchy over 90% of the time for rhythmically produced speech.

In principle, therefore, nested patterns of loudness (nested amplitude modulations) in rhythmic child-directed speech provide sufficient acoustic information for the automatic neural segmentation of phonological units of different grain sizes (stressed syllables, syllables, onset-rime units). This is depicted schematically in Figure 6.3 (see the AM rate column). The slowest band of amplitude modulations, centred on ~2 Hz, provides information relevant to identifying stressed syllables. The next slowest band of amplitude modulations, centred on ~5 Hz, provides information relevant to identifying syllables. Together, these two bands of amplitude modulation can be used to identify the rhythm pattern of a phrase, for example whether it follows a trochaic

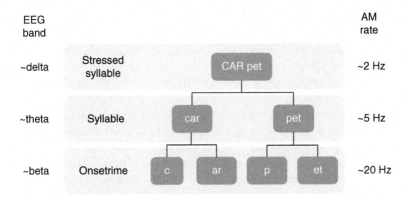

Figure 6.3 The Linguistic Hierarchy for "Carpet" With Associated Bands of Neuro-electric Oscillations Shown on the Left-hand Side and Associated Bands of Amplitude Modulations Shown on the Right-hand Side.

rhythm, with strong and weak syllables alternating ("Doctor Foster went to Gloucester"), or an iambic rhythm, with weak and strong syllables alternating ("As I was going to St Ives"). The faster band of amplitude modulations, centred on ~20 Hz, provides information relevant to identifying the onset-rime division of the syllable (hence for CV syllables, this band of AM could also identify the constituent phonemes). As nursery rhymes are frequently sung rather than spoken, they are automatically timed to an external beat—the beat of the music. This means that sung nursery rhymes are providing reliable amplitude-modulation driven acoustic clues to over 90% of the larger phonological units in the speech that the children are hearing: stressed syllables, syllables and onset-rimes. The linguistic routines of the nursery hence provide optimal acoustic statistical input for children's phonological development.

The Oscillatory Hierarchy

How does the brain encode these acoustic statistics? Auditory neuroscience research shows that the patterns of amplitude modulation nested in the amplitude envelope of speech are extracted automatically by the brain, in a process called oscillatory *entrainment*. Oscillations are essentially "brain waves"—the variability in cell electrical excitability that occurs naturally in the brain, because individual brain cells are either actively firing an electrical pulse (excitation) or recovering from firing a pulse (inhibition). Neurons are arranged in large networks in the brain, and so an entire network will in effect be oscillating or alternating rhythmically between excitation and inhibition. Studies investigating neural speech encoding by adults reveal that these neuroelectric oscillations in cell networks in auditory cortex have four preferred temporal rates (Giraud & Poeppel, 2012, Poeppel, 2014, for recent summaries). The cell networks are naturally active at the speech-relevant rates of *delta* (~1–3 Hz), *theta* (~4–8 Hz), *beta* (~15–30 Hz), and *low gamma* (~30–50 Hz). These labels of delta, theta etc. have long been used to describe neuro-electric oscillations, as these temporal rates of oscillation (plus some others, such as alpha, ~8–12 Hz) are found throughout the brain. Brain waves at these different temporal rates can be observed even when there is no stimulus to encode, for example during sleep. Hence regarding the speech signal, the brain's auditory cortex is naturally fluctuating in excitability at the same timescales identified by the nursery rhyme modelling described—delta, theta, beta and low gamma.

Recent adult neuroimaging studies (Giraud & Poeppel, 2012, for review) have shown how oscillations at the rates of *delta* (fluctuations that occur approximately twice a second, or 2 Hz), *theta* (fluctuations that occur approximately 5 times a second, 5 Hz) and *beta/low gamma* (faster fluctuations) work together to encode the speech signal. The oscillations function both in parallel and in an integrated information hierarchy. As speech enters the brain via the ear, each cell network adjusts the timing of its naturally occurring peaks and troughs in electrical excitability to align with the peaks and troughs in amplitude modulations (energy fluctuations) present in the speech signal.

The cell networks adjust their activity on the basis of the *rise times* of the different amplitude modulations. This is an automatic process, driven by the physical characteristics of the incoming signal, such as its amplitude envelope structure.

For example, as discussed earlier, the "energy arc" of the amplitude modulations associated with the production of each syllable will rise until the vowel is pronounced, and then fall again. Most speakers produce around five syllables a second, and the *rise time* in amplitude up to the vowel provides an acoustic clue to this (*theta*) rate of amplitude modulation. So the amplitude rise times of syllables are used by the brain to re-set the activity of theta cell networks, which are naturally oscillating with a centre frequency of ~5 Hz. This process of alignment, called "phase re-setting" of the cell networks, enables the oscillations to track the amplitude modulations at the syllable rate in speech. We can think of this as the brain using amplitude rise times to discover the rate of incoming information, and then re-setting the activity of its cell networks to align their timing to be *in synchrony* with this incoming information. This process of "phase alignment" enables the brain cells to align their activity to be in synchrony or "in phase" with the amplitude modulations nested in speech (see Giraud & Poeppel, 2012, for a full review).

The same process of phase alignment is happening simultaneously in all the cell networks in auditory cortex, both those oscillating relatively slowly (e.g., delta networks) and those oscillating quickly (e.g., gamma networks). The multi-time information from the different cell networks is then automatically bound together to yield the perception of speech as a seamless single input. Neurally, this binding process is accomplished by an information hierarchy. Neuroimaging studies with adults show that delta phase governs theta phase, and that theta phase governs gamma power (Gross et al., 2013). In other words, the timing of the slowest-oscillating cell network (delta) determines the relative timing of the next slowest-oscillating cell network (theta), and the timing of the theta network determines how strong the firing is in the fastest network (gamma). There is also "motor prediction" of speech, with neural coupling of delta-rate activity in auditory cortex with beta-rate activity in motor cortex (motor cortex is active during movement or when we imagine moving). Here delta phase (timing) governs beta power (firing strength, see Arnal, Doelling, & Poeppel, 2014). In these multiple ways, the brain uses timing information to form a rich representation of the speech signal, encoding information from multiple modalities (auditory, motor and visual) and at multiple time scales simultaneously. When this multi-time and multi-domain process of phase alignment or *phase entrainment* is accurate, the speech signal becomes intelligible.

We can also think about this complex neural process in terms of evolution. As might be expected, the brain has evolved to encode energy at the same timescales provided by the speech signal. Speech is dependent on our physiology, for example the length of our vocal tracts and the size of our tongues. These parts of our body enable us to speak, and thereby determine the characteristics of the sound waves that we are able to produce. The cells in the brain (auditory neurons), operating in large networks, have evolved to encode the characteristics of these sound waves as optimally as possible. Optimal encoding entails taking account of the multi-modal nature of speech (auditory, visual, motor). Automatic neural encoding of the speech signal at these different oscillatory rates also provides a basis for parsing the continuous speech signal into linguistically-relevant—phonological—units (also depicted in Figure 6.3, see EEG band column). Delta oscillations provide a basis for parsing syllable stress patterns, theta oscillations provide a basis for parsing syllables, delta-theta phase alignment enables the rhythm pattern of an utterance (strong and weak syllables) to be determined, and beta oscillations provide a basis for parsing onset-rime units (see Ghitza & Greenberg, 2009; Giraud & Poeppel, 2012). The linguistic hierarchy is preserved neurally because the neuroelectric oscillations are also temporally nested, with a hierarchy of information encoded over multiple timescales (multi-time resolution models of speech processing, Poeppel, 2003; Greenberg, 2006). Acoustically, amplitude rise times specify the rates of change of energy in the speech signal, and govern successful oscillatory entrainment. Accurate discrimination of rise times can be shown experimentally to support the temporal alignment of different oscillatory rhythms with different patterns of amplitude modulation in the speech signal (Doelling, Arnal, Ghitza, & Poeppel, 2014).

At the time of writing, the neural mechanisms underpinning the motor prediction of speech have not been described in similar detail to the mechanisms underpinning auditory entrainment. Nevertheless, speech rhythm is likely to play a central role in motor encoding and motor prediction also, because when we deliberately speak rhythmically, we are timing our motor production of the rise times of syllables (Scott, 1998). As children's phonological representations for speech develop in part from their experience in making speech sounds, individual differences in rhythmic timing in the motor domain may also be important regarding developmental language disorders. Nevertheless, the neural discoveries in the auditory realm already suggest at least two important factors regarding children's phonological development. One is that individual differences in discriminating amplitude envelope rise times may have consequences for the development of phonological awareness. The second is that individual differences in the accuracy of oscillatory phase entrainment may also have consequences for the development of phonological awareness. Both rise time discrimination and oscillatory phase entrainment turn out to be atypical in children with developmental dyslexia, and children with dyslexia indeed have poor phonological skills. We will turn to the evidence regarding atypical development in a later section. First, we will consider how the amplitude modulation structure of natural language may underpin the efficiency of responding in the different oral tasks used to measure phonological awareness in typically developing children.

The Amplitude Modulation Hierarchy and Phonological Awareness Tasks

As noted earlier, acoustic modelling of the speech signal has shown that a unique acoustic statistic, the phase alignment of the very slow (~delta) and slow (~theta) rates of amplitude modulation provides information specifying the prosodic patterning of a phrase like "Doctor Foster went to Gloucester", in which strong and weak syllables alternate. This was discovered in part by experiments with adult listeners, using nursery rhymes that had been filtered to remove phonetic content. In these studies, nursery rhymes had to be iden- tified on the basis of their rhythm patterns alone. Leong, Stone, Turner, and Goswami (2014) found that while delta-rate amplitude modulations indicated the presence of prosodic stress, they did not specify its syllabic location. Mean- while, theta-rate amplitude modulations indicated the number and location of syllables, but not their prosodic status. When considered together, however, the *relative alignment* or *phase alignment* of these slow rates of amplitude modu- lation revealed the syllable stress patterning of each utterance. Accordingly, it is plausible that automatic entrainment of delta and theta cell networks in the brain and the accuracy of their phase alignment provides a sensory/neural underpinning for children's development of prosodic awareness.

Single word phonological awareness tasks can also be analysed in terms of their amplitude modulation structure. Regarding rhyme awareness, one task that has been used widely across languages is the rhyme oddity task (Bradley & Bryant, 1978). In the rhyme oddity task, children are asked to listen to triplets of words such as "good, wood, book" and "nurse, verse, worth", and identify the non-rhyming word ("book", "worth"). Leong and Goswami (2017) ana- lysed the amplitude modulation structure of pairs of words that rhymed in the oddity task, and compared their amplitude modulation structure to pairs of words that did not rhyme. So for example, the amplitude modulation structure of the pair "good-wood" was compared to the amplitude modulation structure of the pair "good-book", and the amplitude modulation structure of the pair "nurse-verse" was compared to the amplitude modulation structure of the pair "nurse-worth". Our approach was to apply the model that we had derived from English nursery rhymes (Leong & Goswami, 2015), which was based on nursery rhyme phrases.

As will be recalled, this modelling had shown that the speech energy in child-directed speech was clustered into three bands of energy varying at dif- ferent temporal rates, amplitude modulations in a very slow band (~2 Hz, delta; labelled Stress AM in the figure), amplitude modulations in a slow band (~5 Hz, theta; labelled Syllable AM in the figure), and amplitude modulations in a faster band (~20 Hz, spanning beta/low gamma; labelled Phoneme AM in the figure). For the oddity task, we accordingly estimated the acoustic similar- ity of the temporal structure of pairs of words by using two different mathemat- ical metrics for estimating informational similarity, mutual information and magnitude squared coherence. Describing these methods is beyond the scope of this chapter, but both metrics gave the same results, which are depicted schematically in Figure 6.4. The significant acoustic correlate of rhyme was *delta phase*—the temporal alignment of the amplitude modulations in each word in a rhyming pair carried by the slowest band, centred on 2 Hz. When two words had similar delta phase, they were perceived as rhyming. As the figure shows, the shape of the modulation (the shapes of the coloured bands) across the spectral range of speech is more similar for the words "nurse" and "verse" for this slowest temporal band. When two words differed in delta phase, they were perceived as non-rhyming. This can also be seen in the figure. The shape of the modulation (the shapes of the coloured bands) across the spectral range of speech for the delta band is less similar for the words "nurse" and "worth". Furthermore, when behavioural data from the rhyme oddity task were analysed (data collected from 101 children with and without dyslexia), the only significant predictor of children's errors was the acoustic information given by amplitude modulations in the delta band across the spectral (~pitch) range of speech—the slowest fluctuations in loudness in the speech signal. These data suggest that the accuracy of entrainment of delta cell networks provides a neural underpinning for the development of rhyme awareness by children.

Single word tasks are also used to measure phoneme awareness. One of the most frequent tasks used across languages has been phoneme deletion. In phoneme deletion tasks, the child is presented orally with a word or a nonword, is given a sound to remove, and is asked for the response. For example, the child might be asked "say glamp without the 'g'", requiring the response "lamp",

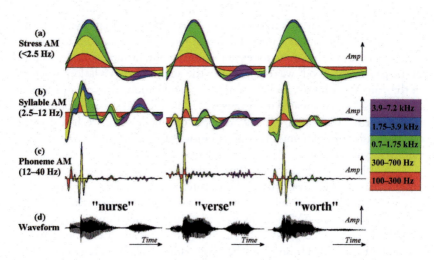

Figure 6.4 Schematic Depiction of the Amplitude Modulation Patterns in the Words "Nurse, Verse, Worth" Over Time. The colours show the different frequencies in speech grouped into five bands.

Source: Figure by Vicky Leong.

or "say hift without the 'f' ", requiring the response "hit". Flanagan and Goswami (2018) modelled the amplitude modulation structure of the items in such phoneme deletion tasks and their correct responses. They applied the model of Leong and Goswami (2015), computing the amplitude modulations for each nonword or word (e.g., "hift", "hit") in the three temporal rate bands (delta, theta, beta/low gamma). They then computed the degree of phase synchronisation between the pairs of bands (delta-theta and theta-beta/low gamma). The analyses showed that the only acoustic measure that changed consistently when a phoneme was deleted from an item was the magnitude of delta-theta phase synchronisation. The magnitude of the synchronisation between very slow (~2 Hz) and slow (~5 Hz) bands of amplitude modulation got systematically larger following phoneme deletion. These data suggest that the automatic entrainment of delta and theta cell networks and the accuracy of their phase alignment within words provides a neural underpinning for successful phoneme awareness.

This result regarding phonemes was unexpected, as multi-time resolution models of speech processing have assumed that faster modulations, especially gamma-rate modulations, are the key acoustic guide to phonemic information. In our modelling, it was changes in the phase alignment of *slower* modulations that was systematically related to phoneme deletion. Nevertheless, we (Flanagan & Goswami, 2018) got the same result when we analysed the plural elicitation task (Berko, 1958). This is a morphological awareness task, in which children are asked to generate the plural forms of nonword items (as in "wug-wugs" and "lun-luns"). The plural elicitation task in this form can be thought of as phoneme addition instead of phoneme deletion. When we analysed the items in this task by modelling the amplitude modulation structure of singular ("wug") and then plural ("wugs") forms, we found that the only acoustic statistic that changed consistently was again the magnitude of delta-theta phase synchronisation. Hence the phase synchronisation or temporal alignment of the two slowest bands of amplitude modulations in speech provides important acoustic information regarding phonemes when considering single words. To check the reliability of this counter-intuitive finding, the amplitude modulation structure of other phoneme awareness tasks should also be modelled, ideally across languages.

Amplitude Rise Times and Phonological Awareness in Developmental Dyslexia

This novel amplitude modulation perspective on phonological awareness, supported by recent neuroimaging data, suggests a number of important factors for children's phonological development. Firstly, in order to develop a mental lexicon of word forms that is phonologically well-structured, children need good amplitude rise time discrimination skills. This is because the brain uses amplitude rise times for the automatic phase-resetting of the cell networks that encode the different patterns of amplitude modulation in the speech signal. Secondly, children's brains need to be entraining *accurately* to these different patterns of amplitude modulation in speech. As the brain uses division of labour, with cell networks that oscillate at the delta rate (~2 Hz) entraining to the slowest amplitude modulations governing stress patterning, cell networks that oscillate at the theta rate (~5 Hz) entraining to the syllable-rate amplitude modulations, and cell networks that oscillate at the beta/low gamma rates (~20 Hz) contributing to the identification of the onset-rime division of syllables, inaccurate entrainment at *any one* of these temporal rates would lead to atypical speech perception. For example, even if only one temporal rate showed inaccurate entrainment, this poorly specified information would automatically bind together with better-specified information at other temporal rates to give the overall speech percept. This percept would thus be of lower informational quality than that created by a brain in which all cell networks were entraining optimally (the phonological representations of speech created by a brain with atypical entrainment would be "degraded" or "poorly specified", see Snowling, 2000). During the past decade, a series of studies of children with developmental dyslexia learning different languages have shown impaired discrimination of amplitude envelope rise times in dyslexia. These acoustic difficulties in rise time discrimination may be expected to contribute to the poor phonological development typically exhibited by children with dyslexia.

Acoustic sensitivity in children can be measured by using psychoacoustic threshold estimation tasks. These are listening tasks that measure the "just noticeable difference" (or *threshold* for noticing a difference) between two simple sounds. For example, one sound might have a higher pitch than another (frequency discrimination), or one sound might be longer than another (duration discrimination). Children with dyslexia consistently show impairments in psychoacoustic threshold estimation tasks measuring amplitude envelope rise times, and they seem to have particular problems with slower rise times (Richardson, Thomson, Scott, & Goswami, 2004, Stefanics et al., 2011). This acoustic insensitivity to amplitude rise time has been shown in many languages—English, Chinese, Hungarian, Finnish, Dutch, Spanish and French (see Goswami, 2015, for a recent summary). Furthermore, the rise time difficulties in amplitude envelope onset discrimination have been correlated with phonological difficulties in these different languages. For example, one study found that poor rise time discrimination was correlated with poor rhyme awareness in English, with poor tone awareness in Chinese, and with poor phoneme awareness in Spanish (Goswami et al., 2011).

In fact, behavioural studies with English children have found that individual differences in rise time perception are related to individual differences in a range of rhythmic and prosodic tasks. Regarding speech rhythm and prosody, we already know that the amplitude envelope of speech carries perceptual information about speech rhythm and prosodic structure. To measure sensitivity to prosodic structure in children with dyslexia, we can use oral tasks in which all syllables in an utterance are replaced by the single syllable "dee", either stressed ("DEE") or unstressed ("dee"; Whalley & Hansen 2006). In this "DeeDee" task, most of the phonetic information in an utterance is removed while the stress and rhythm patterns of the original words and phrases are retained. Goswami et al. (2010) created novel DeeDee measures for children with dyslexia in a picture recognition task, based on celebrity names (e.g., *David Beckham*) and film and book titles (e.g., *Harry Potter*). In their task, the child was shown a picture whose name was 'spoken in DeeDees' (for example, "Harry Potter" would be "DEEdeeDEEdee"). The name hence retained the metrical phrasal-level structure of the original utterances, but the phonetic information distinguishing each word was removed. In a variation of the DeeDee task, this phrasal-level information was also removed, by utilising speech tokens synthesised by a computer, "DEE" and "dee". This served to emphasise syllable stress only (strong or weak). The selected film and book titles were then created by combining the synthetic "Dees" in the appropriate strong-weak syllable sequence.

Goswami et al. (2010) reported that both versions of the DeeDee task were performed significantly more poorly by 12-year-old children with developmental dyslexia compared to 12-year-old control children. In a second study, Goswami et al. (2013) found that 9-year-old children with dyslexia performed significantly more poorly in the synthetic DeeDee task than 7-year-old typically developing control children—a "reading-level match" experimental design. The reading-level match design is methodologically important, as it holds reading level constant between groups rather than chronological age. The reading-level match design thus approximately equates the reading experience received by the brain. It also gives a mental age advantage to the children with dyslexia. The finding that the children with dyslexia were significantly less accurate than *younger* controls in the DeeDee task suggests that the prosodic difficulty in dyslexia is a profound one.

Direct measures of lexical stress perception have yielded similar results. Working with dyslexic adults, Leong, Hämäläinen, Soltész, and Goswami (2011) designed a direct measure of syllable stress perception, using a task based on four-syllable words. The words selected either had first syllable primary stress, like "COMfortable", or second syllable primary stress, like "deBAteable". Participants were required to make a same-different judgement about pairs of words that were either pronounced with the same stress template, or with a correct and an incorrect stress template. For example, a pronunciation like "comFORtable" is incorrect. Highly compensated adults with dyslexia (undergraduate students at the University of Cambridge) showed significantly lower sensitivity to syllable stress than adults without dyslexia (other Cambridge students) in this task. Reduced stress sensitivity was found *both* when different lexical templates had to be compared (e.g., "*maternity-ridiculous*" [same]), and when the same word repeated twice had to be compared (e.g., "*difficulty-diFFIculty*" [different]). The unique auditory predictor of individual differences in the direct stress perception task was rise time discrimination. The children with developmental dyslexia who received the DeeDee task at age 9 were also given the "same word" version of the direct stress perception task (*"difficulty-diFFIculty"*) when they were aged 13 years. Significant impairments in the perception of syllable stress were again found for these children, and the degree of impairment was again related to individual differences in rise time perception (Goswami et al., 2013). Accordingly, we can conclude that the impaired discrimination of amplitude rise time that characterises children with developmental dyslexia affects their ability to extract prosodic structure from speech.

Oscillatory Phase Entrainment in Children With Developmental Dyslexia

We saw earlier that the patterns of amplitude modulation in the speech signal yield acoustic information relevant to identifying rhymes and phonemes as well as prosodic patterning. For example, delta phase governs rhyme similarity between words, and delta-theta phase synchronisation changes with phoneme deletion. To date, studies of children with developmental dyslexia have not investigated the auditory processing of delta phase and delta-theta phase synchronisation. Rather, they have investigated directly oscillatory entrainment to delta- and theta-band speech information by the brain.

In the first study ever conducted to investigate neural entrainment to speech by typically developing children (Power, Mead, Barnes, & Goswami, 2012), we decided to use a rhythmic speech paradigm. This was repetition of the syllable "ba" at a 2 Hz rate ("ba . . . ba . . . ba . . .") by a native female speaker of British English. In order to study both auditory and visual entrainment independently, children either watched a video of a "talking head" repeating the syllable (auditory-visual measure, AV), heard the auditory soundtrack without a visual stimulus (auditory measure, A), or watched the talking head producing syllables without hearing the speech (visual measure, V). Power et al. (2012) found both auditory and visual oscillatory entrainment to rhythmic speech by the participating children, with significant entrainment in all conditions at the stimulation rate (2 Hz, delta) and also (for A and AV entrainment) at the theta rate (the syllable rate, ~5 Hz). In addition, we found that *preferred phase* in the theta band was altered by predictive visual speech information. Preferred phase reflects the point in time during a temporal cycle when most neurons discharge their electrical pulses. The information about speech that was provided visually (seeing the person's mouth opening, ready to produce a syllable) thus made the electrical discharge of the auditory cells more temporally accurate. This effect is well-documented in adults (e.g., Schroeder, Lakatos, Kajikawa, Partan, & Puce, 2008). In essence, visual rhythmic information automatically modulates auditory oscillations to the optimal phase for the auditory processing of speech, providing an additional (cross-modal) cue to that provided by acoustic rise times. Interestingly, we found that individual differences in auditory theta entrainment were related to individual differences in reading development in our sample of children.

We next tested children with dyslexia in the same rhythmic paradigm (Power, Mead, Barnes, & Goswami, 2013). In general the dyslexic children's brains behaved very similarly to the typically developing group, with significant entrainment in all conditions, and visual information phase re-setting the auditory cell networks in the same way as for non-dyslexic children. The only group difference that we found was when the auditory modality was involved. Children with dyslexia showed a significant difference in preferred phase in the delta band compared to control children in both the A and the AV conditions. This difference has potentially serious consequences for the neural encoding of speech. It suggests that most neurons in the dyslexic brain are discharging their electrical pulses at a non-optimal phase for speech processing (at this particular temporal rate, delta, corresponding to the "stressed syllable" rate of amplitude modulation). The effects are depicted schematically in Figure 6.5. The figure shows the raw speech signal for the nursery rhyme phrase "Doctor Foster went to Gloucester", with an imaginary 2 Hz modulation super-imposed over the speech. For typically developing children, the neural response (solid line) is in time with the speech, with peak electrical activity coinciding with the most informative parts of the speech signal. For children with dyslexia, the neural response (dotted line) is out of time with the speech, with peak electrical activity coinciding with less informative parts

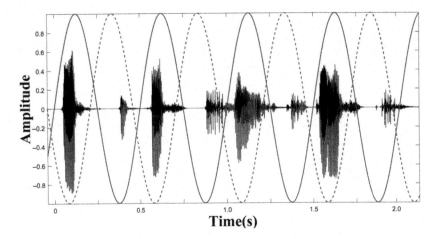

Figure 6.5 The Raw Speech Waveform for the Nursery Rhyme Phrase "Doctor Foster Went to Gloucester", With a Schematic of a Delta-band (2 Hz) Neuroelectric Oscillation Overlaid. The solid line represents a brain whose peak response is "in phase" with the signal, thereby capturing most of the important speech information. The dotted line represents a brain whose peak response is "out of phase" with the signal, thereby missing most of the important speech information. Both are exaggerated, and recall that simultaneous oscillations at faster rates will also be occurring.

Source: Figure by Sheila Flanagan.

of the speech signal. The effect has been exaggerated in the figure (the average phase delay in our study was 12.8 ms). Note also that, at least in this experiment, theta phase was in time for the children with dyslexia (i.e., no group difference). Nevertheless, the studies by Power and colleagues suggest that for English-speaking children with developmental dyslexia, the phase entrainment of networks of cells that respond to rhythmic speech input at the delta rate is "out of time".

In subsequent work we have used semantically unpredictable sentences (e.g., "Arcs blew their cough") and a sentence repetition task to study phase entrainment in the delta band in dyslexia further. Semantically unpredictable sentences are used to avoid children guessing the correct repetition on the basis of context. We have then reverse-engineered children's electrical brain responses to re-create the amplitude modulation patterns in the sentences that they were listening to. This enables a direct measure of the neural quality of children's speech envelope representations. Power, Colling, Mead, Barnes, and Goswami (2016) reported that the envelopes in the 0–2 Hz (delta) band were encoded significantly less accurately by the brains of the children with dyslexia. This significant difference was found even when the children with dyslexia were compared to a reading-level matched control group, who were 2 years younger in age. Both groups of children could report the same number of words in the sentences correctly; however, the neural data suggests that they were achieving this by different means. The RL-match comparison suggests a fundamental encoding deficit for very slow amplitude modulation information in speech for English-speaking children with dyslexia. Individual differences in envelope encoding were also significantly related to individual differences in lexical stress perception (the "difficulty-diFFIculty" same-different judgement task).

As previous sections in this chapter make clear, inaccurate encoding of delta-band amplitude modulations is likely to have a number of detrimental effects regarding phonological development. Firstly, the acoustic information required for extracting the linguistic hierarchy shown in Figure 6.1 is likely to be degraded at the top level—the governing level of delta-band amplitude modulation information, relevant to perceiving strong-weak syllable patterning. Secondly, the finding that delta *phase* is atypical would have consequences for the extraction of rhyme similarity, as delta phase makes a significant perceptual contribution to children's identification of rhyming words. Thirdly, if delta phase is atypical, then the accuracy of neural delta-theta phase alignment will necessarily also be affected. This is likely to impair children's ability to extract both prosodic and phonemic information from the speech signal. The fact that these neural processes are automatic and occur without conscious awareness suggests that children with dyslexia will face a real struggle to develop the high-quality phonological representations required to become efficient readers. This will be true across languages, as all languages use prosodic structure as the bedrock of their phonological systems. Nevertheless, education can always make a difference developmentally, and this is also true regarding children's ability to develop awareness of linguistic prosodic structures.

Remediating the Rhythmic Difficulties in Dyslexia

Indeed, the educational neuroscience discoveries outlined in this chapter have suggested a number of novel avenues regarding remediation, some of which look very promising. As will be recalled, slow amplitude modulations in speech contribute to our perception of speech rhythm and prosodic structure. Accordingly, children with dyslexia may also have general acoustic difficulties with rhythm. One of the simplest ways of measuring rhythmic skills is to ask a child to tap in time to a beat. Thomson and Goswami (2008) asked children with dyslexia to tap to a metronome which either delivered a beat every 600 ms, or every 500 ms or every 400 ms. Compared to age-matched controls, the children with dyslexia showed significantly more variability in tapping at the two faster rates (500 ms, or 2 Hz, and 400 ms, or 2.5 Hz). All the children were very variable when tapping to the slowest rate (600 ms). Statistical analyses showed that individual differences in tapping accuracy contributed significant unique variance to individual differences in reading (15% unique variance) and in spelling (21% unique variance).

Another way of measuring rhythmic sensitivity is to ask children to listen to simple musical tunes and decide which tunes contain notes played "out of time". In a study of children with dyslexia carried out by Huss and her colleagues (Huss et al., 2011), simple tunes were created on a chime bar using a single note (G). Children listened to pairs of tunes, which were either both the same, or in which one tune had notes played "out of time". The children with dyslexia found this same-different judgement task significantly more difficult, even when compared to reading-level matched younger controls (Goswami et al., 2013). Statistical analyses showed that individual differences in the musical rhythm task accounted for 42% of unique variance in reading skills and were a significant predictor of individual progress in reading a year later.

These behavioural studies suggest that explicitly matching external beats to language rhythms, for example via tapping/drumming or utilising musical rhythms, may confer linguistic benefits. Rhythmic interventions may help children with reading difficulties by improving their rhythm perception, their perception of rhythm patterns in language, and accordingly, their phonological awareness. In a small-scale exploratory study, Bhide, Power, and Goswami (2013) investigated the possible phonological benefits of a music, poetry and rhythm intervention with 6- to 7-year-old poor readers. The children carried out oral tasks with rhythm, such as playing beat patterns on bongo drums to match strong syllables in nursery rhymes and practicing the DeeDee task. Children also made rhythm judgements with different tempi, played marching and clapping games that matched motor rhythms to language rhythms, and learned to recite rhythmic oral poetry. Following 10 weeks of oral/motor training, significant improvements in phonological awareness, reading and spelling were found, with large effect sizes (e.g., $d = 1.01$ for rhyme awareness). Circular statistics showed that individual improvements in tapping to a beat over the 10 weeks were significantly related to improvements in reading. Hence rhythmic timing and phonology are intimately related developmentally. For older children, rapping games or bongo drumming to pop songs may provide similar benefits.

Conclusions

What Has Neuroscience Added to Our Understanding Over and Above Psychology?

In the past decade, educational neuroscience has made a unique contribution to our understanding of phonological development in children. Growing understanding of the physiological mechanisms comprising the neural oscillatory hierarchy has revealed novel information concerning the successful encoding of speech. Related work has shown the importance of the accurate discrimination of amplitude rise times for successful neural oscillatory entrainment. In particular, successful neural encoding of the statistical patterns of acoustic information nested in the amplitude envelope of speech, identified by their amplitude rise times (the rhythmic energy patterns that occur at slow and faster rates), and successful encoding of their phase relations (or relative timing), has been found to provide a basis for the successful and automatic extraction of phonological units such stressed syllables, syllables, onsets, rimes and phonemes. Similarly, neuroscience studies have shown that when oscillatory encoding is "out of phase" or out of time for one rhythmic rate, the slowest rate (delta, 2 Hz), then children have difficulty in processing phonological information at all levels of the linguistic hierarchy. Educational neuroscience has thus identified a new sensory/neural basis for developmental dyslexia across languages—impaired amplitude envelope rise time discrimination, impaired perception of the amplitude modulation structure of the speech envelope, and atypical oscillatory phase synchronisation to amplitude modulation information (Goswami et al., 2002; Power et al., 2013, 2016).

What Are the Concrete Implications of Research and Opportunities for Translation?

These novel insights offer concrete opportunities for educational translation. Firstly, activities based on rhythm, particularly activities involving more than one modality (as when synchronising drumming and reciting a poem), can improve children's rhythmic behaviour, with significant effects on phonology. Secondly, children can practice synchronising rhythms at more than one rate, for example tapping on every second beat of a metronome (Colling, Noble, & Goswami, 2017), or clapping to the strong syllables in a song while shaking fingers to the weak syllables. This could potentially enhance neural phase synchronisation by "entraining the oscillators" (see Goswami & Szűcs, 2011). Thirdly, the importance of metrical language activities with young children (nursery rhymes, poetry out loud, singing) as a core foundation for phonological development and therefore literacy is supported. Indeed, as infant-directed speech (IDS) is also known to contain enhanced delta-rate amplitude modulations (see Leong, Kalashnikova, Burnham, & Goswami, 2017), the use of IDS for longer with children at family risk for dyslexia may be helpful.

Finally, and most exciting of all, it may be possible to adapt the speech signal in light of our discoveries about the amplitude modulation hierarchy. For example, the amplitude envelope cues in speech that are perceived poorly by children with dyslexia could be synthetically amplified or exaggerated. Indeed, our current research funding aims to do exactly this. A clear prediction from the studies discussed in this chapter would be that receiving adapted speech from a young age would improve the language processing skills of children at family risk for dyslexia, so that their phonological systems can develop age-appropriately, and so that phonological representations for words are not "under-specified". Although technically complex, such adaptations are within the reach of current technology (for example, some of the processing done by the electrodes in cochlear implants has the effect of enhancing the amplitude envelope of speech). We take it for granted that children who are born short-sighted can be fitted with glasses. Within the next decade, it is possible that children who are born at risk for phonological impairments may be offered a listening device that makes developmental dyslexia unnoticeable or a minor inconvenience, rather than a major learning difficulty.

Further Resources for the Reader to Learn More About the Topic

Goswami, U. (2014). *Child psychology: A very short introduction.* Oxford: Oxford University Press.

Goswami, U. (2015). Sensory theories of developmental dyslexia: Three challenges for research. *Nature Reviews Neuroscience, 16,* 43–54.

Goswami, U., & Bryant, P. E. (2016). *Phonological skills and learning to read.* Reissue of 1990 research monograph in the Classics in Psychology series. Hove: Psychology Press.

Acknowledgements

Usha Goswami's dyslexia research is funded by the Botnar Foundation.

References

Anthony, J. L., Lonigan, C. J., Burgess, S. R., Driscoll, K., Phillips, B. M., & Cantor, B. G. (2002). Structure of preschool phonological sensitivity: Overlapping sensitivity to rhyme, words, syllables, and phonemes. *Journal of Experimental Child Psychology, 82,* 65–92.

Anthony, J. L., Lonigan, C. J., Driscoll, K., Phillips, B. M., & Burgess, S. R. (2003). Phonological sensitivity: A quasi-parallel progression of word structure units and cognitive operations. *Reading Research Quarterly, 38*(4), 470–487.

Arnal, L. H., Doelling, K. B., & Poeppel, D. (2014). Delta-beta coupled oscillations underlie temporal prediction accuracy. *Cerebral Cortex, 25*(9), 3077–3085.

Berko, J. (1958). The child's learning of English morphology. *Word, 14,* 150–177.

Bhide, A., Power, A. J., & Goswami, U. (2013). A rhythmic musical intervention for poor readers: A comparison of efficacy with a letter-based intervention. *Mind Brain & Education, 7*(2), 113–123.

Bradley, L., & Bryant, P. E. (1978). Difficulties in auditory organisation as a possible cause of reading backwardness. *Nature, 271,* 746–747.

Bryant, P. E., Bradley, L., Maclean, M., & Crossland, J. (1989). Nursery rhymes, phonological skills and reading. *Journal of Child Language, 16,* 407–428.

Colling, L. J., Noble, H. L., & Goswami, U. (2017). Neural entrainment and sensorimotor synchronization to the beat in children with developmental dyslexia: An EEG study. *Frontiers in Neuroscience, 11,* 360.

Doelling, K. B., Arnal, L. H., Ghitza, O., & Poeppel, D. (2014). Acoustic landmarks drive delta-theta oscillations to enable speech comprehension by facilitating perceptual parsing. *Neuroimage, 85,* 761–768.

Flanagan, S. A., & Goswami, U. (2018). The role of phase synchronisation between low frequency amplitude modulations in child phonology and morphology speech tasks. *Journal of the Acoustical Society of America, 143*(3), 1366–1375.

Frith, U., Wimmer, H., & Landerl, K. (1998). Differences in phonological recoding in German- and English-speaking children. *Scientific Studies of Reading, 2,* 31–54.

Ghitza, O., & Greenberg, S. (2009). On the possible role of brain rhythms in speech perception: Intelligibility of time-compressed speech with periodic and aperiodic insertions of silence. *Phonetica, 66,* 113–126.

Giraud, A. L., & Poeppel, D. (2012). Cortical oscillations and speech processing: Emerging computational principles and operations. *Nature Neuroscience, 15,* 511–517.

Goswami, U. (2015). Sensory theories of developmental dyslexia: Three challenges for research. *Nature Reviews Neuroscience, 16,* 43–54.

Goswami, U., & Bryant, P. E. (1990). *Phonological skills and learning to read.* Hillsdale, NJ: Lawrence Erlbaum Associates.

Goswami, U., Gerson, D., & Astruc, L. (2010). Amplitude envelope perception, phonology and prosodic sensitivity in children with developmental dyslexia. *Reading and Writing, 23,* 995–1019.

Goswami, U., Mead, N., Fosker, T., Huss, M., Barnes, L., & Leong, V. (2013). Impaired perception of syllable stress in children with dyslexia: A longitudinal study. *Journal of Memory and Language, 69*(1), 1–17.

Goswami, U., & Szűcs, D. (2011). Educational neuroscience: Developmental mechanisms; Towards a conceptual framework. *Neuroimage, 57,* 651–658.

Goswami, U., Thomson, J., Richardson, U., Stainthorp, R., Hughes, D, Rosen, S., & Scott, S. K. (2002). Amplitude envelope onsets and developmental dyslexia: A new hypothesis. *Proceedings of the National Academy of Sciences, 99*(16), 10911–10916.

Goswami, U., Wang, H.-L., Cruz, A., Fosker, T., Mead, N., & Huss, M. (2011). Language-universal sensory deficits in developmental dyslexia: English, Spanish and Chinese. *Journal of Cognitive Neuroscience, 23,* 325–337.

Greenberg, S. (2006). A multi-tier framework for understanding spoken language. In S. Greenberg & W. Ainsworth (Eds.), *Understanding speech—an auditory perspective* (pp. 411–434). Mahwah, NJ: LEA.

Gross, J., Hoogenboom, N., Thut, G., Schyns, P., Panzeri, S., Belin, P., & Garrod, S. (2013). Speech rhythms and multiplexed oscillatory sensory coding in the human brain. *PLoS Biology*, *11*(12), e1001752.

Huss, M., Verney, J. P., Fosker, T., Mead, N., & Goswami, U. (2011). Music, rhythm, rise time perception and developmental dyslexia: Perception of musical meter predicts reading and phonology. *Cortex*, *47*, 674–689.

Leong, V., & Goswami, U. (2015). Acoustic-emergent phonology in the amplitude envelope of child-directed speech. *PLoS One*, *10*(12), e0144411.

Leong, V., & Goswami, U. (2017). Difficulties in auditory organization as a cause of reading backwardness? An auditory neuroscience perspective. *Developmental Science*, *20*, e12457.

Leong, V., Hämäläinen, J., Soltész, F., & Goswami, U. (2011). Rise time perception and detection of syllable stress in adults with developmental dyslexia. *Journal of Memory and Language*, *64*, 59–73. doi:10.1016/j.jml.2010.09.003

Leong, V., Kalashnikova, M., Burnham, D., & Goswami, U. (2017). The temporal modulation structure of infant-directed speech. *Open Mind*, *1*(2), 78–90.

Leong, V., Stone, M., Turner, R. E., & Goswami, U. (2014). A role for amplitude modulation phase relationships in speech rhythm perception. *Journal of the Acoustical Society of America*, *136*, 366–381.

Liberman, I. Y., Shankweiler, D., Fischer, F. W., & Carter, B. (1974). Explicit syllable and phoneme segmentation in the young child. *Journal of Experimental Child Psychology*, *18*, 201–212.

Mehler, J., Jusczyk, P., Lambertz, G., Halsted, N., Bertoncini, J., & Amiel-Tison, C. (1988). A precursor of language acquisition in young infants. *Cognition*, *29*, 143–178.

Opie, I., & Opie, P. (1987). *The lore and language of schoolchildren*. Oxford: Oxford University Press.

Poeppel, D. (2003). The analysis of speech in different temporal integration windows: Cerebral lateralization as "asymmetric sampling in time". *Speech Communication*, *41*, 245–255.

Poeppel, D. (2014). The neuroanatomic and neurophysiological infrastructure for speech and language. *Current Opinion in Neurobiology*, *28c*, 142–149.

Power, A. J., Colling, L. C., Mead, N., Barnes, L., & Goswami, U. (2016). Neural encoding of the speech envelope by children with developmental dyslexia. *Brain & Language*, *160*, 1–10.

Power, A. J., Mead, N., Barnes, L., & Goswami, U. (2012). Neural entrainment to rhythmically-presented auditory, visual and audio-visual speech in children. *Frontiers in Psychology*, *3*, 216.

Power, A. J., Mead, N., Barnes, L., & Goswami, U. (2013). Neural entrainment to rhythmic speech in children with developmental dyslexia. *Frontiers in Human Neuroscience*, *7*, 777.

Richardson, U., Thomson, J. M., Scott, S. K., & Goswami, U. (2004). Auditory processing skills and phonological representation in dyslexic children. *Dyslexia*, *10*, 215–233.

Schroeder, C. E., Lakatos, P., Kajikawa, Y., Partan, S., & Puce, A. (2008). Neuronal oscillations and visual amplification of speech. *Trends in Cognitive Sciences*, *12*, 106–113. https://doi.org/10.1016/j.tics.2008.01.002

Scott, S. K. (1998). The point of P-centres. *Psychological Research*, *61*, 4–11.

Shannon, R., Zeng, F.-G., Kamath, V., Wygonski, J., & Ekelid, M. (1995). Speech recognition with primarily temporal cues. *Science*, *270*, 303–304.

Siok, W. T., & Fletcher, P. (2001). The role of phonological awareness and visual-orthographic skills in Chinese reading acquisition. *Developmental Psychology*, *37*, 886–899.

Snowling, M. J. (2000). *Dyslexia* (2nd ed.). Oxford: Blackwell.

Stefanics, G., Fosker, T., Huss, M., Mead, N., Szűcs, D., & Goswami, U. (2011). Auditory sensory deficits in developmental dyslexia, a longitudinal ERP study. *Neuroimage, 57*(3), 723–732.

Thomson, J. M., & Goswami, U. (2008). Rhythmic processing in children with developmental dyslexia: Auditory and motor rhythms link to reading and spelling. *Journal of Physiology (Paris), 102*, 120–129.

Turner, R. E. (2010). *Statistical models for natural sounds* (Doctoral dissertation), University College London. Retrieved from www.gatsby.ucl.ac.uk/~turner/Publications/Thesis.pdf

Whalley, K., & Hansen, J. (2006). The role of prosodic sensitivity in children's reading development. *Journal of Research in Reading, 29*, 288–303. https://doi.org/10.1111/j.1467-9817.2006.00309.x

Wood, C., & Terrell, C. (1998). Poor readers' ability to detect speech rhythm and perceive rapid speech. *British Journal of Developmental Psychology, 16*, 397–413.

Ziegler, J. C., & Goswami, U. (2005). Reading acquisition, developmental dyslexia, and skilled reading across languages: A psycholinguistic grain size theory. *Psychological Bulletin, 131*, 3–29.

7 Sources of Variability in Mathematical Development

Bert De Smedt

Introduction

Mathematics represents a key component of the educational curriculum of children and adolescents and remains quintessential in our daily adult life. There are large individual differences in the way children acquire mathematical skills (Dowker, 2005; Vanbinst & De Smedt, 2016), and these individual differences are very stable predictors of later mathematical development (Duncan et al., 2007) and real-life outcomes, such as employment (Rivera-batiz, 1992), socioeconomic status (Ritchie & Bates, 2013) or medical decision making (Reyna, Nelson, Han, & Dieckmann, 2009). This raises the question as to why learning mathematics is so easy for some but so difficult for others (e.g., Berch, Geary, & Mann-Koepke, 2016). Characterizing these individual differences is a first step in understanding different learners' profiles, so that education can be suitably tailored to each individual. This understanding represents an interdisciplinary area of inquiry where cognitive neuroscientists, psychologists and educators can work together. It has the potential to result in new effective interventions and diagnostic approaches. In addition, mathematics is in essence a symbolic, culturally acquired skill that needs to be learned via formal education and schooling. It therefore offers an exciting test case to understand how the developing brain reorganizes itself in response to the demands of education (Dehaene & Cohen, 2007) and how brain networks of school-taught abilities are gradually *constructed* via experience and interaction with the (educational) environment (e.g., *neuro*constructivism, see Westermann, Thomas, & Karmiloff-Smith, 2011).

While there are general explanations for individual differences that affect learning more broadly, such as sensory dysfunction, intelligence, socioeconomic status or general environmental factors, the present chapter focuses on variables that are somewhat (more) specific to individual differences in mathematics learning. In doing so, the focus of this chapter is on the role of neurocognitive factors, because these are on a theoretical level of analysis closer to the study of neurobiological factors, such as brain structure and function (Hulme & Snowling, 2009). This does not, however, underestimate the importance of environmental factors, such as the home environment or parental expectations and attitudes towards mathematics (Chang & Beilock, 2016) in these differences, but their roles have not (yet) been studied at the neurobiological level in children.

The current chapter reviews what is known about children's development of arithmetic and its neurocognitive correlates. It will also discuss atypical development of arithmetic, a condition referred to as dyscalculia (e.g., De Smedt, Peters, & Ghesquiere, 2019). Dyscalculia is described as a specific *neurodevelopmental learning disorder* (American Psychological Association, 2013), suggesting that the cause of the difficulties lies at the neurobiological level, and brain imaging studies have tried to elucidate this. The chapter ends with a discussion about the value added of neuroscience to our understanding of children's arithmetic development and its individual differences.

Arithmetic

A key feature of mathematics learning is that it consists of a wide range of components (Kilpatrick, Swafford, & Findell, 2001), such as arithmetic, geometry, measurement, algebra etc., which are all likely to have different neurocognitive determinants and neural substrates. This echoes observations in neuropsychological studies with brain-damaged patients (Dowker, 2005), where it is not uncommon to observe very selective impairments in different yet specific areas of mathematical performance (e.g., deficits in subtraction but not multiplication, or vice versa), depending on the type of lesion (Dehaene & Cohen, 1997). This fractionation is also evident in the development of educational interventions, where these components have been used as starting points to tailor interventions to the specific strengths and weaknesses of children in mathematics (Dowker, 2008). Unfortunately, many neurocognitive studies have used general standardized mathematics tests, which summarize performance on a wide variety of mathematical abilities into one composite score, as their main dependent variable of interest. The outcome of these studies is, however, difficult to interpret, as the observed neurocognitive correlates of mathematics achievement will depend on the types of mathematical abilities that are included in these standardized tests, and these vary over countries and ages (see Vanbinst & De Smedt, 2016, for a discussion). Recent meta-analyses on the association between cognitive factors and individual differences in mathematical performance have indeed shown that these associations are significantly moderated by the mathematical ability under study (Peng, Namkung, Barnes, & Sun, 2016; Schneider et al., 2017).

Against this background, the current chapter focuses on one domain of mathematics learning, namely arithmetic or the ability to add, subtract, multiply and divide whole numbers. This was done because arithmetic constitutes one of the first components of mathematics that children learn at school and it receives a high amount of instructional time (National Mathematics Advisory Panel, 2008). It is also a building block for learning more complex mathematical skills, such as algebra (Kilpatrick et al., 2001). Persistent and lifelong difficulties in arithmetic constitute the hallmark problem of children with dyscalculia (American Psychiatric Association, 2013), and many studies in the field of educational neuroscience have tried to elucidate the neurocognitive origins of these difficulties, as is reviewed in the following. On the other hand, arithmetic, rather than more complex mathematical abilities, has been the major focus of cognitive neuroscience studies on mathematics learning (De Smedt & Grabner, 2015; Peters & De Smedt, 2018). This is because more complex mathematical abilities involve a multitude of steps and require domain-specific and domain-general processes at various points during the task. This represents a technical constraint for neuroimaging methods, such as ERP or fMRI, because the more cognitive processes are involved in a task the more difficult it becomes to disentangle them at the neurophysiological level (De Smedt & Grabner, 2015).

The development of arithmetic has been the subject of decades of cognitive developmental research (Geary, 2011; Siegler, 1996). The main finding from this work is that arithmetic development is characterized by a change in mix of strategies that children use to solve a particular problem. Using counting strategies, children can already calculate the answer to simple sums (if presented non-symbolically or with counting words) before the start of formal mathematics instruction (Jordan, Kaplan, Olah, & Locuniak, 2006). This counting is initially executed with external aids, such as fingers or manipulatives, but children gradually move to counting strategies without these aids (verbal counting). The first stages of arithmetic learning in primary school are further characterized by an increasing efficiency of these counting strategies, where children evolve from counting all numbers in the problem (counting-all; counting 1,2,3–4,5,6,7,8,9 to solve 3 + 6), to counting on from the larger number (counting-on-larger; stating 6 and counting 7,8,9 to solve 3 + 6) (Geary, Bow-Thomas, & Yao, 1992; Siegler & Jenkins, 1989). Through the repeated use of these counting procedures, these procedures become automatized and children develop associations between problems and their answers, the so-called arithmetic facts, which are stored in long-term memory (but see, Baroody, 1984; Thevenot, Barrouillet, Castel, & Uittenhove, 2016, for alternative views). The availability of these facts is important because fact retrieval is more efficient (i.e., faster and less error-prone) and cognitively less demanding (i.e., it requires less working memory and attentional resources) than counting. These facts are also needed to learn the more complex decomposition strategy, which requires children to decompose a problem into smaller ones (i.e., facts) as is needed when calculating with larger numbers (e.g., 8 + 7 can be solved via 8 + 2 = 10 and 10 + 5 = 15) and in (mental) multi-digit calculation.

The change in children's mix of strategies is not an abrupt shift from one strategy to the other. Rather, different strategies remain available over development, even in adulthood, but the frequency with which they are used changes at different time points, with the more efficient strategies becoming more dominant over time, as has been outlined in the so-called overlapping waves model (Siegler, 1996). For example, children show a decreasing reliance on procedural strategies, such as counting and decomposition, but they develop an increasing reliance on fact retrieval. These changes are accompanied by changes in brain activity, as is reviewed in the following, and they have also been documented in other academic domains, such as reading (Eden, Olulade, Evans, Krafnick, & Alkire, 2016), at both behavioral and neural levels. In reading, for example, children show a decreasing reliance on phonological strategies (letter-by-letter decoding) and an increasing reliance on direct word recognition and this is coupled with a shift in brain activity from temporoparietal to occipitotemporal brain networks (Eden et al., 2016).

It is important to emphasize that children's strategy use will be heavily dependent on the way arithmetic is taught in the classroom. For example, multiplication is typically learned by extensive (rote) training of multiplication tables rather than by counting or decomposing a problem into its sub-parts. On the other hand, subtraction is often instructed via counting or decomposing and much less frequently memorized, explaining why fact retrieval is less common in subtraction than in multiplication. Furthermore, there are critical differences between countries in the way arithmetic strategies are instructed, ranging from a continuing emphasis on counting strategies in some countries to a prohibition of counting from an early point on in others (De Smedt, 2016). There are also cross-cultural differences in how much the mathematics curriculum emphasizes the need to develop a reliance on fact retrieval (e.g., the so-called math wars, Schoenfeld, 2004). It is without doubt that these environmental factors will have a high impact on the emergence and organization of the arithmetic network in the brain as well as on the sources of variability in children's arithmetic performance. These cross-cultural differences have been largely ignored in brain imaging studies, and in neurocognitive studies too, but they represent a critical area of collaboration where neuroscientists and educators should work together to gain a better understanding of children's arithmetic development.

This section ends with a brief note on how children's strategies are measured (see De Smedt, 2016; Siegler, 1987, for a more elaborate discussion). In behavioral studies, these strategies are investigated via verbal reports, in which children are asked after the solution of a particular problem to indicate how they solved this problem. If collected on a problem-by-problem basis, these reports can be reliably and validly classified into categories, such as procedures (counting or decomposition) or fact retrieval (I just knew it). Technical issues (i.e., the loud noise during fMRI acquisition; the increase of movements during verbally reporting about the used strategy) have made the collection of verbal reports very difficult in brain imaging studies. For this reason, these studies have used designs in which they compared the brain activity when the use of a particular strategy was expected on the basis of the characteristics of the problem, such as its problem size (De Smedt, Holloway, & Ansari, 2011) or operation (Prado, Mutreja, & Booth, 2014). The interpretation of these data is not without limitations (De Smedt, 2016), because not all problems of the same type are solved by the same strategy and because there are huge individual differences in the strategies children use to solve a particular problem type (Siegler, 1987), an issue that is particularly at stake in the context of atypical development or when comparing different countries. Recent brain imaging studies in both adults (Grabner & De Smedt, 2011; Tschentscher & Hauk, 2014) and children (Polspoel, Peters, Vandermosten, & De Smedt, 2017) show that it is possible to analyze brain activity as a function of the self-reported strategy and they indicate that it is the strategy and not the problem type that modulates the arithmetic network in the brain.

Neural Basis of Arithmetic

The investigation of the neural basis of arithmetic has a long history and dates back to the descriptions of patients with brain damage, who exhibited difficulties in calculation after lesions in the parietal cortex (e.g., Henschen, 1919). Conventional non-invasive methods, such as fMRI, have been able to delineate in the last two decades the different areas of the network underlying arithmetic in adults (for reviews see Arsalidou & Taylor, 2011; Menon, 2015; Zamarian & Delazer, 2015). In adults, this network is dependent on strategy use (Grabner et al., 2009; Tschentscher & Hauk, 2014), expertise (Grabner et al., 2007) and training (Zamarian & Delazer, 2015).

In the context of this volume, the current chapter focuses on developmental imaging data. This is critical because studies in adults cannot be merely generalized to the developing brain (Ansari, 2010; Karmiloff-Smith, 2010). Indeed, adult studies only provide information on the end state of arithmetic development and do not inform us about how these skills develop. These adult data could mistakenly suggest that brain structure and functions are static. This is not the case as the developing brain is highly plastic and its structure and function changes dramatically during development, a process driven by environmental input, such as (math) education (Johnson & de Haan, 2011). Against this background, this chapter mainly discusses developmental imaging data, which have pointed to communalities as well as important differences in the arithmetic network compared to what has been observed in adults (Peters & De Smedt, 2018, for a detailed review).

Developmental brain imaging studies have shown that a widespread bilateral network of interconnected areas shows increases in brain activity during arithmetic (Peters & De Smedt, 2018; Figure 7.1). This network includes the bilateral intraparietal sulci (IPS) and posterior superior parietal lobe (PSPL), the temporo-parietal cortex (including the angular (AG) and supramarginal (SMG) gyri), dorsal and ventral lateral prefrontal cortex (PFC), occipitotemporal regions (comprising the fusiform gyrus) and the medial temporal lobe (including the hippocampus). As is observed in adults, the activity in this network is modulated by strategy use (Polspoel et al., 2017), operation (Prado et al., 2014), and the level of arithmetic fluency (De Smedt et al., 2011). The network undergoes developmental changes in its function (Qin et al., 2014; Rivera, Reiss, Eckert, & Menon, 2005), connectivity and structure, which are not yet fully understood (Peters & De Smedt, 2018).

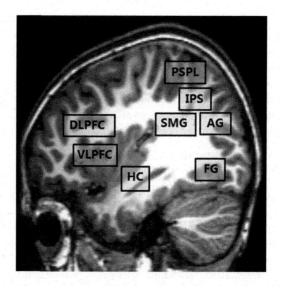

Figure 7.1 Sagittal Slice Showing the Arithmetic Network. The black boxes indicate the most relevant areas implicated in arithmetic, including DLPFC =
dorsolateral prefrontal cortex, VLPFC = ventrolateral prefrontal cortex,
HC = hippocampus, PSPL = posterior superior parietal lobe, IPS = intraparietal sulcus, SMG = supramarginal gyrus, AG = angular gyrus and
FG = fusiform gyrus.

Consistent with data in adults (Arsalidou & Taylor, 2011; Menon, 2015) a
bilateral fronto-parietal network, comprising the bilateral IPS and prefrontal
cortex (Figure 7.1), shows increased activity during the use of procedural strategies (Polspoel et al., 2017), which are more common early in development,
during calculation with larger numbers and in operations such as subtraction
(Prado et al., 2014). Activity in the IPS suggests the involvement of numerical magnitude processing during these strategies (Arsalidou & Taylor, 2011;
Menon, 2015), which may be needed to decompose a problem into smaller
problems. For example, when one is solving 8 + 7, one could understand that
7 can be decomposed of 2 and 5, and consequently solve 8 + 7 via 8 + 2 = 10
and 10 + 5 = 15; another possibility could be to understand that 7 is close to
8, and that 8 + 8 = 16 of which 1 needs to be subtracted to obtain 15. Both
strategies require a good understanding of the magnitude of the numbers and
this might explain why the IPS shows increased activity during these kinds
of problems and strategies. It needs to be noted that increased activity in the
IPS has also been associated with domain-general cognitive functions, such
as visuospatial working memory, and consequently activity in this area might
reflect both domain-specific and domain-general processes (Fias, 2016; Matejko & Ansari, 2017), a possibility that clearly needs to be verified in future
studies. Increased activity in the PFC has been attributed to the involvement

of auxiliary cognitive functions, such as working memory and attentional processes. These cognitive functions are also more needed during procedural strategies as compared to fact retrieval, because the application of procedures is cognitively more demanding, particularly in multi-digit arithmetic where solving a problem requires the sequence of different steps.

Increases in activity in the temporo-parietal cortex (Figure 7.1) have been typically associated with the retrieval of arithmetic facts from memory, at least in adults (Arsalidou & Taylor, 2011; Menon, 2015), as activity in this region typically increases during the solution of multiplications. Training studies in adults have also shown that, as a consequence of training, brain activity in the parietal cortex increases in the AG, potentially reflecting the increasing reliance on fact retrieval (Zamarian & Delazer, 2015), for a review). These training studies offer an interesting window onto how brain activity changes as a function of learning, yet these studies in adults are not merely transferable to children as children's brains are not simply smaller versions of highly skilled adults (Ansari, 2010). In children, data have been mixed with regard to the involvement of the temporo-parietal cortex in fact retrieval (Peters & De Smedt, 2018, for a discussion).

In contrast to studies in adults, there is now an increasing number of studies pointing to the involvement of the medial temporal lobe, and in particular the hippocampus (Figure 7.1), in the retrieval of arithmetic facts in children (De Smedt et al., 2011; see Menon, 2016, for a recent review). The activity in the hippocampus might reflect the formation of long-term memories of arithmetic facts. More specifically, brain imaging studies investigating memory have revealed that the hippocampus has a time-limited role in the consolidation of information in long-term memory (Smith & Squire, 2009), with its role being particularly prominent in the early stages of memory consolidation. This might explain why brain activity in this area has been observed in children, rather than adults. It might be that arithmetic fact retrieval is a protracted process, with the early stages of fact retrieval being associated with brain activity in the hippocampus, and the more advanced stages of automatization being correlated with brain activity in the AG. Although an age-related decrease in activity in the hippocampus has been observed (Qin et al., 2014), longitudinal data are needed to verify this possibility. In all, this emphasizes the need for taking a developmental perspective and exemplifies that adult brain imaging data are not merely generalizable to children.

The mere comparison of adults and children indicates that brain activity during arithmetic changes over time but it does not inform us about how and when these brain networks change. There is only a handful of studies that have specifically investigated this question (Peters & De Smedt, 2018). Most of these studies have investigated developmental change by correlating brain activity with age or by comparing different age groups. These studies have observed that brain activity in the prefrontal cortex decreased with age, reflecting the decreasing involvement of attentional resources and working memory. However, they have also revealed increased activity in the parietal cortex with age and this might point to an increasing functional specialization of this area over developmental time. It is important to emphasize that these findings should be interpreted with great caution. Studies that have correlated brain activity with age typically comprise samples with wide age ranges, which makes it difficult to pinpoint precisely when developmental changes occur. On the other hand, findings from studies that compare different age groups might be explained by cohort differences, rather than developmental effects. One way to solve this problem is to conduct longitudinal studies, in which brain activity in one sample of children is investigated over developmental time. Only one study has done this so far (Qin et al., 2014), revealing that over one year of development, brain activity increases in the hippocampus and decreases in the prefrontal cortex and superior parietal lobe (Figure 7.1). This change was associated with verbal report data, which indicated these neural changes coincide with an increase in fact retrieval strategies and a decrease in counting. More longitudinal brain imaging studies are clearly needed to further replicate and refine these findings.

Adult brain imaging data have revealed that the brain activity during arithmetic is modulated by individual differences (Grabner et al., 2007), but are such individual differences also observed in children? Only a few studies have investigated this question (Peters & De Smedt, 2018), revealing that typically developing children with lower arithmetical fluency show increased activity in the IPS compared to their more arithmetically fluent peers. This observation can be interpreted in different ways. For example, it could reflect individual differences in numerical magnitude processing or it might point to differences in strategy use between children with low and high arithmetical fluency, with the former children relying more and longer on procedural strategies, which require more numerical magnitude processing, and the latter children having shifted earlier to arithmetic fact retrieval. The brain imaging data currently available do not allow us to disentangle between these two possibilities.

Neurocognitive Factors

The above-reviewed brain networks might provide additional hints as to which neurocognitive functions are crucial for understanding individual differences in arithmetic development. In some cases, brain imaging data have confirmed what was already known from psychological studies, but they have also refined these findings and made them plausible at the biological level. In other cases, brain imaging data have provided biological hypotheses that were subsequently tested in psychological studies.

These neurocognitive correlates can be categorized as domain-specific and domain-general factors. Domain-specific refers to factors that are exclusively relevant for learning arithmetic, for example numerical magnitude processing (e.g., De Smedt, Noel, Gilmore, & Ansari, 2013; Merkley & Ansari, 2016; Schneider et al., 2017). Domain-general refers to factors that are also relevant for other domains of academic learning, such as reading, i.e., phonological processing (De Smedt, 2018a), or to more general cognitive abilities that are relevant for all types of cognitive learning, such as working memory (Peng et al., 2016). The use of domain-specific and domain-general categories does not imply that these two are independent of one another. Numerical magnitude processing also depends on working memory, and relatedly, brain activity in the IPS has been interpreted as reflecting not only numerical but also other cognitive functions, such as (visuospatial) working memory (Fias, 2016).

Numerical Magnitude Processing

The consistent activation of the IPS during mathematical tasks has triggered a large number of behavioral studies that examined the role of numerical magnitude processing in arithmetic (De Smedt et al., 2013). Various studies have shown that children's understanding of the meaning of numbers, i.e., that they represent numerical magnitudes, explains individual differences in their arithmetic development (De Smedt et al., 2013; Merkley & Ansari, 2016; Schneider et al., 2017; Siegler, 2016). This understanding of numerical magnitudes has been investigated by means of number comparison tasks, during which children have to indicate the larger of two presented numbers (Schneider et al., 2017), and by number line estimation tasks, in which children have to locate a number on an empty number line (Schneider et al., 2018). Both types of measures can be administered in symbolic (Arabic digits) and non-symbolic (dot arrays) formats, and each of these has been related to individual differences in mathematics achievement across the life span, as is shown by recent meta-analyses (Schneider et al., 2017, 2018). These meta-analyses also revealed that symbolic numerical magnitude processing is a significantly stronger and more consistent predictor of individual differences in mathematics achievement than non-symbolic abilities. While both non-symbolic and symbolic magnitude processing have been related to brain activity in the IPS (Ansari, 2008, for a review), the association between non-symbolic and symbolic magnitude processing constitutes one of the most debated topics in the field of numerical cognition (Ansari, 2016; Leibovich, Katzin, Harel, & Henik, 2017). The dominant view posits that the understanding of symbolic numbers is grounded in pre-existing representations of non-symbolic magnitudes. This dominant and unidirectional view has been questioned against the background of developmental and brain imaging data, and alternative models suggest that both types of representations develop independently from each other, or even that symbolic representations shape the development of non-symbolic abilities (Ansari, 2016, for an extensive discussion). Whichever view holds, it is clear that symbolic number processing constitutes an important source of variability in individual differences in mathematics.

Symbolic numerical magnitude processing has been related to individual differences in arithmetic and strategy use (Vanbinst & De Smedt, 2016, for a review). For example, symbolic number comparison at primary school entrance predicted future competence in arithmetic and reliance on fact retrieval use (Vanbinst, Ghesquiere, & De Smedt, 2015): Children who were able to identify the larger of two Arabic digits more quickly were subsequently more accurate, faster and used more retrieval in arithmetic in grade 1 and 2, and, their arithmetic performance improved faster from grade 1 to grade 2. This predictive value of symbolic numerical magnitude processing was unique and not accounted for by intellectual ability, processing speed or working memory. This has been further confirmed in later stages of primary school, and it has been suggested that symbolic numerical magnitude processing is as important to arithmetic as phonological awareness is to reading (Vanbinst, Ansari, Ghesquiere, & De Smedt, 2016).

At the theoretical level, it remains to be determined through which mechanisms symbolic numerical processing affects the development of arithmetic. One explanation could be that understanding number symbols provides a scaffold for developing more advanced procedural strategies. Being able to quickly identify the larger digit in an addition problem might help the development of the counting-on-larger strategy (e.g., in 2 + 9, starting to count from 9). This advanced counting strategy could in turn lead to a faster consolidation of arithmetic facts in memory. Another explanation could be that arithmetic facts are stored in memory along a meaningful dimension, i.e., according to their magnitude (Butterworth, Zorzi, Girelli, & Jonckheere, 2001; Campbell, 1995; Robinson, Menchetti, & Torgesen, 2002). Finally, it could be that symbolic number processing is affected by children's arithmetic development and that the association between the two is bidirectional, as has been observed for phonological awareness and reading (Perfetti, Beck, Bell, & Hughes, 1987), a possibility that should be explored in future research.

Phonological Processing

The most influential (adult) neurocognitive model of number processing, the triple-code model (Dehaene & Cohen, 1995) postulated, against the background of neuropsychological case studies of brain damaged patients, an association between phonological processing, i.e., the ability to understand that words consist of different sounds, and arithmetic. More specifically, the model stipulated that arithmetic facts, particularly multiplication, are stored in a phonological way in memory. Cognitive neuroimaging research has pointed to shared neural correlates between arithmetic and reading in the temporo-parietal cortex (De Smedt, Taylor, Archibald, & Ansari, 2010, for a discussion), which includes the angular and supramarginal gyri (Figure 7.1). Studies on reading have shown that the temporo-parietal cortex is particularly active during phonological tasks and phonological reading strategies (Schlaggar & McCandliss, 2007). Studies on arithmetic have shown that the left temporo-parietal cortex is active during arithmetic fact retrieval (e.g., Grabner et al., 2007; Peters & De Smedt, 2018). This neural overlap predicts an association between reading and arithmetic fact retrieval, due to a common reliance on phonological codes. This has fueled a series of developmental behavioral studies (De Smedt, 2018a, for a review) which have tested via psychological and educational research this prediction derived from brain imaging data.

Summarizing the existing body of data, De Smedt (2018a) concluded that behavioral studies point to an association between phonological processing and individual differences in arithmetic. This association is most prominent in the context of arithmetic fact retrieval, as was predicted on the basis of brain imaging data (De Smedt et al., 2010). The association is most frequently observed in multiplication, probably due to the way multiplication is usually taught (i.e., via recitation of multiplication tables, a verbally based process). Some studies have shown that these associations disappear when other relevant correlates of arithmetic fact retrieval, such as numerical magnitude processing, are taken into account (Vanbinst et al., 2016). On the other hand, studies in children with specific learning disorders have observed that difficulties in phonological processing and arithmetic fact retrieval co-occur frequently (De Smedt, 2018a, for a review). For example, individuals with dyslexia without dyscalculia, who are known to be impaired in phonological processing, have difficulties in arithmetic fact retrieval, despite otherwise no difficulties in mathematics (De Smedt & Boets, 2010). This has also been observed at the neural level (Evans, Flowers, Napoliello, Olulade, & Eden, 2014): Children with dyslexia showed less brain activity in the left supramarginal gyrus during arithmetic fact retrieval and this region is within the temporo-parietal cortex area that shows overlap between arithmetic and phonological processing (Figure 7.1). Conversely, children with dyscalculia without dyslexia, who are known to be impaired in arithmetic fact retrieval, show weaker performance in phonological processing, despite having no difficulties in reading (De Smedt, 2018a, for a review). The existing body of data therefore indicates that poor phonological processing might constitute one risk factor for difficulties in arithmetic fact retrieval, even though the association might not always be prominent in typically developing children (De Smedt, 2018a).

Working Memory and Executive Function

It has been shown for decades that working memory and executive function play an important role in arithmetic and its development (e.g., Alloway & Passolunghi, 2011; Destefano & Lefevre, 2004; Friso-van den Bos, van der Ven, Kroesbergen, & van Luit, 2013; Gathercole & Pickering, 2000; Holmes & Adams, 2006; Peng et al., 2016; Raghubar, Barnes, & Hecht, 2010). This is particularly prominent in solving more complex mental arithmetic problems, which require the maintenance of intermediate results and involve different steps that should be executed in a given order. As a consequence, the consistent brain activity in the prefrontal cortex during the solution of these more complex problems has been typically interpreted as reflecting working memory and executive resources. Core executive functions include working memory, inhibition and cognitive flexibility (Diamond, 2013) and they all have been connected to brain activity in the prefrontal cortex in children

(Diamond, 2013; Houde, Rossi, Lubin, & Joliot, 2010). As these executive functions are interrelated (Diamond, 2013) and the most consistent associations with individual differences in arithmetic have been observed for working memory (Friso-van den Bos et al., 2013), this section focuses mainly on the role of working memory.

Most of the studies on the association between working memory and arithmetic have used Baddeley's multicomponent model of working memory as their theoretical framework (Baddeley, 2003). The core of this model encompasses the central executive, which is responsible for the attention-driven control and monitoring of complex cognitive processes. This central executive is sometimes fractionated into interrelated functions such as updating, inhibition and shifting (or cognitive flexibility) (Baddeley, 1996; Friso-van den Bos et al., 2013). The model additionally consists of two so-called slave systems of limited capacity, which are similar to the concept of short-term memory. These systems are used for the temporary storage of phonological and visuospatial information, i.e., the phonological loop and visuospatial sketchpad respectively (Baddeley, 2003). Many studies have examined the predictive value of working memory for learning arithmetic (Friso-van den Bos et al., 2013; Peng et al., 2016; Vanbinst & De Smedt, 2016), but the evidence remains inconclusive as to which components of the Baddeley working memory model are critical predictors of individual differences.

The most consistent associations with arithmetic have been observed for measures of the central executive. These measures are typically complex span tasks, such as repeating a sequence of words or digits in a backward order, during which children have to simultaneously store and process information. Performance on these measures has been related to individual differences in arithmetic (e.g., Bailey, Littlefield, & Geary, 2012). It also has been shown that children with poor central executive capacities rely longer on immature counting strategies (Geary, Hoard, Byrd-Craven, & Desoto, 2004) and rely less frequently on arithmetic fact retrieval (Barrouillet & Lepine, 2005). Findings on the involvement of the visuospatial sketchpad and the phonological loop are less clear. Some studies have suggested a time-limited role of these slave systems in predicting arithmetic, with the visuospatial sketchpad being more predictive in the initial stages of arithmetic development (e.g., when children rely on (visuospatial) manipulatives such as fingers), and the phonological loop being more predictive of later stages, when fact retrieval, a process that might be related to verbal abilities, plays a more prominent role (De Smedt et al., 2009; McKenzie, Bull, & Gray, 2003). However, other studies have not been able to replicate this (Andersson & Lyxell, 2007; Szucs, Devine, Soltesz, Nobes, & Gabriel, 2013; Vanbinst et al., 2015).

It is important to emphasize that the load placed on working memory resources is highly dependent on the complexity and novelty of the task that needs to be performed (e.g., Raghubar et al., 2010). Working memory is therefore specifically important in the early learning stages, when new skills are acquired and when more demanding calculation strategies are being used; on the other hand, the role of working memory might be less important during later learning stages when calculation becomes more automatized. This aligns with the observations from the aforementioned brain imaging studies that have observed age-related decreased in brain activity in the prefrontal cortex during calculation (Rivera et al., 2005), reflecting the decreasing involvement of working memory.

Most of the studies have used a correlational approach to study the role of working memory in arithmetic, leaving it open as to whether the influence of working memory is causal or not. There are experimental data available, such as dual-task studies, which have only been rarely applied to children (McKenzie et al., 2003). These studies show a clear causal influence of working memory on arithmetic performance (i.e., arithmetic performance decreases when the working memory load is too high). This does not, however, necessarily imply that variability in working memory abilities contributes to variability in working memory performance. For example, it might be possible that some minimum level of working memory is needed to perform an arithmetic task (of a given complexity).

The existing body of evidence indicates that working memory clearly plays a role in learning arithmetic, yet the precise associations between working memory and arithmetic are highly complex. These associations are dependent on the type of working memory, but even more critically on the skill level (early vs. advanced) as well as the strategies (e.g., counting all numbers requires more working memory resources than counting on from the larger) children apply during arithmetic, both of which have an impact on the amount of information that needs to be kept in working memory during arithmetic processing. The complexity of this association also explains why working memory training does not lead to improvements in arithmetic performance (Melby-Lervag & Hulme, 2013).

Discussion

This section has focused on the neurocognitive factors numerical magnitude processing, phonological processing and working memory, as these have received the largest amount of attention in research on individual differences in arithmetic and their roles in arithmetic can be predicted on the basis of brain imaging data. It is important to note that most of the existing evidence is correlational, which leaves unresolved the question of whether the association between these neurocognitive factors is causal or not. The use of the term neurocognitive sometimes mistakenly suggests a direction of associations, such that neurocognitive variables are being more easily perceived as predictive of or causal in learning to calculate. However, it also might be that learning to calculate itself changes related neurocognitive processes. This possibility has been clearly shown in the field of reading (Bradley & Bryant, 1983), but has remained relatively unexplored in research on mathematical ability. Importantly, and the same applies to brain imaging research, it is the research design and not the type of data (e.g., neurocognitive or brain imaging) that determines its predictive value or causality. This should be kept in mind, when evaluating the existing body of data. Intervention studies that manipulate a given neurocognitive factor are needed to further determine which factors are causal or not. Carefully controlled longitudinal studies (i.e., cross-lagged designs) can test the directions of associations between learning to calculate and its neurocognitive correlates.

It is also clear that the relative contribution of these neurocognitive factors changes with the level of expertise, and consequently with age, although at this point it remains unclear when a particular neurocognitive factor exerts its largest effects on arithmetic. Furthermore, it is highly likely that different pathways contribute to individual differences in children's arithmetic (see Lefevre et al., 2010, for a similar rationale) and therefore, these domain-specific and domain-general neurocognitive factors should be considered in concert when studying sources of variability in arithmetic development. Impairments in these neurocognitive factors might all constitute risk factors for developing deficits in learning to calculate. The study of variability between children in these factors might therefore constitute a lens for understanding atypical development. Indeed, deficits in symbolic numerical magnitude processing (Schwenk et al., 2017) and working memory (Peng & Fuchs, 2016) have been consistently observed in children with dyscalculia, yet the evidence on phonological processing is less clear (De Smedt, 2018a). As has been argued in the context of other developmental disorders (Peterson & Pennington, 2015), it is unlikely that one single deficit accounts for the emergence of such a disorder (Pennington, 2006), and consequently, future studies on atypical development in arithmetic should consider the relative contribution of each of these risk factors.

Understanding Atypical Development: Dyscalculia

Approximately 5% to 8% of children experience lifelong difficulties in learning to calculate, a condition that has been referred to as dyscalculia (American Psychiatric Association, 2013; Butterworth, Varma, & Laurillard, 2011; Geary, 2011). These difficulties are not merely explained by uncorrected sensory problems, intellectual disabilities, other mental disorders or inadequate instruction (American Psychiatric Association, 2013). This specific learning disorder, and the same applies to dyslexia (a disorder in learning to read), has been grouped under the category *neuro*developmental disorders (American Psychological Association, 2013), which refers to the idea that the origin of these disorders might result from aberrant brain structure or function. This idea was already prominent in the first definition of dyscalculia in the scientific literature (Kosc, 1974), where it was proposed that this disorder was brain-based and that it was the consequence of an "impairment in the growth dynamics of brain centers, which are the organic substrate of mathematical abilities" (p. 166). At that time, however, the brain imaging techniques that we currently have at our disposal to investigate brain structure and function were not available. Understanding this neurobiological origin has been put forward as one of the areas in which neuroscience can been applied to education (Butterworth et al., 2011; De Smedt, 2018b; Gabrieli, 2009). There are, however, only a handful of neuroimaging studies that have investigated this neural basis of dyscalculia, leaving the precise neurobiological origin of this disorder currently unknown.

Despite their highlighted potential, surprisingly few studies have examined brain activity during arithmetic in children with dyscalculia and the findings of these studies are mixed (Peters & De Smedt, 2018, for a review). Some studies have observed increased activity as well as connectivity in the aforementioned brain network that is active during arithmetic in children, particularly in and between fronto-parietal areas (Davis et al., 2009; Rosenberg-Lee et al., 2015). These increases in activity and connectivity have been interpreted as reflecting compensatory processes, but these processes remain poorly understood. Other studies have observed decreased activity in the arithmetic network in children with dyscalculia compared to matched control children, particularly in prefrontal cortex as well as posterior parietal areas, such as the IPS (Ashkenazi, Rosenberg-Lee, Tenison, & Menon, 2012; Berteletti, Prado, & Booth, 2014; De Smedt et al., 2011; Peters, Bulthe, Daniels, Op de Beeck, & De Smedt, 2018). Structural brain imaging studies have reported significantly less grey matter (Isaacs, Edmonds, Lucas, & Gadian, 2001; Rotzer et al., 2008) and white matter (Rykhlevskaia, Uddin, Kondos, & Menon, 2009) in these fronto-parietal areas compared to typically developing children.

There is some emerging evidence to suggest that children with dyscalculia show differences in the brain networks that support arithmetic in children, but the present number of studies is currently too few to draw strong definitive conclusions. An important limitation of the current literature is that there are no longitudinal brain imaging data in children with dyscalculia available. This leaves it currently unresolved as to whether the observed differences in brain activity and structure are the cause or the consequence (or both) of the observed difficulties in learning to calculate. For example, it is possible that the observed brain abnormalities in children with dyscalculia are simply the consequence of less experience with arithmetic, and therefore are not the origin of the difficulties. We also do not know if the observed brain abnormalities were already present in children with dyscalculia before they learned to calculate, in which case these abnormalities would represent a neurobiological cause of their disorder. This can be investigated by studying at-risk children before they go to school, an approach that has been used in investigating the neurobiological cause of dyslexia (Vandermosten, Hoeft, & Norton, 2016, for a review) but which has not been applied to the study of dyscalculia so far. As already highlighted when discussing the roles of neurocognitive factors in individual differences, brain imaging data are more easily perceived as being causal (Beck, 2010), yet it is the research design and not the type of data or level of analysis (biological vs. behavioral) that determines causality (De Smedt, 2018b).

The possibility of a neurobiological origin in dyscalculia does not imply that these difficulties in calculation are hardwired or unchangeable. It also does not mean that the aforementioned brain networks and abnormalities in these networks are static and do not change over time. For example, two recent intervention studies, although preliminary, suggest that it is possible to change brain activity in children with dyscalculia via a specific intervention focused on number lines (Michels, O'Gorman, & Kucian, 2018) or on calculation (Iuculano et al., 2015). These two studies only represent baby steps and many more studies are needed in order to fully elucidate the effects of remedial interventions on brain function, structure and connectivity.

The potential neurobiological origin of dyscalculia also does not mean that at this point in time, brain imaging data can be used to determine whether a child has dyscalculia or not. The observed brain abnormalities in children with dyscalculia are very subtle and cannot be observed on a clinical brain scan. These abnormalities are not visible in an individual child, but they only occur when the data of several children are grouped together. In the wider educational neuroscience community, there is currently an active interest in the possibility of using such neurobiological measures or biomarkers to predict which children will develop learning disorders and how they will respond to interventions (Black, Myers, & Hoeft, 2015), but these avenues have not yet been explored in the context of mathematics learning and dyscalculia.

Conclusion

What Neuroscience Has Added to Our Understanding Over and Above Psychology

The brain imaging studies reviewed in this chapter allow us to understand school-taught skills at the biological level. This adds a new level of analysis to educational theories about mathematics learning (see Lieberman, Schreiber, & Ochsner, 2003, for a similar application in political science). These brain imaging studies complement and extend the existing knowledge that has been largely obtained via psychological or educational research. If a particular mental process, such as arithmetic and its associated strategies, has an identified biological substrate, then the theoretical understanding of this process will have more explanatory power if it is constrained by both behavioral and biological data, as obtained via psychology and neuroscience, respectively (Howard-Jones et al., 2016). In other words, the integration of different levels of analysis and data has the potential to generate a better explanatory model of mechanisms underlying a particular educational phenomenon, i.e., arithmetic, its strategies and its development over time. This might then constitute a better base for grounding diagnostic approaches and educational interventions related to arithmetic learning.

One of the major connections between neuroscience and education lies in the understanding of very basic cognitive processes that underlie individual differences in academic achievement (De Smedt, 2018b; Goswami, 2012; Howard-Jones et al., 2016). In view of the tight connection between cognitive neuroscience and cognitive (developmental) psychology, it is not easy to disentangle, if at all possible, the independent contribution of each of these two disciplines. This is exemplified in the use of the concept of *neurocognitive* correlates, which merges neuroscience and psychology, to explain individual differences. The literature reviewed here suggests that symbolic numerical magnitude processing, phonological processing and working memory are critical processes in learning arithmetic and in individual differences in arithmetic skills. While these studies are behavioral and do not include brain imaging data per se, many of them have been inspired by or predicted from brain imaging data. One example is the focus on numerical magnitude processing, against the background of the consistent activation of the IPS during arithmetic (De Smedt et al., 2013). Another example is the association between phonological processing and arithmetic fact retrieval, against the background of overlapping brain networks between reading and arithmetic (De Smedt et al., 2010; De Smedt, 2018a). These are examples of how cognitive neuroscience studies indirectly can help to understand the basic cognitive processes that underlie academic achievement (De Smedt, 2018b).

An often-cited application of neuroscience to education is that it contributes to our understanding of atypical development or learning disorders by providing a causal model of these disorders, i.e., a biological cause, such as aberrant brain structure or function (Butterworth et al., 2011). As reviewed in this chapter, a handful of brain imaging studies on dyscalculia have started to investigate this. The available brain imaging data point to structural and functional abnormalities in the brain networks underlying arithmetic in dyscalculia. The current body of evidence is only nascent and we are far from a complete understanding of how these abnormalities contribute to difficulties in learning to calculate in children with dyscalculia.

Concrete Implications of Research and Opportunities for Translation to Education

The research reviewed in this chapter has two major implications. These implications are both relevant to education and to neuroscience, and, as a result, provide opportunities for translation and collaboration. One application deals with the development of early and accurate methods of identification of children at risk for difficulties in learning to calculate. Another application lies in the design and evaluation of effective educational interventions.

Studies on the neurocognitive correlates of individual differences in arithmetic development (third section) provide hints as to which variables should be included in diagnostic measures that aim to identify children at risk for developing mathematical learning difficulties. The development of such measures of early identification represents an area where researchers in neuroscience and education can work together. The evidence reviewed in this chapter suggests that symbolic numerical processing is a very strong and stable predictor of arithmetic, more so than working memory or phonological processing. This research on symbolic magnitude processing has led to development of easy-to-use diagnostic instruments (Brankaer, Ghesquiere, & De Smedt, 2017; Nosworthy, Bugden, Archibald, Evans, & Ansari, 2013) that can be used by teachers to screen children at risk for subsequent mathematical difficulties in their classrooms. For example, Brankaer et al. (2017) developed the Symbolic Magnitude Processing test, in which children have to cross out the larger of two single- or two-digit numbers, and evaluated its psychometric characteristics. This measure has good test-retest reliability, it correlates with performance on curriculum-based standardized mathematics tests and discriminates children with and without mathematical difficulties throughout the entire primary school. That said, one might wonder how at-risk children could already be identified before they are behaviorally able to take the test. The use of neural measures or biomarkers could be a solution to this problem (Goswami, 2009). These have not been investigated in the context of mathematics learning, so this represents an area for future translation. Importantly, the sensitivity (percentage of at-risk children who are correctly identified as having mathematical learning difficulties) and specificity (percentage of typically developing children who are identified as not being at risk) of these measures needs to be evaluated and needs to be high. These indices should be pitted against the predictive value of behavioral measures, such that the most cost-effective measures can be selected.

The identification of at-risk children only makes sense if adequate remedial interventions are available. This represents a second implication of the previously reviewed studies and an area of translation. The neurocognitive studies reviewed previously can provide starting points for developing educational interventions, with the strongest neurocognitive predictors of arithmetic being the most likely candidates for (preventive) interventions. For example, the consistent observation of number processing as a critical correlate of children's mathematics learning has led to the development of remedial interventions, which aim to improve children's numerical skills (Jordan, Fuchs, & Dyson, 2015, for a review). It is important to emphasize that the mere identification of a neural correlate or neurocognitive factor does not readily answer questions about effective teaching and curriculum design. This requires a nuanced translation and an integration of findings from neurocognitive studies with educational theories and frameworks of effective instructional design. Ignoring the context in which learning takes place, i.e., the curriculum, how a skill is taught, and what pedagogical approaches are used, runs the risk of misinterpretations. Some neuroscientists might be easily tempted to simply convert an experimental task that is sensitive to individual differences in brain activity into an intervention. One example is the training of working memory, during which individuals have to repeat easy working memory tasks that have been used in scientific research, to improve arithmetic performance. Although these interventions improve performance on the trained working memory task, they do not result in better arithmetic skills (Melby-Lervag & Hulme, 2013). Taken together, neurocognitive studies that pinpoint a key variable in children's arithmetic development should be coupled with applied educational research, including the design and evaluation of interventions to optimally foster this development. It is imperative that teachers and educators play a critical role in the design and evaluation of these interventions.

The development of these interventions is also crucial on a more theoretical level. As discussed in a preceding section, such interventions are needed to verify if the aforementioned neurocognitive correlates of mathematics learning are causal or not. However, the learning of symbolic mathematics only occurs via education and schooling through which it leads to the construction and reorganization of brain circuits that support arithmetic. Understanding this process of brain plasticity requires a good understanding and characterization of the context in which learning takes place (e.g., learning histories, teaching materials). This might additionally be investigated via neuroscientific studies that evaluate the outcomes of educational interventions via brain imaging data. The success of this approach will stand or fall on the quality of educational interventions that are being investigated. It necessitates the involvement of both educational researchers and neuroscientists. Without this collaboration, it is a serious risk that the outcome of these studies is meaningless to both education and to neuroscience.

Further Resources for the Reader to Learn More About the Topic

Berch, D. B., Geary, D. C., & Mann-Koepke, K. (2016). *Development of mathematical cognition: Neural substrates and genetic influences.* San Diego, CA: Elsevier Academic Press.

De Smedt, B. (2018). Language and arithmetic: The potential role of phonological processing. In A. Henik & W. Fias (Eds.), *Heterogeneity of function in numerical cognition* (pp. 51–74). San Diego, CA: Elsevier Academic Press.

De Smedt, B., & Grabner, R. (2015). Applications of neuroscience to mathematics education. In. A. Dowker & R. Cohen Kadosh (Eds.), *Oxford handbook of mathematical cognition* (pp. 613–636). Oxford: Oxford University Press.

Peters, L., & De Smedt, B. (2018). Arithmetic in the developing brain: A review of brain imaging studies. *Developmental Cognitive Neuroscience, 30*, 265–279.

References

Alloway, T. P., & Passolunghi, M. C. (2011). The relationship between working memory, IQ and mathematical skills in children. *Learning and Individual Differences, 21*, 133–137.

American Psychiatric Association. (2013). *Diagnostic and statistical manual of mental disorders* (5th ed.). Washington, DC: American Psychiatric Association.

Andersson, U., & Lyxell, B. (2007). Working memory deficit in children with mathematical difficulties: A general or specific deficit? *Journal of Experimental Child Psychology, 96*(3), 197–228. doi:10.1016/j.jecp.2006.10.001

188 Bert De Smedt

Ansari, D. (2008). Effects of development and enculturation on number representation in the brain. *Nature Reviews Neuroscience*, 9(4), 278–291.

Ansari, D. (2010). Neurocognitive approaches to developmental disorders of numerical and mathematical cognition: The perils of neglecting the role of development. *Learning and Individual Differences*, 20(2), 123–129.

Ansari, D. (2016). Number symbols in the brain. In D. B. Berch, D. C. Geary, & K. Mann-Koepke (Eds.), *Development of mathematical cognition: Neural substrates and genetic influences* (pp. 27–50). San Diego, CA: Elsevier Academic Press.

Arsalidou, M., & Taylor, M. J. (2011). Is 2 + 2 = 4? Meta-analyses of brain areas needed for numbers and calculations. *Neuroimage*, 54(3), 2382–2393. doi:10.1016/j.neuroimage.2010.10.009

Ashkenazi, S., Rosenberg-Lee, M., Tenison, C., & Menon, V. (2012). Weak task-related modulation and stimulus representations during arithmetic problem solving in children with developmental dyscalculia. *Developmental Cognitive Neuroscience*, 2, S152–S166. doi:10.1016/j.dcn.2011.09.006

Baddeley, A. (1996). Exploring the central executive. *Quarterly Journal of Experimental Psychology Section a-Human Experimental Psychology*, 49(1), 5–28.

Baddeley, A. (2003). Working memory: Looking back and looking forward. *Nature Reviews Neuroscience*, 4(10), 829–839.

Bailey, D. H., Littlefield, A., & Geary, D. C. (2012). The codevelopment of skill at and preference for use of retrieval-based processes for solving addition problems: Individual and sex differences from first to sixth grades. *Journal of Experimental Child Psychology*, 113(1), 78–92. doi:10.1016/j.jecp.2012.04.014

Baroody, A. J. (1984). A reexamination of mental arithmetic models and data—a reply *Developmental Review*, 4(2), 148–156. doi:10.1016/0273-2297(84)90004-2

Barrouillet, P., & Lepine, R. (2005). Working memory and children's use of retrieval to solve addition problems. *Journal of Experimental Child Psychology*, 91(3), 183–204.

Beck, D. M. (2010). The appeal of the brain in the popular press. *Perspectives on Psychological Science*, 5(6), 762–766.

Berch, D. B., Geary, D. C., & Mann-Koepke, K. M. (2016). *Development of mathematical cognition: Neural substrates and genetic influences*. San Diego, CA: Elsevier Academic Press.

Berteletti, I., Prado, J., & Booth, J. R. (2014). Children with mathematical learning disability fail in recruiting verbal and numerical brain regions when solving simple multiplication problems. *Cortex*, 57, 143–155.

Black, J. M., Myers, C. A., & Hoeft, F. (2015). The utility of neuroimaging studies for informing-educational practice and policy in reading disorders. *New Directions for Child and Adolescent Development*, 147, 49–56. doi:10.1002/cad.20086

Bradley, L., & Bryant, P. E. (1983). Categorizing sounds and learning to read—a causal connection. *Nature*, 301(5899), 419–421.

Brankaer, C., Ghesquiere, P., & De Smedt, B. (2017). Symbolic magnitude processing in elementary school children: A group administered paper-and-pencil measure (SYMP Test). *Behavior Research Methods*, 49(4), 1361–1373. doi:10.3758/s13428-016-0792-3

Butterworth, B., Varma, S., & Laurillard, D. (2011). Dyscalculia: From brain to education. *Science*, 332(6033), 1049–1053.

Butterworth, B., Zorzi, M., Girelli, L., & Jonckheere, A. R. (2001). Storage and retrieval of addition facts: The role of number comparison. *Quarterly Journal of Experimental Psychology Section A: Human Experimental Psychology*, 54(4), 1005–1029.

Campbell, J. I. D. (1995). Mechanisms of simple addition and multiplication: A modified network-interference theory and simulation. *Mathematical Cognition*, *1*(2), 121–164.

Chang, H., & Beilock, S. L. (2016). The math anxiety-math performance link and its relation to individual and environmental factors: A review of current behavioral and psychophysiological research. *Current Opinion in Behavioral Sciences*, *10*, 33–38. doi:10.1016/j.cobeha.2016.04.011

Davis, N., Cannistraci, C. J., Rogers, B. P., Gatenby, J. C., Fuchs, L. S., Anderson, A. W., & Gore, J. C. (2009). The neural correlates of calculation ability in children: An fMRI study. *Magnetic Resonance Imaging*, *27*(9), 1187–1197.

De Smedt, B. (2016). Individual differences in arithmetic fact retrieval. In D. Berch, D. Geary, & K. Mann-Koepke (Eds.), *Mathematical cognition and learning* (Vol. 2, pp. 219–243). San Diego, CA: Elsevier Academic Press.

De Smedt, B. (2018a). Language and arithmetic: The potential role of phonological processing. In A. Henik & W. Fias (Eds.), *Heterogeneity of function in numerical cognition* (pp. 51–74). San Diego, CA: Elsevier Academic Press.

De Smedt, B. (2018b). Applications of (cognitive) neuroscience in educational research. In G. Noblit (Ed.), *Oxford handbook of educational research*. New York: Oxford University Press. doi:10.1093/acrefore/9780190264093.013.69

De Smedt, B., & Boets, B. (2010). Phonological processing and arithmetic fact retrieval: Evidence from developmental dyslexia. *Neuropsychologia*, *48*(14), 3973–3981. doi:10.1016/j.neuropsychologia.2010.10.018

De Smedt, B., & Grabner, R. (2015). Applications of neuroscience to mathematics education. In A. Dowker & R. Cohen-Kadosh (Eds.), *Oxford handbook of mathematical cognition* (pp. 613–636). Oxford: Oxford University Press.

De Smedt, B., Holloway, I. D., & Ansari, D. (2011). Effects of problem size and arithmetic operation on brain activation during calculation in children with varying levels of arithmetical fluency. *Neuroimage*, *57*(3), 771–781. doi:10.1016/j.neuroimage.2010.12.037

De Smedt, B., Janssen, R., Bouwens, K., Verschaffel, L., Boets, B., & Ghesquiere, P. (2009). Working memory and individual differences in mathematics achievement: A longitudinal study from first grade to second grade. *Journal of Experimental Child Psychology*, *103*(2), 186–201. doi:10.1016/j.jecp.2009.01.004

De Smedt, B., Noel, M. P., Gilmore, C., & Ansari, D. (2013). The relationship between symbolic and non-symbolic numerical magnitude processing and the typical and atypical development of mathematics: A review of evidence from brain and behavior. *Trends in Neuroscience and Education*, *2*, 48–55. doi:10.1016/j.tine.2013.06.001

De Smedt, B., Peters, L., & Ghesquiere, P. (2019). Neurobiological origins of mathematical learning disabilities or dyscalculia: A review of brain imaging data. In A. Fritz-Stratmann, V. Haase, & P. Räsänen (Eds.), *The international handbook of mathematical learning difficulties* (pp. 367–384). New York, NY: Springer.

De Smedt, B., Taylor, J., Archibald, L., & Ansari, D. (2010). How is phonological processing related to individual differences in children's arithmetic skills? *Developmental Science*, *13*(3), 508–520. doi:10.1111/j.1467-7687.2009.00897.x

Dehaene, S., & Cohen, L. (1995). Towards an anatomical and functional model of number processing. *Mathematical Cognition*, *1*(1), 83–120.

Dehaene, S., & Cohen, L. (1997). Cerebral pathways for calculation: Double dissociation between rote verbal and quantitative knowledge of arithmetic. *Cortex*, *33*(2), 219–250.

Dehaene, S., & Cohen, L. (2007). Cultural recycling of cortical maps. *Neuron, 56*(2), 384–398. doi:10.1016/j.neuron.2007.10.004

Destefano, D., & Lefevre, J. A. (2004). The role of working memory in mental arithmetic. *European Journal of Cognitive Psychology, 16*(3), 353–386.

Diamond, A. (2013). Executive functions. *Annual Review of Psychology, 64,* 135–168.

Dowker, A. (2005). *Individual differences in arithmetic: Implications for psychology, neuroscience, and education.* Hove: Psychology Press.

Dowker, A. (2008). Individual differences in numerical abilities in preschoolers. *Developmental Science, 11*(5), 650–654. doi:10.1111/j.1467-7687.2008.00713.x

Duncan, G. J., Claessens, A., Huston, A. C., Pagani, L. S., Engel, M., Sexton, H., . . . Duckworth, K. (2007). School readiness and later achievement. *Developmental Psychology, 43*(6), 1428–1446. doi:10.1037/0012-1649.43.6.1428

Eden, G. F., Olulade, O. A., Evans, T. M., Krafnick, A. J., & Alkire, D. A. (2016). Developmental dyslexia. In G. Hickok & S. Small (Eds.), *Neurobiology of language* (pp. 815–826). Oxford: Elsevier Academic Press.

Evans, T. M., Flowers, D. L., Napoliello, E. M., Olulade, O. A., & Eden, G. F. (2014). The functional anatomy of single-digit arithmetic in children with developmental dyslexia. *Neuroimage, 101,* 644–652. doi:10.1016/j.neuroimage.2014.07.028

Fias, W. (2016). Neurocognitive components of mathematical skills and dyscalculia. In D. B. Berch, D. C. Geary, & M.-K. K. (Eds.), *Development of mathematical cognition: Neural substrates and genetic influences* (pp. 195–218). San Diego, CA: Elsevier Academic Press.

Friso-van den Bos, I., van der Ven, S. H. G., Kroesbergen, E. H., & van Luit, J. E. H. (2013). Working memory and mathematics in primary school children: A meta-analysis. *Educational Research Review, 10,* 29–44. doi:10.1016/j.edurev.2013.05.003

Gabrieli, J. D. E. (2009). Dyslexia: A new synergy between education and cognitive neuroscience. *Science, 325*(5938), 280–283. doi:10.1126/science.1171999

Gathercole, S. E., & Pickering, S. J. (2000). Working memory deficits in children with low achievements in the national curriculum at 7 years of age. *British Journal of Educational Psychology, 70,* 177–194.

Geary, D. C. (2011). Consequences, characteristics, and causes of mathematical learning disabilities and persistent low achievement in mathematics. *Journal of Developmental and Behavioral Pediatrics, 32*(3), 250–263. doi:10.1097/DBP.0b013e318209edef

Geary, D. C., Bow-Thomas, C. C., & Yao, Y. H. (1992). Counting knowledge and skill in cognitive addition—a comparison of normal and mathematically disabled children. *Journal of Experimental Child Psychology, 54*(3), 372–391.

Geary, D. C., Hoard, M. K., Byrd-Craven, J., & Desoto, M. C. (2004). Strategy choices in simple and complex addition: Contributions of working memory and counting knowledge for children with mathematical disability. *Journal of Experimental Child Psychology, 88*(2), 121–151.

Goswami, U. (2009). Mind, brain, and literacy: Biomarkers as usable knowledge for education. *Mind Brain and Education, 3*(3), 176–184. doi:10.1111/j.1751-228X.2009.01068.x

Goswami, U. (2012). Neuroscience and education: Can we go from basic research to translation? A possible framework from dyslexia research. *British Journal of Educational Psychology Monograph Series, 1,* 129–142.

Grabner, R. H., Ansari, D., Koschutnig, K., Reishofer, G., Ebner, F., & Neuper, C. (2009). To retrieve or to calculate? Left angular gyrus mediates the retrieval of arithmetic facts during problem solving. *Neuropsychologia, 47*(2), 604–608. doi:10.1016/j.neuropsychologia.2008.10.013

Grabner, R. H., Ansari, D., Reishofer, G., Stern, E., Ebner, F., & Neuper, C. (2007). Individual differences in mathematical competence predict parietal brain activation during mental calculation. *Neuroimage, 38*(2), 346–356. doi:10.1016/j. neuroimage.2007.07.041

Grabner, R. H., & De Smedt, B. (2011). Neurophysiological evidence for the validity of verbal strategy reports in mental arithmetic. *Biological Psychology, 87*(1), 128–136. doi:10.1016/j.biopsycho.2011.02.019

Henschen, S. E. (1919). Über sprach-, musik- und rechenmechanismen und ihre lokalisationen im großhirn. *Zeitschrift Für Die Gesmate Neurologie Und Psychiatrie, 52*(1), 273–298.

Holmes, J., & Adams, J. W. (2006). Working memory and children's mathematical skills: Implications for mathematical development and mathematics curricula. *Educational Psychology, 26*, 339–366.

Houde, O., Rossi, S., Lubin, A., & Joliot, M. (2010). Mapping numerical processing, reading, and executive functions in the developing brain: An fMRI meta-analysis of 52 studies including 842 children. *Developmental Science, 13*(6), 876–885.

Howard-Jones, P. A., Varma, S., Ansari, D., Butterworth, B., De Smedt, B., Goswami, U., . . . Thomas, M. S. C. (2016). The principles and practices of educational neuroscience: Comment on Bowers (2016). *Psychological Review, 123*(5), 620–627. doi:10.1037/rev0000036

Hulme, C., & Snowling, M. J. (2009). *Developmental disorders of language learning and cognition.* Malden, MA: Wiley-Blackwell.

Isaacs, E. B., Edmonds, C. J., Lucas, A., & Gadian, D. G. (2001). Calculation difficulties in children of very low birthweight—a neural correlate. *Brain, 124*, 1701–1707. doi:10.1093/brain/124.9.1701

Iuculano, T., Rosenberg-Lee, M., Richardson, J., Tenison, C., Fuchs, L., Supekar, K., & Menon, V. (2015). Cognitive tutoring induces widespread neuroplasticity and remediates brain function in children with mathematical learning disabilities. *Nature Communications, 6*. doi:10.1038/ncomms9453

Johnson, M. H., & de Haan, M. (Eds.). (2011). *Developmental cognitive neuroscience* (3rd ed.). Malden, MA: Wiley-Blackwell.

Jordan, N. C., Fuchs, L. S., & Dyson, N. (2015). Early number competencies and mathematical learning: Individual variation, screening, and intervention. In R. Cohen-Kadosh & A. Dowker (Eds.), *The Oxford handbook of numerical cognition* (pp. 1079–1098). Oxford: Oxford University Press.

Jordan, N. C., Kaplan, D., Olah, L. N., & Locuniak, M. N. (2006). Number sense growth in kindergarten: A longitudinal investigation of children at risk for mathematics difficulties. *Child Development, 77*(1), 153–175.

Karmiloff-Smith, A. (2010). Neuroimaging of the developing brain: Taking "developing" seriously. *Human Brain Mapping, 31*(6), 934–941. doi:10.1002/hbm.21074

Kilpatrick, J., Swafford, J., & Findell, B. (2001). *Adding it up: Helping children learn mathematics.* Washington, DC: National Academies Press.

Kosc, L. (1974). Developmental dyscalculia. *Journal of Learning Disabilities, 7*(3), 164–177.

Lefevre, J. A., Fast, L., Skwarchuk, S. L., Smith-Chant, B. L., Bisanz, J., Kamawar, D., & Penner-Wilger, M. (2010). Pathways to mathematics: Longitudinal predictors of performance. *Child Development, 81*(6), 1753–1767.

Leibovich, T., Katzin, N., Harel, M., & Henik, A. (2017). From "sense of number" to "sense of magnitude": The role of continuous magnitudes in numerical cognition. *Behavioral and Brain Sciences, 40*, 1–16. doi:10.1017/s0140525x16000960

Lieberman, M. D., Schreiber, D., & Ochsner, K. N. (2003). Is political cognition like riding a bicycle? How cognitive neuroscience can inform research on political thinking. *Political Psychology*, 24(4), 681–704.

Matejko, A. A., & Ansari, D. (2017). How do individual differences in children's domain specific and domain general abilities relate to brain activity within the intraparietal sulcus during arithmetic? An fMRI study. *Human Brain Mapping*, 38(8), 3941–3956. doi:10.1002/hbm.23640

McKenzie, B., Bull, R., & Gray, C. (2003). The effects of phonological and visual-spatial interference on children's arithmetic performance. *Educational and Child Psychology*, 20(3), 93–108.

Melby-Lervag, M., & Hulme, C. (2013). Is working memory training effective? A meta-analytic review. *Developmental Psychology*, 49(2), 270–291. doi:10.1037/a0028228

Menon, V. (2015). Arithmetic in the child and adult brain. In R. Cohen-Kadosh & A. Dowker (Eds.), *Oxford handbook of numerical cognition* (pp. 502–530). Oxford: Oxford University Press.

Menon, V. (2016). A neurodevelopmental perspective on the role of memory systems in children's math learning. In D. B. Berch, D. C. Geary, & K. Mann-Koepke (Eds.), *Development of mathematical cognition: Neural substrates and genetic influences* (pp. 79–108). San Diego, CA: Elsevier Academic Press.

Merkley, R., & Ansari, D. (2016). Why numerical symbols count in the development of mathematical skills: Evidence from brain and behavior. *Current Opinion in Behavioral Sciences*, 10, 14–20. doi:10.1016/j.cobeha.2016.04.006

Michels, L., O'Gorman, R., & Kucian, K. (2018). Functional hyperconnectivity vanishes in children with developmental dyscalculia after numerical intervention. *Developmental Cognitive Neuroscience*, 30, 291–303. doi:10.1016/j.dcn.2017.03.005

National Mathematics Advisory Panel. (2008). *Foundations for success: The final report of the national mathematics advisory panel*. Washington, DC: US Department of Education.

Nosworthy, N., Bugden, S., Archibald, L., Evans, B., & Ansari, D. (2013). A two-minute paper-and-pencil test of symbolic and nonsymbolic numerical magnitude processing explains variability in primary school children's arithmetic competence. *PloS One*, 8(7). doi:10.1371/journal.pone.0067918

Peng, P., & Fuchs, D. (2016). A meta-analysis of working memory deficits in children with learning difficulties: Is there a difference between verbal domain and numerical domain? *Journal of Learning Disabilities*, 49(1), 3–20. doi:10.1177/0022219414521667

Peng, P., Namkung, J., Barnes, M., & Sun, C. Y. (2016). A meta-analysis of mathematics and working memory: Moderating effects of working memory domain, type of mathematics skill, and sample characteristics. *Journal of Educational Psychology*, 108(4), 455–473. doi:10.1037/edu0000079

Pennington, B. F. (2006). From single to multiple deficit models of developmental disorders. *Cognition*, 101(2), 385–413. doi:10.1016/j.cognition.2006.04.008

Perfetti, C. A., Beck, I., Bell, L. C., & Hughes, C. (1987). Phonemic knowledge and learning to read are reciprocal—a longitudinal study of 1st grade children *Merrill-Palmer Quarterly-Journal of Developmental Psychology*, 33(3), 283–319.

Peters, L., Bulthe, J., Daniels, N., Op de Beeck, H., & De Smedt, B. (2018). Dyscalculia and dyslexia: Different behavioral, yet similar brain activity profiles during arithmetic. *Neuroimage: Clinical*, 18, 663–674. doi:10.1016/j.nicl.2018.03.003

Peters, L., & De Smedt, B. (2018). Arithmetic in the developing brain: A review of brain imaging studies. *Developmental Cognitive Neuroscience*, 30, 265–279. doi:10.1016/j.dcn.2017.05.002

Peterson, R. L., & Pennington, B. F. (2015). Developmental dyslexia. *Annual Review of Clinical Psychology, 11*, 283–307. doi:10.1146/annurev-clinpsy-032814-112842

Polspoel, B., Peters, L., Vandermosten, M., & De Smedt, B. (2017). Strategy over operation: Neural activation in subtraction and multiplication during fact retrieval and procedural strategy use in children. *Human Brain Mapping.* doi:10.1002/hbm.23691

Prado, J., Mutreja, R., & Booth, J. R. (2014). Developmental dissociation in the neural responses to simple multiplication and subtraction problems. *Developmental Science, 17*(4), 537–552.

Qin, S. Z., Cho, S., Chen, T. W., Rosenberg-Lee, M., Geary, D. C., & Menon, V. (2014). Hippocampal-neocortical functional reorganization underlies children's cognitive development. *Nature Neuroscience, 17*(9), 1263–1269. doi:10.1038/nn.3788

Raghubar, K. P., Barnes, M. A., & Hecht, S. A. (2010). Working memory and mathematics: A review of developmental, individual difference, and cognitive approaches. *Learning and Individual Differences, 20*(2), 110–122.

Reyna, V. F., Nelson, W. L., Han, P. K., & Dieckmann, N. F. (2009). How numeracy influences risk comprehension and medical decision making. *Psychological Bulletin, 135*(6), 943–973.

Ritchie, S. J., & Bates, T. C. (2013). Enduring links from childhood mathematics and reading achievement to adult socioeconomic status. *Psychological Science, 24*(7), 1301–1308. doi:10.1177/0956797612466268

Rivera, S. M., Reiss, A. L., Eckert, M. A., & Menon, V. (2005). Developmental changes in mental arithmetic: Evidence for increased functional specialization in the left inferior parietal cortex. *Cerebral Cortex, 15*(11), 1779–1790.

Rivera-Batiz, F. L. (1992). Quantitative literacy and the likelihood of employment among young adults in the United States. *Journal of Human Resources, 27*(2), 313–328. doi:10.2307/145737

Robinson, C. S., Menchetti, B. M., & Torgesen, J. K. (2002). Toward a two-factor theory of one type of mathematics disabilities. *Learning Disabilities Research and Practice, 17*, 81–89.

Rosenberg-Lee, M., Ashkenazi, S., Chen, T. W., Young, C. B., Geary, D. C., & Menon, V. (2015). Brain hyper-connectivity and operation-specific deficits during arithmetic problem solving in children with developmental dyscalculia. *Developmental Science, 18*(3), 351–372. doi:10.1111/desc.12216

Rotzer, S., Kucian, K., Martin, E., Von Aster, M., Klaver, P., & Loenneker, T. (2008). Optimized voxel-based morphometry in children with developmental dyscalculia. *Neuroimage, 39*(1), 417–422.

Rykhlevskaia, E., Uddin, L. Q., Kondos, L., & Menon, V. (2009). Neuroanatomical correlates of developmental dyscalculia: Combined evidence from morphometry and tractography. *Frontiers in Human Neuroscience, 3.* doi:10.3389/neuro.09.051.2009

Schlaggar, B. L., & McCandliss, B. D. (2007). Development of neural systems for reading *Annual Review of Neuroscience, 30*, 475–503.

Schneider, M., Beeres, K., Coban, L., Merz, S., Schmidt, S., Stricker, J., & De Smedt, B. (2017). Associations of non-symbolic and symbolic numerical magnitude processing with mathematical competence: A meta-analysis. *Developmental Science, 20*, e12372. doi:10.1111/desc.12372

Schneider, M., Merz, S., Stricker, J., De Smedt, B., Torbeyns, J., Verschaffel, L., & Luwel, K. (2018). Associations of number line estimation with mathematical competence: A meta-analysis. *Child Development, 89*, 1467–1484. doi:10.1111/cdev.13068

Schoenfeld, A. L. (2004). The math wars. *Educational Policy, 18*(1), 253–286. doi:10. 1177/0895904803260042

Schwenk, C., Sasanguie, D., Kuhn, J. T., Kempe, S., Doebler, P., & Holling, H. (2017). (Non-)symbolic magnitude processing in children with mathematical difficulties: A meta-analysis. *Research in Developmental Disabilities, 64,* 152–167. doi:10.1016/j. ridd.2017.03.003

Siegler, R. S. (1987). The perils of averaging data over strategies—an example from children's addition. *Journal of Experimental Psychology-General, 116*(3), 250–264.

Siegler, R. S. (1996). *Emerging minds: The process of change in children's thinking.* New York, NY: Oxford University Press.

Siegler, R. S. (2016). Magnitude knowledge: The common core of numerical development. *Developmental Science, 19*(3), 341–361. doi:10.1111/desc.12395

Siegler, R. S., & Jenkins, E. (1989). *How children discover new strategies.* Hillsdale, NJ: Lawrence Erlbaum Associates.

Smith, C. N., & Squire, L. R. (2009). Medial temporal lobe activity during retrieval of semantic memory is related to the age of the memory. *Journal of Neuroscience, 29*(4), 930–938.

Szucs, D., Devine, A., Soltesz, F., Nobes, A., & Gabriel, F. (2013). Developmental dyscalculia is related to visuo-spatial memory and inhibition impairment. *Cortex, 49*(10), 2674–2688.

Thevenot, C., Barrouillet, P., Castel, C., & Uittenhove, K. (2016). Ten-year-old children strategies in mental addition: A counting model account. *Cognition, 146,* 48–57. doi:10.1016/j.cognition.2015.09.003

Tschentscher, N., & Hauk, O. (2014). How are things adding up? Neural differences between arithmetic operations are due to general problem solving strategies. *Neuroimage, 92,* 369–380. doi:10.1016/j.neuroimage.2014.01.061

Vanbinst, K., Ansari, D., Ghesquiere, P., & De Smedt, B. (2016). Symbolic numerical magnitude processing is as important to arithmetic as phonological awareness is to reading. *PloS One, 11*(3). doi:10.1371/journal.pone.0151045

Vanbinst, K., & De Smedt, B. (2016). Individual differences in children's mathematics achievement: The roles of symbolic numerical magnitude processing and domain-general cognitive functions. *Progress in Brain Research, 227,* 105–130. doi:10.1016/ bs.pbr.2016.04.001

Vanbinst, K., Ghesquiere, P., & De Smedt, B. (2015). Does numerical processing uniquely predict first graders' future development of single-digit arithmetic? *Learning and Individual Differences, 37,* 153–160. doi:10.1016/j.lindif.2014.12.004

Vandermosten, M., Hoeft, F., & Norton, E. S. (2016). Integrating MRI brain imaging studies of pre-reading children with current theories of developmental dyslexia: A review and quantitative meta-analysis. *Current Opinion in Behavioral Sciences, 10,* 155–161. doi:10.1016/j.cobeha.2016.06.007

Westermann, G., Thomas, M. S. C., & Karmiloff-Smith, A. (2011). Neuroconstructivism. In U. Goswami (Ed.), *Childhood cognitive development* (2nd ed., pp. 723–748). Malden, MA: Wiley-Blackwell.

Zamarian, L., & Delazer, M. (2015). Arithmetic learning in adults—evidence from brain imaging. In R. Cohen-Kadosh & A. Dowker (Eds.), *The Oxford handbook of numerical cognition* (pp. 821–850). Oxford: Oxford University Press.

8 Lifespan Conceptual Development in Science
Brain and Behaviour

Andy Tolmie and Selma Dündar-Coecke

What Does Understanding Science Involve?

Science is complex, and precise definitions of it are contentious (Jenkins, 2007; Reiss, 2003), though it may be said to be about understanding the reality of the universe and constructing accurate knowledge of how it functions in terms of causal processes through observation and experimentation. Reflecting this complexity, scientific reasoning and academic science in particular require a broad range of different skills (see Zimmerman, 2007), which past research has gathered under two main strands: 'science as problem solving' and 'science as concept formation' (Dunbar & Klahr, 1988; Klahr, 2000). This chapter mainly focuses on the second, concept formation, as the core of scientific *understanding*, where concepts are the carriers of meanings that allow the abstraction of commonalities across natural phenomena.

The chapter is made up of five sections, each of which brings together relevant theory, experimental evidence, and, where available, recent neuroscience research focusing on certain periods of life. In **early years**, we briefly focus on the relationships between perceptual processes and the initial formation of concepts. In **childhood**, the focus is on the growth of more elaborated causal concepts that capture the processes that lead from cause to effect, and the role of external social influences in the development of these. The **late childhood and adolescence** section addresses the cognitive changes—and sources of individual variation in these—that take place as children and teenagers encounter formal instruction in science. The **adulthood** section elaborates the more sophisticated resources adults employ depending on greater or lesser science expertise. This is followed by a discussion on **language induced thoughts vs inadequacy of language in science,** since although by late childhood language-based concepts become dominant and remain so, these are often only partially accurate compared to more implicit perceptual representations and later emerging abstract models, from which they commonly appear to be distinct. Taken together, the chapter aims to set a clearer agenda for the work of science educators, focused on better integration of these different levels of representation.

Early Years

Debates on conceptual development have been dominated historically by stage theories. Within these, the fundamental stages of concept development are typically distinguished as sensory-motor/perceptual, representational, and abstract (that is, concepts which are not accessible in sensory-motor/perceptual mode). The products of these stages gradually increase in complexity. Theorists who in contrast believe in continual growth argue that developmental processes never follow stages tied to certain times of life. However, both camps agree that humans are born with the capacity to sense their immediate environment. From very early on, senses continuously submit data about the internal and external world, which may provide the basis of later conceptual thought (see Piaget, 1929; Wellman, 1990; Wellman & Gelman, 1992; Gopnik & Meltzoff, 1997).

According to nativists (e.g., Spelke, Baillargeon, Leslie) infants have objective knowledge of the physical properties of the world by 4 months. Knowledge emerges early in development, driven by innate structures, appears to be domain-specific (i.e., tied to particular areas of understanding), and initial knowledge matures over the course of development (see e.g., Spelke, Breinlinger, Macomber, & Jacobson, 1992; Spelke, Phillips, & Woodward, 1995). Stage theorists (e.g., Piaget), on the other hand, argue that this is a slower process of construction. As movement starts to be directed by desire, sensory-motor activity (starting with hands, feet, legs, and gradually the body) allows the newborn to experience objects and events in egocentric fashion,[1] and gradually build up concrete ideas about the physical world and the effects of actions upon it. A reciprocal feedback system (interact and construct) mediates conceptual development through these activities, giving rise to pre-logical thought. Piaget and Inhelder (1971) call this process sensory-motor conceptual development, and argue it produces considerable growth prior to the appearance of speech and symbolic images. During this stage, children are believed to (re)construct their conceptual repertoire directly via contact and perception in its widest sense. Mental representations become evident with the emergence of language and drawing skills, and concepts then become not only perceptual but also imaginal, and accessible in the absence of events themselves.

The transition from sensory to mental representations is not clearly mapped out, however, as these different positions illustrate, and *how* concepts emerge is a matter of considerable debate. What is clear in this debate is that knowledge, concepts, and categories are highly interrelated in nature (see Lamberts & Shanks, 1997), but the origin of these relationships is disputed. This has important implications for the nature and development of scientific concepts.

Early representations of the physical world and associated categories of events arguably provide a foundation for scientific concepts. Categories refer to sets of objects/events, and the mental representations of these sets are referred to as concepts (see Murphy, 2010). Computational modelling research that simulates cognitive development (French, Mareschal, Mermillod, & Quinn, 2004; Mareschal, Quinn, & French, 2002) suggests category representations emerge in bottom-up fashion, based on statistical sensitivity to co-occurring attributes (correlation-based categories and concepts) or the most commonly occurring attributes (prototypes) of similar objects. Rakinson and Lupyan (2008) extend this to dynamic events, finding that artificial networks show increased sensitivity to causal relations as they gain experience, with motion playing a specific role in linking cause and effect. This suggests that early causal awareness has perceptual roots.

However, the key issue is whether and how these early representations become linked to language, since concepts are commonly indexed by words. Vygotsky (1962) argued that thought and language are initially separate systems, but become joined around three years of age, producing verbal thought that is mostly shaped by social and cultural precursors. Mandler (2004) went further, arguing that infants do not have concepts as such, only perceptual representations, derived by building categories of similar objects and then events. Conceptual representations are a *separate*, language-dependent development. Others (see Carey, 2009) suggest a more direct connection, arguing that the acquisition of concepts can be explained by the operation of a set of innate primitives, phylogenetically pre-tuned to the external world, which provide the building blocks for complex concepts. Wagner and Lakusta (2009) argue that preverbal representations must relate to the semantic structures of language from the beginning to support language acquistion, and report (Lakusta & Wagner, 2016) that as early as 10 months, infants have rich representations of the observed world that involve both perceptual and conceptual information.

The uncertainties captured by these different positions apply to the emergence of scientific concepts. The focus of early science concepts is on events (single occurrences associated with a subsequent outcome, such as a stone dropped into water, followed by the stone falling rapidly through the water). These early concepts seem likely to take the form of causal event schemas that map observed co-occurrences and allow anticipation of outcomes when the child encounters known examples (cf. Rakinson & Lupyan, 2008) i.e., they rest on perceptual information. They may also depend centrally on language structures, though: Nelson (1996) and Tomasello (1999) argue the construction of event representations is strongly influenced by language that codes temporal sequences (i.e., syntagmatics), as in 'the stone . . . falls through . . . the water'. These schemas then provide the basis for more abstract event representations as different instances of similar episodes are experienced. These replace specific objects and contexts with 'slot-fillers' i.e., *variables* (see e.g., Tomasello, 1999), and become indexed by relational language terms (e.g., 'sinking') that refer to the core transition from one state to another (cf. Nelson, 1996). Relational abstraction and language-derived segmentation of causal sequences may help, then, to explain why children's conceptual representations show an early focus on the role of variables (see Howe, 1998; Wilkening & Cacchione, 2011).

At the same time, it is significant that infants show sensitivity to causal connections prior to acquisition of language (Leslie, 1982; Leslie & Keeble, 1987; Oakes & Cohen, 1990), treating events in which one shape makes contact with another and the second then moves as causal in nature. Crucially, these results are consistent with Michotte's (1963) findings with adults, also taken to suggest that perception of causality is direct and immediate, without the assistance of language. This means that perception of rapid causal events at least appears to occur without involving language structures. The emergence of causal concepts may therefore reflect an initial *alignment* between perceptual representations and distinct language-based conceptual structures that draw on perceptual information, as Mandler argued, rather than deriving directly from earlier representations. Note that similar arguments have been made in the context of number development—relevant because of the later use of numerical and other symbolic representations in science. Rips, Bloomfield, and Asmuth (2008), for instance, acknowledged the evidence that infants possess quantitative abilities, but argued that despite obvious parallels, their early perceptual representations provide an insufficient basis for natural number and arithmetical concepts, which they suggested are instead top-down constructions.

Although there is no neuroscience evidence available from infants, the view that perceptual and conceptual systems are separate from the outset is consistent with adult evidence from the neurobiology of category learning. Ashby and Crossley (2010) detail the competition between verbal and implicit systems; and the differential role in these of various brain regions such as the prefrontal cortex, the basal ganglia, the hippocampus and other medial temporal lobe structures, and the anterior cingulate. The strong implication of this work is that humans have *multiple* category-learning systems that function in different ways.

To summarise:

1. There is general agreement that from early infancy children form a variety of perceptual representations from their interactions with the world. These include representations relating to causal events, based on statistical sensitivity to co-occurring causes and effects.
2. Although these representations provide a plausible foundation for causal concepts, it is unclear whether conceptual level representations do in fact build directly upon them. Various strands of theory and evidence suggest that causal—and numerical—concepts may be a distinct development, though initially aligned with perceptual data, rather than an elaboration of perceptual representations following language acquisition.

Childhood

There are therefore doubts as to whether children's causal concepts are based in any direct fashion on their early causal representations. There is growing behavioural evidence from primary-age children (though scant neuroscience evidence due to the difficulty in keeping young participants still enough to avoid movement artefacts) that supports the notion that they are indeed separate, though initially aligned. For example, Hast and Howe (2015) compared 5- to 11-year-olds' ability to explicitly predict (a conceptually driven response) or simply recognise (a perceptual response) depictions of the correct relative rate of fall of a heavy and light ball through a vertical tube. Prediction responses were characterised by a growing tendency with age to anticipate that the heavier ball would fall faster: same-speed predictions were made in under 10% of trials. In contrast, same-speed *depictions* were selected as correct on 80% of relevant trials, while heavier-faster depictions were rejected on a majority of trials. Recognition responses did not alter in pattern with age, but became significantly faster, and were also faster where correct decisions were made. Since prediction and recognition responses were if anything better aligned among younger children, this indicates not only that there is a gap between conceptual and perceptual representations, but that the gap actually increases across this age range. Wilkening and Cacchione (2011) noted similar dissociations between conceptually driven and action-based task responses in a range of contexts.

This does not mean that perceptual representations remain static. Howe, Tolmie, and Sofroniou (1999) assessed 9- to 14-year-olds' understanding of four topic areas (object flotation, water pressure, shadow size and motion down an incline). They found participants rarely discounted as causally irrelevant any variable that actually affected outcome, regardless of whether and how they explained their influence. This accuracy could only be attributed to children having previously tracked the effects they had experienced with a high degree of sensitivity, since the study provided no opportunity for observation prior to response. diSessa (1988) reported similar findings. In the context of motion down an incline, Symons (2017) found 6- to 11-year-olds showed increasingly accurate calibration of the relative strength of the effects of slope angle, start position and surface friction—although this was accompanied by inaccurate beliefs that object weight also affects outcome. In general, then, by the time they have reached the age of 11 children show acute perceptual awareness of variables that genuinely affect outcomes, even if this is conflated with false beliefs about other factors.

Perceptual representations therefore appear to have a separate trajectory of development during this period. This kind of awareness may relate to distinct visual and spatial systems (cf. Ashby & Crossley, 2010): Harris (2014) reported that accuracy on a spatial task predicted understanding of force and motion at 5 years—when perceptual representations appear to be more dominant—but not later. Interestingly, Link, Moeller, Huber, Fischer, and Nuerk (2013) reported that training which required first graders to physically walk a number line had a range of benefits for estimation and related tasks compared to controls, especially among those with lower cognitive ability. This suggests that in number, too, embodied spatial representations derived from direct experience may have a separate developmental trajectory (see also Rips et al., 2008, on the perceptual basis of initial arithmetic skills). Consistent with this, Deheane, Spelke, Pinel, Stanescu, and Tsivkin (1999) reported a series of behavioural and brain-imaging experiments that indicate exact arithmetic is acquired in a language-specific format, and recruits networks involved in word-association processes. In contrast, approximate arithmetic shows language independence, and recruits bilateral areas of the parietal lobes involved in visuospatial processing.

Consistent with the argument that there is initial alignment between perception and causal concepts, by 5 years of age children can accurately report variations in outcomes for a range of phenomena, including the impact of start point and surface friction on objects rolling down a slope (Ape, Flottmann, & Leuchter, 2015) and of watering on plant growth (Inagaki & Hatano, 1996; see Howe, 1998; Wilkening & Cacchione, 2011, for other examples). It appears to be the emergence of *explanatory* ideas that opens up a gap. Even if science concepts initially take the form of representations of covarying events and outcomes (cf. the event schema account in the previous section), they eventually need to incorporate some idea of the causal mechanisms that connect them—it is the introduction of mechanism that turns representations of covariation into genuinely causal concepts (Koslowski & Masnick, 2011). Since causal mechanisms have inherently invisible factors (cf. Piaget, 1972), this cannot be achieved on the basis of perception. This implies a process of enrichment of basic event schemas into what Keil (1994) termed theory-based representations, which are not reliant on direct perception (see also Carey, 1985). Howe (1998) argues there is consistent evidence that these theory-like ideas are slow to emerge, and do so *after* children have grasped many relationships between variables and outcomes. The period from 6 years on is focal, and marked by growth of explanatory language across a wide range of areas—in line with the growing disjunction between perceptual and conceptual performance noted earlier.

This raises the question of how these more elaborated causal concepts develop. A number of authors (e.g., Howe, 1998; Tolmie, Ghazali, & Morris, 2016; Tomasello, 1999) have pointed to a key role here for everyday experiences and the conversations in which these are embedded—and the consequent observed impact of language skills on science. Harris and colleagues (e.g., Harris & Koenig, 2006; Harris & Corriveau, 2014) have shown that children readily attend to the knowledge implications of others' statements (especially their parents), making refined judgments about the reliability of different sources; and that these effects extend to learning about aspects of science. In line with this, Howe (1998) found that topics where children exhibit more theory-like ideas (e.g., heating and forces) correspond with those that are more commonly referred to in everyday conversation. In the context of motion down an incline, Symons, Tolmie, and Oaksford (2015) found that 6- to 11-year-olds exhibited sensitivity to source reliability in being told that weight did not affect outcome, changing their predictions more when that information ostensibly came from a teacher as opposed to another child. Interestingly, a final shift to dismissing weight as a relevant variable only came when children subsequently tested outcomes themselves, suggesting that it was the combination of external information and personal observation—in that order—that had the greatest impact.

Rips et al. (2008) argued in parallel fashion that arithmetical principles cannot be arrived at by induction from perceptual knowledge, since, for example, the commutativity principle (a + b = b + a) applies of necessity to *all* numbers, and could not therefore be determined from restricted direct experience with objects. They suggest instead that children acquire inherently abstract schemas about arithmetical principles in top-down fashion, and extend the operation of these to physical objects (cf. theory-based causal representations). Although they did not explore the idea in detail, they too pointed to a key role for natural language in the acquisition of these schemas.

Philips and Tolmie (2007) argued that the process by which dialogue with others generates more organised causal concepts can be understood in terms of the representational redescription (RR) model proposed by Karmiloff-Smith (1992) (see also Tomasello, 1999). In the RR model, conceptual development commences with the acquisition of fragmentary implicit representations of action-event relationships (cf. the event schema account). Over time, these representations are coordinated into more general and accessible structures as the connections between them are made explicit, initially via heightened cognitive awareness, and eventually via encoding in language. Karmiloff-Smith portrays this as a solely internal process. However, Philips and Tolmie found that parents' explanatory language while supporting 8-year-olds' performance on a balance task had exactly this effect. By directing children's attention to the key factors underlying balance and providing a sense of the causal mechanism at work, it helped them construct more coordinated, theory-like structures focused on the effects of torque and the application of the torque rule (if weight × distance is equal on both sides of the fulcrum, then balance will be achieved). Children subsequently applied these ideas with increasing consistency in solving and explaining similar problems in the absence of parental support—again indicating that the combination of external input followed by personal observation is particularly effective in promoting the growth of more theoretical concepts.

This socially driven RR account carries a number of important implications. *Firstly*, according to the RR model, at the initial stage of coordination, much of the detail contained in implicit representations is lost and the resulting structures become ideas that are detached from data (Karmiloff-Smith, 1992), in much the same way as noted earlier. As the process of explicit coordination progresses, there is renewed attention to data and mapping of this to language-based structures, but now with that attention being driven by concepts rather than deriving from perceptual information (i.e., it shifts to being top-down instead of bottom-up). This suggests that concepts and perceptual information undergo a shift in relationship from (1) connected but steered by perceptual data; to (2) unconnected, or only loosely connected; to (3) connected again but driven by concepts (cf. Keil, 1994). In line with this shift, Karmiloff-Smith and Inhelder (1974) found that children exhibited a U-shaped pattern in performance when balancing weight-asymmetric objects: 4- and 8-year-olds both performed better than 6-year-olds, but the younger children relied on proprioceptive feedback (bottom-up), and the older on more theoretical conceptions (top-down).

Secondly, since the shift to concept-driven awareness is influenced by external input, its timing varies according to topic. In the context of heating and cooling, for instance, Howe (1998) found that from 6 years on, greater understanding of mechanism was associated with narrowing of attention to the effects of theoretically plausible variables. This influence of concepts on ideas about variables was not apparent till past the age of 10 in the context of flotation, which is less a focus of conversation (see also Wilkening & Cacchione, 2011). Everyday dialogue has an influence not just on emergence of ideas of mechanism, therefore, but also on conceptually driven attention to variables.

Thirdly, once theory-driven representations have emerged, what children explicitly attend to may differ considerably from the information picked up by perceptual representations. Howe, McWilliam, and Cross (2005) found the biggest effect of explanatory dialogue with others (albeit in the context of collaborative group work) was to re-sensitize children's attention to variables, promoting attention to some and reducing it to others. If the ideas children acquire from dialogue are inaccurate or incorrect—as may frequently be the case—this is likely to result in the distortion of deliberate *observations* to fit those ideas, while tacit *perception* remains accurate. In some task contexts, this may produce a complex mix of influence on responses. In Symons' (2017) work on motion down an incline, for instance, responses regarding the effects of genuinely operative variables seemed to be perceptually driven, but the 'observed' effects of weight were a theoretical addition. As Wilkening and Cacchione (2011) noted, "children's intuitive physics is a non-trivial blend of sensorimotor action and operational thought, to use Piagetian terms" (p. 483).

To summarise:

1. Childhood sees the growth of more elaborated concepts of causal processes that increasingly lose alignment with perceptual representations, though they drive more deliberate attention to variables. Arithmetical concepts exhibit a similar pattern.
2. Brain imaging studies confirm the distinctions of the various types of representations constituting conceptual knowledge—in the context of number, at least—which involves various parts of developing brain.
3. These elaborated causal concepts emerge at different rates in different areas, according to the extent and nature of environmental input. The combination of explanatory language from trusted sources and subsequent observation is central to this growth.

4. According to the social RR account, these more theory-driven concepts lead to selective observation to fit ideas, sometimes resulting in inaccuracies that are absent in tacit perceptions.
5. Perceptual and conceptual systems not only appear to have distinct developmental trajectories, but to be differentially activated according to task characteristics even when this leads to conflicting responses.

Late Childhood and Adolescence

As children become exposed to more formal science curricula, instruction takes over from everyday experience as the dominant context for development, and they enter a period of growth of increasingly detailed and refined concepts (Kind, 2013). This requires them to rebuild their existing concepts and the relations between them, though there are different ideas about what this involves.

Theories of *conceptual change* emphasise the restructuring of concepts in response to mismatch between existing ideas and new experiences or ideas (cf. Piaget, 1932, 1985, on the creation of more advanced concepts as a result of conflict-driven re-equilibration of cognitive structures). Carey and colleagues (Carey, 2009; Zaitchik, Solomon, Tardiff, & Bascandziev, 2016) described this in terms of a process of 'Quinian bootstrapping' (i.e., filling out the conceptual content of initially empty or limited symbolic placeholders) that commences in childhood. When conflict is experienced, existing representations—placeholder structures—are extended by deliberate efforts to map between them, draw analogies, and make inductive inferences that link them together. The appeal of this as a process that might explain development over time is that it indicates an inherent pressure towards more refined and complex meta-ideas, and increasing *coherence* between concepts, first in related areas and then more widely.

A second approach, *theory replacement*, also sees a role for conflict with existing structures in promoting change, but via substitution rather than restructuring. According to Vosniadou (2014), learners first construct organised knowledge structures—'framework theories'—on the basis of their everyday experiences and under the influence of everyday culture, before exposure to systematic science instruction starts. Initially, students assimilate the new information this provides into their existing but incompatible knowledge base, creating fragmented conceptions in the process. When the conflict between old and new becomes evident, students resolve this either by accepting the new input over their existing framework or ignoring the novel concepts. Vosniadou and Ioannides (1998) argued that meta-representation (awareness of representations across related areas) is key to recognising conflict, and the need to accept instructed ideas. In contrast to Carey's model, this account suggests that increased coordination is the trigger for change, rather than a result of it, and earlier concepts do not get revised but are simply suppressed.

A third approach sees change as occurring through *conceptual elaboration*. The RR model outlined in the previous section (Karmiloff-Smith, 1992) suggests conceptual growth is largely a gradual and cumulative process of coordination. This is driven by increased breadth of experience and the role of language and more abstract symbols in making connections between representations explicit. Recent work on understanding of physical state change (Tolmie et al., 2016, in preparation) suggests that language relating to mechanism serves an important function in linking concepts together. This work found that explicit references to the role of heat emerged first in the context of melting, but were then extended to both evaporation and freezing. Osborne and Cosgrove (1983) also found that heat becomes recognised in early adolescence as a common mechanism across different types of physical state change, and is increasingly understood to involve the transmission of energy. Coherence between related concepts may therefore take the form of ideas of causal mechanisms being extended from more to less developed cognate areas as they become more refined. The social RR model (Philips & Tolmie, 2007) suggests external input plays a key role in this, by providing more elaborated language and symbolic expressions (cf. the torque rule example) to capture and describe mechanisms, and drawing out the connections between concepts. Ideas about variables become tied to these concepts of mechanism (i.e., become theory-driven; cf. Keil, 1994), and variables that fail to fit (e.g., shape in the context of flotation) are discounted (Wilkening & Cacchione, 2011). This also leads to greater understanding of the joint operation of variables (e.g., the role of density in flotation as the combined impact of weight and size; Janke, 1995).

Changes of this kind occur on a wide scale. Science learning during this period requires a massive and *organised* increase in subject knowledge and conceptual understanding. Amin, Smith, and Wiser (2014) framed this in terms of the growth of *knowledge networks*. These are comprised of a range of heterogeneous elements, including propositional representations captured first in language and then in more abstract mathematical symbols and expressions, as well as image schematic representations (cf. the role of perceptual structures), and eventually models that integrate these to provide coherent and generalised understanding of causal mechanisms. Moreover, increased conceptual understanding now becomes combined with procedural skills that can be used to systematically explore mechanisms, especially in the context of project work and problem solving. Ability in science during this period therefore becomes increasingly a matter of the *use* of subject knowledge, leaving conceptual understanding as one element of a much wider skill set (Amin et al., 2014). This usage affects the growth of knowledge networks, and the coherence of perceptual, language-based and mathematical/symbolic representations within these, since it influences how much experience and effort is put into developing them. Note too the implication that mathematical and symbolic representations acquired in other contexts become repurposed to serve causal understanding as part of this process of interconnectivity (cf. Rips et al., 2008, on the extension of abstract schemas to different contexts).

This is the point at which students most obviously diverge into more and less expert.

The three approaches to conceptual development just described suggest differing ways in which education contributes to this process. Accounts of *Quinian bootstrapping* portray conceptual growth as being essentially driven by learners' own efforts, although science curricula may provide a stimulus for conflict and exposure to the elements that help resolve it. However, Wiser and Smith (2016) argued that Quinian bootstrapping is inadequate on its own to explain the scale of change that occurs (the 'incommensurability problem'). This is only possible via ordered external assistance that promotes successive approximations to more advanced concepts. *Theory replacement* assumes external input from education but provides no account of what determines when instructed concepts are chosen in preference to earlier framework theories, or what happens cognitively when they are. Conceptual *elaboration* actively embraces a role for education if the impact of external influence is accepted. The argument that the combination of language/symbolic representations that define mechanisms more precisely with subsequent direct experience helps learners to build out incrementally from initial core concepts resembles Wiser and Smith's (2016) learning progression model. Within this, instruction proceeds by supporting development of successive stepping stones via a similar combination of conceptual input and direct experience.

The increasing interconnectivity underpinning the growth of knowledge networks (Amin et al., 2014) may be supported by the formation of associative conceptual networks at a neurocognitive level, with language and other forms of symbolic representation serving as the bridging device (see Rips, Smith, & Medin, 2012; Thomas, Purser, & Mareschal, 2012). Mechanism-related language or symbolic representations acquired in one context initially activate concepts related to that context most strongly. When the same language or symbols are encountered in a different context, it creates linked activations that facilitate the connection of ideas regarding mechanism and variables from the initial context to the new one. The growth of knowledge networks may not only be a product of this increasing connectivity, but also a resource that makes further interconnection possible when students are required to address novel problems. This process has similarities to the connection by analogy described by Carey (2009), but the implication is that it occurs more automatically as a product of repeated linked experiences, driven by education.

The development of more refined and integrated concepts—and eventually models—may also be supported by other types of core cognitive activity. One particular area of interest has been the role of executive function (EF), the ability to shift focus of attention, inhibit previously dominant activations and update understanding (Miyake et al., 2000). Zaitchik et al. (2016) argued that improvements in EF (see Zelazo, Carlson, & Kesek, 2008) are a key facilitator of bootstrapping. Consistent with this, data from a meta-analysis of functional magnetic resonance imaging (fMRI) with more than 800 children and adolescents (Houde, Rossi, Lubin, & Joliot, 2010) showed that children engage the frontal cortex when dealing with numerical tasks, placing greater demands on EF; but with age, a shift to the parietal cortex is observable, as processing becomes more automated. This leads to a reduction in cognitive load, making it possible to engage in more complex operations. Vosniadou (2014) similarly saw EF as central to both meta-representational awareness and the inhibition of framework theories once these have been replaced. She also argued that maturation of the anterior cingulate plays an important role in conflict detection (cf. Fugelsang & Dunbar, 2005). Conceptual elaboration less obviously requires EF, though it may enable deliberate extension of ideas across contexts and the suppression of inappropriate connections.

However, the evidence of EF effects in science learning is inconsistent. In line with theory replacement, Brookman-Byrne, Mareschal, Tolmie, and Dumontheil (2018) found that individual differences in 11- to 15-year-olds' inhibitory control predicted their ability to identify accurate science concepts in preference to common misconceptions (see Mareschal, 2016, for a broader review). Latzman, Elkovitch, Young, and Clark (2010) found that measures of the EF ability of shifting also predicted adolescent science attainment. However, there is little evidence that updating ability—theoretically the most relevant aspect of EF in terms of conceptual integration—has any impact. Moreover, not all kinds of learning can be explained by the inhibition of prior (false) beliefs. In line with this, inhibition was not a significant influence on performance on a general science measure in Mayer, Sodian, Koerber, and Schwippert's (2014) study of 11-year-olds; or on biology and chemistry attainment in two studies by Rhodes with 12–13-year-olds (Rhodes et al., 2014, 2016). These variations in reported findings are not explicable in terms of the importance of EF growing with age, either, since other studies have found evidence of positive EF influence with younger children (e.g., Zaitchik, Iqbal, & Carey, 2014). Overall, the picture is of certain aspects of EF having an effect that is restricted to certain aspects of performance, in keeping with the conceptual elaboration account. These may include use of controlled tests, where adolescents manifest problems in maintaining a stable focus on individual variables because of the cognitive load involved (Howe et al., 1999; Kuhn, Iordanou, Pease, & Wirkala, 2008; Schauble, Klopfer, & Raghavan, 1991).

There is more consistent evidence of the influence of spatial abilities, although these have been less well researched. Spatial ability during adolescence is a strong predictor of following a STEM pathway after school, with 45% of those holding STEM PhDs in the top 4% of spatial ability 11 years previously (Wai, Lubinksi, & Benbow, 2009). Delialioğlu and Aşkar (1999) found that spatial ability (rotation and visualisation) accounted for 9% of the variance in physics test scores in high school students. Stavridou and Kakana (2008) found a high correlation in 14-year-olds between science performance and spatial ability, as assessed by a drawing task, a mental rotation task and a block design task. More recent work (Dündar-Coecke & Tolmie, 2018; Dündar-Coecke, Tolmie, & Schlottmann, submitted) has focused on the specific role of spatial-temporal ability (mental transformations of spatial properties over *time*) in understanding of naturally occurring causal processes, and found that by 11 years of age, this is the strongest predictor of causal understanding itself (up to 16% explained variance), as well as a unique predictor of grasp of causal mechanisms. This suggests that greater ability to map these temporal transformations provides learners with direct insight into the operation of mechanisms, taking their understanding beyond language-based explanations, and supplementing symbolic representations.

To summarise:

1. There are different accounts explaining how scientific concepts become more refined and mechanism-focused during late childhood and adolescence, as learners encounter formal science curricula, with theories of conceptual change, theory replacement and conceptual elaboration proposing the involvement of contrasting processes in terms of deliberate individual effort and external input.
2. Development in this period can be characterised as involving the growth of knowledge networks that comprise increasingly interconnected schematic, linguistic, and abstract symbolic representations, especially among those who are becoming more expert in science. This growth—and the role of education within it—appears to be best explained by the conceptual elaboration account. This argues that external input of explanatory language and symbolic representations alongside practical experience (cf. the social RR model) is central, providing a tool for conceptual activation and organisation.
3. The growth of knowledge networks may be supported by the formation of associative networks at the neurocognitive level. It is less clear how far executive function has an impact, although suppression of misconceptions through inhibitory control may be helpful under some circumstances.
4. Evidence is more robust on the role of spatial, in particular spatial-temporal analysis of causal processes, and this may be distinct from language-based and symbolic representations in important ways.

Adulthood

By adulthood, humans have developed a sophisticated and flexible system for forming categories and concepts at levels from the perceptual to the abstract, according to need. As we shall see, this flexibility is a hallmark of adult reasoning, but is often unacknowledged. For instance, despite the evidence of separation between levels of representation discussed in the first two sections, the consensus remains that most concepts are inferred from perceptual properties. Because of this, although categories imply a broader class than lexicalized concepts (i.e., are not dependent on words to mark them), many cognitive theories draw no distinction between category learning and concept acquisition (see Sloutsky, 2010), and simply attempt to explain both aspects of learning through the same mechanisms (e.g., rule-based categories, prototype theory, exemplar theory, family resemblance, decision bound theory, information integration). However, when the focus shifts to how adults use existing representations in other tasks—in this case reasoning about scientific phenomena—we venture into less established territory. In this context, theories have begun to move away from single approaches to address the full complexity of human representation (see e.g., Ashby & Maddox, 2005; Close, Hahn, Hodgetts, & Pothos, 2010; Kruschke, 2005).

The neuroscience of adult category learning considers the role of multiple systems even within conceptual categorization (e.g., Ashby, Alfonso-Reese, Turken, & Waldron, 1998; Nomura et al., 2007), in line with the existence of a more diverse set of cognitive processes. For instance, investigating the neurobiology of category learning, Ashby and Crossley (2010) suggest that various brain regions (basal ganglia, striatum, hippocampus, prefrontal cortex) and neural pathways mediate category learning, underpinned by two distinct memory systems: declarative (i.e., explicit) working memory, with activity focused in the head of the caudate nucleus; and procedural or nondeclarative (i.e., tacit) memory, with activity in the body and tail of the caudate and putamen. Though there is ongoing debate on the structures involved in category learning, most studies have indicated activity in the cortex, basal ganglia, thalamus, and medial temporal lobe (see e.g., Ashby & Waldron, 2000; Sloutsky, 2010, for a broad review).

One body of research also indicates maturation of the prefrontal cortex from childhood to adulthood—resulting in more efficient executive function—is relevant to abstract category learning (Diamond, 2002; Fan, McCandliss, Sommer, Raz, & Posner, 2002). This suggests there are substantial developmental differences in abstract concept formation. Consistent with this, behavioural data indicate that, for instance, children and adults differ in the use of category labels. For adults, a label is a symbol that represents a category; for children, labels often function as features (i.e., they are treated as equivalent to colour, shape, size etc.) contributing to similarity-based thinking (Sloutsky & Fisher, 2004; Yamauchi & Markman, 2000; Yamauchi & Yu, 2008). As suggested previously, this implies that early in development learning processes are subserved by different systems, probably more perceptually driven; in contrast to this, later learning systems can integrate more elaborate representational and abstract operations, which are crucial to the acquisition of abstract mathematical and scientific concepts.

Adults themselves also differ in level of expertise. The period of post-compulsory education and shift into work sees a continued divergence between the more and the less 'expert' in terms of formal engagement in science learning and involvement in science careers. At the same time, though, one of the consequences of modern schooling is that an increasing proportion of adults are scientifically literate. Even if they are not scientists, adults often acquire a refined set of concepts from relevant scientific literature. Many of them continue to learn science in their informal environment (self-directed, practical, goal-oriented learning), and tend to consider a wide variety of sources rather than relying on a single source (e.g., see Miller's 2010, 'civic scientific literacy' model).

Despite these different elements of increased sophistication, however—and the growth of knowledge networks outlined in the previous section—many adults still appear to show compartmentalization between formal and less formal understanding. Under some circumstances, they revert to the use of more intuitive concepts, regardless of the training that they have received. This suggests that conceptual organization—and activation—post-adolescence may in fact not be that different in some fundamental ways, with new layers being added on top of existing ones rather than the latter being transformed (cf. Vosniadou, 2014, on the replacement of earlier framework theories with ideas received via instruction, without those earlier concepts being overwritten or lost).

For instance, McCloskey (1983) reports a series of studies with undergraduate students in which they were asked to make predictions about the paths that would be followed by falling objects that were already in motion at the point of descent. Errors were frequent, even among students taking a college physics course. A subsequent study by Anderson, Howe, and Tolmie (1996) using the same problems as McCloskey found a similar mixture of prediction errors. Interestingly, though, explanation responses were more consistent, and the correlation of explanation quality with prediction quality was close to zero, suggesting participants made use of two distinct levels of representation for different aspects of the task. Prediction responses appeared to have commonly followed from activation of less integrated, fragmentary, and often incorrect simulations of expected outcomes (cf. Vosniadou's framework theories). Explanations, on the other hand, seemed to have been based on more coherent and explicit mental models of the forces at work.

An EEG study by Kallai and Reiner (2010) employing a trajectory task based on McCloskey (1983), indicates a third level of representation in addition to these two. Participants viewed animations of an object exiting (1) straight versus circular tubes with (2) normal parabolic versus circular motion. In their behavioural judgments of whether the displayed motion was accurate, participants made more errors for the circular tube, in line with McCloskey's results. However, EEG data on the same trials showed a negative activation peak at 400 ms (associated with perceptual violations) for displays of circular motion, irrespective of tube type. This suggests that participants held an accurate perceptual expectation about the trajectory shape that was overruled by the behavioural judgment in the case of the circular tube. Importantly, there were no differences in response patterns among participants who had taken physics courses.

Taken alongside the data from McCloskey (1983) and Anderson et al. (1996), this suggests such problems result in three levels of activity: (1) a perceptual level corresponding to the N400 pattern noted by Kallai and Reiner, and perhaps a continuing manifestation of the tacit perceptual representations discussed in earlier sections; (2) partially explicit rule-based frameworks of cause-effect relationships, tied to particular event types; and (3) fully explicit and coordinated concepts of cause-effect relations that can be applied across different events, corresponding to products of the knowledge networks described previously. These three levels appear to be largely unintegrated for many people, and the third may vary across individuals according to exposure to formal instruction in or personal engagement with science, providing the main source of difference between experts and novices.

The data also suggest that these different levels of representation are not just largely separated, but that conflicts between them are effectively ignored by many participants in favour of the intuitive and dominant middle level. However, Fugelsang and Dunbar (2005) found that processing of patterns of data that were inconsistent with an otherwise plausible theory led to activation of (1) conflict detection mechanisms in the anterior cingulate, and (2) executive function mechanisms in the dorsolateral prefrontal cortex. In other words, conflicts between representations and data apparently activate alert mechanisms (cf. the N400 pattern) and, on Fugelsang and Dunbar's interpretation, suppression of the inconsistent information, in order to maintain existing beliefs. The implication is that the preference for the intuitive middle level is the result of active management of conflicts rather than a passive process—and that there is some degree of connection between the levels otherwise the conflict would not be detected.

Moreover, there is evidence that for some individuals conflict between the different levels of representation leads to inhibition of intuitive expectations rather than of inconsistent data or accurate tacit perceptions. Masson, Potvin, Riopel, and Brault Foisy (2014) report that when presented with diagrams of non-functional electric circuits that nevertheless correspond to common misconceptions, physics experts who accurately judged the stimuli to be incorrect showed increased activation in the dorsolateral and ventrolateral prefrontal cortex and anterior cingulate cortex. These activations were absent among novices who judged the circuits to be functional. Masson et al. conclude that these brain activations reflect the experts' inhibition of misconceptions or naïve responses to the stimuli—i.e., the middle level in the specification outlined earlier—and corresponding attention to the relationship between data and theoretical models.

The implication is that experts deal with conflict in a different way to novices, explaining why, despite the proliferation of errors, many responses in the McCloskey (1983) and Kallai and Reiner (2010) studies were actually scientifically accurate; and why, in the McCloskey studies at least, these accurate responses were more likely to be made by those with formal training in science. Such individuals may differ in the extent of connection between levels, with greater coordination in particular between perceptual systems and theoretical models, i.e., they exhibit fuller integration of the elements comprising knowledge networks.

For this reason, we distinguish between non-experts, experts, and highly experienced experts in a particular field rather than focusing on age as such. We propose that adults who are more expert not only have more detailed knowledge in their chosen areas than children and adolescents, but know things *in a different way.* In order to illustrate the nature of this difference, consider the contrast between a teenager learning to drive a car and an experienced adult driver. The teenager may possess an array of concepts related to driving—the parts of the vehicle and what they do, the position of vehicles on the road in different contexts, the signals that other drivers may make to indicate upcoming movements, and so on. However, these concepts are as yet essentially individual elements, and the task of driving is highly taxing because each has to be laboriously connected to others, and the implications computed. What experienced drivers have acquired is a mental *system* of how traffic environments function that automatically interconnects the constituent concepts, representations, and relationships between them into a dynamic and (mostly) predictable superordinate process, that can be tracked and interacted with at a fraction of the cognitive load (cf. Durkin & Tolmie, 2010). Note too that this system is *shared* with other drivers, otherwise coordinated behaviour would not be possible. Similarly, in science, as compared to laymen, experts utilise many diverse representations in practice. Therefore, they must develop the skills of structuring, interpreting, translating between various representations, and meta-representational competence for specific problems (see Stull, Hegarty, Dixon, & Stieff, 2012). The growth of increasingly automated associative networks (see earlier) may assist in this.

We therefore argue that highly experienced experts in science rely on detailed and shared causal models of how the different elements within systems operate and interact with each other. They also use more and more abstract representations in order to be precise in their communications about these. Moreover, these concepts may convey different meanings within these models and may mislead non-experts with less contextual knowledge. For instance, in statistics, concepts such as correlation, regression, and likelihood do not have implications within causal models. On the other hand, causal concepts like influence, effect, confounding, intervention, and so on suggest more structural relations, making it possible to distinguish between 'the effects of applied cause' and 'the causes of observed effects' (see Pearl, 2000). Therefore, models guide experts to categorize, predict, explain, and act to achieve their goals in more refined ways, as they provide knowledge about both causal and acausal processes.

These causal relations are also critical for categorization (Sloman, 2005). For instance, the most natural explanation of 'why a kitten is a cat but not a dog' is that it has cat parents, their genetic structure, and behaviour. In other words, categories inherit causal relations that can be used to determine membership, as in Sloman's example of resolving perception of a winged shape in the sky making a roaring sound via an airplane causal model rather than a bird or car model (Sloman, 2005, pp. 126–127). The implication is that adults are active problem solvers and hypothesis testers during the concept formation and identification process, and this involves reasoning about both actuals and counterfactuals. They use a set of logical tools, what Smith and Medin (1981) called 'necessary and sufficient conditions', in order to determine their decisions regarding membership of a category (Mathews, Stanley, Buss, & Chinn, 1984–1985). For instance, if the relation between two events is causal, a causal model is employed (e.g., mathematical equations; social models such as schemas and attitudes). If it is not, a search for analogies or associations is considered. The further corollary is that experts categorize and conceptualise phenomena *differently* to non-experts because they operate models at a more abstract level.

To summarise:

1. Adults—especially those with greater scientific expertise—continue to build more sophisticated, elaborated, and integrated conceptual systems, and exhibit greater flexibility in the application of these.
2. Nevertheless, many still show evidence of distinct representational systems, at the perceptual level, a partially explicit conceptual level corresponding to earlier framework theories, and a more fully explicit conceptual level based on causal models derived from knowledge networks. In general, the intermediate level—based on initial language-based representations—appears to dominate in many task contexts, with perceptual representations in particular effectively reduced to low-level neural activations that are actively ignored.
3. This dominance of language-based representations appears to be less the case for those with well-developed scientific expertise, possibly because they have acquired better integrated causal models or strategies to deal with abstract phenomena. We consider the implications of this further after the following section.

Language Induced Thoughts Versus Inadequacy of Language in Science

The formation of concepts in science is complex. On the basis of what has been considered in the previous sections there is no doubt that language has a ubiquitous influence on understanding of science. It plainly provides a basis for capturing ideas about causal processes through accounts received from others, whether deliberately or in passing. Perhaps more importantly, it provides a tool for coordinating experiences into more general representations and plays an active role in the way even scientists communicate to each other and with others. This communication relies on the body of concepts and categories that are used for not just verbal descriptions of objects or events but also as a mental strategy to deal with different forms of representations, including their semantic functions. However, solely language-based analysis of causal understanding is limited and also implausible, given the role of both perceptual representations and abstract models discussed previously.

Neural analyses of human thinking suggest that we are multimodal reasoners, and our thinking abilities are not constrained solely by language. Looking at brain organization and processes, research has suggested that although there is a close relationship between language and logical thinking, human thought uses a network system comprised of multiple functions (see e.g., Gazzaniga, 1967, on functional laterality). Reber, Stark, and Squire (1998a, 1998b) scanned participants while they carried out explicit prototype-extraction and implicit category recognition tasks. The recognition task resulted in increased activations in numerous brain areas which were *not* activated in the explicit task. In particular, an area of the visual cortex involved in early visual processing was activated in recognition but deactivated in explicit categorization. Ashby and Crossley (2010) also reported that category learning in explicit rule-based and implicit information integration tasks differentially activated areas in the caudate and striatum. Moreover, success in the implicit task but not the explicit one required immediate feedback, took substantially longer, and the results were not amenable to verbalisation. Rips et al. (2012) argued that these implicit structures are more akin to sensations, and not available to communication. They concluded that since different perceptual modalities are processed in different brain regions, "perceptual-conceptual knowledge" must be represented by a distributed network of brain regions, again implying that these different elements are distinct. Similarly, Hayward and Tarr (1995) asserted that there are various visual percepts that we cannot put into words. For example, we are very accurate at perceiving differences between faces and yet often find it extremely difficult to describe why one face is different from another.

The inadequacies of natural language become more prominent in the context of adult science. One difficulty arises from *scientific clarification*. Since the concepts of ordinary language are mostly imprecise and context-dependent, general laws are formulated by means of mathematical language or statistical models that aim to achieve complete precision. Accuracy, precision, and efficiency of information and meaning are addressed by specialised symbolic systems (e.g., numbers, axioms, equations) which rely to a high degree on abstract thinking. By using these specialised systems, scientific research should deal with the need for *consistent* disambiguation.

These systems are not static, either. Understanding of phenomena in science evolves and changes discontinuously (cf. Kuhn's, 1970, notion of 'paradigm shift'), with the result that older concepts cease to apply and are replaced by new ways of thinking. In Heisenberg's (1958–1989) expression, words and concepts that are familiar in daily life become *increasingly* distant from science, and lose their meanings when they are applied to, for instance, general relativity and quantum mechanics. There is no way of speaking about atoms in ordinary language, and in consequence their underlying ontology. Therefore, the translation of mathematical symbols to common concepts of ordinary language is highly problematic. What is translated is not the notion representing the phenomena itself, but the eventual modification of that logic in natural language. In Bohr's example (see Peterson, 1968), words like 'position', 'momentum', 'space' and 'time', which refer to classical conceptual representations, have no sense in quantum theory. These examples underline the fact that concepts and words may become meaningless or constrain human thinking when new understanding of phenomena is required.

To summarise, then:

1. There are different levels or forms of human thinking, many of which cannot be articulated properly, such as symbols/numbers, diagrams, imagery, or imageless thoughts that aid this, and as our use of music, pictorial arts, ballet, signs and gestures illustrates, we often use alternative channels to send and receive sophisticated meanings, feelings, or interpretations, so as to avoid missing information in our communications. These may take longer to understand, but the convenience of language does not mean that we are tied strictly to language-driven concepts in science, whether formal or informal understanding.

2. An integrated understanding of causality requires some translation of qualitative and quantitative features, and their representations in linguistic knowledge. However, this comes with an inevitable information loss in thought/feelings/knowings (cf. Dündar-Coecke, 2014; Dündar-Coecke, submitted). The linguistic outcomes of this translation (between senses, experience, thought) cannot cover at least some part of the information. Other levels of representation must be maintained, therefore.

3. Highly experienced experts in science appear in fact to be able to maintain or recover a combination of perceptual and conceptual representations—especially in abstract causal models—that appears commonly to become lost during typical development; how they achieve this is not as yet well understood.

Conclusions

What Has Neuroscience Added to Our Understanding Over and Above Psychology?

Neuroscience research relevant to conceptual development in science has led to a richer, if more complex, understanding of what this development involves. Previously dominant Piagetian and information processing approaches to the development of science understanding have portrayed this as a process of coordination of concepts into more coherent overarching structures. Within these, conflicts and inconsistencies are gradually resolved. Neuroscience, and behavioural work informed by it, reveals instead that fragmented—or at best loosely connected—representations and concepts of different types and degrees of accuracy are present from early childhood and persist into adulthood, each with its own trajectory of development. Apparent gains in understanding result from new layers of representation being added on top of existing ones. This typically happens without earlier representations being altered or replaced, and as a result, different tasks activate different representational levels. By late childhood, though, partially explicit—and often only partially accurate— language-based concepts have become central to behavioural responses, and commonly remain so. Greater connection between implicit perceptual representations and more fully explicit concepts and causal models does occur, and results in more accurate and flexible understanding. However, this is more usually the case for those with higher levels of expertise.

Concrete Implications of Research and Opportunities for Translation

Recognition of this complexity helps set a clearer agenda for the work of science educators. The neuroscience account suggests that good understanding of science requires the building of *bridges*—not fully integrated structures, given the different neural systems involved—between perceptual (in the widest sense), conceptual and abstract capacities. The first supplies an implicit sense of 'how things are' that serves as a resource for new insights. The second provides initial frameworks for thinking explicitly about the logic of causal sequences. The last underpins grasp of established scientific ideas and ways of representing these accurately and consistently, allowing room for alternatives. Educators need to support development of all three strands of representation, and connections between them, as a cumulative exercise from preschool towards high school. This support involves: activities encouraging implicit and explicit processes in learning, as connected to verbal concepts and operative variables and their outcomes; encouraging imaginative thinking about the causal processes that facilitates use of non-linguistic representations of causal mechanisms (e.g., spatial-temporal awareness); and exposure to accurate models through the scientific language that children hear, using these for building abstract levels of representations. Note that these ideas can then be taken as a *start* point for the development of richer knowledge networks.

Further Resources for the Reader

While we have identified a wide range of relevant literature in each of the sections of this chapter, the interested reader may wish to look further at the following sources, which cover in greater depth the focal issues that we have addressed:

Mandler (2004) provides one of the key arguments for the separation of perceptual and conceptual representations.
Mareschal, Quinn, and Lea (2010) is a collection of chapters by leading researchers in the field of human concepts, many of which have direct relevance to the points

that we have discussed, including the neuroscience evidence on multiple representational systems.

Deheane et al. (1999) provide key behavioural and neuroscience evidence on the separation of language-based and visuospatial systems in the context of mathematics.

Wilkening and Cacchione (2011) provide a very detailed overview of evidence relating to the shift from variable-based to explanatory concepts in primary age children's understanding of science.

Klahr (2000) contains a detailed account of work relating to the way in which activity in science relates to children's growing understanding.

Philips and Tolmie (2007) contains both the detailed theoretical argument in favour of the social RR model of conceptual elaboration, and evidence relating to this in the context of balance.

Amin et al. (2014) provide a wide-ranging and carefully assembled overview of theories and evidence relating to student conceptions and conceptual growth through the primary and secondary school years.

Mareschal (2016) provides an important holistic view on recent neuroscience work relating to science concepts.

Sloman (2005) is a detailed and very readable account of causal systems and causal reasoning in adults.

Note

1. NB Gibbs (2003) suggests that embodiment contributes extensively to concept formation and conceptual representations beyond the sensory-motor stage, a point we will return to.

References

Amin, T. G., Smith, C., & Wiser, M. (2014). Student conceptions and conceptual change: Three overlapping phases of research. In N. Lederman and S. Abell (Eds.), *Handbook of research in science education* (Vol. II, pp. 57–81). New York: Routledge.

Anderson, A., Howe, C. J., & Tolmie, A. (1996). Interaction and mental models of physics phenomena: Evidence from dialogues between learners. In J. Oakhill & A. Garnham (Eds.), *Mental models in cognitive science: Essays in honour of Phil Johnson-Laird* (pp. 247–273). London: Psychology Press.

Ape, M., Flottmann, J., & Leuchter, M. (2015). *Coherence between science content and process knowledge in preschool age.* EARLI Biennial Conference, Limassol.

Ashby, F. G., Alfonso-Reese, L. A., Turken, A. U., & Waldron, E. M. (1998). A neuropsychological theory of multiple systems in category learning. *Psychological Review*, *105*, 442–481.

Ashby, F. G., & Crossley, M. J. (2010). The neurobiology of categorization. In D. Mareschal, P. C. Quinn, & S. E. G. Lea (Eds.), *The making of human concepts* (pp. 75–98). New York: Oxford University Press.

Ashby, F. G., & Maddox, T. W. (2005). Human category learning. *Annual Review of Psychology*, *56*, 149–178.

Ashby, F. G., & Waldron, G. M. (2000). The neuropsychological bases of category learning. *Current Directions in Psychological Science*, *9*(1), 10–14.

Brookman-Byrne, A., Mareschal, D., Tolmie, A. K., & Dumontheil, I. (2018). Inhibitory control and counterintuitive science and math reasoning in adolescence. *PLOS One*, *13*(6), e0198973.

Carey, S. (1985). *Conceptual change in childhood.* Cambridge, MA: MIT Press.

Carey, S. (2009). *The origins of concepts.* New York: Oxford University Press.

Close, J., Hahn, U., Hodgetts, C. J., & Pothos, E. M. (2010). Rules and similarity in adult concept learning. In D. Mareschal, P. C. Quinn, & S. E. G. Lea (Eds.), *The making of human concepts* (pp. 29–52). Oxford: Oxford University Press.

Deheane, S., Spelke, E., Pinel, P., Stanescu, R., & Tsivkin, S. (1999). Sources of mathematical thinking: Behavioral and brain-imaging evidence. *Science, 284,* 970–974.

Delialioğlu, Ö., & Aşkar, P. (1999). Contribution of students' mathematical skills and spatial ability of achievement in secondary school physics. *Hacettepe Üniversitesi Eğitim Fakültesi Dergisi, 16.*

Diamond, A. (2002). Normal development of prefrontal cortex from birth to young adulthood: Cognitive functions, anatomy, and biochemistry. In D. T. Stuss & R. T. Knight (Eds.), *Principles of frontal lobe function* (pp. 466–503). Oxford: Oxford University Press.

diSessa, A. A. (1988). Knowledge in pieces. In G. Forman & P. Pufall (Eds.), *Constructivism in the computer age* (pp. 49–70). Hillsdale, NJ: Lawrence Erlbaum Associates.

Dunbar, K., & Klahr, D. (1988). Developmental differences in scientific discovery strategies. In D. Klahr & K. Kotovsky (Eds.), *Complex information processing: The impact of Herbert A. Simon. Proceedings of the 21st Carnegie-Mellon symposium on cognition* (pp. 109–144). Hillsdale, NJ: Lawrence Erlbaum Associates.

Dündar-Coecke, S. (2014). Ramifications of quantum physics for education. *Problems of Education in the 21st Century, 58,* 53–66.

Dündar-Coecke, S. (submitted). What quantum physicists can tell educators: A mixed-methods study. *American Journal of Physics.*

Dündar-Coecke, S., & Tolmie, A. (2018). *What skills predict children's understanding of causal processes?* EARLI SIG 22: Neuroscience & Education, London.

Dündar-Coecke, S., Tolmie, A., & Schlottmann, A. (submitted). The development of reasoning and the role of spatial-temporal abilty. *Cognition.*

Durkin, K., & Tolmie, A. (2010). *The development of children's and young people's attitudes to driving: A critical review of the literature.* London: Department for Transport.

Fan, J., McCandliss, B. D., Sommer, T., Raz, A., & Posner, M. I. (2002). Testing the efficiency and independence of attentional networks. *Journal of Cognitive Neuroscience, 14,* 340–347.

French, R. M., Mareschal, D., Mermillod, M., & Quinn, P. C. (2004). The role of bottom-up processing in perceptual categorization by 3- to 4-month-old infants: Simulations and data. *Journal of Experimental Psychology: General, 133,* 382–397.

Fugelsang, J. A., & Dunbar, K. N. (2005). Brain-based mechanisms underlying complex causal thinking. *Neuropsychologia, 43,* 1204–1213.

Gazzaniga, M. S. (1967). The split brain in man. *Scientific American, 217*(2), 24–29.

Gibbs, R. (2003). Embodied experience and linguistic meaning. *Brain and Language, 84*(1), 1–15.

Gopnik, A., & Meltzoff, A. N. (1997). *Words, thoughts, and theories.* Cambridge, MA: MIT Press.

Harris, J. (2014). *Where will it go? Concepts of motion in complex events* (Unpublished PhD thesis), Temple University.

Harris, P. L., & Corriveau, K. H. (2014). Learning from testimony about religion and science. In E. J. Robinson & S. Einav (Eds.), *Trust and skepticism: Children's selective learning from testimony* (pp. 28–41). Hove: Psychology Press.

Harris, P. L., & Koenig, M. (2006). Trust in testimony: How children learn about science and religion. *Child Development, 77,* 505–524.

Hast, M., & Howe, C. (2015). Children's predictions and recognition of fall: The role of object mass. *Cognitive Development, 36,* 103–110.

Hayward, W. G., & Tarr, M. J. (1995). Spatial language and spatial representation. *Cognition, 55,* 39–84.

Heisenberg, W. (1958/1989). *Physics and philosophy: The revolution in modern science.* New York: Harper & Brothers Publishers.

Houde, O., Rossi, S., Lubin, A., & Joliot, M. (2010). Mapping numerical processing, reading, and executive functions in the developing brain: An fMRI meta-analysis of 52 studies including 842 children. *Developmental Science, 13,* 876–885.

Howe, C. J. (1998). *Conceptual structure in childhood and adolescence.* London: Routledge.

Howe, C. J., McWilliam, D., & Cross, G. (2005). Chance favours only the prepared mind: Incubation and the delayed effects of peer collaboration. *British Journal of Psychology, 96,* 67–93.

Howe, C. J., Tolmie, A., & Sofroniou, N. (1999). Experimental appraisal of personal beliefs in science: Constraints on performance in the 9 to 14 age group. *British Journal of Educational Psychology, 69,* 243–274.

Inagaki, K., & Hatano, G. (1996). Young children's recognition of commonalities between animals and plants. *Child Development, 67,* 2823–2840.

Janke, B. (1995). Entwicklung naiven Wissens ü ber den physikalischen Auftrieb: Warum schwimmen Schiffe? *Zeitschrift für Entwicklungspsychologie und Pädagogische Psychologie, 27,* 122–138.

Jenkins, E. (2007). School science: A questionable construct? *Journal of Curriculum Studies, 39,* 265–282.

Kallai, A. Y., & Reiner, M. (2010). *The source of misconceptions in physics: When event-related potential components N400 and P600 disagree.* Paper presented at the 2010 Meeting of the European Association for Research on Learning and Instruction Neuroscience and Education Special Interest Group, Zurich.

Karmiloff-Smith, A. (1992). *Beyond modularity: A developmental perspective on cognitive science.* Cambridge, MA: MIT Press.

Karmiloff-Smith, A., & Inhelder, B. (1974). If you want to get ahead, get a theory. *Cognition, 3,* 195–212.

Keil, F. C. (1994). The birth and nurturance of concepts by domain: The origins of concepts of living things. In L. A. Hirschfeld & S. A. Gelman (Eds.). *Mapping the mind: Domain specificity in cognition and culture* (pp. 234–254). Cambridge: Cambridge University Press.

Kind, P. M. (2013). Conceptualizing the science curriculum: 40 years of developing assessment frameworks in three large-scale assessments: Conceptualizing the science curriculum. *Science Education, 97,* 671–694.

Klahr, D. (2000). *Exploring science: The cognition and development of discovery process.* Cambridge, MA: MIT Press.

Koslowski, B., & Masnick, A. (2011). Causal reasoning and explanation. In U. Goswami (Ed.), *The Wiley-Blackwell handbook of childhood cognitive development* (2nd ed., pp. 377–398). Oxford: Wiley-Blackwell.

Kruschke, J. K. (2005). Category learning. In K. Lamberts & R. L. Goldstone (Eds.), *The handbook of cognition* (pp. 183–201). London: Sage Publications Ltd.

Kuhn, D., Iordanou, K., Pease, M., & Wirkala, C. (2008). Beyond control of variables: What needs to develop to achieve skilled scientific thinking? *Cognitive Development, 23,* 435–451.

Kuhn, T. (1970). *The structure of scientific revolutions.* Chicago: University of Chicago Press.

Lakusta, L., & Wagner, L. (2016). Conceptualising the event. In D. Barner & A. S. Baron (Eds.), *Core knowledge and conceptual change* (pp. 245–260). Oxford: Oxford University Press.

Lamberts, K., & Shanks, D. (1997). *Knowledge, concepts and categories*. Cambridge, MA: MIT Press.

Latzman, R. D., Elkovitch, N., Young, J., & Clark, L. A. (2010). The contribution of executive functioning to academic achievement among male adolescents. *Journal of Clinical and Experimental Neuropsychology, 32*, 455–462.

Leslie, A. M. (1982). The perception of causality in infants. *Perception, 11*, 173–186.

Leslie, A. M., & Keeble, S. (1987). Do six-month-old infants perceive causality? *Cognition, 25*, 265–288.

Link, T., Moeller, K., Huber, S., Fischer, U., & Nuerk, H.-C. (2013). Walk the number line—an embodied training of numerical concepts. *Trends in Neuroscience and Education, 2*, 74–84.

Mandler, J. M. (2004). *The foundations of mind*. Oxford: Oxford University Press.

Mareschal, D. (2016). The neuroscience of conceptual learning in science and mathematics. *Current Opinion in Behavioral Sciences, 10*, 14–18.

Mareschal, D., Quinn, P. C., & French, R. M. (2002). Asymmetric interference in 3- to 4-month-olds' sequential category learning. *Cognitive Science, 26*, 377–389.

Mareschal, D., Quinn, P. C., & Lea, S. E. G. (Eds.). (2010). *The making of human concepts: Oxford series in developmental cognitive neuroscience*. Oxford: Oxford University Press.

Masson, S., Potvin, P., Riopel, M., & Brault Foisy, L.-M. (2014). Differences in brain activation between novices and experts in science during a task involving a common misconception in electricity. *Mind, Brain and Education, 8*, 44–55.

Mathews, R. C., Stanley, W. B., Buss, R. R., & Chinn, R. (1984–1985, Winter). Concept learning: What happens when hypothesis testing fails? *The Journal of Experimental Education, 53*(2), 91–96.

Mayer, D., Sodian, B., Koerber, S., & Schwippert, K. (2014). Scientific reasoning in elementary school children: Assessment and relations with cognitive abilities. *Learning and Instruction, 29*, 43–55.

McCloskey, M. (1983). Naïve theories of motion. In D. Gentner & A. L. Stevens (Eds.), *Mental models* (pp. 299–324). Hillsdale, NJ: Lawrence Erlbaum Associates.

Michotte, A. (1963). *The perception of causality* (Translated from the French by T. R. Miles & E. Miles). New York: Basic Books.

Miller, J. D. (2010). Adult science learning in the internet era. *Curator, 53*(2), 191–208.

Miyake, A., Friedman, N. P., Emerson, M. J., Witzki, A. H., Howerter, A., & Wager, T. D. (2000). The unity and diversity of executive functions and their contributions to complex "frontal lobe" tasks: A latent variable analysis. *Cognitive Psychology, 41*, 49–100.

Murphy, G. L. (2010). What are categories and concepts? In D. Mareschal, P. C. Quinn, & S. E. G. Lea (Eds.), *The making of human concepts* (pp. 11–28). Oxford: Oxford University Press.

Nelson, K. (1996). *Language in cognitive development: The emergence of the mediated mind*. Cambridge: Cambridge University Press.

Nomura, E. M., Maddox, W. T., Filoteo, J. V., Ing, A. D., Gitelman, D. R., Parrish, T. B., . . . Reber, P. J. (2007). Neural correlates of rule-based and information-integration visual category learning. *Cerebral Cortex, 17*, 37–43.

Oakes, L., & Cohen, L. B. (1990). Infant perception of a causal event. *Cognitive Development, 5*, 193–207.

Osborne, R. J., & Cosgrove, M. M. (1983). Children's conception of the changes of state of water. *Journal of Research in Science, 20,* 825–838.

Pearl, J. (2000). *Causality: Models, reasoning, and inference.* New York: Cambridge University Press.

Peterson, A. (1968). *Quantum physics and the philosophical tradition.* Cambridge, MA: MIT Press.

Philips, S., & Tolmie, A. (2007). Children's performance on and understanding of the balance scale problem: The effects of parental support. *Infant and Child Development, 16,* 95–117.

Piaget, J. (1929). *The child's conception of the world.* London: Routledge & Kegan Paul.

Piaget, J. (1932). *The moral judgement of the child.* London: Routledge & Kegan Paul.

Piaget, J. (1972). *The principles of genetic epistemology.* New York: Basic Books.

Piaget, J. (1985). *The equilibration of cognitive structures.* Chicago: Chicago University Press.

Piaget, J., & Inhelder, B. (1971). *The child's conception of space* (F. J. Langdon & J. L. Lunzer, Trans). London: Routledge & Kegan Paul.

Rakinson, D. H., & Lupyan, G. (2008). Developing object concepts in infancy: An associative learning perspective. *Monographs of Society for Research in Child Development, 73*(1), 1–110.

Reber, P. J., Stark, C. E. L., & Squire, L. R. (1998a). Cortical areas supporting category learning identified using functional MRI. *Proceedings of the National Academy of Sciences of the USA, 95,* 747–750.

Reber, P. J., Stark, C. E. L., & Squire, L. R. (1998b). Contrasting cortical activity associated with category memory and recognition memory. *Learning and Memory, 5,* 420–428.

Reiss, M. (2003). What is science? Teaching science in secondary schools. In E. Scanlon, P. Murphy, J. Thomas, & A. Whitelegg (Eds.), *Reconsidering science learning* (pp. 3–12). London: Routledge Farmer.

Rhodes, S. M., Booth, J. N., Campbell, L. E., Blythe, R. A., Wheate, N. J., & Delibegovic, M. (2014). Evidence for a role of executive functions in learning biology: Executive functions and science. *Infant and Child Development, 23,* 67–83.

Rhodes, S. M., Booth, J. N., Palmer, L. E., Blythe, R. A., Delibegovic, M., & Wheate, N. J. (2016). Executive functions predict conceptual learning of science. *British Journal of Developmental Psychology, 34,* 261–275.

Rips, L. J., Bloomfield, A., & Asmuth, A. (2008). From numerical concepts to concepts of number. *Behavioral and Brain Sciences, 31,* 623–687.

Rips, L. J., Smith, E. E., & Medin, D. L. (2012). Concepts and categories: Memory, meaning, and metaphysics. In K. J. Holyoak & R. G. Morrison (Eds.), *The Oxford handbook of thinking and reasoning* (pp. 177–209). Oxford: Oxford University Press.

Schauble, L., Klopfer, L. E., & Raghavan, K. (1991). Students' transition from an engineering model to a science model of experimentation. *Journal of Research in Science Teaching, 28,* 859–882.

Sloman, S. (2005). *Causal models: How people think about the world and its alternatives.* Oxford: Oxford University Press.

Sloutsky, V. M. (2010). From perceptual categories to concepts: What develops? *Cognitive Science, 34,* 1244–1286.

Sloutsky, V. M., & Fisher, A. V. (2004). Induction and categorization in young children: A similarity-based model. *Journal of Experimental Psychology: General, 133,* 166–188.

Smith, E. E., & Medin, D. L. (1981). *Categories and concepts*. Cambridge, MA: Harvard University Press.

Spelke, E. S., Breinlinger, K., Macomber, J., & Jacobson, K. (1992). Origins of knowledge. *Psychological Review, 99*, 605–632.

Spelke, E. S., Phillips, A., & Woodward, A. L. (1995). Infants' knowledge of object motion and human action. In D. Sperber, D. Premack, & A. J. Premack (Eds.), *Causal cognition: A multidisciplinary debate*. Oxford: Clarendon Press.

Stavridou, F., & Kakana, D. (2008). Graphic abilities in relation to mathematical and scientific ability in adolescents. *Educational Research, 50*, 75–93.

Stull, A. T., Hegarty, M., Dixon, B., & Stieff, M. (2012). Representational translation with concrete models in organic chemistry. *Cognition and Instruction, 30*(4), 404–434.

Symons, G. (2017). *The effect of source reliability on the understanding of causal systems in primary and secondary school children* (Unpublished PhD thesis), University of London, Birkbeck.

Symons, G., Tolmie, A., & Oaksford, M. (2015). *Source reliability in the development of children's understanding of causal systems*. EuroAsianPacific Joint Conference on Cognitive Science, Turin.

Thomas, M. S. C., Purser, H. R. M., & Mareschal, D. (2012). Is the mystery of thought demystified by context-dependent categorisation? Towards a new relation between language and thought. *Mind & Language, 27*(5), 595–618.

Tolmie, A., Ghazali, Z., & Morris, S. (2016). Children's science learning: A core skills approach. *British Journal of Educational Psychology, 86*(3), 481–497.

Tolmie, A., Tenenbaum, H., Pino-Pasternak, D., Reynolds, R., Simes, J., & Messenger, A. (in preparation). *Language and generalization in children's explanations of physical state changes*.

Tomasello, M. (1999). *The cultural origins of human cognition*. Cambridge, MA: Harvard University Press.

Vosniadou, S. (2014). Examining cognitive development from a conceptual change point of view: The framework theory approach. *European Journal of Developmental Psychology, 11*, 1–17.

Vosniadou, S., & Ioannides, C. (1998). From conceptual development to science education: A psychological point of view. *International Journal of Science Education, 20*, 1213–1230.

Vygotsky, L. S. (1962). *Thought and language*. Cambridge, MA: MIT Press.

Wagner, L., & Lakusta, L. (2009). Using language to navigate the infant mind. *Perspectives on Psychological Science, 4*(2), 177–184.

Wai, J., Lubinski, D., & Benbow, C. P. (2009). Spatial ability for STEM domains: Aligning over 50 years of cumulative psychological knowledge solidifies its importance. *Journal of Educational Psychology, 101*, 817–835.

Wellman, H. M. (1990). *The child's theory of mind*. Cambridge, MA: MIT Press.

Wellman, H. M., & Gelman, S. A. (1992). Cognitive development: Foundational theories of core domains. *Annual Review of Psychology, 43*, 337–375.

Wilkening, F., & Cacchione, T. (2011). Children's intuitive physics. In U. Goswami (Ed.), *The Wiley-Blackwell handbook of childhood cognitive development* (2nd ed., pp. 473–496). Oxford: Wiley-Blackwell.

Wiser, M., & Smith, C. L. (2016). How is conceptual change possible? Insights from science education. In D. Barner & A. S. Baron (Eds.), *Core knowledge and conceptual change* (pp. 29–52). Oxford: Oxford University Press.

Yamauchi, T., & Markman, A. B. (2000). Inference using categories. *Journal of Experimental Psychology: Learning, Memory, and Cognition, 26,* 776–795.

Yamauchi, T., & Yu, N.-Y. (2008). Category labels versus feature labels: Category labels polarize inferential predictions. *Memory & Cognition, 36,* 544–553.

Zaitchik, D., Iqbal, Y., & Carey, S. (2014). The effect of executive function on biological reasoning in young children: An individual differences study. *Child Development, 85,* 160–175.

Zaitchik, D., Solomon, G. E. A., Tardiff, N., & Bascandziev, I. (2016). Conceptual change: Where domain-specific learning mechanisms meet domain-general cognitive resources. In D. Barner & A. S. Baron (Eds.), *Core knowledge and conceptual change* (pp. 73–88). Oxford: Oxford University Press.

Zelazo, P. D., Carlson, S. M., & Kesek, A. (2008). The development of executive function in childhood. In C. A. Nelson & M. Luciana (Eds.), *Handbook of developmental cognitive neuroscience* (2nd ed., pp. 533–574). Cambridge, MA: MIT Press.

Zimmerman, C. (2007). The development of scientific thinking skills in elementary and middle school. *Developmental Review, 27,* 172–223.

Section 3

Discipline-General Abilities

Executive Functions, Social
and Affective Development

9 The Development of Executive Functions in Childhood and Adolescence and Their Relation to School Performance

Sabine Peters

In order for a child to be successful in school, there are many skills to master aside from academic skills alone. For instance, children must be able to think about and manipulate information, avoid being distracted by irrelevant stimuli and stay focused on a certain task for a prolonged period. These kinds of cognitive skills are often grouped under the umbrella term of 'executive functions'. Broadly, executive functions (often used synonymously with the term cognitive control) refer to the ability to control and regulate one's behavior so that certain goals (such as performing well in school) can be reached. Executive functions are not a unitary process, but, as the name implies, consist of different subfunctions. There are higher-order executive functions such as planning, multitasking and performance monitoring, which rely on the building blocks of lower-order executive functions. The most important lower-order executive functions are generally thought to be (1) working memory, (2) inhibition, and (3) cognitive flexibility (Huizinga, Dolan, & van der Molen, 2006; Miyake et al., 2000). *Working memory* refers to the ability to keep relevant information 'online' in your mind, such as when performing arithmetic problems: Working memory is necessary to keep the problem in mind, to perform the necessary calculation steps and to remember the outcomes of previous steps. *Inhibition* is the ability to only attend to the relevant task and disregard irrelevant distractions, such as from other students or smartphones. *Cognitive flexibility* means being able to quickly adapt and adjust behavior when the current behavior is no longer working, such as when receiving negative feedback from a teacher, or when switching from addition to subtraction arithmetic problems.

Studying executive functions is important for school settings for several reasons. First, in many cases educational programs are not well-tailored to the specific level of neural development and executive functions a child or adolescent possesses at that age. Knowing about executive functions and neural development can help to adjust educational programs to a pupil's current developmental stage. Second, it has been shown that measures of executive functions and neural measures can help to predict future school performance. This may help with early identification of students who will potentially run into problems. Third, training programs targeting executive functions might be able to improve school performance. This is especially interesting given its potential efficiency: What if instead of training a specific skill (e.g., mathematics), we could train executive functions and improve performance on multiple school subjects?

In this chapter, I will provide an overview of adolescent brain development and its implications for the development of executive functions. The development of working memory, inhibition and cognitive flexibility will be described separately, as well as their neural underpinnings, trainability and relevance for school settings.

Adolescent Brain Development and Executive Functioning

Adolescence is a period that is especially interesting to study in the context of executive functioning. Biologically, adolescence starts with the onset of puberty around age 10 (Shirtcliff, Dahl, & Pollak, 2009), and continues until the early twenties (Steinberg, 2008). A key finding from research on adolescent brain development has indicated that the frontal cortex develops for much longer than was previously thought, until the age of around 22 years old (Giedd et al., 1999; Gogtay et al., 2004). This is important in the context of cognitive performance and school performance, because the frontal cortex is a crucial brain region for executive functioning (Diamond, 2013). These and other studies set the stage for the most prominent theory on adolescent brain development: the imbalance model (also referred to as the dual-systems model; Ernst, Pine, & Hardin, 2006; Somerville & Casey, 2010; Steinberg, 2008). This theory states that brain regions for cognitive control (such as the frontal cortex) develop more slowly compared to 'emotional' brain regions (such as the striatum), resulting in an imbalance between the emotional and cognitive control systems in adolescence. Moreover, many studies have shown that there is even a peak in the activity of emotional brain regions in adolescence, especially for activity in brain regions associated with reward (e.g., the striatum; for a meta-analysis see Silverman, Jedd, & Luciana, 2015). The adolescent brain has therefore been compared to a car in which the gas pedal is working overtime, but in which the brakes and steering wheel are not yet strong enough to keep the car under control (Payne, 2012). The imbalance model has been used to explain (stereo)typical adolescent behaviors such as impulsivity and risk-taking, but also difficulties with executive functioning, such as problems with planning and organizing. This is one example of how neuroimaging findings have led to a better understanding of adolescent behaviors by providing a neurobiological explanation for reduced executive functioning capacity in adolescence. This is highly relevant for school settings because it suggests that the adolescent brain simply functions differently from the adult brain, and consequently educational programs should take into account this reduced capacity for executive functioning to help optimize school settings for adolescents. In the next sections, the development of specific executive functions (working memory, inhibition and cognitive flexibility) and their importance for school learning will be described in more detail.

In the final section, I will describe more recent research which emphasizes not only vulnerabilities, but also unique opportunities of the adolescent brain.

The Development of Working Memory

Given its critical role in all aspects of cognition, multiple studies have investigated whether working memory skills are related to school performance. A possible way in which low working memory may have consequences for school learning is that it constitutes a bottleneck which limits the amount of information that children can keep in mind, ultimately impacting upon school learning (Alloway, 2006). Several studies have indeed shown that working memory performance is related to both reading and mathematics performance (Blair & Razza, 2007; Bull & Scerif, 2001; Raghubar, Barnes, & Hecht, 2010; Van der Sluis, De Jong, & Van der Leij, 2004).

Recently, interest has emerged into whether neural activity during working memory tasks can be used to predict (future) school performance. The idea is that neuroimaging measures of working memory can provide additional information for predicting school performance that cannot be gathered with behavioral testing alone. Indeed, a study in 8- to 10-year-old children showed that reduced neural activity during a working memory task in the intraparietal sulcus (IPS), a brain region that is also important for numerical cognition, was linked to poorer mathematical skills (Rotzer et al., 2009). Another study showed that neural activity in the IPS during a working memory task could even be used to predict mathematics performance two years later (Dumontheil & Klingberg, 2012). Moreover, when the researchers tried to predict which children would later demonstrate low mathematical skills, they found that using both behavioral and neural predictors resulted in a twofold better prediction compared to behavioral measures alone (Dumontheil & Klingberg, 2012).

Aside from these results demonstrating that individual differences in working memory performance are related to academic achievement, there is also evidence for a general increase in working memory skills from childhood into adulthood. Behavioral research shows that even in very young infants, basic forms of working memory (keeping information in mind) are already present (Diamond, 1995). Studies in children and adolescents, however, have revealed that working memory capacity, measured using a wide range of tasks, continues to develop well into adolescence (Crone, Wendelken, Donohue, van Leijenhorst, & Bunge, 2006; Luciana, Conklin, Hooper, & Yarger, 2005; Peters, Van Duijvenvoorde, Koolschijn, & Crone, 2016). In addition, neuroimaging studies have investigated how brain regions important for working memory develop across adolescence. The brain regions involved in working memory include regions in the prefrontal cortex (PFC), such as ventrolateral PFC and dorsolateral PFC, but also parts of the parietal cortex (Crone, Wendelken, Donohue, van Leijenhorst et al., 2006). Neuroimaging studies on age-related changes in brain activity during working memory tasks have mostly shown that activity in frontal and parietal areas is still immature in children, and increases with age through adolescence (Crone, Wendelken, Donohue, van Leijenhorst et al., 2006; Jolles, Kleibeuker, Rombouts, & Crone, 2011; Klingberg, Forssberg, & Westerberg, 2002). For instance, Crone, Wendelken, Donohue, van Leijenhorst et al. (2006) compared a group of 8- to 12-year-olds, 13- to 17-year-olds and 18- to 25-year-olds on a working memory task requiring both maintenance (recalling a set of pictures) and manipulation (recalling a set of pictures in reverse order). As expected, behavioral performance was lower for manipulation compared to maintenance, as this is the more difficult condition. Moreover, adults generally performed better than both children and adolescents. The fMRI results showed that in contrast to adolescents and adults, children did not activate the DLPFC and parietal cortex during the maintenance trials, suggesting functional immaturity of these brain regions. A study on structural development in these regions revealed that not only activity, but also the anatomical structure of these brain regions is important for working memory development (Tamnes et al., 2013). In this study, children and adolescents (8 to 22 years old) were followed longitudinally over a period of two years. The behavioral results showed continued improvements in working memory performance well into adolescence, similar to other studies. Changes in cortical thickness in prefrontal and posterior parietal cortices were related to performance improvements in working memory. Together, these results show that working memory is still developing into adolescence and that this development is related to underlying immaturities in both the structure and the function of the neural system for working memory.

Given the relation between working memory and school performance, there has recently been a surge of interest in working memory training programs in schools. Many of the 'brain training games' that are already commercially available also train aspects of working memory. However, it is very important to remain critical when implementing a working memory training program, as although evidence to their efficacy is promising, there are still many mixed findings reported in the current scientific literature. When studying the effects of training, a crucial question is always whether training results not only in better performance on the trained task, or a very similar task (near transfer), but also leads to improvements on other types of cognitive tasks (far transfer). Achieving far transfer would be a crucial prerequisite for working memory training to be useful for improving school performance.

Current reviews and meta-analyses have generally concluded that working memory training is effective in terms of near transfer, but results on far transfer are mixed (Gathercole, Dunning, & Holmes, 2012; Shipstead, Hicks, & Engle, 2012), showing either no far transfer or limited far transfer to attention tasks (Shinaver, Entwistle, & Söderqvist, 2014). As a consequence, researchers have set out to discover what needs to change in working memory training programs to achieve far transfer. One possibility is that working memory training becomes too repetitive after a number of repetitions, because the difficulty of the task is not adjusted to the performance level of the participant.

This results in the training program being too easy for some participants, but too challenging for others. It has been hypothesized that in order to achieve far transfer, training needs to be complex, novel and continually adapted to the participant's performance (Moreau & Conway, 2014). So far, this type of adaptive working memory training has shown promising effects for far transfer. For instance, a study in 28 7- to 9-year-old children (Karbach, Strobach, & Schubert, 2015) divided children into adaptive working memory training and non-adaptive low-level training. The children in the adaptive group showed larger gains in performance on near-transfer tasks, and in addition showed far transfer to improvements in general reading ability.

A remaining question for working memory training research is whether training and transfer effects are different depending on the type of working memory task that is trained. A distinction can be made between verbal working memory and visuospatial working memory (Baddeley & Hitch, 1994), which refer to the temporary maintenance of verbal and visual information, respectively. This is important because in students it has been found that there can be discrepancies in verbal vs. visuospatial working memory skills (Alloway, Gathercole, & Pickering, 2006) and they differentially predict later academic achievement (Bull, Espy, & Wiebe, 2008).

Another question for working memory training research is to figure out *why* exactly training improves performance. It could be that working memory capacity simply becomes larger, but it could also be that children learn to use a new strategy (such as 'chunking' information: remembering a string of numbers '316' rather than the numbers '3', '1', '6' individually). It is often difficult to disentangle these processes based on behavioral research alone, and here neuroimaging studies can come in useful. That is, training could lead to changes (increases or decreases) in the same brain network that was already active before training, but could also lead to recruitment of new brain regions. It has been argued that simple types of training (non-adaptive; not teaching children to employ new strategies) results in activity differences within the same network, whereas more complex adaptive training emphasizing acquiring new strategies results in recruitment of new brain regions after training (Jolles & Crone, 2012). The majority of simple working memory training studies have shown that activity in frontal and parietal brain regions is reduced after training, suggesting a reduced need for cognitive effort (Landau, Schumacher, Garavan, Druzgal, & D'Esposito, 2004; Sayala, Sala, & Courtney, 2005). This makes sense given that due to the non-adaptive nature of the training, the task will have become easier over time. However, when training was adapted to the performance level of the participants (and would therefore be expected to result in the same cognitive effort both before and after training), there were increases in frontal and parietal activity after training (Olesen, Westerberg, & Klingberg, 2004). This increase in activity within the same network led the authors to hypothesize that training had increased the capacity of working memory. Other working memory training programs have instead centered on teaching new strategies to children, such as chunking, verbally rehearsing to-be-remembered items, or using mnemonics. Studies using this type of training have indeed observed that new brain regions are recruited after training (Chein & Schneider, 2005; Kelly & Garavan, 2004). Together, these studies provide an example of how neuroimaging studies give additional information over behavioral studies alone, providing insights into which working memory training programs work, and also why they work. Ultimately, this contributes to the continued development and improvement of working memory training programs.

The Development of Inhibition

Another important executive function in the context of child and adolescent development is inhibition. There are so many potential distractions in school that staying focused on a single task is one of the most challenging skills that a student needs to master. However, this skill is often not explicitly addressed in school curricula. This is surprising given that better inhibition in childhood has been associated with a range of positive outcomes in later life, such as better grades, less substance dependence, and fewer criminal offences in adulthood, and better health outcomes (Moffitt et al., 2011; Tangney, Baumeister, & Boone, 2004).

To study the development of inhibition, several different experimental tasks have been employed. A distinction can be made between inhibition in 'hot' and 'cold' contexts. In hot contexts, motivational and affective tendencies must be regulated (e.g., 'do not eat this chocolate'), whereas in 'cold' contexts, inhibition is more abstract (e.g., 'do not press this button'). Perhaps the most famous task that has been used to study inhibition in hot contexts is the marshmallow task (Mischel, Ebbesen, & Zeiss, 1972). In this task, children (around age 4) were presented with a marshmallow. The experimenter leaves the room and the child is told that if she does not eat the marshmallow until the experimenter has returned, she will receive two marshmallows instead. Several follow-up studies were performed to investigate how participants from the original marshmallow experiment performed on a range of tasks and questionnaires years later. The results showed that children who were better able to wait for the second marshmallow (high delayers) when they were 4 years old had obtained higher Standardized Academic Testes (SAT) scores and better social-emotional skills in adolescence (Mischel, Shoda, & Peake, 1988; Shoda, Mischel, & Peake, 1990). Twenty years later, these participants had obtained higher educational achievements, reported less cocaine/crack use, better self-worth and better stress-coping skills (Ayduk et al., 2000). Several researchers followed these same participants up 40 years later with a neuroimaging study (Casey et al., 2011). They compared participants who were high delayers with participants who were low delayers at age 4 using a Go-NoGo task in an MRI scanner. In the Go-Nogo task (an example of inhibition in a cold context), participants are instructed to continually make a certain response (e.g., press a button when a green square appears). However, sometimes the stimulus suddenly changes and a stop-signal is presented, indicating that participants must inhibit the response they were preparing (e.g., they were preparing to press the button for the green square, but suddenly it turned red). Casey et al. (2011) showed that in participants who were high delayers at age 4, the inferior frontal gyrus (an important brain region for inhibition in the prefrontal cortex) showed more activity 40 years later during inhibition trials (NoGo) compared to Go trials. On the other hand, the ventral striatum (a region associated with reward processing) showed increased activity in participants who were low delayers at age 4, suggesting heightened reward sensitivity and reduced inhibition skills in low delayers. Together, these studies show that inhibition is a relatively stable trait with important consequences for daily functioning and school performance and is associated with differential functioning of brain regions involved during executive functioning and reward processing.

Aside from these individual differences in inhibition skills, there are also developmental changes in inhibition. Studies in children and adolescents using a variety of inhibition tasks have shown that performance on inhibition tasks continues to improve over childhood and into mid- or late adolescence (Luna, Garver, Urban, Lazar, & Sweeney, 2004; Ridderinkhof, van der Molen, Band, & Bashore, 1997; Williams, Ponesse, Schachar, Logan, & Tannock, 1999). Inhibition relies on a network of brain regions, including the motor response control circuit (including supplementary motor area, posterior parietal cortex, putamen), the executive control network (including dorsal and ventral lateral prefrontal cortex) and the error-processing network (including dorsal anterior cingulate cortex) (Ordaz, Foran, Velanova, & Luna, 2013). Research on how activity in these regions changes between childhood and adolescence have so far shown both increases (Bunge, Dudukovic, Thomason, Vaidya, & Gabrieli, 2002; Rubia et al., 2006) and decreases with age (Durston et al., 2006; Velanova, Wheeler, & Luna, 2008). A possible reason for these inconsistent findings is that these studies did not use longitudinal designs, but compared children of different ages with each other. A longitudinal design is important because it allows for the investigation of within-person development and is robust to between-subject differences such as cohort effects. To date, one large-scale longitudinal study tested how neural activity changes during child and adolescent development (Ordaz et al., 2013). The results revealed that different types of inhibition showed a different pattern of neural changes with age. Activity in executive control regions showed decreases with age in activity, whereas activity in the error-monitoring system increased with age. Activity in the motor control circuit showed no changes with age, suggesting that this circuit is already mature at a young age, whereas the error processing system continues to develop into adolescence. The decrease in activity with age in executive control regions may mean that executive control regions temporarily compensate for the immature error-processing activity in adolescence. Together, the behavioral and neural evidence so far indicates that similar to working memory, inhibition is a skill that is still developing into adolescence.

Despite the demonstrated importance of inhibition for school and life outcomes, the number of studies on the trainability of inhibition skills is relatively scarce compared to the wealth of literature on working memory training. So far, a study in children showed that inhibition training using a playground-inhibition game (in 8–12-year-old children) resulted in improved performance on a computerized Go-NoGo task, but there was no increase in performance on a Stroop task (Zhao, Chen, Fu, & Maes, 2015). The Stroop task is a well-known psychological task in which participants are instructed to name the color of a written word, rather than the word itself. Thus, participants need to inhibit their automatic tendency to read out the word, which is a form of semantic inhibition. The fact that there was only transfer to a Go-NoGo task (a response inhibition task) but not to the Stroop task (a semantic inhibition task) could be because the Go-NoGo task is more similar to the trained playground-inhibition game, indicating near but not far transfer after training. Another study in younger children (4–5 years) also found improvements on the inhibition tasks that were trained, but no far transfer effects to working memory or attention tasks (Thorell, Lindqvist, Bergman Nutley, Bohlin, & Klingberg, 2009). Finally, a study in 10–12-year-old children and 18–24-year-old adults showed that there were near transfer effects to another inhibition task in both age groups. Moreover, in the children there was also a far transfer effect to working memory updating and task switching performance, although this improvement was not long-lasting (Zhao, Chen, & Maes, 2016). A neuroimaging study in adults (Berkman, Kahn, & Merchant, 2014) sheds light on why inhibition training seems to mostly result in near but not far transfer. In this study, participants received either inhibitory control training using an adaptive stop-signal reaction time task or active sham training. In the sham training group, participants performed the same task as the training group, but without the stop signals. The behavioral results indicated, as expected, that the inhibitory training group showed more improvement on the inhibition task compared to the sham training group. The neuroimaging results showed that in the inhibition training group, neural activity in the inferior frontal gyrus increased during preparation for an inhibitory action (stopping), whereas activity during the actual inhibition decreased. This may explain why there is mostly evidence for near but not far transfer, as transfer to a different type of task may require a different preparatory process which appears not to be changed by inhibition training.

The Development of Cognitive Flexibility

Aside from keeping relevant information online (working memory) and blocking irrelevant information and controlling impulses (inhibition), it is important to keep behavior flexible and to constantly monitor whether behavior is still adequate for the current situation. Real-life examples include being able to learn from mistakes, changing from speaking Spanish to speaking French when switching classes, and alternating between sending texts and paying attention in class. If a child did not possess any cognitive flexibility, she would keep performing the same actions repeatedly and would not be able to respond to changing demands from the environment, and use new information, such as negative feedback from parents or teachers. Unsurprisingly, increased cognitive flexibility is linked to better school performance. In preschoolers, cognitive flexibility predicts better mathematics performance and more advanced phonemic awareness (Blair & Razza, 2007). A longitudinal study in both preschoolers and primary schoolers also found evidence for a relation between cognitive flexibility and reading and mathematics performance (Bull et al., 2008).

A task that has often been used to measure cognitive flexibility is the Wisconsin Card Sorting Task (WCST) (Chelune & Baer, 1986). In this task, participants are instructed to sort cards with images (e.g., blue houses, red animals) according to a certain rule (e.g., by color), and they receive positive or negative feedback after each sort. After a number of sorts, the rule changes without warning (e.g., from color to shape) so that the child suddenly receives negative feedback for an answer that was correct before. The child needs to flexibly adapt to this new situation and use performance feedback to figure out the new sorting rule. Performance on the WCST relies heavily on the prefrontal cortex, as patients with damage to the prefrontal cortex tend to show perseveration behavior: They have severe difficulties with switching to a new sorting rule (Barcelo & Knight, 2002). Interestingly, children also have difficulty switching to new sorting rules, which is why performance on the WCST in children has been compared to that of patients with damage to the PFC (Chelune & Baer, 1986). Although the WCST is a great tool for assessing general cognitive flexibility, it also recruits many other cognitive processes, which cannot easily be disentangled. Therefore researchers have designed simpler tasks to investigate separately task-switching (without the need to infer a switch from feedback), and learning from feedback. The Dimensional Change Card Sort (DCCS) is a task suitable for measuring task-switching in children (Zelazo, 2006). This task is similar to the WCST but instead of children having to infer from negative feedback that the sorting rule has changed, they are explicitly instructed to change the sorting rule (e.g., now sort the pictures by color instead of shape). Interestingly, despite these explicit instructions, young children still show inflexible persevering behavior on this task (Zelazo, 2006). A meta-analysis on 69 reports studies using the DCCS showed that there is a robust improvement in performance with age (Doebel & Zelazo, 2015). At the age of 4 years, around 50% of children can successfully switch on the DCCS (Doebel & Zelazo, 2015).

Computerized task-switching paradigms are often used to study cognitive flexibility in older children, adolescents and adults. In such tasks, participants are generally trained to switch back and forth between two simple tasks (e.g., judge whether a letter is a consonant/vowel, and decide whether a letter is odd/even). After a while, an explicit pre-learned cue (a verbal instruction or sound) is given which indicates a switch to the other task. From these tasks, the 'switch cost' can be calculated, which is the difference in performance and accuracy when repeating the same task (e.g., two consecutive tasks with letter judgements) vs. when switching to a different task (first letter judgements, then number judgements). Studies on how task switching develops have shown that adults generally perform better on these tasks than children (Crone, Bunge, van der Molen, & Ridderinkhof, 2006; Huizinga et al., 2006). The most pronounced performance improvements appear to occur between ages 7–12, but there are also continued improvements in adolescence (Huizinga et al., 2006). Developmental fMRI studies on task-switching performance have generally reported increased frontal and parietal activity in adults compared to children or adolescents in switch trials (Christakou et al., 2009; Crone, Wendelken, Donohue, & Bunge, 2006; Rubia et al., 2006).

Another aspect of cognitive flexibility that has been investigated in childhood and adolescence is the ability to learn from positive and negative feedback. A large study in participants aged 8 to 25 years (Peters, Braams, Raijmakers, Koolschijn, & Crone, 2014) showed that in adults, brain regions in the feedback learning network (dorsolateral prefrontal cortex and parietal cortex) were more active after negative feedback compared to positive feedback. However, in children and adolescents, these same regions were more active after receiving positive feedback compared to negative feedback. This shows that children and adolescents can in fact use these brain regions (which were previously thought to be 'underdeveloped' based on predictions from the imbalance model), but instead use them in different situations compared to adults. A follow-up study in this sample showed that feedback learning performance could be used to predict reading and mathematics performance two years later (Peters, Van der Meulen, Zanolie, & Crone, 2017). Moreover, neural activity during feedback learning could be used to predict reading and mathematics performance even better than using these behavioral measures alone. That is, increased activity in the dorsolateral prefrontal cortex predicted how well a participant performed on a standardized reading task two years later. Similarly, increased activity in the supplementary motor area/anterior cingulate cortex (a medial region in the prefrontal cortex) was linked to better mathematics performance two years later.

To date, only a few studies have investigated whether training cognitive flexibility has benefits for cognitive performance in childhood and adolescence. A study by Zinke, Einert, Pfennig, and Kliegel (2012) in adolescents (10 to 14 years old) investigated the effects of task-switching training. They demonstrated that performance on the trained task improved, and that there was near transfer to another task-switching paradigm. Far transfer effects were also found, but only for performance on a choice reaction time task. Another study tested the effects of task-switching training in children (8–10 years), young adults and older adults (Karbach & Kray, 2009). They found near transfer effects to a similar task-switching paradigm in all age groups. There were also far transfer effects in all age groups to fluid intelligence and other executive functioning tasks. This study also revealed that when training tasks were more variable, there were enhanced near transfer effects in adults, but impaired near transfer effects in children. Importantly, this shows that the impact of training may be different for different age groups and underlines the need for further studies on cognitive flexibility training in childhood and adolescence.

Adolescent-Specific Opportunities for Executive Functioning

To date, most research on executive functioning in adolescence has emphasized how executive functioning performance and the underlying neural mechanisms are still underdeveloped in adolescents compared to adults. This fits with imbalance models of adolescence, which hypothesized an imbalance between immature activity in executive control regions (e.g., frontal cortex) and hyperactivity in affective brain regions (e.g., striatum), resulting in reduced executive functioning capacity and heightened reward sensitivity (Steinberg, 2008). This model has been used to explain negative aspects of adolescence, such as increased risk-taking behavior and adverse health outcomes. More recent research is less negative and also highlights that there may be unique benefits of being an adolescent for executive functioning. Given that the striatum is not only a reward-related region, but also an important brain region for cognitive learning (Liljeholm & O'Doherty, 2012), one study tested whether adolescents also show heightened striatum responses during cognitive learning. In a large longitudinal study, participants (aged 8 to 25 years) were followed longitudinally over three time points (N = 736 scans from 299 participants) while they performed a cognitive feedback learning task (Peters & Crone, 2017). The neuroimaging results revealed that the striatum peaks in sensitivity to the learning value of feedback in late adolescence (around 17 to 20 years of age) compared to children and young adolescents. That is, in late adolescence, the striatum differentiated the most between feedback that was valuable for learning (early in the learning process, when the correct rule had not yet been learned) compared to feedback without learning value (feedback for a rule that was already learned). Moreover, participants whose striatum was more sensitive to learning value generally showed better learning performance on the feedback task, and performance on this task was linked to reading and mathematics performance in a prior study (Peters et al., 2017). This may mean that adolescents are uniquely sensitive to new information from their environment and that late adolescence is a window-of-opportunity for learning.

Other studies on adolescent-specific opportunities for executive functioning have emphasized how heightened emotional responsiveness in adolescence can sometimes be beneficial for executive functioning performance. That is, the heightened emotional and social sensitivity of adolescents may, in the right context, result in a higher motivation for cognitive performance (Crone & Dahl, 2012). As an example, think of how adolescents may have difficulty planning their homework assignments, often leaving everything to the last minute and missing deadlines. However, when they are planning a birthday party, they may suddenly have excellent planning and organizing skills, because of heightened motivation and the potential for social reward if they throw a successful party. Although participants from all ages may perform better in contexts of high motivation, it is possible that this effect is even stronger in adolescents. If this is true than that would mean that the adolescent brain is more flexible or variable: the range of cognitive outcomes is larger because it is influenced more by the affective and social context compared to other ages (Crone & Dahl, 2012). Until recently, executive functions were often studied in isolation from a social environment. However, schools are inherently a social environment and this may pose challenges for adolescents (such as distraction), but also opportunities due to the potential rewards a social environment offers. So far only a few studies have investigated the effect of a social or rewarding context on cognitive performance in adolescence relative to other age groups. A study using an inhibitory anti-saccade task compared performance with and without a monetary reward in adults and adolescents (Geier, Terwilliger, Teslovich, Velanova, & Luna, 2010). For adults, a monetary reward did in most circumstances not influence performance. But for adolescents, financial rewards led to increases in performance. Neuroimaging results provided clues as to why performance increased. During the preparation for rewarded trials, adolescents showed relatively more activity in the striatum (a region associated with reward processing) and the frontal cortex. This suggests that the increased striatum response in adolescence leads to an upregulation of cognitive control and thus better performance when rewards are at stake.

Another research line focuses on whether the supposed increased flexibility of adolescents (Crone & Dahl, 2012) means that adolescents are more receptive to executive functions training. The idea that training is more effective in certain age groups is supported by a meta-analysis (Melby-Lervåg & Hulme, 2012) which showed that training benefits after working memory training were influenced by the participant's age: younger children benefited more from training than older children. Another large meta-analysis investigated the effects of working memory and attentional control in a very broad age range (1–90 years). It was found that the amount of transfer achieved during training was largest in childhood and adolescence but showed declines with increasing age (Wass, Scerif, & Johnson, 2012).

In sum, these recent findings highlight that the adolescent brain offers not only disadvantages, but also potential opportunities for executive functioning.

To conclude this chapter, I will provide an overview of the advances a neuroscience perspective can bring to the understanding of executive functioning in childhood and adolescence.

What Has Neuroscience Added to Our Understanding Over and Above Psychology?

Neuroscientific and behavioral findings together have provided us with important insights into the development of executive functions. Key aspects in which neuroscience has added to our understanding over behavioral research alone are as follows: (1) Neuroscience has led to the discovery of age-related vulnerabilities and opportunities in childhood and adolescence based on underlying brain development; (2) a combination of neural and behavioral measures predicts future academic outcomes better than behavioral measures alone; and (3) neuroscience can provide us with insights into the mechanisms of training and why some training programs work better than others.

First, research on age-related changes in brain development has provided a neurobiological explanation for the results of most behavioral studies, that executive functioning performance shows protracted development until well into adolescence. The imbalance model of adolescent brain development hypothesized that frontal brain regions (important for executive functioning) develop relatively slowly, whereas emotional brain regions show heightened activity in adolescence (Steinberg, 2008). This research has contributed to the understanding that adolescents are not 'small adults' who are simply misbehaving, but has emphasized that their brains function differently from adults. In part as a result of this research, schools have become increasingly interested in adjusting their teaching programs in age-appropriate ways, to ensure an optimal fit with the developmental stage of a pupil. As an example, keeping lessons short and varied, and helping adolescents plan their homework may help to reduce the effort placed on executive functioning skills, which can then hopefully be invested in the actual learning process. Aside from these shortcomings in how the adolescent brain functions, more recent research has also provided hints that adolescent-specific sensitivities in the brain could potentially be used to improve cognitive performance. Heightened striatum activity for rewards (Silverman et al., 2015) and during cognitive feedback learning (Peters & Crone, 2017) points to a unique period in development where adolescents are optimally sensitive to their environments. Providing adolescents with affective or social rewards may work to improve cognitive performance (Geier et al., 2010), although more research is needed to confirm whether this translates to school settings.

Second, neuroscientific measures have also been shown to make predictions about future academic outcomes more accurate (Dumontheil & Klingberg, 2012; Hoeft et al., 2007; Peters et al., 2017). It is possible that neuroimaging offers a way to measure a pupil's capacity for growth and may capture a potential for cognitive performance that is not yet measurable at the behavioral level. For instance, take the situation where two children obtain the same score on a reading test, but one child is already performing at her maximum level, whereas the other child is not yet performing at her full capacity. It is possible that neuroscience measures can help to signal early on which students will benefit most from interventions, although this needs to be confirmed in further studies.

Third, neuroscience allows us to investigate the underlying mechanisms of training effects. Although arguably the most important question in training research is *whether* a training program works, understanding *why* a training program works can help to improve existing programs or can inspire the development of new training programs. For instance, if training results in enhanced recruitment of the same neural network that was active before training, this could indicate that capacity is increased by training. If new brain regions are recruited after training, this may point to a different strategy being employed (Olesen et al., 2004). Disentangling these processes may inform future training programs to specifically target working memory capacity or instead explicitly train strategy. Moreover, neuroscientific measures could eventually be used to tailor interventions to individual students. Understanding which strategies and neural networks a student currently uses during a cognitive task could potentially indicate which type of intervention may work to bring their performance to a higher level.

What Are Concrete Implications of Research and Opportunities for Translation?

Together, the results from these studies on the development of executive functioning may have implications for school learning. The understanding that the brains of children and adolescents function differently from adults could inform changes in school curricula, as it underlines the importance of adjusting course programs to the specific skill level of pupils. Both behavioral and neural research revealed that executive functioning skills do not reach adult levels until well into adolescence. Therefore it is probably good practice to organize school programs in such a way that they place no unnecessary burden on executive functioning. With regard to the adolescent-specific opportunities for executive functioning, the unique sensitivity of adolescents to rewards and their (social) environment could possibly be used to advance their cognitive skills. That is, rewards for good performance and the heightened salience of peer feedback could be used to help students to become more motivated to perform well. However, it is important to take into account that these approaches may work well for some but not all students.

Given the cautious optimism on the effectiveness of executive functioning training programs, schools and teachers could consider implementing training of executive functions into the school curriculum. Currently several schools are already experimenting with working memory training programs (Holmes & Gathercole, 2014). The finding that adaptive types of training work especially well could also be important for school settings. When teaching a class (rather than a one-on-one teaching situation), it is inevitable that the lesson is not challenging enough for some students, but too advanced for others. Individualized assignments or computerized programs which are adaptive to the individual student's performance may help to train students at their optimal level.

Further Resources for the Reader to Learn More About the Topic

More information on this topic can be found in the following articles:

Constantinidis, C., & Klingberg, T. (2016). The neuroscience of working memory capacity and training. *Nature Reviews Neuroscience, 17*(7), 438–449.

Crone, E. A., & Steinbeis, N. (2017). Neural perspectives on cognitive control development during childhood and adolescence. *Trends in Cognitive Sciences*, 3(21), 205–215.

Titz, C., & Karbach, J. (2014). Working memory and executive functions: Effects of training on academic achievement. *Psychological Research*, 78(6), 852–868.

Van Duijvenvoorde, A. C. K., Peters, S., Braams, B. R., & Crone, E. A. (2016). What motivates adolescents? Neural responses to rewards and their influence on adolescents' risk taking, learning, and cognitive control. *Neuroscience and Biobehavioral Reviews*, 70, 135–147.

References

Alloway, T. P. (2006). How does working memory work in the classroom? *Educational Research and Reviews*, 1, 134–139.

Alloway, T. P., Gathercole, S. E., & Pickering, S. J. (2006). Verbal and visuospatial short-term and working memory in children: Are they separable? *Child Development*, 77, 1698–1716.

Ayduk, O., Mendoza-Denton, R., Mischel, W., Downey, G., Peake, P. K., & Rodriguez, M. (2000). Regulating the interpersonal self: Strategic self-regulation for coping with rejection sensitivity. *Journal of Personality and Social Psychology*, 79, 776–792.

Baddeley, A. D., & Hitch, G. J. (1994). Developments in the concept of working memory. *Neuropsychology*, 8, 485–493.

Barcelo, F., & Knight, R. T. (2002). Both random and perseverative errors underlie WCST deficits in prefrontal patients. *Neuropsychologia*, 40, 349–356.

Berkman, E. T., Kahn, L. E., & Merchant, J. S. (2014). Training-induced changes in inhibitory control network activity. *The Journal of Neuroscience*, 34, 149–157.

Blair, C., & Razza, R. P. (2007). Relating effortful control, executive function, and false belief understanding to emerging math and literacy ability in kindergarten. *Child Development*, 78, 647–663.

Bull, R., Espy, K. A., & Wiebe, S. A. (2008). Short-term memory, working memory, and executive functioning in preschoolers: Longitudinal predictors of mathematical achievement at age 7 years. *Developmental Neuropsychology*, 33, 205–228.

Bull, R., & Scerif, G. (2001). Executive functioning as a predictor of children's mathematics ability: Inhibition, switching, and working memory. *Developmental Neuropsychology*, 19, 273–293.

Bunge, S. A., Dudukovic, N. M., Thomason, M. E., Vaidya, C. J., & Gabrieli, J. D. E. (2002). Immature frontal lobe contributions to cognitive control in children: Evidence from fMRI. *Neuron*, 33, 301–311.

Casey, B. J., Somerville, L. H., Gotlib, I. H., Ayduk, O., Franklin, N. T., Askren, M. K., . . . Shoda, Y. (2011). Behavioral and neural correlates of delay of gratification 40 years later. *Proceedings of the National Academy of Sciences of the United States of America*, 108, 14998–5003.

Chein, J. M., & Schneider, W. (2005). Neuroimaging studies of practice-related change: fMRI and meta-analytic evidence of a domain-general control network for learning. *Brain Research. Cognitive Brain Research*, 25, 607–623.

Chelune, G. J., & Baer, R. A. (1986). Developmental norms for the Wisconsin card sorting test. *Journal of Clinical and Experimental Neuropsychology*, 8, 219–228.

Christakou, A., Halari, R., Smith, A. B., Ifkovits, E., Brammer, M., & Rubia, K. (2009). Sex-dependent age modulation of frontostriatal and temporo-parietal activation during cognitive control. *NeuroImage*, 48, 223–236.

Crone, E. A., Bunge, S. A., van der Molen, M. W., & Ridderinkhof, K. R. (2006). Switching between tasks and responses: A developmental study. *Developmental Science, 9*, 278–287.

Crone, E. A., & Dahl, R. E. (2012). Understanding adolescence as a period of social—affective engagement and goal flexibility. *Nature Reviews Neuroscience, 13*, 636–650.

Crone, E. A., Wendelken, C., Donohue, S. E., & Bunge, S. A. (2006). Neural evidence for dissociable components of task-switching. *Cerebral Cortex, 16*, 475–486.

Crone, E. A., Wendelken, C., Donohue, S., van Leijenhorst, L., & Bunge, S. A. (2006). Neurocognitive development of the ability to manipulate information in working memory. *Proceedings of the National Academy of Sciences, 103*, 9315–9320.

Diamond, A. (1995). Evidence of robust recognition memory early in life even when assessed by reaching behavior. *Journal of Experimental Child Psychology, 59*, 419–456.

Diamond, A. (2013). Executive functions. *Annual Review of Psychology, 64*, 135–168.

Doebel, S., & Zelazo, P. D. (2015). A meta-analysis of the dimensional change card sort: Implications for developmental theories and the measurement of executive function in children. *Developmental Review, 38*, 241–268.

Dumontheil, I., & Klingberg, T. (2012). Brain activity during a visuospatial working memory task predicts arithmetical performance 2 years later. *Cerebral Cortex, 22*, 1078–1085.

Durston, S., Davidson, M. C., Tottenham, N., Galvan, A., Spicer, J., Fossella, J. A., & Casey, B. J. (2006). A shift from diffuse to focal cortical activity with development. *Developmental Science, 9*, 1–8.

Ernst, M., Pine, D. S., & Hardin, M. (2006). Triadic model of the neurobiology of motivated behavior in adolescence. *Psychological Medicine, 36*, 299–312.

Gathercole, S. E., Dunning, D. L., & Holmes, J. (2012). Cogmed training: Let's be realistic about intervention research. *Journal of Applied Research in Memory and Cognition, 1*, 201–203.

Geier, C. F., Terwilliger, R., Teslovich, T., Velanova, K., & Luna, B. (2010). Immaturities in reward processing and its influence on inhibitory control in adolescence. *Cerebral Cortex, 20*, 1613–1629.

Giedd, J. N., Blumenthal, J., Jeffries, N. O., Castellanos, F. X., Liu, H., Zijdenbos, A., . . . Rapoport, J. L. (1999). Brain development during childhood and adolescence: A longitudinal MRI study. *Nature Neuroscience, 2*, 861–863.

Gogtay, N., Giedd, J. N., Lusk, L., Hayashi, K. M., Greenstein, D., Vaituzis, A. C., . . . Thompson, P. M. (2004). Dynamic mapping of human cortical development during childhood through early adulthood. *Proceedings of the National Academy of Sciences of the United States of America, 101*, 8174–8179.

Hoeft, F., Ueno, T., Reiss, A. L., Meyler, A., Whitfield-Gabrieli, S., Glover, G. H., . . . Jo, B. (2007). Prediction of children's reading skills using behavioral, functional, and structural neuroimaging measures. *Behavioral Neuroscience, 121*, 602.

Holmes, J., & Gathercole, S. E. (2014). Taking working memory training from the laboratory into schools. *Educational Psychology, 34*, 440–450.

Huizinga, M., Dolan, C. V., & van der Molen, M. W. (2006). Age-related change in executive function: Developmental trends and a latent variable analysis. *Neuropsychologia, 44*, 2017–2036.

Jolles, D. D., & Crone, E. A. (2012). Training the developing brain: A neurocognitive perspective. *Frontiers in Human Neuroscience, 6*, 76.

Jolles, D. D., Kleibeuker, S. W., Rombouts, S. A. R. B., & Crone, E. A. (2011). Developmental differences in prefrontal activation during working memory maintenance and manipulation for different memory loads. *Developmental Science, 14*, 713–724.

Karbach, J., & Kray, J. (2009). How useful is executive control training? Age differences in near and far transfer of task-switching training. *Developmental Science, 12*, 978–990.

Karbach, J., Strobach, T., & Schubert, T. (2015). Adaptive working-memory training benefits reading, but not mathematics in middle childhood. *Child Neuropsychology, 21*, 285–301.

Kelly, A. M. C., & Garavan, H. (2004). Human functional neuroimaging of brain changes associated with practice. *Cerebral Cortex, 15*, 1089–1102.

Klingberg, T., Forssberg, H., & Westerberg, H. (2002). Increased brain activity in frontal and parietal cortex underlies the development of visuospatial working memory capacity during childhood. *Journal of Cognitive Neuroscience, 14*, 1–10.

Landau, S. M., Schumacher, E. H., Garavan, H., Druzgal, T. J., & D'Esposito, M. (2004). A functional MRI study of the influence of practice on component processes of working memory. *Cerebral Cortex, 15*, 1089–1102.

Liljeholm, M., & O'Doherty, J. P. (2012). Contributions of the striatum to learning, motivation, and performance: An associative account. *Trends in Cognitive Sciences, 16*, 467–475.

Luciana, M., Conklin, H. M., Hooper, C. J., & Yarger, R. S. (2005). The development of nonverbal working memory and executive control processes in adolescents. *Child Development, 76*, 697–712.

Luna, B., Garver, K. E., Urban, T. A., Lazar, N. A., & Sweeney, J. A. (2004). Maturation of cognitive processes from late childhood to adulthood. *Child Development, 75*, 1357–1372.

Melby-Lervåg, M., & Hulme, C. (2012). Is working memory training effective? A meta-analytic review. *Developmental Psychology.* doi:10.1037/a0028228

Mischel, W., Ebbesen, E. B., & Zeiss, A. R. (1972). Cognitive and attentional mechanisms in delay of gratification. *Journal of Personality and Social Psychology, 21*, 204–218.

Mischel, W., Shoda, Y., & Peake, P. K. (1988). The nature of adolescent competencies predicted by preschool delay of gratification. *Journal of Personality and Social Psychology, 54*, 687–696.

Miyake, A., Friedman, N. P., Emerson, M. J., Witzki, A. H., Howerter, A., & Wager, T. D. (2000). The unity and diversity of executive functions and their contributions to complex "frontal lobe" tasks: A latent variable analysis. *Cognitive Psychology, 41*, 49–100.

Moffitt, T. E., Arseneault, L., Belsky, D., Dickson, N., Hancox, R. J., Harrington, H., . . . Caspi, A. (2011). A gradient of childhood self-control predicts health, wealth, and public safety. *Proceedings of the National Academy of Sciences of the United States of America, 108*, 2693–2698.

Moreau, D., & Conway, A. R. A. (2014). The case for an ecological approach to cognitive training. *Trends in Cognitive Sciences, 18*, 334–336.

Olesen, P. J., Westerberg, H., & Klingberg, T. (2004). Increased prefrontal and parietal activity after training of working memory. *Nature Neuroscience, 7*, 75–79.

Ordaz, S. J., Foran, W., Velanova, K., & Luna, B. (2013). Longitudinal growth curves of brain function underlying inhibitory control through adolescence. *Journal of Neuroscience, 33*, 18109–18124.

Payne, M. A. (2012). All gas and no brakes! *Journal of Adolescent Research, 27*, 3–17.

Peters, S., Braams, B. R., Raijmakers, M. E. J., Koolschijn, P. C. M. P., & Crone, E. A. (2014). The neural coding of feedback learning across child and adolescent development. *Journal of Cognitive Neuroscience, 26*, 1705–1720.

Peters, S., & Crone, E. A. (2017). Increased striatal activity in adolescence benefits learning. *Nature Communications, 8*, 1983.

Peters, S., Van der Meulen, M., Zanolie, K., & Crone, E. A. (2017). Predicting reading and mathematics from neural activity for feedback learning. *Developmental Psychology, 53*, 149–159.

Peters, S., Van Duijvenvoorde, A. C. K., Koolschijn, P. C. M. P., & Crone, E. A. (2016). Longitudinal development of frontoparietal activity during feedback learning: Contributions of age, performance, working memory and cortical thickness. *Developmental Cognitive Neuroscience, 19*, 211–222.

Raghubar, K. P., Barnes, M. A., & Hecht, S. A. (2010). Working memory and mathematics: A review of developmental, individual difference, and cognitive approaches. *Learning and Individual Differences, 20*, 110–122.

Ridderinkhof, K. R., van der Molen, M. W., Band, G. P. H., & Bashore, T. R. (1997). Sources of interference from irrelevant information: A developmental study. *Journal of Experimental Child Psychology, 65*, 315–341.

Rotzer, S., Loenneker, T., Kucian, K., Martin, E., Klaver, P., & von Aster, M. (2009). Dysfunctional neural network of spatial working memory contributes to developmental dyscalculia. *Neuropsychologia, 47*, 2859–2865.

Rubia, K., Smith, A. B., Woolley, J., Nosarti, C., Heyman, I., Taylor, E., & Brammer, M. (2006). Progressive increase of frontostriatal brain activation from childhood to adulthood during event-related tasks of cognitive control. *Human Brain Mapping, 27*, 973–993.

Sayala, S., Sala, J. B., & Courtney, S. M. (2005). Increased neural efficiency with repeated performance of a working memory task is information-type dependent. *Cerebral Cortex, 16*, 609–617.

Shinaver, C. S., Entwistle, P. C., & Söderqvist, S. (2014). Cogmed WM Training: Reviewing the Reviews. *Applied Neuropsychology: Child, 3*, 163–172.

Shipstead, Z., Hicks, K. L., & Engle, R. W. (2012). Cogmed working memory training: Does the evidence support the claims? *Journal of Applied Research in Memory and Cognition, 1*, 185–193.

Shirtcliff, E. A., Dahl, R. E., & Pollak, S. D. (2009). Pubertal development: Correspondence between hormonal and physical development. *Child Development, 80*, 327–337.

Shoda, Y., Mischel, W., & Peake, P. K. (1990). Predicting adolescent cognitive and self-regulatory competencies from preschool delay of gratification: Identifying diagnostic conditions. *Developmental Psychology, 26*, 978–986.

Silverman, M. H., Jedd, K., & Luciana, M. (2015). Neural networks involved in adolescent reward processing: An activation likelihood estimation meta-analysis of functional neuroimaging studies. *NeuroImage, 122*, 427–439.

Somerville, L. H., & Casey, B. J. (2010). Developmental neurobiology of cognitive control and motivational systems. *Current Opinion in Neurobiology, 20*, 236–241.

Steinberg, L. (2008). A social neuroscience perspective on adolescent risk-taking. *Developmental Review, 28*, 78–106.

Tamnes, C. K., Walhovd, K. B., Grydeland, H., Holland, D., Østby, Y., Dale, A. M., & Fjell, A. M. (2013). Longitudinal working memory development is related to structural maturation of frontal and parietal cortices. *Journal of Cognitive Neuroscience, 25*, 1611–1623.

Tangney, J. P., Baumeister, R. F., & Boone, A. L. (2004). High self-control predicts good adjustment, less pathology, better grades, and interpersonal success. *Journal of Personality, 72*, 271–324.

Thorell, L. B., Lindqvist, S., Bergman Nutley, S., Bohlin, G., & Klingberg, T. (2009). Training and transfer effects of executive functions in preschool children. *Developmental Science, 12*, 106–113.

Van der Sluis, S., De Jong, P. F., & Van der Leij, A. (2004). Inhibition and shifting in children with learning deficits in arithmetic and reading. *Journal of Experimental Child Psychology, 87*, 239–266.

Velanova, K., Wheeler, M. E., & Luna, B. (2008). Maturational changes in anterior cingulate and frontoparietal recruitment support the development of error processing and inhibitory control. *Cerebral Cortex, 18*, 2505–2522.

Wass, S. V., Scerif, G., & Johnson, M. H. (2012). Training attentional control and working memory—is younger, better? *Developmental Review, 32*, 360–387.

Williams, B. R., Ponesse, J. S., Schachar, R. J., Logan, G. D., & Tannock, R. (1999). Development of inhibitory control across the life span. *Developmental Psychology, 35*, 205–213.

Zelazo, P. D. (2006). The dimensional change card sort (DCCS): A method of assessing executive function in children. *Nature Protocols, 1*, 297–301.

Zhao, X., Chen, L., Fu, L., & Maes, J. H. R. (2015). Wesley says: A children's response inhibition playground training game yields preliminary evidence of transfer effects. *Frontiers in Psychology, 6*, 207.

Zhao, X., Chen, L., & Maes, J. H. R. (2016). Training and transfer effects of response inhibition training in children and adults. *Developmental Science.* doi:10.1111/desc. 12511

Zinke, K., Einert, M., Pfennig, L., & Kliegel, M. (2012). Plasticity of executive control through task switching training in adolescents. *Frontiers in Human Neuroscience, 6*, 41.

10 Understanding Emotional Thought Can Transform Educators' Understanding of How Students Learn

Mary Helen Immordino-Yang and Rebecca J.M. Gotlieb

The way students feel affects how they learn—a fact developmental psychologists and master educators have known long and well (e.g., Bruner, 1990; Montessori, 1914, 2009; Nasir, 2012). Indeed, students' abilities to recognize, understand, and manage their emotions; to build and maintain a sense of interest and curiosity; to persist through challenges and uncertainty; to embrace new experiences; to imagine alternative futures for themselves and their communities; and to feel purposeful . . . all of these powerfully influence personal and academic success (Damon, 2008; Duckworth & Seligman, 2005; Kaufman, 2013; Oyserman, 2015). Why is learning such an emotion-dependent process, and what does this mean for teachers and schools?

Education research has for the past century, and with increasing empirical evidence more recently, explored the contributions of social-emotional feelings to students' learning and achievement (Durlak, Weissberg, Dymnicki, Taylor, & Schellinger, 2011; Osher et al., 2016; Pekrun, Goetz, Titz, & Perry, 2002; Yeager & Walton, 2011). Terms referring to the impact of beliefs and feelings in learning contexts have become widely used even in the non-academic lexicon. For example, educators routinely speak of "stereotype threat" (the phenomenon in which individuals' fear of conforming to stereotypes negatively influences their performance; Steele, 2011), "growth mindset" (the belief that intelligence and talent can be changed with hard work; Dweck, 2006) and "grit" (the ability to persist in the face of frustrations; Duckworth, 2016). Popular press coverage of social-emotional learning (SEL) has burgeoned, and major consensus reports have focused on outlining the state of the evidence on how SEL programs impact academic achievement (Jones & Kahn, 2017). In the United States, the value of supporting the "whole child" has even been codified into law at the national level: the 2015 *Every Student Succeeds Act* (Public Law No. 114–95, 2015) allows curriculum funds to be used to support social-emotional programming. Even the business community has argued for the economic value of supporting the growth of students' social-emotional skills to prepare them for the collaborations, frustrations, and social relations of the adult workplace (Brackett, Divecha, & Stern, 2015; Deming, 2017).

And yet, despite the growing recognition that emotions are central to the learning process, many educators and policy makers still implicitly believe that engaging students' interests and curiosities is a luxury that cannot be afforded to students who are struggling academically, or to students who have trouble appropriately managing their behavior and therefore require strict, prescripted interventions that disregard and negate their feelings (Immordino-Yang, 2016; Okonofua, Paunesku, & Walton, 2016). Too often, social-emotional learning is viewed either as a luxury for those with the opportunity and the means, or as a remediation strategy for the underprivileged or underperforming, rather than as a universal need of all people. Others incorrectly view emotions as "interfering" with clear-headed thinking—akin to an emotional toddler running amuck with a baseball bat in a store that sells glassware (Immordino-Yang & Damasio, 2007). Still others misunderstand the role of emotions, believing that as long as students are "having fun," teachers are adequately attending to students' wellbeing and deep learning (Immordino-Yang, 2015a).

Each of these perspectives gives way to a more nuanced and accurate view once educators understand what emotions actually are from a developmental, neuropsychological perspective, and what "learning", in the broad, developmental sense in which we mean it in education, actually entails. Why do we have emotions, and how do emotions organize thinking? How is emotional development influenced by the social and cultural context, including by the micro-cultural context of the classroom? The purpose of this chapter is to equip educators and those who work with young people with basic answers to these questions, with the dual aims of helping them become more strategic in how they leverage emotions in their work, and of helping them more convincingly advocate for policies consistent with the science.

The Making of an Emotion: Body, Brain, Mind, and Consciousness in a Social World

Consider the experience of Alan, a 15-year-old from a crime-riddled neighborhood in Los Angeles. In a radio interview he explained that three of his friends, who were not involved in gangs, died because of separate instances of gang violence. He recalls that he cried when his first friend died, and cried when his second friend died, but by the third friend, he reported not being able to believe that it had happened yet again. He described a feeling of shock and disbelief, and was unable to mount any emotional response (KPCC Southern California Public Radio, story by F. Stoltze [Ed.], 5–22–08).

Alan's story is one of fear and sadness, of turning from compassion and embodied, tearful awareness to numbness and shock. It is a story of empathy come and gone, of emotion felt and lost, of consciousness altered by engagement changed to disbelief. Alan speaks of his life in Los Angeles, but he could be telling the story of many young people caught in urban violence, war or abuse worldwide.

In explaining his story, Alan gives away what social-affective neuroscience is also uncovering: that the mind and body are tied together in emotional experience. Alan cries for the deaths of his first two friends, innocent bystanders caught in criminal violence. He subjectively feels the sadness of their loss as an emotion that changes his body state, through crying as well as other physiological changes, which typically include loss of energy, lowered heart rate, and a sad facial expression and physical posture, among other things. Other more subtle changes would also be present as a result of his reaction (Butler, Yang, Laube, Kühn, & Immordino-Yang, 2018). If we measured, we would expect to find changes in blood pressure, breathing patterns, sleep patterns, and even digestion and immune responding (Barrett, 2017; Sapolsky, 2017; Van der Kolk, 2015). These physiological changes, in turn, would alter his mind in characteristic ways, potentially causing him to dwell on the event (in effect, to continually use up cognitive resources thinking about it), to have trouble concentrating on other topics, and perhaps even shaking his ability to relate well to the other people he loves for fear that he will lose them.

As we can see from Alan's story, cognition and emotion each play a role in Alan's response to the tragic news, and his reaction reflects the interdependence of his body, brain, and mind. Alan learns (cognitively) of his friends' deaths. His (cognitive) interpretation of the significance of these events automatically triggers the (emotional) reaction of sadness. This reaction plays out in part by modulating basic physiological life-regulatory processing in his body and brain. These physiological changes are, in turn, sensed or "felt" by the brain, where they have the possibility of shifting and shaping the kinds of mental processing Alan is likely to engage going forward. In this way, what Alan feels influences and is influenced by what he thinks and what he knows. His cognitions and emotional responses are intertwined, not separate, and his evolving understanding and affective experience become two dimensions of the same mental process (Fischer & Bidell, 2006; Immordino-Yang, 2010), a concept that we have previously termed "emotional thought" (Immordino-Yang & Damasio, 2007). In this body ↔ brain ↔ mind cycle, emotions and cognitions are intertwined in processes of thinking and learning, and to varying degrees influence and are influenced by changes in body state. (See also Figure 10.1.)

Beyond the emotions that Alan reports for his first two friends' deaths, Alan's experience illustrates another feature of the interdependence between the mind and body in emotion. When his third friend dies, Alan's reaction breaks past his previous feeling of sadness to instead induce a state of shock. That is, unable to reconcile the events he knows are true (his friends' deaths) with his knowledge about what ought to be true based on his previous expectations (his friends' presence), his emotion, cognition, and sense of self are temporarily stunned. He does not cry for his third friend's death because he cannot connect his current knowledge to his past experiences in order to engage his body and mind in an appropriate emotional reaction. Unable to

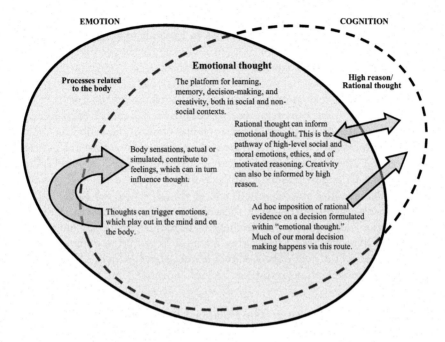

Figure 10.1 Social and Affective Neuroscientists Are Describing the Interrelatedness of Emotion, Cognition, and the Body in Thinking and Consciousness. The thought processes that educators care about—among them learning, memory, creativity, and critical thought—involve both emotional and cognitive aspects, and can involve the body as well as the mind. In the diagram, the solid ellipse represents emotion; the dashed ellipse represents cognition. The extensive overlap between the two ellipses represents the domain of "emotional thought." Emotional thought can be conscious or non-conscious (below the level of conscious awareness) and is the means by which bodily reactions influence the mind, and vice versa. High reason is a small section of the diagram and refers to the most disembodied and logical of thought processes, which are nevertheless informed by emotional thought.

Source: Reprinted with permission from Immordino-Yang and Damasio (2007).

make meaning of what happened, the resulting state feels to him like shock, or the sense of numbness and disembodiment that many people report following traumatic events and fear.

From a scientific perspective, Alan's reaction to his third friend's death illustrates the neuropsychological connection between affect and mechanisms of consciousness (Damasio, 1994/2005). Alan is describing the altered state of awareness he experienced at such an overwhelming event and alluding to the *cognitive* disconnect between his previous experiences and this new occurrence, by describing his disbelief about what had just happened. When Alan is unable to assimilate the knowledge of his third friend's death into the rest of what he knows about how the world ought to work, he cannot mount an appropriate, coherent emotional response in his body and mind, and shows no overt emotional display. He notices a change in his perceived level of consciousness—a state of detachment or disembodiment—which he describes as shock and disbelief.

Finally, though we do not know more about how these effects played out for Alan over time, it is common for survivors of this kind of trauma to later have altered memories of the event and surrounding context. Typically they hold either highly crystalline, vivid, and focused memories of one moment in time that are unresolvable (the kind of memories that can be intrusive and lead to syndromes such as post-traumatic stress disorder; Harris, 2018), or they have very vague memories and amnesia (Lynn et al., 2014; Van der Kolk, 2015). Either way, survivors of trauma or those experiencing undue stress illustrate how emotion and cognition are interdependent in the formation of memories. They also illustrate how, when either emotion or cognition dominates the thinking process too much, the resulting learning tends either to be less flexible and transferable to new contexts, or weaker overall.

Emotions Steer Thinking: The Balanced Interdependence of Cognition and Emotion, and the Importance of Emotional Relevance

How does the discussion of Alan help us understand how emotions relate to learning in school? Though Alan's tragic situation is extreme compared to the emotions most students and teachers experience daily in classrooms, nonetheless the principles are the same in both cases. In essence, emotion plays a role in engaging the neural substrate for thinking by helping people attend to, evaluate and react to stimuli, situations, and happenings, and then to integrate what they have attended to and evaluated into their knowledge structures and memory in a coordinated way going forward. It may be helpful to understand emotions as *steering* thinking, like a rudder steers a ship (Damasio, 1994/2005; Immordino-Yang & Damasio, 2007). Thinking, in turn, promotes learning, as thoughts are compared with previous knowledge called up from memory, and integrated and reconciled to build updated understanding. Unsurprisingly given the interdependence of these processes, extensive research now makes clear that the brain networks supporting emotion and bodily sensation, and those supporting learning and memory, are functionally intertwined (Immordino-Yang, Christodoulou, & Singh, 2012; Panksepp & Biven, 2012), even for expertise in technical domains like mathematics (Zeki, Romaya, Benincasa, & Atiyah, 2014). Emotions are an essential and ubiquitous dimension of thought, important for shifting thought patterns and for forming and recalling memories (Immordino-Yang & Singh, 2013; Perry, Hendler, & Shamay-Tsoory, 2011; Phelps, 2004; Yang, Pavarini, Schnall, & Immordino-Yang, 2018).

As we can see, though the emotions and cognitions from an episode can be analyzed separately, emotions are not separate from cognition in the mind, as earlier generations of cognitive science researchers believed (Gardner, 1985). It is much more conducive to think deeply about or remember information about which we have had genuine emotion, because the healthy brain does not waste energy processing information that does not matter to the individual (Immordino-Yang, 2015a). However, this means that for emotions to enhance and drive academic achievement and deep learning in school, the emotions induced need to be, as directly as possible, relevant to the ideas being engaged with (Immordino-Yang & Faeth, 2010; Mather, 2007). In other words, people mostly think about and remember the topic that the emotion pertains to—in Alan's case, relationships, insecurity, death, and loss. Alan's emotions could help him learn deeply about the injustices of gang violence, or about the importance of safety for building trusting attachments and friendships, but they would likely interfere with his ability to learn math or some other academic subject.

To sum up, emotions promote thinking which in turn promotes learning—but the vital question for educators is, "about what?" If the emotions being felt during scholarly activities pertain not to disciplinary, intellectual ideas but instead to something else (e.g., the trauma one has experienced, the football match later, the grade one hopes for, or what others will think about my performance), then the emotion will likely interfere with the learning that teachers intend to foster in their classrooms. This is why overuse of extrinsic rewards like prizes and payment in exchange for completed schoolwork tends not to improve learning and even to undermine deep understanding, interest, and enjoyment of learning over time (Allan & Fryer, 2011; Kuhbandner, Aslan, Emmerdinger, & Murayama, 2016; Murayama, Matsumoto, Izuma, & Matsumoto, 2010); why high-arousal "fun" and exciting school activities tend not to result in improved understanding of the underlying concepts (Okan, 2003; Meinhardt & Pekrun, 2003); and why children who don't feel safe in school have trouble learning from their classes (Glew, Fan, Katon, Rivara, & Kernic, 2005). In each of these cases, the emotions students are experiencing do not enrich the nature of their conceptual understanding. By contrast, students grow and achieve more over time if the emotions they are experiencing pertain to ideas and skills they are meant to be learning (Perkins, 2014). For example, students may feel pride and satisfaction at truly understanding something new and explaining it successfully to classmates, feel interest or curiosity about why a science experiment works, or feel inspired to create a touching essay that truly expresses their perspective and moves those who read it (Hantzopoulos, 2016; Taylor, 2017). Each of these situations promotes deeper engagement and learning because the student feels emotionally connected to the intellectual endeavor or *process* of meaningful learning, rather than to superficial, immediate, distracting or irrelevant outcomes or circumstances (Hubberman, Duffy, Mason, Zeiser, & O'Day, 2016; Immordino-Yang & Faeth, 2010; Savery, 2015).

During learning, emotions help us set goals, tell us when to keep working and when to stop, when we are on the right path to solve a problem and when we need to change course, what we should remember and what is not important, etc. (Immordino-Yang & Damasio, 2007). People are willing to work harder to learn the content and skills they are emotionally engaged with, and they are emotionally engaged when the content and skills they are learning seem useful for understanding the world or are connected to their curiosities, motivations, and future goals (Engel, 2015). Conversely, emotions like anxiety can undermine learning by causing worrying, which depletes cognitive resources and activates thought patterns (and neural activity patterns) associated with fear and escape rather than with academic thinking (Beilock, 2010). (The most effective fix, not surprisingly, is not to ignore the anxiety or to try to suppress it. It is, instead, to reappraise what the bodily sensations associated with arousal and nervousness actually imply about one's ability to succeed, which probably is not much [Brady, Hard, & Gross, 2018]). Thinking begets emotion, and emotion begets thinking, and when these processes feed off each other and *pertain to core ideas implicit in the work at hand*, then high-quality learning is more likely to happen.

Many Emotions in Education Are Social and Cultural, Even When Working Alone

Think again of the reactions that Alan described in his interview. His reactions involve perceived changes to his own body and mind. And yet, perhaps least obvious but most important, these reactions are induced by Alan's thoughts about events that happened to other people with whom he had relationships. In this way, Alan illustrates how, from a neuropsychological perspective, the mechanisms involved in the feeling and regulation of the body and consciousness also double as a platform for the social mind (Fiske, 2014; Immordino-Yang, Chiao, & Fiske, 2010).

Many of the emotions most relevant for learning are either implicitly or explicitly social. They often pertain to the self in relation to other people, to one's interpretations of others' beliefs, or to socially constructed values and morals that guide decision making, goal setting, and outcome evaluation (Damasio, 2018; Kaplan et al., 2017; Pekrun et al., 2002). Children come prepared to observe, imitate, and learn from those around them (Bandura, 1977; Gopnik, 2016; Moll, 2018; Tomasello, 2009). As they grow, they search to identify the tools, skills, and concepts that seem most relevant to their future, and they naturally want to adapt to the norms and expectations of their social context (Montessori, 1914/2009; Rogoff, 2003; Vygotsky, 1929). In this way, brain development and functioning, like the learning they support, are socially and culturally contextualized—they happen in the context of cultural experiences, social relationships, and cognitive opportunities, as subjectively perceived and emotionally experienced by the learner. This is true even when the person is working alone or independently, because the emotion-related cultural norms and goals the person has previously internalized shape how she interprets situations, builds goals, and remembers the situation into the future (Rogoff, 2003; Bruner, 1972).

Neuropsychological research has even revealed that, cumulatively, socio-cultural experience shifts which brain regions' activations correlate with experiences of emotions (as described on pages 254–255; Immordino-Yang & Yang, 2017; Immordino-Yang, Yang, & Damasio, 2014, 2016). Interpreted in a developmental light, such data suggest that individuals may learn to rely on different cues and thought patterns to know how they are emotionally feeling. For example, a person struggling to calm himself and focus may come to realize that he is deeply angered by a situation, or a person may feel her heart pounding and interpret this as evidence that she is excited or, alternately, afraid. Over time, the person's interpretation of socially situated experiences contributes to the development of cultural identity, as broader patterns emerge across interactions and situations, and one's responses take on significance related to personal meaning, values, and group memberships (Gutiérrez & Rogoff, 2003; Immordino-Yang & Gotlieb, 2017; Nasir, 2012). Here, the person who is angered may decide that he does not fit in the cultural group of peers who triggered his anger and is not "like them," or the person feeling excited may decide to further pursue and devote work to the issue at hand, perhaps making that issue her life's work. In both cases, the person is interpreting social-emotional cues and deciding what these feelings mean for his or her roles, skills, and identities. This, in turn, impacts what the person does, believes, and values, and who they become.

Figure 10.2 summarizes these mechanisms in a graphic illustration. As the framework illustrates, individuals' thoughts about themselves and other people, and their interpretations and beliefs about situations, result in and are shaped by emotions. These emotions can play out as activation patterns or simulations in the "feeling" (somatosensory) systems of the brain—the regions in the brain responsible for sensing the body (see also Figure 10.3). They can also leak down onto the actual body, causing physiological changes in systems important for survival, such as changes to heart rate, skin sweating, breathing, and digestion (the "Emotion Induction" arrow in the figure). As is represented by the "Feeling Construction" arrow in the figure, bodily arousal patterns are mapped by the "feeling" systems of the brain, where they have the possibility of influencing how a person feels emotionally—nervous, for example—and hence what they are likely to think about next. For example, if a person going into a math test interpreted their arousal as a nervous feeling, they may think next about how they might fail their math exam, and how embarrassing and demeaning that would be. Such a thought pattern would not be conducive to thinking about math concepts and procedures and could therefore undermine performance.

The thoughts we have about ourselves and other people, termed the "social mind," are intermediate between perceived bodily sensations and the meaning an individual makes of a situation (Barrett, 2017; Damasio, 1999). Following

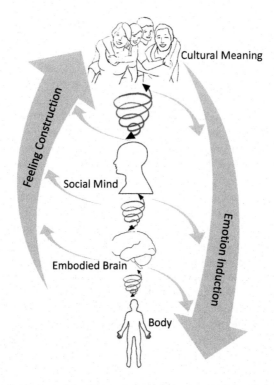

Figure 10.2 A Depiction of the Dynamic Interdependence of the Body and Embodied Brain, the Social Mind, and Processes of Cultural Meaning-making During Experiences of Emotion.

Source: Figure reprinted with permission from Immordino-Yang & Gotlieb, 2017.

the math test/nervousness example, a person could interpret that a math test is important for social standing and future goals. He could also interpret that his teacher doesn't have high expectations for him, based on who his friends and family are, what ethnic group he belongs to, or his past history. Even if he were capable of doing the math, the meaning he would have made about the test's importance, coupled with the meaning he makes of the teacher's expectations, would likely cause him to release stress hormones into his body and brain. These would cause his heart to beat faster, his blood pressure to rise and his digestion to slow (hence, the "dry mouth" that accompanies stress; Sapolsky, 2017). The feeling of his pounding heart, light-headedness, and dry mouth could be sensed by the brain and that arousal could be interpreted as reflecting threat, which in turn could reinforce his belief that, even though he knows the math outside of the testing situation, in the test he is likely to "freeze" and fail. This could in turn push him to think more about how

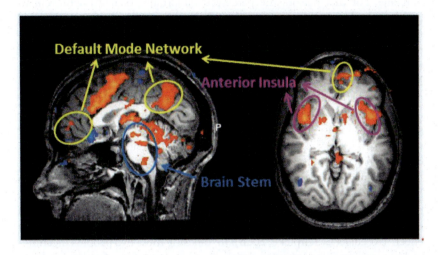

Figure 10.3 Social Emotions Recruit Brain Systems Essential for Survival and Consciousness, in Addition to Those Involved in High-level Cognition.

The figure shows a sagittal (left image; x = +2) and transverse (right image; z = +5) slice of the brain that maps brain areas (in orange) that are more active as individuals are reporting feeling inspired after learning of another person's virtue and triumph over adversity, compared to when they report no strong emotional reaction. The insula is visceral somatosensory cortex, which is involved not only in feeling the guts but also in processing self-awareness and subjective emotional experience. The default-mode network is a constellation of regions that functionally communicate during narrative-like processing that moves the thinker out of the "here and now," for example during daydreaming, thinking about moral values, prospecting about the future, and remembering past experiences. The brainstem lies between the body and the rest of the brain and contains densely packed fiber tracts and nuclei essential for basic physiological regulation, consciousness, and survival. Figure reprinted with permission from Immordino-Yang & Gotlieb, 2017. Data are from Immordino-Yang et al., 2009. The image is thresholded at the False Discovery Rate q < 0.05.

important the test is and how failing will reinforce his teacher's low expectations for "people like him." Cycling through these frantic thoughts, in turn, will use up working memory resources, further depleting his ability to think about math (Beilock, 2010). The result is a downward spiral in performance— a self-perpetuating cycle of social thoughts, emotions, and meaning termed "stereotype threat" that undermines cognitive performance as well as scholarly agency, self-efficacy and identity development, not to mention health and wellbeing (Aronson, Burgess, Phelan, & Juarez, 2013; Spencer, Logel, & Davies, 2016; Steele, 2011).

In an alternative scenario, a person with the same cultural interpretation of the importance of the test but a different way of making meaning about her own academic potential and her teacher's expectations could have a different outcome. For that person, the perceived importance of math achievement and her need for math to pursue broader questions that interest her could lead to arousal during the test-taking situation. But, this person could interpret or "feel" her bodily arousal as indicating that she is "up for the challenge and interested" rather than "nervous and worried about failure" (Beilock & Maloney, 2015; Jamieson, Mendes, & Nock, 2013). Such an interpretation would be facilitated by positive cultural norms in the school and family around math achievement and ability, strong supports and expectations for such growth-oriented achievement in the school, and teaching practices that reinforce students' becoming curious about math (Baehr, 2013). This person's challenge-oriented meaning-making process would help her recall information pertaining to math (Beilock, 2010; Engel, 2015), as well as strengthen her willingness to try hard, helping strengthen her performance. In addition, this person's test-taking experience would bolster and reinforce her math learning through successful recall practice via a process termed the "testing effect" (Roediger & Karpicke, 2006). Juxtaposing these two people's meaning-making, one interpreting arousal as nervousness and fear of failure and one interpreting arousal as an experience of healthy challenge and interest, highlights one way that emotional, social, and cultural processes impact cognition, and by extension, academic performance (Pekrun, Elliott, & Maier, 2009). Interestingly, the physiological manifestations of arousal interpreted as stress can be differentiated from those associated with arousal interpreted as challenge, and have different implications as well for bodily health (Blascovich, 2008; Blascovich & Tomaka, 1996).

Brain Systems for Feeling the Gut Are Co-opted for Emotional Experiences, but "Gut Feelings" Reflect Extensive Learning Rather Than Naïve Intuitions

Ample research now supports that we understand and mount social-emotional reactions like the nervousness versus challenged reactions described in the previous section by feeling (or mentally simulating) our subjective responses (Immordino-Yang, 2010). This process recruits the visceral somatosensory cortex that senses our own "gut" in the direct sense—the same brain region implicated when we experience a stomachache or a pounding heart (Immordino-Yang, McColl, Damasio, & Damasio, 2009; Damasio et al., 2000). In that sense, we really do live with "gut feelings" (Immordino-Yang, 2011; see also Figure 10.3). Critical for educators to realize, though, is that we develop the ability to have complex gut feelings through learning and experience (Immordino-Yang, 2015a), because feelings of this sort require elaborated, culturally shaped cognition (Barrett, Mesquita, Ochsner, & Gross, 2007; Immordino-Yang, 2010; Immordino-Yang & Yang, 2017; Kaplan et al., 2017). Though more basic emotions like disgust to spoiled food require much less learning if any (Ekman, 1973), an emotional appreciation for art, moral righteousness, or mathematical equations each require extensive opportunities for thinking, engaging, and problem solving within the domain. Yet, these complex emotions still engage neural systems for visceral somatosensation and autonomic (bodily physiological) regulation, just as do more basic emotions like disgust to spoiled food or attraction to delicious food (Immordino-Yang et al., 2009; Vessel, Starr, & Rubin, 2013; Wicker et al., 2003; Zeki, Romaya, Benincasa, & Atiyah, 2014). In turn, as we mentally perceive and cognitively deliberate on feelings associated with objects, people, situations, and their implications, brain networks involved in the processing of memories and narratives are increasingly coordinated and engaged (Immordino-Yang & Singh, 2013; Kaplan et al., 2017; Yang, Bossmann, Schiffhauer, Jordan, & Immordino-Yang, 2013). Memories, mental simulations in the form of plans and imaginings, cognitions and sensations come together into concerted mental states that make our experiences feel coherent and "like they matter" (Barrett, 2017; Damasio, 1999).

It is this subjective feeling—the feeling that what one is experiencing and thinking about matters—that effective educational practices leverage. Consider, for example, the impact on learning of a student's feeling of wonder when he comes to appreciate that all life on earth evolved from a single-celled organism, or consider the powerful benefits for learning of a student's anger as she reads about a country's history of voter suppression techniques. Individuals' emotional reactions to the content they learn can precipitate further thinking and reflection, which enhances memory formation (Craik & Tulving, 1975) and furthers learning. This has powerful implications for educators. It suggests that facilitating students' affective processing is not something to do merely so that students attend in the moment or exercise control over their inappropriate negative emotions; rather, attending to students' affective processing about task-relevant information is also a powerful way to strengthen their learning. Teachers who cultivate students' empathies, curiosities, and interests relative to academic subjects can help at-risk students to achieve on par with their low-risk peers (Hamre & Pianta, 2005; Hantzopoulos, 2016). Rigorous randomized experimental studies and meta-analyses of hundreds of studies suggest that investing in social-emotional learning does not merely produce better behaved students or kinder citizens; it also helps students achieve greater long-term academic success (Durlak, Weissberg, Dymnicki, Taylor, & Schellinger, 2011; Jones, Brown, & Aber, 2011; Taylor, Oberle, Durlak, & Weissberg, 2017).

It is also important for educators to understand that emotional feelings are subjective experiences. As such, they vary across people. The neuropsychological work on feelings suggests that individuals may vary not only in which emotions come up in particular situations, but, reminiscent of the math student who feels challenged rather than threatened, potentially individuals may vary also in the processes they invoke to know exactly how they are feeling. This idea is founded in data on emotion-related activation patterns in the insula, a brain region important for emotional experience and evaluative aspects of cognition that is also involved in feeling visceral sensations like heartbeats and stomachache (Craig, 2002; Damasio et al., 2000; Kurth, Zilles, Fox, Laird, & Eickhoff, 2010; Zaki, Davis, & Ochsner, 2012). Our longitudinal and cross-cultural data suggest that people may learn from cultural and social experiences how to translate physiological activation patterns into conscious emotional feelings, as insula activity can correspond to emotional feelings differently depending on social, cultural, and developmental factors (Immordino-Yang, 2015b; Immordino-Yang & Yang, 2014, 2017).

For example, in one study we found that the words people use to describe their emotional feelings in an interview predict differences in the neural activity patterns they show when reacting to emotional stories in the fMRI scanner. In this study, people who described their feelings using a higher proportion of cognitive words, like "think", "know", and "believe," did not report feeling weaker emotions than individuals who used affective words such as "sad," "cry" or "warm". But those who used more cognitive words showed relatively less activation in somatosensory cortices for the same reported strength of feeling, compared to the activation levels for those who used a higher proportion of affective words (Saxbe, Yang, Borofsky, & Immordino-Yang, 2013). The findings suggest that participants varied in the degree to which their feelings were neurally embodied. The implication from these neural data, which could not have been known from the psychological measures alone, is that while some individuals' emotions seem to play out in bodily, sensory feelings, others' emotional feelings may be less bodily and more cognitive in nature. In other words, people can vary in the processes by which they feel their emotions, even when they all claim to be experiencing strong emotion.

In another set of studies, we aimed to test whether such differences could be partly learned. To do this, we set out to test whether cultural differences may exist in the neural correlates of emotional feelings. If individuals from different cultural groups report feeling the same emotions when reacting to a set of stories, for example, but show different patterns of correspondence between brain activity and their reported feelings, it would suggest that individuals in the two groups are potentially processing the *same* emotion in a *different* way. If a bicultural group of individuals, who have been exposed to both cultural contexts, show an intermediate or mixed pattern of results, this would suggest that the newly discovered cultural group difference is not genetic or racial, but *learned*. Because differences in emotion processing could have implications for behavior, decision making, and learning, such findings would have important implications for education. They would potentially provide new insights into appropriate educational cultural accommodations, and open the possibility that the cultural environments of schools may also be shaping the processes by which young people come to experience their social-emotional lives—both topics that would warrant further research.

A series of experiments carried out in Los Angeles and Beijing with university students uncovered cultural patterns of activity during emotional experiences, as we had suspected (Immordino-Yang et al., 2014, 2016; Immordino-Yang & Yang, 2017). Chinese, American, and bicultural

Chinese-American participants were asked to explain their feelings about each of a series of true social stories to an experimenter in a private interview, and then to watch the stories again during fMRI scanning and to report again their feelings as they watched. We found that the groups did not differ in how strongly they reported feeling in response to the stories, or in how much brain activation they showed. However, the Chinese and American groups did differ in how their brain activity corresponded in real-time to their reported feelings. While American participants' feelings tended to track with the dorsal, more somatosensory and cognitive sector of the insula, Chinese participants' feelings tended to track with the ventral sector, which is evolutionarily older and more autonomic regulatory (Kurth et al., 2010). Supporting the interpretation that this difference was learned rather than genetic, the bicultural Chinese-American participants showed an intermediate pattern that fell between the Chinese and the American norms. The findings were replicated.

A follow-up study suggested that the cultural differences may follow from Americans' learned emphasis on expressiveness and Chinese people's learned emphasis on suppressing overt emotional displays. We found that cultural differences in the correlations between insula activity and feelings were mediated by participants' emotional expressiveness in the interview: Americans tended to be more emotionally demonstrative in their interview behavior than had been the Chinese participants, in accordance with American and Chinese cultural expressiveness norms (Tsai, 2007). And it was actually these individual differences in expressiveness, regardless of cultural group, that explained the neural findings. More expressive people in all three cultural groups tended toward the average American neural pattern (Immordino-Yang et al., 2016), as if their more pronounced bodily changes during emotion had "taught" them to attend more to the feeling of their body in deciding how they feel emotionally. (For those interested in the details, we also measured psychophysiological reactions on participants' bodies as they felt emotions, allowing us to analyze the degree to which emotional feelings were related to patterns of bodily reactions like sweating, breathing, and heart rate increases.)

Essentially, we interpreted these findings to suggest that the way in which people had translated their neurophysiological responses into conscious feelings, or how they had become aware of what they were feeling, was different based on cultural norms for expressiveness that participants in every group had adopted to varying degrees. One implication is that how schools teach young people to behave may shape over time the processes by which they feel their bodily reactions and emotions, and such shaping may interact with home-culture norms—a topic that is the focus of current research.

Bringing the research closer to education-relevant questions, we next asked: if cultural experience may shape how individuals feel their emotions, and if emotions in social situations influence social-emotional identity development, how might differences in adolescents' natural visceral sensation sensitivity impact their identities? To begin to examine this, we investigated how bicultural American youths' sensitivity to heartbeat sensations would be related to their ethnic identity development. Heartbeat sensitivity naturally varies among people, and is known to be associated with the thickness of cortex in the insula (visceral somatosensory cortex; Craig, 2002). Ethnic identity reflects young peoples' subjective decision about the degree to which their core identity is from their home culture versus from the mainstream culture outside their home, in this case mainstream American culture. We studied adolescents from East-Asian and Latino immigrant families, because these cultural groups have different ideals for expressiveness, with East Asians being on average less expressive than mainstream American ideals, and Latinos being more so (Spencer & Markstrom-Adams, 1990; Tsai, 2007). We reasoned that individuals with greater sensitivity to heartbeat sensations would find the feeling of bodily emotional expressions more salient. Therefore, we hypothesized that more sensitivity would align with Latino ideals and reinforce home-culture identity for the Latino participants, but potentially undermine home-culture identity for the East Asians because of the desired suppression of emotional expressiveness by that cultural group.

We found that the adolescents' reported home culture identity grew stronger as youths grew older, and was stronger in youths who had witnessed less ethnically motivated violence and who had reported higher quality relationships with their parents. Controlling for these effects, though, identity also interacted with natural variance in visceral interoceptive sensitivity (studied using electrocardiograms to test the accuracy of participants' reported heartbeat rhythm after running up and down sets of stairs). As hypothesized, among youths from Latino families, *greater* sensitivity predicted stronger identification with home culture values in a questionnaire and an interview, while among youths from East-Asian families, *less* sensitivity to heartbeat sensations was associated with stronger endorsement of home culture (Cheng, Yang, Hobeika, & Immordino-Yang, 2015; Immordino-Yang & Gotlieb, 2017). We interpreted these findings to mean that in addition to known social factors like family relationships, natural variation in the neural processing of embodied experience may have influenced these bicultural youths' adoption of cultural identities by influencing how strongly they "feel like" a "Latino" or an "Asian" person versus like an "American".

As educators know, ethnic identity has implications not only for social relationships but, for example, for vulnerability to stereotypes around achievement goals (Gonzales, Blanton, & Williams, 2002; Steele, 2011; Tine & Gotlieb, 2013). Notably, the aim of this work is not to document cultural group differences—and indeed, there were no differences in the degree to which the two groups identified with home versus American culture, and no differences in their heartbeat detection accuracy. Instead, our aim was to document how visceral somatosensory sensitivity in the brain may interact with exposure to cultural norms, values, and expectations to shape identity development over time. Individual differences in bodily feelings experienced in social-emotional situations appeared to have been interpreted by these adolescents as either reinforcing or undermining home cultural identity based on whether those feelings align with the largely unstated values and norms of that culture. In addition to shifting the kinds of stereotypes for achievement that students apply to themselves, which can differ between Latino and Chinese-American culture, one implication for education, still being tested, is that embodied experiences of emotion in school settings may influence how young people learn to identify with school and feel like a "scholar," similar to how social-emotional experiences in the home influence how young people develop home-culture identity. Feelings of belonging are critical to academic persistence and success in school (Walton & Cohen, 2007), but the role of emotional experiences in the development of scholarly identity, though a powerful force, is not fully understood.

What Has Neuroscience Added to Our Understanding Over and Above Psychology?

One might ask how neuroscience supports our understanding of students' psychological need to learn how to feel. As explained earlier, our neural development, psychological development, and enculturation are entwined processes and shape one another. The biopsychosocial framework for affective processing (Figure 10.2) and several examples throughout this chapter suggest that to understand the relation between emotion and learning we need to consider the body, embodied brain, social mind, cultural context, and their mutual interdependences. Analyzing development from multiple perspectives, including from a neuroscientific perspective, gives a new window into the hidden complexities of the interactions that undergird learning.

What the neural data, taken together with the psychological and behavioral data, reveal is that the paths by which students come to know how they feel about academically relevant content may differ in ways that reflect individual experiences, inherent proclivities and cultural shaping, and cognitive development (Immordino-Yang, 2015a). This variability is real and adaptive and should be explained and leveraged rather than explained away. Educators, then, need to be sensitive not only to what emotions students have, which is increasingly a focus of education research (e.g., Pekrun & Linnenbrink-Garcia, 2012), but also to the variability in how they interpret those emotions to construct experiences that both reflect past learning and shape future learning. Such models of emotional-cognitive mechanisms could only be possible with an interdisciplinary, developmental combination of approaches that capture aspects of the biological as well as psychological dimensions (Thomas, Ansari, & Knowland, 2019), and test the implications for educational contexts.

What Are the Concrete Implications of Research and Opportunities for Translation?

The research implications for policy and practice concern effective educational environments that can promote the development of scholarly thinking and belonging by leveraging emotion. The studies described in this chapter focus on social and cultural forces that shape development. Though these studies do not directly test the effects of schooling, they teach us about the power of emotional experiences and embodied sensations in organizing neural systems involved in psychological growth and learning. Schools certainly induce emotional reactions from students and from teachers, and schools are a form of cultural setting (Gutiérrez, 2002). Bringing this neural level of explanation to bear can enrich the conversation about the impacts of emotions in school, and in particular help teachers and policy makers appreciate the deep interdependence of emotional and cognitive development over time. Because this work has begun to document developmental effects, research that specifically targets academic experience in schools can now build onto these findings. One branch of such research, just launching in Immordino-Yang's laboratory and collaborating public schools, is targeting the role of school- and classroom-level emotional enculturation, specifically in the development of so-called "intellectual virtues" (e.g., interest, curiosity, intellectual humility, intellectual agency, etc.; Baehr, 2013) on both students' and teachers' psychological and neural development and learning.

Though the empirical evidence from schools is mainly psychological rather than neural at this point, the educational research findings are better understood when taken together with the neural laboratory work that reveals the hidden neurobiological mechanisms (Immordino-Yang & Christodoulou, 2014; Immordino-Yang & Gotlieb, 2017). For example, there are still debates over the centrality of emotion to learning among policy makers, administrators, and practitioners (especially among practitioners who work with adolescents and young adults). The neural work helps make clear why ignoring the roles of cultural and emotional processes to instead focus overly on standardized "learning outcomes" is misled, and unlikely to produce satisfying explanations for learning underperformance or actionable improvement strategies (Immordino-Yang, Darling-Hammond, & Krone, 2018; Immordino-Yang, Darling-Hammond, & Krone, 2019). Optimal pedagogical practices foster engagement, thinking, and meaning-making by leveraging opportunities to strengthen, balance, and mutually reinforce the cognitive and emotional dimensions of thinking and problem solving (Erickson & Gutiérrez, 2002), in part because these dimensions are mutually reinforcing in the brain. The work suggests that to do education well requires maximizing use of culturally relevant, meaningful, and generative tasks (Hantzopoulos, 2016; Immordino-Yang, 2016)—tasks where the emotions being experienced are relevant to the concepts being learned. In these sorts of tasks, students' emotions are driving further thinking so that students are process oriented, experiencing productive emotions as they work, rather than end-point oriented, experiencing their strongest emotions only after the work is complete (Immordino-Yang, 2015a; Kuhn, 2007).

Such high-quality educational practices share various features. They place the learners' subjective emotional and social experience at the forefront, and help people build scholarly and social identities that incorporate their new skills and knowledge. They help people to feel safe and purposeful, and to believe that their work is important, relevant, and valuable. They support age-appropriate exploration and discovery, followed by cognitive elaboration for deeper understanding. And, they support the learners in pacing themselves to iteratively and authentically move between these modes of engagement as they pursue meaningful learning goals. Mounting evidence suggests that when students are working hard because they are steering toward intrinsic, problem-centered goals, and not primarily because they are trying to satisfy some relatively arbitrary milestone to be "done" or "successful," deep thinking and transfer of knowledge are more likely to happen (Kuhbandner, Aslan, Emmerdinger, & Murayama, 2016; Marsh, Pekrun, Lichtenfeld, Guo, Arens, & Murayama, 2016; Ryan & Deci, 2000).

Effective pedagogical approaches also strategically alternate activities that encourage flexible and exploratory thinking with those that encourage mastery of necessary building-block skills. Doing so attends to the trade-off between plasticity and efficiency in brain and cognitive development (Immordino-Yang, 2007, 2015a), and taps into the emotions associated with each mode. When individuals rehearse and automate skills, they come to experience the satisfaction of mastery and build self-efficacy in scholarship (Bandura, 1993; Schunk & Zimmerman, 2007). However, doing this too much leads to boredom and a lack of intellectual ambition (Pekrun, Hall, Goetz, & Perry, 2014), and can undermine transfer and persistence when encountering new material (Ainley, Hidi, & Berndorff, 2002; Marsh et al., 2016). When individuals explore and investigate in a more open-ended way, they invoke emotions like curiosity that lead to motivation and the formation of more durable memories for the new information (Engel, 2015; Spelke & Schulz, 2011). Experiencing such emotions helps students acquire habits of mind that facilitate acquisition of age-appropriate knowledge and skills, reasoning, and ethical reflectiveness (Gardner, Csikszentmihalyi, & Damon, 2008; Perkins, 2014). These habits of mind—in effect, cultural ways of thinking and feeling—become tools for navigating the world as a learner, bringing curiosity, interest, persistence, and a deep thirst for understanding (Baehr, 2013). Educators and education policy makers' responsibility is to foster the conditions, emotional as well as cognitive, that support the development of these habits of mind (Perkins, 2014).

Exploring Additional Resources

Recent discussions in education underscore that young people's social, emotional, and academic development (SEAD) are intertwined (Jones & Kahn, 2017; Osher, Cantor, Berg, Steyer, & Rose, 2018). An overview of affective processing helps explain why this is so, and what it means for effective educational practices and policies. In the vein of supporting educators in thinking about student's social-emotional development from a holistic, interdisciplinary perspective, we offer several recommendations about further resources that may be of interest:

- An online masters-level course about affective and social neuroscience and education, entitled "Neuroscience and the Classroom: Making Connections". The course is freely available at www.learner.org/courses/neuroscience/ (Immordino-Yang was content director.) (Schneps [Producer], 2011).

- *Emotions, learning and the brain: Exploring the educational implications of affective neuroscience*, (2015) http://books.wwnorton.com/books/Mary-Helen-Immordino-Yang/
  The book presents ten years of work building social-affective neuroscience, and forges connections to education. Each chapter begins with a set of orienting notes and framing for educators. The book has been translated into Italian by Cortina Press, Spanish by AIQUE Publishing House in Argentina, and Mandarin by Tsinghua University Press.

- "Embodied brains, social minds, cultural meaning: Integrating neuroscientific and educational research on social-affective development," (2017) by Immordino-Yang and Gotlieb, published in the *American Education Research Journal*. http://journals.sagepub.com/doi/abs/10.3102/0002831 216669780

- "Emotion, Sociality, and the Brain's Default Mode Network: Insights for Educational Practice and Policy," (2016) by Immordino-Yang, published in *Policy Insights from the Behavioral and Brain Sciences*. http://journals. sagepub.com/doi/abs/10.1177/2372732216656869

- The Alliance for Excellent Education has various resources available, including a 2018 consensus report on the Science of Adolescent Learning. https://all4ed.org/

- The Aspen Institute has launched a National Commission on Social, Emotional and Academic Development (SEAD): www.aspeninstitute. org/programs/national-commission-on-social-emotional-and-academic-development/
  In particular, the consensus report entitled, "The Evidence Base for How We Learn: Supporting Students' Social, Emotional, and Academic Development" is particularly relevant. www.aspeninstitute.org/publications/ evidence-base-learn/. So is a new brief on the science of brain development and implications for educational policy and practice, written by Mary Helen Immordino-Yang, Linda Darling Hammond and Christina Krone: www.aspen institute.org/publications/the-brain-basis-for-integrated-social-emotional-and-academic-development/

- A new edition of *How People Learn: Brain, Mind, Experience and School* was published in 2018 by the National Academies of Sciences, Engineering, and Medicine. The new edition, *How People Learn II: Learners, Contexts, and Cultures*, has a focus on emotions and culture in learning. For access to the new edition, go to: www.nap.edu/catalog/24783/ how-people-learn-ii-learners-contexts-and-cultures

- *School of the Future* is a NOVA program produced in 2016 that documents how current knowledge in the learning sciences and best practices in select schools provide insights into how we can improve education (Bertelsen & Teeling [Producers], 2016). To view the program visit: www.pbs.org/wgbh/nova/body/school-of-the-future.html
- Readers may wish to join the International Mind, Brain and Education Society, an interdisciplinary community of researchers and practitioners from around the world that publishes a journal and holds biannual conferences. https://imbes.org/
- For those interested in reading more broadly about affective neuroscience, Antonio Damasio's *Descartes' Error: Emotion, Reason and the Human Brain* is a foundational work. He explains how neuroscience has led us to understand that affect and cognition are entwined.
- Lisa Feldman Barrett's 2017 book, *How Emotions are Made: The Secret Life of the Brain*, is an accessible read for those wishing to understand better what emotions are, how they manifest in our brains and bodies, and how we can harness the science of emotion to address a range of societal challenges, including challenges related to youth.

Acknowledgements

Support was provided by NSF CAREER 11519520 and a Spencer Foundation Mid-Career to Fellowship to MHIY; NSF GRFP Fellowship to RG, USC Provost's Research and Teaching Fellowship to RG.

References

Ainley, M., Hidi, S., & Berndorff, D. (2002). Interest, learning, and the psychological processes that mediate their relationship. *Journal of Educational Psychology, 94*(3), 545–561.

Allan, B. M., & Fryer, R. G. (2011). *The power and pitfalls of education incentives.* Brookings Institution, Hamilton Project.

Aronson, J., Burgess, D., Phelan, S. M., & Juarez, L. (2013). Unhealthy interactions: The role of stereotype threat in health disparities. *American Journal of Public Health, 103*(1), 50–56.

Baehr, J. (2013). Educating for intellectual virtues: From theory to practice. *Journal of Philosophy of Education, 47*(2), 248–262.

Bandura, A. (1977). Self-efficacy: Toward a unifying theory of behavioral change. *Psychological Review, 84*(2), 191–215.

Bandura, A. (1993). Perceived self-efficacy in cognitive development and functioning. *Educational Psychologist, 28*(2), 117–148.

Barrett, L. F. (2017). *How emotions are made: The secret life of the brain.* Boston, MA: Houghton Mifflin Harcourt.

Barrett, L. F., Mesquita, B., Ochsner, K. N., & Gross, J. J. (2007). The experience of emotion. *Annual Review of Psychology, 58,* 373–403.

Beilock, S. L. (2010). *Choke: What the secrets of the brain reveal about getting it right when you have to.* New York: Simon & Schuster.

Beilock, S. L., & Maloney, E. A. (2015). Math anxiety: A factor in math achievement not to be ignored. *Policy Insights from the Behavioral and Brain Sciences, 2*(1), 4–12.

Bertelsen, P., & Teeling, J. (Producers). (2016, September 14). *NOVA- school of the future* [Television broadcast]. WGBH Boston. Retrieved from www.pbs.org/wgbh/nova/body/school-of-the-future.html

Blascovich, J. (2008). Challenge and threat. In A. J. Elliot (Ed.), *Handbook of approach and avoidance motivation* (pp. 431–445). New York, NY: Psychology Press.

Blascovich, J., & Tomaka, J. (1996). The biopsychosocial model of arousal regulation. *Advances in Experimental Social Psychology, 28*, 1–51. doi:10.1016/S0065-2601(08)60235-X

Brackett, D., Divecha, D., & Stern, R. (2015, May 19). Teaching teenagers to develop their emotional intelligence. *Harvard Business Review Digital Articles*, 2–4. Retrieved from https://hbr.org/2015/05/teaching-teenagers-to-develop-their-emotional-intelligence

Brady, S. T., Hard, B. M., & Gross, J. J. (2018). Reappraising test anxiety increases academic performance of first-year college students. *Journal of Educational Psychology, 110*(3), 395–406.

Bruner, J. S. (1972). The nature and uses of immaturity. *American Psychologist, 27*(8), 687–708.

Bruner, J. S. (1990). *Acts of meaning* (The Jerusalem-Harvard lectures). Cambridge, MA: Harvard University Press.

Butler, O., Yang, X. F., Laube, C., Kühn, S., & Immordino-Yang, M. H. (2018). Community violence exposure correlates with smaller gray matter volume and lower IQ in urban adolescents. *Human Brain Mapping, 39*(5), 2088–2097.

Cheng, T., Yang, X.-F., Hobeika, L., & Immordino-Yang, M. H. (2015, April). *Interoceptive awareness and acculturation in bicultural adolescents* [Abstract]. Poster presented at the 2015 Meeting of the Social and Affective Neuroscience Society, Boston, MA.

Craig, A. D. (2002). How do you feel? Interoception: The sense of the physiological condition of the body. *Nature Reviews Neuroscience, 3*(8), 655–666.

Craik, F. I. M., & Tulving, E. (1975). Depth of processing and the retention of words in episodic memory. *Journal of Experimental Psychology: General, 104*(3), 268–294.

Damasio, A. (1999). *The feeling of what happens.* New York, NY: Harcourt Brace.

Damasio, A. (2005). *Descartes' error: Emotion, reasoning and the human brain.* New York, NY: Random House. (Original work published in 1994).

Damasio, A. (2018). *The strange order of things: Life, feeling, and the making of cultures.* New York: Pantheon Books.

Damasio, A., Grabowski, T. J., Bechara, A., Damasio, H., Ponto, L. L. B., Parvizi, J., & Hichwa, R. D. (2000). Subcortical and cortical brain activity during the feeling of self-generated emotions. *Nature Neuroscience, 3*(10), 1049–1056.

Damon, W. (2008). *The path to purpose: How young people find their calling in life.* New York: The Free Press.

Deming, D. J. (2017). The growing importance of social skills in the labor market. *The Quarterly Journal of Economics, 132*(4), 1593–1640.

Duckworth, A. L. (2016). *Grit: The power of passion and perseverance.* New York: Simon & Schuster.

Duckworth, A. L., & Seligman, M. E. (2005). Self-discipline outdoes IQ in predicting academic performance of adolescents. *Psychological Science, 16*(12), 939–944.

Durlak, J. A., Weissberg, R. P., Dymnicki, A. B., Taylor, R. D., & Schellinger, K. B. (2011). The impact of enhancing students' social and emotional learning: A meta-analysis of school-based universal interventions. *Child Development, 82*(1), 405–432.

Dweck, C. S. (2006). *Mindset: The new psychology of success.* New York: Random House Incorporated.

Ekman, P. (1973). Cross cultural studies of emotion. In P. Ekman (Ed.), *Darwin and facial expression: A century of research in review* (pp. 169–222). New York: Academic Press.

Engel, S. (2015). *The hungry mind: The origins of curiosity in childhood.* Cambridge, MA: Harvard University Press.

Erickson, F., & Gutiérrez, K. (2002). Culture, rigor, and science in educational research. *Educational Researcher, 31*(8), 21–24.

Fischer, K. W., & Bidell, T. R. (2006). Dynamic development of action and thought. In W. Damon & R. Lerner (Eds.), *Handbook of child psychology. Vol. 1: Theoretical models of human development* (6th ed., pp. 313–399). Hoboken, NJ: Wiley.

Fiske, S. T. (2014). *Social beings* (4th ed.). New York: Wiley.

Gardner, H. E. (1985). *The mind's new science: A history of the cognitive revolution.* New York: Basic Books.

Gardner, H. E., Csikszentmihalyi, M., & Damon, W. (2008). *Good work: When excellence and ethics meet.* New York: Basic Books.

Glew, G. M., Fan, M. Y., Katon, W., Rivara, F. P., & Kernic, M. A. (2005). Bullying, psychosocial adjustment, and academic performance in elementary school. *Archives of Pediatrics and Adolescent Medicine, 159*(11), 1026–1031.

Gonzales, P. M., Blanton, H., & Williams, K. J. (2002). The effects of stereotype threat and double minority status on the test performance of Latino women. *Personality and Social Psychology Bulletin, 28*(5), 659–670.

Gopnik, A. (2016). *The gardener and the carpenter: What the new science of child development tells us about the relationship between parents and children.* New York: Palgrave Macmillan.

Gutiérrez, K. D. (2002). Studying cultural practices in urban learning communities. *Human Development, 45*(4), 312–321.

Gutiérrez, K. D., & Rogoff, B. (2003). Cultural ways of learning: Individual traits or repertoires of practice. *Educational Researcher, 32*(5), 19–25.

Hamre, B. K., & Pianta, R. C. (2005). Can instructional and emotional support in the first-grade classroom make a difference for children at risk of school failure?. *Child Development, 76*(5), 949–967.

Hantzopoulos, M. (2016). *Restoring dignity in public schools: Human rights education in action.* New York: Teachers College Press.

Harris, N. B. (2018). *The deepest well: Healing the long-term effects of childhood adversity.* Boston, MA: Pan Macmillan.

Huberman, M., Duffy, H., Mason, J., Zeiser, K. L., & O'Day, J. (2016). *School features and student opportunities for deeper learning what makes a difference?* Washington, DC: American Institutes for Research.

Immordino-Yang, M. H. (2010). Toward a microdevelopmental, interdisciplinary approach to social emotion. *Emotion Review, 2*(3), 217–220.

Immordino-Yang, M. H. (2011). Implications of affective and social neuroscience for educational theory. *Educational Philosophy and Theory, 43*(1), 98–103.

Immordino-Yang, M. H. (2015a). *Emotions, learning and the brain: Exploring the educational implications of affective neuroscience.* New York, NY: W.W. Norton & Co.

Immordino-Yang, M. H. (2015b). Embodied brains, social minds: Toward a cultural neuroscience of social emotion. In J. Chiao, S.-C. Li, R. Seligman, & R, Turner (Eds.), *Oxford handbook of cultural neuroscience* (pp. 129–142) Oxford: Oxford University Press.

Immordino-Yang, M. H. (2016). Emotion, sociality, and the brain's default mode network: Insights for educational practice and policy. *Policy Insights from the Behavioral and Brain Sciences*, 3(2), 211–219.

Immordino-Yang, M. H., Chiao, J. Y., & Fiske, A. P. (2010). Neural reuse in the social and emotional brain. *Behavioral and Brain Sciences*, 33(4), 275–276.

Immordino-Yang, M. H., & Christodoulou, J. A. (2014). Neuroscientific contributions to understanding and measuring emotions in educational contexts. In R. Pekrun & L. Linnenbrink-Garcia (eds.), *International handbook of emotions in education* (pp. 607–624) New York, NY: Taylor & Francis, Routledge.

Immordino-Yang, M. H., Christodoulou, J. A., & Singh, V. (2012). Rest is not idleness: Implications of the brain's default mode for human development and education. *Perspectives on Psychological Science*, 7(4), 352–364.

Immordino-Yang, M. H., & Damasio, A. R. (2007). We feel, therefore we learn: The relevance of affective and social neuroscience to education. *Mind, Brain and Education*, 1(1), 3–10.

Immordino-Yang, M. H., Darling-Hammond, L., & Krone, C. (2018). *The brain basis for integrated social, emotional and academic development: How emotions and social relationships drive learning.* Brief published by the Aspen Institute National Commission on Social, Emotional and Academic Development. Retrieved from www.aspeninstitute.org/publications/the-brain-basis-for-integrated-social-emotional-and-academic-development/

Immordino-Yang, M. H., Darling-Hammond, L., & Krone, C. R. (2019). Nurturing nature: How brain development is inherently social and emotional, and what this means for education. *Educational Psychologist*, 54(3), 185–204.

Immordino-Yang, M. H., & Faeth, M. (2010). The role of emotion and skilled intuition in learning. In D. A. Sousa (Ed.), *Mind, brain, and education: Neuroscience implications for the classroom* (pp. 66–81). Bloomington, IN: Solution Tree Press.

Immordino-Yang, M. H., & Gotlieb, R. (2017). Embodied brains, social minds, cultural meaning: Integrating neuroscientific and educational research on social-affective development. *American Educational Research Journal*, Centennial Issue, 54(1), 344–367.

Immordino-Yang, M. H., McColl, A., Damasio, H., & Damasio, A. R. (2009). Neural correlates of admiration and compassion. *Proceedings of the National Academy of Sciences*, 106(19), 8021–8026.

Immordino-Yang, M. H., & Singh, V. (2013). Hippocampal contributions to the processing of social emotions. *Human Brain Mapping*, 34(4), 945–955.

Immordino-Yang, M. H., & Yang, X. F. (2014, November). *Adolescents' age and emotional home life predict the acquisition of strong and culture-specific patterns of correlation between neural activity and social-emotional feelings.* Poster presented at the bi-annual conference of the International Mind, Brain and Education Society, Fort Worth, TX.

Immordino-Yang, M. H., & Yang, X. F. (2017). Cultural differences in the neural correlates of social—emotional feelings: An interdisciplinary, developmental perspective. *Current Opinion in Psychology*, 17, 34–40.

Immordino-Yang, M. H., Yang, X. F., & Damasio, H. (2014). Correlations between social-emotional feelings and anterior insula activity are independent from visceral states but influenced by culture. *Frontiers in Human Neuroscience*, 8, 728.

Immordino-Yang, M. H., Yang, X. F., & Damasio, H. (2016). Cultural modes of expressing emotions influence how emotions are experienced. *Emotion*, 16(7), 1033–1039.

Jamieson, J. P., Mendes, W. B., & Nock, M. K. (2013). Improving acute stress responses: The power of reappraisal. *Current Directions in Psychological Science*, 22(1), 51–56.

Jones, S. M., Brown, J. L., & Aber, J. L. (2011). Two-year impacts of a universal school-based social-emotional and literacy intervention: An experiment in translational developmental research. *Child Development, 82*(2), 533–554.

Jones, S. M., & Kahn, J. (2017, September 3). *The evidence base for how we learn: Supporting students' social, emotional, and academic development.* Retrieved from www.aspeninstitute.org/publications/evidence-base-learn/

Kaplan, J. T., Gimbel, S. I., Dehghani, M., Immordino-Yang, M. H., Sagae, K., Wong, J. D., . . . Damasio, A. (2017). Processing narratives concerning protected values: A cross-cultural investigation of neural correlates. *Cerebral Cortex, 27*(2), 1428–1438.

Kaufman, S. B. (2013). Opening up openness to experience: A four-factor model and relations to creative achievement in the arts and sciences. *The Journal of Creative Behavior, 47*(4), 233–255.

Kuhbandner, C., Aslan, A., Emmerdinger, K., & Murayama, K. (2016). Providing extrinsic reward for test performance undermines long-term memory acquisition. *Frontiers in Psychology, 7*, 79.

Kuhn, D. (2007). How to produce a high-achieving child. *Phi Delta Kappan, 88*, 757–763.

Kurth, F., Zilles, K., Fox, P. T., Laird, A. R., & Eickhoff, S. B. (2010). A link between the systems: Functional differentiation and integration within the human insula revealed by meta-analysis. *Brain Structure and Function, 214*(5–6), 519–534.

Lynn, S. J., Lilienfeld, S. O., Merckelbach, H., Giesbrecht, T., McNally, R. J., Loftus, E. F., . . . Malaktaris, A. (2014). The trauma model of dissociation: Inconvenient truths and stubborn fictions. Comment on Dalenberg et al., 2012. *Psychological Bulletin, 140*(3), 896–910.

Marsh, H. W., Pekrun, R., Lichtenfeld, S., Guo, J., Arens, A. K., & Murayama, K. (2016). Breaking the double-edged sword of effort/trying hard: Developmental equilibrium and longitudinal relations among effort, achievement, and academic self-concept. *Developmental Psychology, 52*(8), 1273–1290.

Mather, M. (2007). Emotional arousal and memory binding: An object-based framework. *Perspectives on Psychological Science, 2*(1), 33–52.

Meinhardt, J., & Pekrun, R. (2003). Attentional resource allocation to emotional events: An ERP study. *Cognition and Emotion, 17*(3), 477–500.

Moll, H. (2018). The transformative cultural intelligence hypothesis: Evidence from young children's problem-solving. *Review of Philosophy and Psychology, 9*(1), 161–175.

Montessori, M. (2009). *Dr. Montessori's own handbook.* New York, NY: F.A. Stokes Company Publishers. (Original work published 1914). Retrieved from http://www.gutenberg.org/files/29635/29635-h/29635-h.htm

Murayama, K., Matsumoto, M., Izuma, K., & Matsumoto, K. (2010). Neural basis of the undermining effect of extrinsic reward on intrinsic motivation. *Proceedings of the National Academy of Sciences, 107*, 20911–20916.

Nasir, N. I. S. (2012). *Racialized identities: Race and achievement among African American youth.* Palo Alto, CA: Stanford University Press.

National Academies of Sciences, Engineering, and Medicine. (2018). *How people learn II: Learners, contexts, and culture.* Washington, DC: National Academies Press. https://doi.org/10.17226/24783

Okan, Z. (2003). Edutainment: Is learning at risk? *British Journal of Educational Technology, 34*(3), 255–264.

Okonofua, J. A., Paunesku, D., & Walton, G. M. (2016). Brief intervention to encourage empathic discipline cuts suspension rates in half among adolescents. *Proceedings of the National Academy of Sciences, 113*(19), 5221–5226.

Osher, D., Cantor, P., Berg, J., Steyer, L., & Rose, T. (2018). Drivers of human development: How relationships and context shape learning and development. *Applied Developmental Science*, 1–31. doi:10.1080/10888691.2017.1398650

Osher, D., Kidron, Y., Brackett, M., Dymnicki, A., Jones, S., & Weissberg, R. P. (2016). Advancing the science and practice of social and emotional learning: Looking back and moving forward. *Review of Research in Education*, 40(1), 644–681.

Oyserman, D. (2015). *Pathways to success through identity-based motivation*. Oxford: Oxford University Press.

Panksepp, J., & Biven, L. (2012). *The archaeology of mind: Neuroevolutionary origins of human emotions*. New York: W.W. Norton & Co.

Pekrun, R., Elliot, A. J., & Maier, M. A. (2009). Achievement goals and achievement emotions: Testing a model of their joint relations with academic performance. *Journal of Educational Psychology*, 101(1), 115–135.

Pekrun, R., Goetz, T., Titz, W., & Perry, R. P. (2002). Academic emotions in students' self-regulated learning and achievement: A program of qualitative and quantitative research. *Educational Psychologist*, 37(2), 91–105.

Pekrun, R., Hall, N. C., Goetz, T., & Perry, R. P. (2014). Boredom and academic achievement: Testing a model of reciprocal causation. *Journal of Educational Psychology*, 106, 696–710.

Pekrun, R., & Linnenbrink-Garcia, L. (2012). Academic emotions and student engagement. In *Handbook of research on student engagement* (pp. 259–282). Boston, MA: Springer.

Perkins, D. (2014). *Future wise: Educating our children for a changing world*. John Wiley & Sons.

Perry, D., Hendler, T., & Shamay-Tsoory, S. G. (2011). Projecting memories: The role of the hippocampus in emotional mentalizing. *Neuroimage*, 54(2), 1669–1676.

Phelps, E. A. (2004). Human emotion and memory: Interactions of the amygdala and hippocampal complex. *Current Opinion in Neurobiology*, 14(2), 198–202.

Public Law No. 114–195. *Every student succeeds act*, December 10, 2015.

Roediger III, H. L., & Karpicke, J. D. (2006). Test-enhanced learning: Taking memory tests improves long-term retention. *Psychological Science*, 17(3), 249–255.

Rogoff, B. (2003). *The cultural nature of human development*. Oxford: Oxford University Press.

Ryan, R. M., & Deci, E. L. (2000). Intrinsic and extrinsic motivations: Classic definitions and new directions. *Contemporary Educational Psychology*, 25(1), 54–67.

Sapolsky, R. M. (2017). *Behave: The biology of humans at our best and worst*. New York, NY: Penguin Press.

Savery, J. R. (2015). Overview of problem-based learning: Definitions and distinctions. In A. Walker, H. Leary, C. E. Hmelo-Silver, & P. A. Ertmer (Eds.), *Essential readings in problem-based learning* (pp. 5–15). West Lafayette, IN: Purdue University Press.

Saxbe, D., Yang, X., Borofsky, L., & Immordino-Yang, M. H. (2013). The embodiment of emotion: Language use during the feeling of social emotions predicts cortical somatosensory activity. *Social Cognitive and Affective Neuroscience*, 8(7), 806–812.

Schneps, M. H. (Producer). (2011). *Neuroscience and the classroom: Making connections*. Retrieved from www.learner.org/courses/neuroscience/about/credits.html

Schunk, D. H., & Zimmerman, B. J. (2007). Influencing children's self-efficacy and self-regulation of reading and writing through modeling. *Reading & Writing Quarterly*, 23(1), 7–25.

Spelke, E., & Schulz, L. (2011). The double-edged sword of pedagogy: Instruction limits spontaneous exploration and discovery. *Cognition*, 120(3), 322–330.

Spencer, M. B., & Markstrom-Adams, C. (1990). Identity processes among racial and ethnic minority children in America. *Child Development, 61*(2), 290–310.

Spencer, S. J., Logel, C., & Davies, P. G. (2016). Stereotype threat. *Annual Review of Psychology, 67*, 415–437.

Steele, C. M. (2011). *Whistling Vivaldi: How stereotypes affect us and what we can do.* New York: W.W. Norton & Co.

Stoltze, F. (Ed.). (2008, May 22). Children in violent neighborhoods can suffer post-traumatic stress disorder [Radio Program]. In *US & world*. Los Angeles: KPCC Southern California Public Radio.

Taylor, E. W. (2017). Transformative learning theory. In *Transformative learning meets bildung* (pp. 17–29). Rotterdam: Sense Publishers.

Taylor, R., Oberle, E., Durlak, J., & Weissberg, R. (2017). Promoting positive youth development through school-based social and emotional learning interventions: A meta-analysis of follow-up effects. *Child Development, 88*(4), 1156–1171. https://doi.org/10.1111/cdev.12864

Thomas, M. S., Ansari, D., & Knowland, V. C. (2019). Annual research review: Educational neuroscience: Progress and prospects. *Journal of Child Psychology and Psychiatry, 60*(4), 477–492.

Tine, M., & Gotlieb, R. (2013). Gender-, race-, and income-based stereotype threat: The effects of multiple stigmatized aspects of identity on math performance and working memory function. *Social Psychology of Education, 16*(3), 353–376.

Tomasello, M. (2009). *The cultural origins of human cognition.* Cambridge, MA: Harvard University Press.

Tsai, J. L. (2007). Ideal affect: Cultural causes and behavioral consequences. *Perspectives on Psychological Science, 2*, 242–259.

Van der Kolk, B. A. (2015). *The body keeps the score: Brain, mind, and body in the healing of trauma.* New York, NY: Penguin Books.

Vessel, E. A., Starr, G. G., & Rubin, N. (2013). Art reaches within: Aesthetic experience, the self and the default mode network. *Frontiers in Neuroscience, 7*, 258.

Vygotsky, L. S. (1929). II: The problem of the cultural development of the child. *The Pedagogical Seminary and Journal of Genetic Psychology, 36*(3), 415–434.

Walton, G. M., & Cohen, G. L. (2007). A question of belonging: Race, social fit, and achievement. *Journal of Personality and Social Psychology, 92*(1), 82–96.

Wicker, B., Keysers, C., Plailly, J., Royet, J. P., Gallese, V., & Rizzolatti, G. (2003). Both of us disgusted in my insula: The common neural basis of seeing and feeling disgust. *Neuron, 40*(3), 655–664.

Yang, X. F., Bossmann, J., Schiffhauer, B., Jordan, M., & Immordino-Yang, M. H. (2013). Intrinsic default mode network connectivity predicts spontaneous verbal descriptions of autobiographical memories during social processing. *Frontiers in Psychology, 3*, 592.

Yang, X. F., Pavarini, G., Schnall, S., & Immordino-Yang, M. H. (2018). Looking up to virtue: Averting gaze facilitates moral construals via posteromedial activations. *Social Cognitive and Affective Neuroscience.* https://doi.org/10.1093/scan/nsy081

Yeager, D. S., & Walton, G. M. (2011). Social-psychological interventions in education: They're not magic. *Review of Educational Research, 81*(2), 267–301.

Zaki, J., Davis, J. I., & Ochsner, K. N. (2012). Overlapping activity in anterior insula during interoception and emotional experience. *Neuroimage, 62*(1), 493–499.

Zeki, S., Romaya, J. P., Benincasa, D. M., & Atiyah, M. F. (2014). The experience of mathematical beauty and its neural correlates. *Frontiers in Human Neuroscience, 8*, 68.

Section 4

Leading Methods for Cognitive Enhancement

11 Action Video Games

From Effects on Cognition and the Brain to Potential Educational Applications

Irene Altarelli, C. Shawn Green, and Daphne Bavelier

Video games are now played extensively around the world (155 million adult players in the US only—ESA, 2015). Indeed, defying the common stereotype of video games being "just for kids" or "just for boys", video games are played by an exceptionally broad swath of the population. For instance, amongst US video game players 44% are female and 44% are above 35 years old (ESA, 2015). While historically most video games have been developed for purely entertainment purposes, such games have nonetheless found themselves to be of increasing interest in laboratory settings. The research to-date suggests that video games have the capacity to powerfully alter the brain and behavior, leading researchers to further probe whether games can be developed or utilized for positive ends. In the following we review the research in the domain of cognitive neuroscience surrounding the impact of one genre of video games, termed action video games. We then examine developments in potentially translating this basic science into real-world applications, and in particular for use in the educational system. We conclude by discussing open questions—the answers to which would likely further accelerate the rate at which games can be harnessed for practical good.

When discussing the impact that video games have on the brain and cognition, it is important to recognize that the label "video games" encompasses an incredibly wide variety of experiences. Any scientifically useful description of the consequences of video game play needs to take this diversity into account. A helpful analogy is the label of "drugs". An enormous selection of chemical agents falls under the superordinate category label of "drugs"—everything from over-the-counter antacids to doctor prescribed pharmaceuticals to recreational drugs of abuse. Given this diversity in composition, hopefully it is intuitively obvious that it wouldn't be sensible to ask broad questions like, "How do drugs affect the body?" Instead, it is necessary to drill down to ask questions about smaller categories of drugs that have similar chemical compositions and possible targets. The same basic idea is true of video games.

Thus far, the vast majority of published scientific studies in the domain of cognitive neuroscience have probed the impact of one specific video game category, known as action video games. These are fast paced, action-packed video games, requiring players to move around in the game environment, to effectively monitor their surroundings, and to make frequent, quick and accurate motor responses to new stimuli. The broader action video game genre is often taken to encompass two main sub-genres known as first-person shooter games and third-person shooter games (with the primary difference between these subgenres being the character viewpoint—first person/third person respectively).

It is important to note that, although action video games are often violent, violence is not a necessary requirement of action video games in the scientific literature. Indeed, although researchers in some domains have occasionally, and inappropriately, fully conflated "violent video games" with "action video games", there are non-violent action video games (e.g., the non-violent action mini-games found in Rayman's Raving Rabbids—see children section ahead). The converse is also true—there are violent non-action video games (e.g., the classic role playing video game Final Fantasy VII involved a great deal of killing but was not an action video game). For a further discussion of this point we refer the interested reader to Bediou et al. (2018), especially p. 25 point 5 "Contextualizing the current results: Potential adverse effects of video game play".

Cognitive Consequences of Action Video Game Play

To investigate the effects of action video game play on behavior, one—often initial—approach has consisted in utilizing a cross-sectional design. In such studies, habitual action video game players (AVGPs), individuals who have spent a great deal of time primarily playing action video games, are contrasted with non-action video game players (NVGPs), individuals who never play action video games and rarely engage in playing any video games. More specifically, AVGPs are most typically defined as individuals who have played action video games for at least 3 hours per week for at least the previous 6 months, with no other game genre being played as much. This latter qualification is necessary given the goal of isolating the impact of action games alone (i.e., if individuals have played many types of games beyond action games, it can be difficult, or even impossible, to attribute any differences to action games alone). NVGPs meanwhile are typically defined as individuals who have played essentially no action games and less than 3 hours per week across all video game genres. These two groups are also matched for as many factors as possible. For example, age and gender are of particular concern as differences in these very variables could be the source of group differences instead of game play habits. Although, as noted in the introduction, video games are played by wide swaths of individuals worldwide, there do tend to be differences in the types of games, for instance, played by males and females, or by younger and older individuals. In the case of action games, the individuals who naturally choose to play these games tend to be younger and are predominantly male. This has often resulted in cross-sectional studies utilizing exclusively male participants.

Performance in a set of cognitive tasks of interest is collected and then compared across AVGPs and NVGPs. If a significant difference between the two groups is identified, a second approach is then needed in order to establish whether playing action video games is causally related to the reported cross-sectional group difference. Indeed, possible confounding or lurking variables are always a concern in purely cross-sectional work. For instance, given only cross-sectional results, one might be concerned that individuals born with superior cognitive skills are rewarded for those skills when playing action video games (and thus tend to play more) while those with lesser skills are less successful (and thus tend to play less).

Demonstrating a causal relation requires running an intervention or training study. Intervention studies involve recruiting participants who have at most limited video game experience (e.g., no more than between 1–3 hours weekly for the past year). These individuals are pretested on the cognitive task(s) of interest. Half of the participants are then randomly allocated to the action game group, where they'll be asked to play action video games for a given number of hours. The remaining half of the participants are allocated to the control group. This group will also be requested to play a commercial video game for the same number of hours. The control game will be matched along many dimensions with the action game (i.e., it will be rated as just as engaging), but critically, it will not contain any action characteristics. The number of hours of training utilized in the literature has varied from 8 to 50 hours depending on the skills tested. Critically, training is always distributed across several weeks, as distributed practice is well known to result in the most effective learning—a finding amply documented in the learning literature in a host of domains (Baddeley & Longman, 1978), including video games use specifically (Stafford & Dewar, 2014). Single sessions have typically lasted between 20 minutes and 1 hour with 3–5 such sessions per week being completed. After training is over, following a delay of at least 24 hours (in order to ensure any transient effects of video game play, such as arousal, have disappeared), performance on the cognitive task(s) of interest is measured again (post-test) and compared between the two groups. The critical question is whether the performance of the action group has improved more from pre-test to post-test than the performance of the control group (Figure 11.1). If this is the case, it can be concluded that action video game playing exerts a positive influence on the cognitive domain assessed.

There now exists a sizeable, and ever growing, literature utilizing the study designs described previously to probe the impact of action video games on cognitive skills. Given the breadth and depth of the current literature, Bediou and collaborators (2018) recently examined the impact of action video games via two separate meta-analyses. Both meta-analyses focused on work conducted between the years 2000 and 2015 (prior to the year 2000, there were very few games that would qualify as "action" by today's definitions). One meta-analysis was focused exclusively on cross-sectional studies (N = 3789) and revealed an overall beneficial impact on cognition of Hedges' $g = 0.55$,

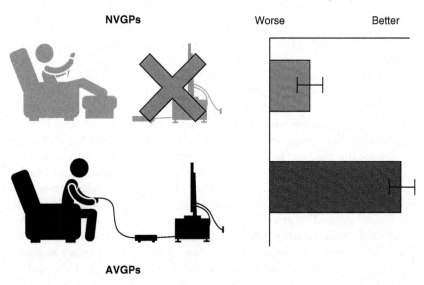

Figure 11.1 Cross-sectional Design

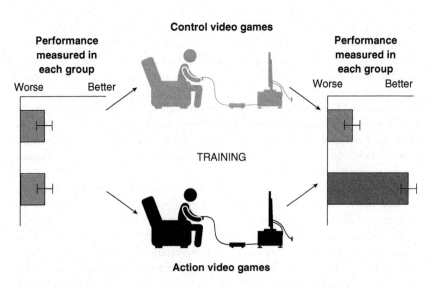

Figure 11.2 True Intervention Design

or an increase of about ½ of a standard deviation. As most studies focused on young male adults, it shows that those individuals who self-select to play action video games show improved cognition as compared to young males who rarely play any video games. The second meta-analysis focused exclusively on intervention studies in young adults (18–35 years of age mostly; N = 609). Importantly, only intervention studies that compared the effects of action video game training with the outcomes of playing other commercially available video games belonging to genres that have non-action mechanics of play such as strategy games, mini-games, puzzle games or social simulation games were included. In doing so, Bediou et al. (2018) enforced that only studies with active control group well-matched in terms of motivation and engagement, and social attention were considered. This intervention meta-analysis revealed an effect of Hedges' g = 0.33, or an increase in overall cognition of about $^1/_3$ of a standard deviation. As a point of comparison, computer-based educational intervention, whether for reading or for mathematics, have been reported to have effect sizes of half that size at about 0.15 when compared to business as usual, and even smaller impact when compared to an active baseline (Cheung & Slavin, 2012, 2013). As expected, the effect size in intervention studies was lower than the effect size for cross-sectional studies. Indeed, the amount of video game play individuals engaged with in intervention studies (most commonly less than 20 hours), is less than a month's worth of gaming for an AVGP since those are selected based on playing 5 or more hours a week for the previous 6 months to a year, and typically have played much more than that. The large difference in amount of action game experience is likely to at least partially explain the lower effect sizes in intervention as compared to cross-sectional studies. As performance following action video game play was evaluated in a number of different cognitive domains, we next discuss the outcome separately for each cognitive domain.

Perception

Perceptual enhancements associated with action video game play have mostly been studied in the visual domain. As an example, Li and colleagues (2009) assessed contrast sensitivity—that is, the ability to detect small changes in shades of grey, such as when trying to identify an object amidst the fog—in AVGPs compared to NVGPs. The authors found significantly higher contrast sensitivity in AVGPs than in NVGPs. They followed up these cross-sectional findings with an intervention study, assessing the impact of 50 hours of action video game training (Unreal Tournament 2004) versus 50 hours of non-action video game training (The Sims 2). At the end of training, the action trained group showed significant gains in contrast sensitivity compared to pre-test levels, while the non-action game training group did not display any changes—suggesting the existence of a causal relation between action video game training and contrast sensitivity enhancement. Other studies explored additional aspects of visual perception, such as the size of central and peripheral visual fields (Buckley, Codina, Bhardwaj, & Pascalis, 2010); visual acuity (Green & Bavelier, 2007); the ability to discriminate objects when presented in cluttered scenes (also known as crowding) (Green & Bavelier, 2007); the capacity to overcome to a large extent the hindering effects of masking (Li, Polat, Scalzo, & Bavelier, 2010; Schubert et al., 2015); or the ability to detect motion (Hutchinson & Stocks, 2013; Green, Pouget, & Bavelier, 2010). All have shown clear benefits of action video game play.

When combining across all the existing studies examining perceptual effects associated with action gaming, Bediou et al.'s meta-analyses (2018) revealed an overall effect of Hedges' g = 0.78, or an increase of about ¾ of a standard deviation in cross-sectional studies and an effect of Hedges' g = 0.23, or an increase of about ¼ of a standard deviation in intervention studies.

Attention

Many studies have now shown that multiple aspects of attention are enhanced following action video game play (see Bavelier & Föcker, 2015 for a review). Briefly, AVGPs have consistently demonstrated greater spatial selective attention, such as is shown in standard search tasks, where a single target appears in the peripheral visual field and must be located from amongst a host of distractors (Green & Bavelier, 2003, 2006a; Feng, Spence, & Pratt, 2007; West, Stevens, Pun, & Pratt, 2008; Sungur & Boduroglu, 2012; Wu et al., 2012). AVGPs also show greater selective attention deployed across time, for instance as is tapped by tasks in which participants have to report the occurrence of two target events that occur very close in time, e.g., 200–400ms (Green & Bavelier, 2003; Oei & Patterson, 2013). Attention deployed to objects is also enhanced as a result of action video game play, as shown by tasks requiring participants to track targets among distractors, while all stimuli move, as in the Multiple Object Tracking task (Green & Bavelier, 2006b; Oei & Patterson, 2013; Trick, Jaspers-Fayer, & Sethi, 2005; Dye & Bavelier, 2010).

In addition to selective attention, sustained attention (i.e., attention exerted for prolonged periods of time) has also been shown to be enhanced in AVGPs (Dye, Green, & Bavelier, 2009). One classic example of a sustained attention task is one condition of the Test of Variables of Attention (TOVA) task. On each trial of this task, participants are shown a square either on the top half or bottom half of the screen. They are asked to press a button as quickly as possible if the square appears on the top half of the screen, but to do nothing (i.e., make no button press) if the square appears on the bottom half of the screen. In the condition of interest here, the statistics are biased such that the square appears on the bottom half of the screen on/in 80% of trials. In other words, on 80% of trials the participant has no action to take (i.e., are "no press" trials). The condition is thus rather boring for participants— thereby taxing sustained attention. The question of interest is whether participants can stay on task and press the button quickly on the rare trials where the square is on the top half of the screen. Interestingly, AVGPs have been found to respond faster than NVGPs in this task, while they do not commit more errors than NVGPs (Dye et al., 2009).

A video game specially designed for older adults to incorporate action mechanics, Neuroracer, was also shown to result in enhanced TOVA performance. In that game, participants had to steer a vehicle on a path while responding to randomly appearing targets along the road. Interestingly, this study has highlighted the importance—for benefits to be noted—of layering, within a same video game experience, both focused and divided attention demands. Indeed, the control group was trained on both the steering task and the target detection task, yet with each task being trained in isolation, and showed no improvements in sustained attention (Anguera et al., 2013).

Consistent with the myriad individual studies in this literature focused on top-down attentional control (e.g., selective/sustained attention), this domain had perhaps the strongest results in Bediou et al.'s meta-analyses (2018). The effect sizes were Hedges' $g = 0.63$ or about $^2/_3$ of a standard deviation improvement in cross-sectional studies and an effect of Hedges' $g = 0.31$ or about $^1/_3$ of a standard deviation improvement in intervention studies.

It should be mentioned that the multiple attentional gains highlighted above only concern aspects of voluntarily exerted top-down attention. In the case of bottom-up attention the field is relatively sparse, as illustrated by the low number of effect sizes for this type of attention in Bediou et al., 2018. The few studies available point to little-to-no effect, with most individual studies failing to find differences between AVGPs and NVGPs in the initial pull exogenous attention exerts (Castel, Pratt, & Drummond, 2005; Hubert-Wallander, Green, Sugarman, & Bavelier, 2011). Accordingly, studies of attentional capture also document similar initial capture in AVGPs as compared to NVGPs (Chisholm & Kingstone, 2012, 2015). Interestingly, however, these same works document a faster re-allocation of attention in AVGPs when wrongly captured, in accord with their greater top-down attentional capabilities. It remains largely unknown why the initial orienting under the control of exogenous attention is not altered by action video game play, despite such abrupt onsets being quite common in action video games. One possible explanation is that orienting develops very early during development and is in a large part mediated by subcortical structures, such as the nucleus basalis or the pulvinar, that may be less plastic later in life than brain regions that support top-down attentional mechanisms (Posner, Rothbart, Sheese, & Voelker, 2012).

Spatial Cognition

Spatial cognition includes the ability to mentally rotate objects (mental rotation) as well as spatial short-term and working memory. This domain is of particular interest with relation to education, as performance on spatial cognitive tasks has been strongly linked with entrance into and performance in science, technology, math, and engineering (STEM) domains. As was true in these domains, multiple research teams have observed enhancements associated with action video game play in the spatial cognitive domain. For instance, Feng and colleagues (2007) demonstrated both a positive cross-sectional and a positive intervention effect of action video games on mental rotation. In the intervention study, an increase in mental rotation accuracy was noted following 10 hours of action video game training, while it was not seen in the case of training in another video game genre. Moreover, enhanced mental rotation in the action trained group was still observed 5 months after the end of training, highlighting that such gain was maintained over that period of time (although note that some of the participants in this study may have continued to play action games in the intervening period).

As regards spatial short-term memory, Sungur and Boduroglu (2012) highlighted AVGPs' greater short-term memory precision in a color memory task, where in each trial participants were presented with three colored squares, the colors of which had been picked at random among 180 options. After the disappearance of the colored squares, participants were asked to retrieve the colors they had just seen, by selecting them from a color wheel. AVGPs outperformed NVGPs in this task, suggesting a greater precision of short-term memory in action gamers. A similar observation was reported by McDermott and collaborators (2014) in a visual short-term memory task, in which participants had to recall the location and orientation of colored bars. Greater accuracy was observed in AVGPs, for larger set sizes.

Concerning working memory, we have reviewed previously the evidence suggesting greater performance of AVGPs in tracking moving objects, as in the Multiple Object Tracking (MOT) task. Interestingly, Eayrs and Lavie (2018) have shown that performance in the MOT is not only related to a perceptual/attentional component, but also to a working memory component. Thus superior performance of AVGPs in the MOT task, as reviewed above, also suggests the possibility of AVGPs having higher working memory. Sungur and Boduroglu (2012) demonstrated greater performance of AVGPs over NVGPs in a modified version of the MOT, requiring participants to recall the final location and identity of moving objects, again supporting the hypothesis of increased working memory ability in action gamers.

When looking at the overall picture of the spatial cognitive domain in Bediou et al.'s meta-analyses (2018), the effect sizes were Hedges' g = 0.75 or ¾ of a standard deviation improvement in cross-sectional studies and an effect of Hedges' g = 0.45 or almost ½ of a standard deviation in intervention studies.

Multitasking and Task-Switching

Multitasking requires participants to concurrently perform at least two individual tasks, such as responding to an auditory target at the same time as memorizing target faces. Task-switching paradigms differ from multitasking in that they require participants to sequentially switch from one task to a different one, as instructed by a cue for example. These two paradigms are, however, intimately related in terms of the cognitive constructs they tap, as they each require a flexible allocation of attentional and/or working memory resources to best schedule task contingencies. Indeed it is most likely that despite the requirement to concurrently manage several tasks of multitasking, this behavior is mediated through internally generated task switches rather than true parallel processing.

Both cross-sectional and intervention studies have shown benefits associated with action gaming on multitasking performance (Strobach, Frensch, & Schubert, 2012; Green & Bavelier, 2006a; Wu & Spence, 2013; but see Donohue, James, Eslick, & Mitroff, 2012; Gaspar et al., 2014). This includes cases where the paradigm closely resembles real-life multitasking, such as mimicking aircraft piloting operations (Chiappe et al., 2013), suggesting the potential for transfer outside the laboratory (although such far transfer studies remain too rare for firm conclusions to be drawn). Similarly, several studies (both cross-sectional and intervention) have shown the benefits of action video games on task switching (Green, Sugarman, Medford, Klobusicky, & Bavelier, 2012; Colzato, van den Wildenberg, & Hommel, 2014; Karle, Watter, & Shedden, 2010; Cain, Landau, & Shimamura, 2012), with a reduction of the cost of switching from one task to another (although the switch cost does not disappear entirely). These findings have also been evaluated in a context closer to real life, namely in a simulated distracted driving situation (Rupp, McConnell, & Smither, 2016).

While in the same direction as the previously reviewed domains, the effect in multitasking/task switching was more variable in the meta-analysis by Bediou et al. (2018) compared to the other domains reviewed earlier. The effect sizes were Hedges' g = 0.55 or about ½ a standard deviation improvement in cross-sectional studies and an effect of Hedges' g = 0.3 or about $^1/_3$ of a standard deviation improvement in intervention studies, but with relatively large error bars.

We have illustrated how action video games modify several different cognitive abilities for the better. Yet not all facets of cognition are equally influenced by action video game play. The meta-analysis by Bediou et al. (2018) suggests that action gaming effects are largest in the case of top-down attention, spatial cognition, and visual perception. This same meta-analysis though highlighted the need for more high-quality intervention studies to further consolidate these findings. Furthermore, a great deal more work is needed in the domains of inhibition (i.e., as probed by tasks in which the participant is required to voluntarily withhold their response on a subset of the trials), verbal cognition and problem solving, as these domains currently have too few studies for firm conclusions to be reached. Finally, video games provide powerful experiences and, as such, it is important to recognize that their impact need not always be positive. In the domains considered in this review, positive impacts have been found. However, other domains, outside of cognition, document potential negative impacts. In particular, there have been numerous published concerns related to violent content (Anderson et al., 2010) as well as problematic interactive media use (Gentile, 2009; Rich, Tsappis, & Kavanaugh, 2017), both of which are highly relevant to video games.

Brain Correlates of Action Video Game Play Training— A Window Into the Underlying Mechanisms?

Given that the impact of action games on top-down attentional skills has been the subject of by far the most behavioral research in the field to-date, it is perhaps not surprising that this domain has also been the subject of the first few research papers probing the potential neural changes induced by action gaming. For example, Mishra and collaborators (2011) presented AVGP and NVGP participants with three concurrent streams of letters (i.e., letters flashing one after another). One stream was presented to the left of fixation, one stream was presented to the right of fixation, and one stream was presented just above fixation. The participants were instructed to attend to just one of the three streams and to report whenever a rare target (a number amongst mostly letters) appeared. Participants' brain responses were recorded through electroencephalography (EEG) throughout the experiment. Importantly, each stream flickered at a distinct temporal frequency, which made it possible to retrieve and isolate the brain signals evoked by each stream. Therefore, brain activity corresponding to both to-be-attended but also to-be-ignored information could be collected. Behaviorally, AVGPs outperformed NVGPs both in terms of accuracy and speed in identifying the targets. Moreover, their brain responses revealed that they suppressed irrelevant, distracting information to a greater extent than NVGPs did. Importantly, these two outcome measures— the behavioral performance and the measured neural suppression—were correlated as the greater the suppression of to-be-ignored information, the greater the speed of response. Thus, investigating the brain responses in this attentional task provided evidence for a potential mechanism of attentional enhancement in AVGPs—more efficient suppression of distracting information. This observation is supported by additional work with EEG (Krishnan, Kang, Sperling, & Srinivasan, 2013; Anguera et al., 2013) and with functional MRI (Bavelier, Achtman, Mani, & Föcker, 2012). In the latter study, it was also reported that the higher-level neural network known to mediate attentional control (comprising frontal and parietal cortices) was recruited to a lesser extent as task demands increased in AVGPs than in NVGPs, suggesting a more automatic allocation of attention in AVGPs. More generally, neural plasticity linked to action video game play seems to be mostly involving high-level brain circuits for attentional control, with modifications of low-level, perceptual information processing remaining elusive (Föcker, Mortazavi, Khoe, Hillyard, & Bavelier, 2018).

Moving From Game Genres to Game Mechanics

Thus far in this chapter, we have examined the cognitive and brain effects of playing a specific game genre—namely action video games. However, as is always the case with rapidly evolving technology, it is worth constantly assessing the extent to which previous definitions and categorizations continue to apply or are in need of updating. In the case of video games, one major trend over the past decade is that many previously distinct genres have melded into what are sometimes called "hybrid genres." For example, twenty years ago there were a host of games that could be called "pure action games" as well as a host of games that could be called "pure role-playing games." Today though a great many games contain elements from both the "action" and the "role-playing" genres—and Consequently, are referred to as "action-role-playing games." Consequently, "pure" action video games, like those tested in the studies mentioned above, are much harder to find (Dale & Green, 2017a). At the same time, new genres have developed that—although not like traditional action games—nonetheless contain some "action-like" elements that could drive similar changes as have been seen to arise from action gaming. This is the case, for instance, of Role Playing games, in particular, an increasingly popular sub-genre of role playing games dubbed action-RPG hybrids (e.g., the *Mass Effect* series), which combine traditional role playing elements with elements of third- or sometimes first-person shooters. This is also found in the case of the Real-Time Strategy genre, especially the sub-genre known as the Multiplayer Online Battle Arena (MOBA), which is also sometimes referred to as the action-RTS genre (e.g., League of Legends) (e.g., Glass, Maddox, & Love, 2013; Dale & Green, 2017b).

In the face of these various mutations, it is clear that a paradigm change is needed whereby rather than focusing on video game genres, the domain will increasingly need to focus on video game mechanics and their impact on brain and cognition. This recognized need does not go without its own challenges. Most commercially available video games provide a rich experience combining many mechanics in a seamless experience. A systematic way of analyzing a given video game experience in terms of its video game mechanics, let alone the cognitive, emotional or social constructs these game mechanics call for, is not within close reach. Yet, we and others have begun to identify key game mechanics in action video games that are hypothesized to enhance attentional control and cognitive flexibility. Although this list is not exhaustive, the main hypothesized mechanics relate to (1) pacing (the need to make decisions under time constraints), (2) putting a load on divided attention (i.e., the need to constantly monitor one's surrounding for possible events of interest), and (3) the need to flexibly switch between such a divided attentional state and a more tightly focused attentional state (e.g., as is needed when carefully aiming at enemies) (Cardoso-Leite, Joessel, & Bavelier, 2020). Of course, as in any well-designed intervention meant to induce learning and neuroplasticity, many other mechanics need to be respected. These include everything from proper tailoring of the game difficulty, to providing an experience that is at once rich and variable, yet sufficiently predictable that there is something to learn. Interestingly, entertainment video games implement this fine balance masterfully, as variety of situations, context and challenges avoids automatization and thus boredom, while some level of predictability ensures playability. It is worth noting that such a balance is one most educational systems have been fighting to achieve for many years. There may be several reasons for this and we review two main possibilities here. First, the game mechanics elaborated on previously are not always naturally aligned with the way academic content is typically delivered in class. Although some educational domains, such as reading or learning geography/history appear ripe for impact, designing educational video games requires careful thought about how to scaffold the introduction of academic content. In addition, it should be acknowledged that commercially available video games are designed and produced by teams of experts encompassing storytellers, graphic artists, game designers, and music experts, just to cite a few, thus calling for budgets that start around $2,000,000 per game title and that can go up to $60,000,000 or beyond. It is unlikely a team of scientists on a small grant budget can match the degree of sophistication and complexity a commercially available product can achieve.

Action Video Games as a General Training in Learning

The range of tasks in which action video gamers show improvements, as we have outlined in the first section, is rather surprising. In the general field of learning, what is far more common is observing performance gains in the trained task, with limited spillover to other types of tasks—in other words, "specificity of learning" or "failure of learning transfer." As an example, repeated training in discriminating whether a horizontal bar is higher or lower than another horizontal bar can result in impressive gains in performance. Yet, as soon as the task is modified even slightly (e.g., having to compare two vertical bars rather than two horizontal ones), performance falls back to initial, pre-training levels. This is a typical observation in perceptual learning (Karni & Sagi, 1991), but the same observation has also been made in many other domains of learning from motor control to cognition. In rehabilitation and/or education, where the ability to generalize what is learned to other contexts and possibly to real-life is key, this phenomenon has been referred to as the "curse" of learning specificity (Owen et al., 2010; Barnett & Ceci, 2002; Fahle, 2005).

In light of such typical specificity of learning, it appears fair to ask why action video game play results in performance gains in tasks that are not directly akin to playing those games. Indeed, typical lab-designed stimuli or task sets do not remotely resemble items that appear in entertainment games (or at a minimum are far more dissimilar than a horizontal bar is to a vertical bar). Why is performance in novel tasks enhanced following action video game training, when typically, we see no transfer of perceptual or cognitive learning?

One key aspect to consider in this context is enhanced attentional control in AVGPs, in particular the ability of AVGPs to suppress distractors more efficiently (Mishra et al., 2011). It has been hypothesized that an enhanced ability to ignore distractors would result in more efficient extraction of the relevant to-be-learned information for the task at hand. In other words, better distractor rejection allows for a refined distinction between signal and noise, leading to better, more informed decisions (Bavelier, Green,

Pouget, & Schrater, 2012). This, in turn, would result in gains in learning that emerge as new tasks unfold. When confronted with a new task, AVGPs would progressively diverge from NVGPs over the course of the task—corresponding to faster *learning*.

While this idea remains to be fully explored (see Bavelier, Green et al., 2012 for a review), there is initial experimental evidence to support these views. Bejjanki et al. (2014) tested AVGPs and NVGPs on a perceptual learning task, where participants were required to discriminate the orientation of Gabor patches (black and white gratings widely used in experimental psychology). While both groups displayed learning, a clear advantage in the rate of learning was seen for the AVGPs. Furthermore, by applying mathematical modeling to participants' behavior, it was shown that AVGPs' enhanced performance during the task could be attributable to better learning of perceptual templates for the task at hand. These results were further confirmed by Bejjanki and colleagues (2014) in an intervention experiment. In the same vein, habitual real-time strategy players have been shown to progressively outperform non-gamers in the initial phases of visual perceptual training (Kim et al., 2015). Similar observations have also been made in the visuo-motor domain, in a cross-modal experiment, with AVGPs improving at a faster rate and eventually outperforming NVGPs (Gozli, Bavelier, & Pratt, 2014). In addition to benefitting from faster learning, frequent AVGPs may also be less subject to interference of learning: when asked to learn two perceptual tasks in a row, where learning the first typically blocks learning of the second, AVGPs overcome to a large part such interference (Berard, Cain, Watanabe, & Sasaki, 2015).

It is important to underline that the hypothesis of better "learning to learn" abilities in action gamers results in practical consequences from an experimental point of view. For instance, somewhat long paradigms may be needed in order for learning performance to emerge. This is not a condition that is commonly met by typical "transfer" experiments, where immediate benefits on new tasks are expected and therefore performance is not always probed in a way that can reveal learning differences.

Overall, the work summarized so far has highlighted how action gaming results in enhanced attentional control and flexible cognition, allowing players to better focus on the tasks at hand and more efficiently filter out irrelevant information. This in turn is proposed to lead to the faster development of perceptual and/or cognitive templates for the task at hand. The potential of such a regimen for training is evident and has led to work in a variety of translational domains, as detailed in the following sections.

Practical Applications of Action Gaming: The Clinical Setting

In the first section, we described positive changes in various cognitive domains following action gaming, including in visual perception and visuospatial attention. It should be noted that in all the studies we mentioned, including intervention studies, participants were healthy adults. This indicates that visual perceptual abilities were enhanced in individuals with normal vision, a finding that has naturally led to striking interest for clinical rehabilitation. Indeed, the scope and scale of the gains observed, combined with the high motivation engendered by video games, make action video games a potentially very seductive option for the treatment of visual conditions.

One example of the use of action games for training in the clinical setting is in the case of amblyopia, a condition also known as "lazy eye". This pathology arises from an early, childhood history of abnormal visual experience (such as strabismus), compromising the quality of the input received by the brain from one of the eyes. This in turn gives rise to cortical maladaptive plasticity: having to deal with incoherent input from the two eyes, the brain develops a "survival strategy", basically leading it to disregard the compromised input arriving from the "lazy" eye. In the absence of any early treatment, amblyopic individuals (2 to 5% of the population in the western world) suffer from two major visual problems—poor vision (e.g., acuity, contrast sensitivity) in the amblyopic eye, as well as poor depth perception (which requires integrating information from both eyes into a coherent whole).

Li and colleagues (2011) were the first to test the effects of action game play on adults with amblyopia. The patients' visual acuity, depth perception and visual attention were evaluated first. Then, similarly to the intervention designs described earlier, patients were divided in two groups. One group played a commercial action video game (N = 10, Medal of Honor) while the other played a control video game (N = 3, SimCity Societies) for 40 hours. Importantly, the patients' "good eye" was patched, forcing them to play with their "lazy eye". As an additional control for the mere effects of patching, an additional group (N = 7) wore a patch while performing daily life activities (noting that patching in adulthood has generally resulted in no changes in vision). Following video game playing or simple patching, the patient's visual abilities were measured again, revealing significant gains in visual acuity in the two video-game-trained groups, and gains in depth perception in a few participants. In contrast, 20 hours of patching alone did not yield any visual improvement. Note that in these patients training on the action video game, but also on the control video game, resulted in visual acuity gains.

A major constraint when using commercially available action video games is that they are designed for young video game players already cognizant of that video game genre. As such, they often make for poorly suited training tools for other populations. Imagine playing an action video game through one blurred eye. The lowest entry level of difficulty is likely already too challenging, potentially leading to frustration and learned helplessness. Indeed, a major lesson from the field of skill learning (Soderstrom & Bjork, 2015; Vygotsky, 1978) is that it is critical that the training regimen be properly calibrated to the learner skill, both in terms of entry-level difficulty and the incremental steps in difficulty as skill progresses. Commercial video games implement these key principles masterfully but do so for the very audience they target (usually young adult video gamers). In this context, it is understandable that older adults asked to train on action video games show few benefits, and even possibly a negative outcome (Bediou et al., 2018). As illustrated by Boot et al. (2013), compliance in particular becomes a major issue when asking older adults to train on commercially designed video games. The same applies to amblyopic patients.

It is for this very reason that other video game studies have taken special care to develop easier, more accessible levels for intervention studies with amblyopic patients (Bayliss et al., 2012; To et al., 2011). Another related approach in the field has been to embody the basic action game mechanics of pacing, divided attention and a concurrent high accuracy, high focus task, yet in a more psychophysics-type of training, as done by Nyquist and colleagues (2016) in visually impaired youth.

In sum, initial exploration of video gaming, and especially action video game play, for the treatment of amblyopia or low vision patients has shown some promising results. There remains, however, a need to develop games specifically tailored to each population's deficits—properly aligning the action video game mechanics and the visual skills to be specifically retrained.

Practical Applications of Action Gaming: Educational Purposes

Considering the cognitive benefits of action video games, as well as their broad appeal, another promising field of application is of course their use for educational purposes in the classroom and/or for job-related training.

As far as educational applications are concerned, the field is still in its infancy. To start with, it should be noted that very few studies have been devoted to examining the cognitive effects of action gaming in child populations. One major concern is, as noted previously, the fact that most (though not all) action video games are violent and thus inappropriate for children. While intervention studies do therefore come with possible ethical issues (although non-violent action games can be found and have been used, as detailed ahead), a few cross-sectional studies comparing children that are habitual action gamers with children that are not action gamers have been reported (see Bediou et al., 2018 for a fuller discussion of this point).

One example is the investigation by Dye and Bavelier (2010) on children aged 7–18 years old. The authors examined the developmental time courses of three facets of visual attention—attention deployed in space, in time and over objects in motion. First, the authors observed that the time course of development for these three sub-domains of visual attention differed, with peak performance being reached at different ages. This finding is in line with the extant literature indicating that (at least partially) different underlying neural resources may be involved, each maturing at a different rate. Second, the authors reported that all aforementioned aspects of visual attention were associated with enhancements in avid action gamers (replicating the findings described in cross-sectional studies in adults). AVGP children displayed performance comparable to older NVGPs in the case of attention directed in time and attention towards moving objects; they also presented higher performance than older NVGPs as concerns attention deployed in space. Intervention studies using non-violent action games will be needed to establish causal links from action games to the enhancement of attentional performance, as has been reported in adults.

In the educational context, the ability of action games to foster attentional control and cognitive flexibility, as well as to potentially facilitate skill learning, is of course of great interest. Greater attentional control—the ability to focus for long windows of time while ignoring sources of disruption or distraction—is potentially highly beneficial to classroom learning (James, 1899; Duckworth & Carlson, 2013). Could action video games and the motivating force they represent be harnessed to support positive changes in the learning of academic skills? The main example of such a proposition so far regards developmental dyslexia—a disorder characterized by difficulties in learning to read. Although the main theoretical account of the underlying cognitive causes of developmental dyslexia involves a phonological deficit, a subsample of dyslexic children appears to be affected by attentional deficits (Bosse & Valdois, 2009).

Franceschini and colleagues (2013) evaluated the ability of action video gaming to enhance attention and reading abilities in a dyslexic population. The authors used a child-friendly video game (Rayman Raving Rabbids) containing both action mini-games and non-action mini-games. They recruited children diagnosed with dyslexia and pre-tested them on attentional skills and reading abilities. Half of the children were then trained on the action mini-games and the other half of the kids played the non-action mini-games, for a total training time for both groups of 12 hours, distributed over the course of several weeks. At the end of training, all children were post-tested using the same attentional and reading measures. The results showed greater improvement in attention for the dyslexic group trained with the action mini-games, as expected from the results described so far. Importantly, greater gains in the action-trained group compared to the non-action-trained group were also observed for reading ability. In particular, reading speed was enhanced, with no cost for reading accuracy. These gains in reading were related to gains in attention, suggesting a potential causal coupling between the two.

It should be noted that these observations were made on Italian children, who learn to read a very transparent orthography, Italian, in which the association between letters or groups of letters and speech sounds is highly consistent. This is not the case in more opaque orthographic systems, such as French or English, where reliance on context is needed to decipher and pronounce irregular words. Interestingly though, similar findings as those described for the Italian sample were reported on dyslexic children learning to read English (Franceschini et al., 2017), with benefits of action mini-games training in terms of reading speed, with no cost for reading accuracy. Overall, these two studies underline the potential that action video gaming holds for training visuo-attentional processing and in turn positively impacts reading-related processes such as the speed of letter string decoding. Further investigations with larger samples will be needed, both to confirm these preliminary observations and to establish whether and how the reported changes could cascade down to other crucial aspects of reading, such as accuracy and comprehension. Considering that children and adolescents can be incredibly avid gamers (ESA, 2015), the challenge of leveraging such enthusiasm and channeling it towards educationally valuable and beneficial experiences is certainly very appealing.

Another aspect of cognition boosted by action video games, which may be relevant for education, is the capacity to precisely enumerate objects (Green & Bavelier, 2003, 2006b). Building on the known relation between this capacity and core skills in mathematics such as the approximate number system (ANS) (Park & Brannon, 2013), one study assessed the possibility that training adults with action video games may result in increased enumeration capacities and in turn may benefit paper and pencil mathematics tests (Libertus et al., 2017). Action video game trained adults showed a small improvement in performance in these latter standardized math tests, compared to participants trained on a control video game. Yet, the two groups did not differ in the ANS task used, indicating possibly other mechanisms than the ANS system for computation improvement after action video game play. More generally, it remains that when video game play competes with time spent on homework, video game play negatively impacts academic achievement as would be expected (Weis & Cerankosky, 2010), calling for caution in time spent on video game play. In fact, the studies reviewed here indicate potential benefits after small distributed doses of about 40 minutes per day of game play, 4–5 times a week over a period of tens of week, rather than the binging consumption typically witnessed when played for entertainment purposes.

Outside of child samples, another possible translational application of action video game training involves job-related training in adults. One example concerns the medical field, more specifically endoscopic surgery. The skills required for endoscopic surgery share several features with skills necessary for succeeding in action video games; in particular, the dexterity in using a handheld device constrained by visual feedback. In line with these observations, a training study by Schlickum and colleagues (2009) demonstrated that, when confronted with realistic simulations of laparoscopic surgery, novice surgeons trained on action video games outperformed their peers trained on a non-action game.

What Is So Special About Video Games as a Training Tool?

Considering all of the positive effects of action video gaming described so far, it appears legitimate to ask what features make video games, and especially action video games, so special as a training tool. While we still lack a definitive answer to the question, a few hypotheses can be drawn.

Overall, it appears that video games, and action games in particular, present several general characteristics of carefully designed learning tools (as described in detail by Gentile & Gentile, 2008). First, a fairly general aspect concerns motivation: by going after gamers' excitement, game designers have come up with solutions that guarantee wide interest and motivation, resulting in prolonged time on task. Several reasons exist for the impressive enthusiasm video games generate, one of which is the skillful reliance on reward: by challenging the gamer at the right level of difficulty and embedding the challenges in the right settings, games have been suggested to successfully evoke the release of key neurotransmitters such as dopamine (Koepp et al., 1998; Mathiak et al., 2011; Kätsyri, Hari, Ravaja, & Nummenmaa, 2013). A first point is therefore that video games could be efficient learning tools because the enjoyment they deliver nourishes the intrinsic motivation to train one's skills more and better.

Second, another general observation is that video games always manage to challenge the gamer by keeping him/her at the right difficulty level: a challenge always exists (so the task is never too easy), yet it is never intractable. Feedback guides the player through what needs to be accomplished. The precise level of difficulty used, not too low nor too high, always guaranteeing that the individual will be playing at the edge of her skill, has been described in the learning literature as the "proximal zone of development" (Vygotsky, 1978). Thus, a second aspect of video games in general that mirrors learning regimens is keeping the individual in a specific zone of difficulty that challenges her without discouraging her and providing feedback for her to monitor her progress.

A third important factor may be the variability of situations comprised within the game (Schmidt & Bjork, 1992; Ackerman & Cianciolo, 2000). Indeed, it has been hypothesized that variability in training is very important, but needs to be finely titrated: too much variability hinders training (imagine that each situation in the game requires a specific response—there would be nothing general or generalizable to learn) yet too little variability leads to a high degree of automaticity, which results in responses being extremely efficient in the trained situation but not being transferrable to any other context (as we have described in the case of perceptual learning resulting from specific, very narrow training). By placing the player under constant challenge, and in ever-changing contexts (yet another of the strategies that game designers have come up with to avoid boredom), video games are designed to maintain the player within the very best amount of variability in order to foster greater generalization.

The aforementioned features are common to all video games. Yet, as discussed in the third section, action video games may be notable in the attentional demands that they create: action games require switching between a highly focused attentional state (e.g., when aiming at a given enemy) and a state of distributed attention (e.g., constantly monitoring the environment while moving around and collecting information or items). Because players need to master the allocation of attention between these two different states, it is possible that this in turn amounts to receiving training in the regulation of attention allocation and the flexible assignment of cognitive resources. As we have suggested in the third section, these very demands on attentional control and cognitive flexibility may be at the heart of action gamers' ability to quickly grasp and learn the specific demands of the task at hand—allowing them to display faster learning of new tasks.

Finally, it is important to point out that by no means do the works presented here suggest that heavy gaming is healthy and desirable. Again, mirroring well-known findings from the learning literature, the training regimens we have described entail playing in short, distributed sessions over relatively long periods of time: rather than 12 hours over two days, a 12 hour training study would typically schedule the training/game play to be distributed over 2–3 weeks. Thus, the optimal training regime is often not the one that would be induced if only guided by the bingeing some video game players like to indulge in.

Final Considerations

What Neuroscience Has Added to Our Understanding Over and Above Psychology

Overall, we have eludicating a body of work, coming from both psychology and neuroscience, eludicating the positive consequences of action video games on a surprisingly wide array of cognitive skills. While behavioral intervention studies have demonstrated the causal role of action gaming on the observed enhancements in performance, neuroimaging studies have identified changes in the fronto-parietal network of attention as a potential mechanism at the source of these behavioral changes. More specifically, neuroimaging studies have shown that the ability to more fully suppress task irrelevant information— at the neural level—may underlie many of the benefits observed after action gaming.

Concrete Implications of Research and Opportunities for Translation to Education

The work we have presented suggests a new pathway for the development of therapeutic or educational video games, at least in the context of interventions that will benefit from enhanced attentional control and cognitive flexibility. The present work calls for designing a game experience that implements the three key mechanics of action video games—pacing, high divided attention load and the need for focused attention challenges—all the while aligning the game play experience with the type of content to be trained. We recognize that the action mechanics considered so far are more naturally aligned with skill training, such as enhancing vision, mental rotation or reading, than with most academic content training. Yet, academic proficiency tends to be anchored in foundational skills, as for example number sense in mathematics (Libertus et al., 2017) or the size of the attentional window in reading (Antzaka et al., 2017) that could benefit from being properly integrated with action video game play. In short, opportunities are manifold, but future developments will require a careful evaluation of both patients' or students' needs, as well as the type of game play mechanics most likely to foster the targeted skills in a seamless true gaming experience.

Further Resources for the Reader to Learn More About the Topic

- Hodent, C. (2017). *The gamer's brain: How neuroscience and UX can impact video game design.* Boca Raton: CRC Press.
- Strobach, T., & Karbach, J. (Eds.). (2016). *Cognitive training: an overview of features and applications.* Cham, Switzerland: Springer.

References

Ackerman, P. L., & Cianciolo, A. T. (2000). Cognitive, perceptual-speed, and psychomotor determinants of individual differences during skill acquisition. *Journal of Experimental Psychology: Applied, 6*(4), 259.

Anderson, C. A., Shibuya, A., Ihori, N., Swing, E. L., Bushman, B. J., Sakamoto, A., Rothstein, H., & Saleem, M. (2010). Violent video game effects on aggression, empathy, and prosocial behavior in Eastern and Western countries: A meta-analytic review. *Psychological Bulletin, 136*(2), 151.

Anguera, J. A., Boccanfuso, J., Rintoul, J. L., Al-Hashimi, O., Faraji, F., Janowich, J., . . . Gazzaley, A. (2013). Video game training enhances cognitive control in older adults. *Nature, 501*(7465), 97.

Antzaka, A., Lallier, M., Meyer, S., Diard, J., Carreiras, M., & Valdois, S. (2017). Enhancing reading performance through action video games: The role of visual attention span. *Scientific Reports, 7*(1), 14563.

Baddeley, A., & Longman, D. (1978). The influence of length and frequency of training sessions on the rate of learning to type. *Ergonomics, 21*, 627–635.

Barnett, S. M., & Ceci, S. J. (2002). When and where do we apply what we learn? A taxonomy for far transfer. *Psychological Bulletin, 128*(4), 612–637.

Bavelier, D., Achtman, R. L., Mani, M., & Föcker, J. (2012). Neural bases of selective attention in action video game players. *Vision Research, 61*, 132–143.

Bavelier, D., & Föcker, J. (2015). Videogames in the spotlight: The case of attentional control. In J. Fawcett, E. Risko, & A. Kingstone (Eds.), *The handbook of attention.* Boston, MA: MIT Press.

Bavelier, D., Green, C. S., Pouget, A., & Schrater, P. (2012). Brain plasticity through the life span: Learning to learn and action video games. *Annual Review of Neuroscience, 35*(1), 391–416.

Bayliss, J., Vedamurthy, I., Nahum, M., Levi, D., & Bavelier, D. (2012). *Lazy eye shooter: A novel game therapy for visual recovery in adult amblyopia.* Games Innovation Conference (IGIC), 2012 IEEE International.

Bediou, B., Adams, D. M., Mayer, R. E., Tipton, E., Green, C. S., & Bavelier, D. (2018). Meta-analysis of action video game impact on perceptual, attentional, and cognitive skills. *Psychological Bulletin, 144*(1), 77.

Bejjanki, V. R., Zhang, R., Li, R., Pouget, A., Green, C. S., Lu, Z. L., & Bavelier, D. (2014). Action video game play facilitates the development of better perceptual templates. *Proceedings of the National Academy of Sciences, 111*(47), 16961–16966.

Berard, A. V., Cain, M. S., Watanabe, T., & Sasaki, Y. (2015). Frequent video game players resist perceptual interference. *PloS One, 10*(3), e0120011.

Boot, W. R., Champion, M., Blakely, D. P., Wright, T., Souders, D., & Charness, N. (2013). Video games as a means to reduce age-related cognitive decline: Attitudes, compliance, and effectiveness. *Frontiers in Psychology, 4*, 31.

Bosse, M., & Valdois, S. (2009). Influence of the visual attention span on child reading performance: A cross-sectional study. *Journal of Research in Reading, 32*, 230–253.

Buckley, D., Codina, C., Bhardwaj, P., & Pascalis, O. (2010). Action video game players and deaf observers have larger Goldmann visual fields. *Vision Research, 50*(5), 548–556.

Cain, M. S., Landau, A. N., & Shimamura, A. P. (2012). Action video game experience reduces the cost of switching tasks. *Attention, Perception, & Psychophysics, 74*(4), 641–647.

Cardoso-Leite, P., Joessel, A., & Bavelier, D. (2020). Games for enhancing cognitive abilities. In J. Plass, R. Mayer, & B. Homer (Eds.), *Handbook of game-based learning*. Boston, MA: MIT Press.

Castel, A. D., Pratt, J., & Drummond, E. (2005). The effects of action video game experience on the time course of inhibition of return and the efficiency of visual search. *Acta Psychologica, 119*(2), 217–230.

Cheung, A. C., & Slavin, R. E. (2012). How features of educational technology applications affect student reading outcomes: A meta-analysis. *Educational Research Review, 7*(3), 198–215.

Cheung, A. C., & Slavin, R. E. (2013). The effectiveness of educational technology applications for enhancing mathematics achievement in K-12 classrooms: A meta-analysis. *Educational Research Review, 9*, 88–113.

Chiappe, D., Conger, M., Liao, J., Caldwell, J. L., & Vu, K. P. L. (2013). Improving multi-tasking ability through action videogames. *Applied Ergonomics, 44*(2), 278–284.

Chisholm, J. D., & Kingstone, A. (2012). Improved top-down control reduces oculomotor capture: The case of action video game players. *Attention, Perception, & Psychophysics, 74*(2), 257–262.

Chisholm, J. D., & Kingstone, A. (2015). Action video games and improved attentional control: Disentangling selection-and response-based processes. *Psychonomic Bulletin & Review, 22*(5), 1430–1436.

Colzato, L. S., van den Wildenberg, W. P., & Hommel, B. (2014). Cognitive control and the COMT Val 158 Met polymorphism: Genetic modulation of videogame training and transfer to task-switching efficiency. *Psychological Research, 78*(5), 670–678.

Dale, G., & Green, C. S. (2017a). The changing face of video games and video gamers: Future directions in the scientific study of video game play and cognitive performance. *Journal of Cognitive Enhancement, 1*(3), 280–294.

Dale, G., & Green, C. S. (2017b). Associations between avid action and real-time strategy game play and cognitive performance: A pilot study. *Journal of Cognitive Enhancement, 1*(3), 295–317.

Donohue, S. E., James, B., Eslick, A. N., & Mitroff, S. R. (2012). Cognitive pitfall! Videogame players are not immune to dual-task costs. *Attention, Perception, & Psychophysics, 74*(5), 803–809.

Duckworth, A. L., & Carlson, S. M. (2013). Self-regulation and school success. In B. W. Sokol, F. M. E. Grouzet, & U. Müller (Eds.), *Self-regulation and autonomy: Social and developmental dimensions of human conduct* (pp. 208–230). New York: Cambridge University Press.

Dye, M. W., & Bavelier, D. (2010). Differential development of visual attention skills in school-age children. *Vision Research, 50*(4), 452–459.

Dye, M. W., Green, C. S., & Bavelier, D. (2009). Increasing speed of processing with action video games. *Current Directions in Psychological Science, 18*(6), 321–326.

Eayrs, J., & Lavie, N. (2018). Establishing individual differences in perceptual capacity. *Journal of Experimental Psychology: Human Perception and Performance, 44*(8), 1240.

Entertainment software association (ESA). (2015). *Essential facts about the computer and video game industry.* Retrieved from www.theesa.com/wp-content/uploads/2015/04/ESA-Essential-Facts-2015.pdf

Fahle, M. (2005). Perceptual learning: Specificity versus generalization. *Current Opinion in Neurobiology, 15*(2), 154–160.

Feng, J., Spence, I., & Pratt, J. (2007). Playing an action video game reduces gender differences in spatial cognition. *Psychological Science, 18*(10), 850–855.

Föcker, J., Mortazavi, M., Khoe, W., Hillyard, S. A., & Bavelier, D. (2018). Neural correlates of enhanced visual attentional control in action video game players: An event-related potential study. *Journal of Cognitive Neuroscience,* 1–15.

Franceschini, S., Gori, S., Ruffino, M., Viola, S., Molteni, M., & Facoetti, A. (2013). Action video games make dyslexic children read better. *Current Biology, 23*(6), 462–466.

Franceschini, S., Trevisan, P., Ronconi, L., Bertoni, S., Colmar, S., Double, K., . . . Gori, S. (2017). Action video games improve reading abilities and visual-to-auditory attentional shifting in English-speaking children with dyslexia. *Scientific Reports, 7*(1), 5863.

Gaspar, J. G., Neider, M. B., Crowell, J. A., Lutz, A., Kaczmarski, H., & Kramer, A. F. (2014). Are gamers better crossers? An examination of action video game experience and dual task effects in a simulated street crossing task. *Human Factors, 56*(3), 443–452.

Gentile, D. A. (2009). Pathological video-game use among youth ages 8 to 18: A national study. *Psychological Science, 20*(5), 594–602.

Gentile, D. A., & Gentile, J. R. (2008). Violent video games as exemplary teachers: A conceptual analysis. *Journal of Youth and Adolescence, 37*(2), 127–141.

Glass, B. D., Maddox, W. T., & Love, B. C. (2013). Real-time strategy game training: Emergence of a cognitive flexibility trait. *PloS One, 8*(8), e70350.

Gozli, D. G., Bavelier, D., & Pratt, J. (2014). The effect of action video game playing on sensorimotor learning: Evidence from a movement tracking task. *Human Movement Science, 38,* 152–162.

Green, C. S., & Bavelier, D. (2003). Action video game modifies visual selective attention. *Nature, 423*(6939), 534.

Green, C. S., & Bavelier, D. (2006a). Effect of action video games on the spatial distribution of visuospatial attention. *Journal of Experimental Psychology: Human Perception and Performance, 32*(6), 1465.

Green, C. S., & Bavelier, D. (2006b). Enumeration versus multiple object tracking: The case of action video game players. *Cognition, 101*(1), 217–245.

Green, C. S., & Bavelier, D. (2007). Action-video-game experience alters the spatial resolution of vision. *Psychological Science, 18*(1), 88–94.

Green, C. S., Pouget, A., & Bavelier, D. (2010). Improved probabilistic inference as a general learning mechanism with action video games. *Current Biology, 20*(17), 1573–1579.

Green, C. S., Sugarman, M. A., Medford, K., Klobusicky, E., & Bavelier, D. (2012). The effect of action video game experience on task-switching. *Computers in Human Behavior, 28*(3), 984–994.

Hubert-Wallander, B., Green, C. S., Sugarman, M., & Bavelier, D. (2011). Changes in search rate but not in the dynamics of exogenous attention in action videogame players. *Attention, Perception, & Psychophysics, 73*(8), 2399–2412.

Hutchinson, C. V., & Stocks, R. (2013). Selectively enhanced motion perception in core video gamers. *Perception, 42*(6), 675–677.

James, W. (1899). *Talks to teachers on psychology and to students on some of life's ideals.* New York, NY: Holt.

Karle, J. W., Watter, S., & Shedden, J. M. (2010). Task switching in video game players: Benefits of selective attention but not resistance to proactive interference. *Acta Psychologica, 134*(1), 70–78.

Karni, A., & Sagi, D. (1991). Where practice makes perfect in texture discrimination: Evidence for primary visual cortex plasticity. *Proc. Natl. Acad. Sci. USA, 88*, 4966–4970.

Kätsyri, J., Hari, R., Ravaja, N., & Nummenmaa, L. (2013). Just watching the game ain't enough: Striatal fMRI reward responses to successes and failures in a video game during active and vicarious playing. *Frontiers in Human Neuroscience, 7*, 278.

Kim, Y. H., Kang, D. W., Kim, D., Kim, H. J., Sasaki, Y., & Watanabe, T. (2015). Real-time strategy video game experience and visual perceptual learning. *Journal of Neuroscience, 35*(29), 10485–10492.

Koepp, M. J., Gunn, R. N., Lawrence, A. D., Cunningham, V. J., Dagher, A., Jones, T., . . . Grasby, P. M. (1998). Evidence for striatal dopamine release during a video game. *Nature, 393*(6682), 266.

Krishnan, L., Kang, A., Sperling, G., & Srinivasan, R. (2013). Neural strategies for selective attention distinguish fast-action video game players. *Brain Topography, 26*, 83–97.

Li, R. W., Ngo, C., Nguyen, J., & Levi, D. M. (2011). Video-game play induces plasticity in the visual system of adults with amblyopia. *PLoS Biology, 9*(8), e1001135.

Li, R. W., Polat, U., Makous, W., & Bavelier, D. (2009). Enhancing the contrast sensitivity function through action video game training. *Nature Neuroscience, 12*(5), 549.

Li, R. W., Polat, U., Scalzo, F., & Bavelier, D. (2010). Reducing backward masking through action game training. *Journal of Vision, 10*(14), 33.

Libertus, M. E., Liu, A., Pikul, O., Jacques, T., Cardoso-Leite, P., Halberda, J., & Bavelier, D. (2017). The impact of action video game training on mathematical abilities in adults. *AERA Open, 3*(4), doi:10.1177/2332858417740857

Mathiak, K. A., Klasen, M., Weber, R., Ackermann, H., Shergill, S. S., & Mathiak, K. (2011). Reward system and temporal pole contributions to affective evaluation during a first person shooter video game. *BMC Neuroscience, 12*(1), 66.

McDermott, A. F., Bavelier, D., & Green, C. S. (2014). Memory abilities in action video game players. *Computers in Human Behavior, 34*, 69–78.

Mishra, J., Zinni, M., Bavelier, D., & Hillyard, S. A. (2011). Neural basis of superior performance of action videogame players in an attention-demanding task. *Journal of Neuroscience, 31*(3), 992–998.

Nyquist, J. B., Lappin, J. S., Zhang, R., & Tadin, D. (2016). Perceptual training yields rapid improvements in visually impaired youth. *Scientific Reports, 6,* 37431.

Oei, A. C., & Patterson, M. D. (2013). Enhancing cognition with video games: A multiple game training study. *PLoS One, 8*(3), e58546.

Owen, A. M., Hampshire, A., Grahn, J. A., Stenton, R., Dajani, S., Burns, A. S., . . . Ballard, C. G. (2010). Putting brain training to the test. *Nature, 465*(7299), 775–778.

Park, J., & Brannon, E. M. (2013). Training the approximate number system improves math proficiency. *Psychological Science, 24*(10), 2013–2019.

Posner, M. I., Rothbart, M. K., Sheese, B. E., & Voelker, P. (2012). Control networks and neuromodulators of early development. *Developmental Psychology, 48*(3), 827.

Rich, M., Tsappis, M., & Kavanaugh, J. R. (2017). Problematic interactive media use among children and adolescents: Addiction, compulsion, or syndrome? In K. S. Young & C. Nabuco De Abreu (Eds.), *Internet addiction in children and adolescents: Risk factors, assessment, and treatment.* New York, NY: Springer Publishing Company.

Rupp, M. A., McConnell, D. S., & Smither, J. A. (2016). Examining the relationship between action video game experience and performance in a distracted driving task. *Current Psychology, 35*(4), 527–539.

Schlickum, M. K., Hedman, L., Enochsson, L., Kjellin, A., & Felländer-Tsai, L. (2009). Systematic video game training in surgical novices improves performance in virtual reality endoscopic surgical simulators: A prospective randomized study. *World Journal of Surgery, 33*(11), 2360.

Schmidt, R. A., & Bjork, R. A. (1992). New conceptualizations of practice: Common principles in three paradigms suggest new concepts for training. *Psychological Science, 3*(4), 207–218.

Schubert, T., Finke, K., Redel, P., Kluckow, S., Müller, H., & Strobach, T. (2015). Video game experience and its influence on visual attention parameters: An investigation using the framework of the theory of visual attention (TVA). *Acta Psychologica, 157,* 200–214.

Soderstrom, N. C., & Bjork, R. A. (2015). Learning versus performance: An integrative review. *Perspectives on Psychological Science, 10*(2), 176–199.

Stafford, T., & Dewar, M. (2014). Tracing the trajectory of skill learning with a very large sample of online game players. *Psychological Science, 25*(2), 511–518.

Strobach, T., Frensch, P. A., & Schubert, T. (2012). Video game practice optimizes executive control skills in dual-task and task switching situations. *Acta Psychologica, 140*(1), 13–24.

Sungur, H., & Boduroglu, A. (2012). Action video game players form more detailed representation of objects. *Acta Psychologica, 139*(2), 327–334.

To, L., Thompson, B., Blum, J. R., Maehara, G., Hess, R. F., & Cooperstock, J. R. (2011). A game platform for treatment of amblyopia. *IEEE Transactions on Neural Systems and Rehabilitation Engineering, 19*(3), 280–289.

Trick, L. M., Jaspers-Fayer, F., & Sethi, N. (2005). Multiple-object tracking in children: The "catch the spies" task. *Cognitive Development, 20*(3), 373–387.

Vygotsky, L. S. (1978). *Mind and society: The development of higher psychological processes.* Cambridge, MA: Harvard University Press.

Weis, R., & Cerankosky, B. C. (2010). Effects of video-game ownership on young boys' academic and behavioral functioning: A randomized, controlled study. *Psychological Science, 21*(4), 463–470.

West, G. L., Stevens, S. A., Pun, C., & Pratt, J. (2008). Visuospatial experience modulates attentional capture: Evidence from action video game players. *Journal of Vision, 8*(16), 13.

Wu, S., Cheng, C. K., Feng, J., D'angelo, L., Alain, C., & Spence, I. (2012). Playing a first-person shooter video game induces neuroplastic change. *Journal of Cognitive Neuroscience, 24*(6), 1286–1293.

Wu, S., & Spence, I. (2013). Playing shooter and driving videogames improves top-down guidance in visual search. *Attention, Perception, & Psychophysics, 75*(4), 673–686.

12 Mindfulness and Executive Function

Implications for Learning and Early Childhood Education

Andrei D. Semenov, Douglas Kennedy, and Philip David Zelazo

Introduction

There is now widespread public recognition that children's developing executive function (EF) skills provide an important foundation for learning and school success (e.g., Zelazo, Blair, & Willoughby, 2016). EF skills are the attention-regulation skills necessary for the top-down, goal-directed modulation of attention (and downstream, reasoning, behavior, and emotion), typically measured as inhibitory control, cognitive flexibility, and working memory (Miyake et al., 2000), as well as the "hot" EF skills needed for emotion regulation and for the flexible, goal-directed reversal of basic approach and avoidance motivations (Zelazo & Müller, 2002; Zelazo & Cunningham, 2007). Together, EF skills make it possible for children to sustain attention, keep goals and information in mind, refrain from responding immediately, resist distraction, tolerate frustration, consider the consequences of different behaviors, reflect on past experiences, and plan for the future (Zelazo et al., 2016). Not surprisingly, better EF skills are reliably linked to better academic outcomes (e.g., Allan, Hume, Allan, Farrington, & Lonigan, 2014, for a meta-analysis). Children with better EF skills have been found to learn more from a given amount of instruction and practice (e.g., Benson, Sabbagh, Carlson, & Zelazo, 2013), and to show larger gains in achievement across school grades (e.g., Hassinger-Das, Jordan, Glutting, Irwin, & Dyson, 2014). In contrast, poor EF skills may interfere with children's own (and others') learning and may lead to behavior problems, suspension, expulsion, or being held back (U.S. Department of Education, 2014).

Both hot and cool EF skills are increasingly a target of instruction in educational settings, especially in early childhood but also across the lifespan. The hope is that it will be relatively easy to teach traditional content (reading, writing, and arithmetic) to children who can control their attention and behavior in the classroom. Efforts to teach EF skills may prepare children to learn more efficiently and effectively in the classroom, reflecting on new material, processing it at a deeper level, and integrating with what is already known (Marcovitch, Jacques, Boseovski, & Zelazo, 2008). In addition, however, these efforts may help children to get along with their teachers and with other students and avoid behavioral problems.

In this chapter, we provide a developmental neuroscience framework for understanding the impact of interventions on children's developing EF skills, and then review research on one increasingly popular approach to EF skills training, *mindfulness*. Mindfulness is a particular way of paying attention—on purpose, in the present moment, and nonjudgmentally (Kabat-Zinn, 1994). Mindful attention involves sustaining attention to one's ongoing experiences, including one's experience of what is happening internally (e.g., thoughts or emotions), without evaluating or making a judgment about each experience (Brown & Ryan, 2003; Kabat-Zinn, 2003; Lutz, Dunne, & Davidson, 2007), and it is often practiced in the context of focused attention (e.g., paying attention to one's breathing and gently redirecting attention back to one's breathing when the mind wanders). We first review research on the neuroscience of mindfulness and potential mechanisms by which mindfulness can facilitate EF skills, then review the efficacy of mindfulness interventions that target children themselves, and, finally, examine interventions targeting teachers, which are designed to produce classroom-level improvements in children's mindfulness, EF, and wellbeing. The emerging evidence suggests that mindfulness practices may be beneficial for children, with concurrent as well as cascading benefits for academic and social success. Clearly, however, more research is needed to demonstrate the efficacy of mindfulness interventions with children in a rigorous fashion. We conclude with recommendations for future research and a summary of implications for learning and education.

A Developmental Neuroscience Perspective on EF skills and Their Development

Research on the developing brain has revealed several principles that together provide a framework for conceptualizing the impact of interventions such as mindfulness on children's developing EF skills. First, interventions targeting children's EF skills are informed by research that has established clearly that the human brain is highly malleable and influenced by experience, a phenomenon called *neural plasticity* (see Dumontheil & Mareschal, this volume). Inspired in part by Hebb's (1949) suggestion that neurons that fire together wire together,[1] and research with nonhuman animals (e.g., Krech, Rosenzweig, & Bennett, 1960; Gibson et al., 2014; Greenough, Black, & Wallace, 1987), more recent research with both human adults (e.g., Bengtsson et al., 2005; Elbert, Pantev, Wienbruch, Rockstroh, & Taub, 1995; Maguire et al., 2000; Scholz et al., 2009; Takeuchi et al., 2010) and children (e.g., Astle, Barnes, Baker, Colclough, & Woolrich, 2015; Espinet, Anderson, & Zelazo, 2013; Rueda, Rothbart, McCandliss, Saccomanno, & Posner, 2005) has found that when particular neural networks in the brain are activated and used, these networks become more efficient, reflecting myelination, dendritic thickening, and synaptic pruning (reduction of connections among neurons that are not used), among other structural and functional changes (see Constantinidis & Klingberg, 2016 for review). Therefore, the repeated engagement and use of EF skills should not only render those skills more efficient, but also increase the efficiency of the corresponding neural circuitry, which may in turn provide children more opportunities for thoughtful reflection prior to overt action or decision making.

Recent reviews confirm that EF skills can indeed be improved by a variety of interventions that engage children's EF skills and provide children with opportunities to practice these skills at increasing levels of challenge (Diamond & Lee, 2011). Although there are questions about the extent to which the benefits of EF training transfer to new situations (e.g., Karbach & Kray, 2009), it has been proposed that most training studies are not optimally designed to promote transfer (e.g., they fail to train skills in a wide range of different contexts), and that supplementing direct EF skills training with reflection training facilitates transfer by inducing metacognitive awareness of the skills and their range of application (Zelazo, 2015). For example, in a study by Espinet et al. (2013), children who failed a widely used measure of EF (the Dimensional Change Card Sort, or DCCS) were given a new DCCS (with different shapes and colors) and taught to pause before responding, reflect on the hierarchical nature of the task, and formulate higher-order rules for responding flexibly: "In the color game, then if it's a red rabbit, then it goes here; but in the shape game that same red rabbit goes there." Compared to children who received only minimal yes/no feedback (without practice in reflection) or mere practice with no feedback at all, children who received reflection training showed significant improvements in performance on a subsequent administration of the DCCS. Improvements were also seen on other tasks, including a measure of perspective taking or theory of mind, and these behavioral changes were accompanied by changes in children's brain activity measured using electroencephalography (a measure of scalp electrical activity that reflects the firing of neurons in cortex).

Second, research on the neural correlates of EF skills and their development is revealing specific neural targets of intervention. Key top-down components of this circuitry include prefrontal cortex (e.g., as part of a fronto-parietal network), one of the last brain regions to mature. Whereas cool EF skills involve regions in lateral prefrontal cortex, hot EF skills rely more on ventral and medial regions of prefrontal cortex. This has been demonstrated in lesion studies (where specific parts of the brain are damaged), and in studies using brain imaging technology (e.g., fMRI) (e.g., Bechara, Damasio, Damasio, & Anderson, 1994; Manes et al., 2002). Case studies of individuals (both children and adults) with lesions to orbitofrontal cortex provide striking evidence that it is possible to do well on clinic-based and laboratory measures of EF, but still have considerable difficulty managing emotionally charged situations in daily life.

Third, more top-down influences on attention and behavior interact in a reciprocal way with more bottom-up influences, which can override one's current goals and attention. This is well illustrated by the Emotional Interference Task (Buodo, Sarlo, & Palomba, 2002). In this task, adult participants are shown emotionally charged pictures, such as a photograph of a bloody car accident, and then while the picture remains visible, played a tone that is either high-pitched or low-pitched. Participants are told to ignore the pictures and categorize the tones as quickly and accurately as possible. Buodo et al. (2002) found that participants were slower to respond to the pitch of the tone if they saw pictures that were arousing or had blood/injury as compared to pictures that were of sporting events, or household objects. This finding demonstrates how emotional reactivity can interfere with goal-directed attention and behavior.

Stress and stress hormones (cortisol) have also been shown to undermine the use of EF skills and interfere with EF development (e.g., Blair et al., 2011; Evans & Schamberg, 2009; Hostinar, Sullivan, & Gunnar, 2014), and this may account in part for differences in EF and academic outcomes in children growing up in poverty (e.g., Noble, Norman, & Farah, 2005) or otherwise exposed to difficult circumstances (e.g., Masten, 2014). Poverty is associated with both lower levels of EF skill and higher levels of stress in childhood, likely because stress impairs EF, and impaired EF in turn leads to more stress (Evans & Schamberg, 2009). There is also evidence, however, that good EF skills can protect against risks associated with poverty and adversity, including the risk of academic failure (Masten et al., 2012).

Finally, fourth, while the human brain is inherently plastic, continually adapting to its environment, research in developmental neuroscience suggest that there are periods of relatively high plasticity (i.e., "sensitive periods") when particular parts of the brain and their corresponding functions are especially susceptible to environmental influences. These periods typically correspond to times of rapid growth in those regions and functions, when the relevant neural regions are adapting especially rapidly to structure inherent in the environment (e.g., Huttenlocher, 2002). Because EF skills undergo a particularly rapid transformation during early childhood, from about 2 to 6 years of age, the preschool period may be a window of opportunity for the cultivation of these skills via well-timed, targeted scaffolding and support (Zelazo, 2015). There is also considerable reorganization of prefrontal systems during the transition to adolescence, however, when gray matter volume in PFC reaches a peak (Giedd et al., 1999), and this too may be an auspicious time for intervention.

The principles of neural plasticity, reciprocal interactions between more top-down (e.g., prefrontal) and more bottom-up (e.g., limbic) influences, and sensitive periods inform efforts to design and optimize interventions to promote the development of EF, and they support the suggestion that age-appropriate mindfulness exercises may be conceptualized as a *neural training regime*. Mindfulness training for children often includes small group activities designed to promote sustained introspective reflection on various experiences, as well as attentive observation of one's surroundings (e.g., awareness of others, awareness of stimuli in the environment; e.g., Broderick & Metz, 2009; Flook et al., 2010; Kaiser Greenland, 2010; Lantieri, 2008; Miller & Butler, 2011; Saltzman, 2014; Willard, 2010). For example, to foster awareness of internal states, children might describe how different parts of their bodies feel from head to toe. Props may scaffold these exercises; for example, holding a hula hoop around their bodies and moving it up and down helps children focus attention to a zone like their shoulders, and a stuffed animal may be placed on children's abdomens to help them pay attention to their breathing as they lie down on a mat and breathe to lift the animal up and down. Practices such as these are increasingly being used in schools (Butzer, Ebert, Telles, & Khalsa, 2015), supported by a small but growing body of evidence that these practices improve children's performance on measures of EF and emotion regulation (e.g., Flook et al., 2010; Flook, Goldberg, Pinger, & Davidson, 2015; Schonert-Reichl et al., 2015; Zelazo, Forston, Masten, & Carlson, 2018; Zenner, Herrnleben-Kurz, & Walach, 2014).

Attending intentionally, and redirecting attention when it wanders, may lead to improvements in executive function (EF) skills (e.g., Carlson, Zelazo, & Faja, 2013; Diamond, 2013; Jacques & Marcovitch, 2010; Zelazo et al., 2017), as well as the reflective, metacognitive skills that underlie and accompany them (e.g., Allen & Bickhard, 2018; Chevalier & Blaye, 2016; Demetriou et al., 2018; Lyons & Zelazo, 2011; Roebers, 2017; Zelazo, 2004, 2015). In addition, however, practice being nonjudgmental may promote calmness and wellbeing, as may focusing on the present moment (e.g., instead of ruminating over a recollected source of anxiety; Kabat-Zinn, 2003). Zelazo and Lyons (2012) suggested that mindfulness training therefore seems well designed to foster the healthy development of EF skills and emotion regulation because it involves practice using top-down influences on attention (e.g., sustained introspective reflection and cognitive flexibility) while simultaneously reducing bottom-up influences that may undermine EF skills (e.g., by reducing anxiety, and emotional reactivity) and promoting bottom-up influences that may facilitate them (e.g., curiosity about what one is observing in the environment). Indeed, as reviewed in the following sections, research indicates that children and youth trained in mindfulness report lower levels of psychological distress, show higher levels of activation in prefrontal cortical regions and lower activation in regions such as the amygdala (Modinos, Ormel, & Aleman, 2010; Tan & Martin, 2013).

What Neuroscience Teaches Us About Mindfulness

Neuroscientific Framework for Understanding Mindfulness and Self-regulation

To date, there has been a paucity of neuroimaging research on the effects of mindfulness in children and adolescents. Instead the majority of research relies on self and other report, as well as performance on cognitive and behavioral tasks. However, a recent review of the adult literature points to the enhancement of self-regulatory attentional networks as the main mechanism of change following mindfulness practice (e.g., Tang, Hölzel, & Posner, 2015). The adult imaging evidence suggests that there are two primary vectors by which mindfulness training may enhance self-regulation. First, mindfulness involves training attention networks to improve top-down cognitive control and help practitioners form more robust problem-solving strategies (e.g., Lewis et al., 2008). Second, mindfulness changes how practitioners experience and respond to bottom-up emotional reactions (e.g., Hajcak & Dennis, 2009). While some neural indices may reveal differential responses following mindfulness training across development (see Lewis et al., 2008), there is reason to believe that the overall benefit of mindfulness on self-regulation skills persists from childhood through adulthood (Kaunhoven & Dorjee, 2017).

Throughout development there is a dynamic, reciprocal "give and take" relation between "top-down" and "bottom-up" influences. With increased maturity and efficiency of the underlying neural networks, children typically come to rely more on more complex forms of top-down attention regulation relative to more limbic bottom-up responses. For example, whereas infants rely more on the parietal attention networks responsible for orienting attention, which allow them to look away from irrelevant or unpleasant stimuli, older children are more likely to engage frontal networks that allow them to form cognitive strategies through which they can reappraise negative experiences and thoughts. This pattern of self-regulation development can be categorized as a shift from short-term and relatively inflexible regulation strategies to more complex and flexible regulation strategies (Kaunhoven & Dorjee, 2017; Petersen & Posner, 2012).

As more complex forms of self-regulation become possible, due to the increased efficiency of networks involving PFC and the development of more complex representations, children are able to develop more effective strategic skills for self-regulation (Rothbart, Sheese, Rueda, & Posner, 2011). It should be noted, however, that recruitment of higher-order top-down strategies can be metabolically and cognitively taxing and therefore not always appropriate. Mindfulness meditation is also directed at the development of bottom-up self-regulation strategies. Bottom-up strategies can be used prior to the recruitment of top-down processes, as a kind of "first pass" at regulating emotions and behavior (Posner, Rothbart, Sheese, & Voelker, 2014; Rothbart et al., 2011). During mindfulness training, students are often taught to notice and let go of emotions as temporary states of mind (Flook et al., 2010), and this approach to emotions indeed has lower cognitive and metabolic costs than more complex strategies (Kaunhoven & Dorjee, 2017; Keng, Robins, Smoski, Dagenbach, & Leary, 2013; Sheppes & Gross, 2011).

One focus of mindfulness practice is to help children to use their attention deliberately, noticing negative experiences, and recognizing successful strategies in dealing with emotions. For example, mindfulness practice may be directed at reframing the meditator's awareness and response to their own

thoughts and emotions, and to that extent, mindfulness practice also involves
the recruitment and training of specific neural networks involved in increased
metacognitive awareness. In the following section, we will look at specific
networks and neural structures involved in mindfulness practice and what
changes in these structures may mean for the development of self-regulation
strategies.

Neural Structures and Indices of Mindfulness-Related Changes to Self-regulation

Mindfulness meditators are often asked to pay focused attention to one thing
(such as one's breathing), and they are also told to notice but not dwell upon
distractors that compete for attention. The primary neural system recruited
by this aspect of mindfulness practice is the executive attention network
(e.g., Posner & Petersen, 1990), important for controlling attention while
ignoring distractors. The recruitment of this fronto-parietal network can be
indexed by increased activation in the anterior cingulate cortex (ACC, van
Veen & Carter, 2002), a region involved in conflict monitoring. Studies looking at the activation of the ACC during meditation showed greater activation
of rostral ACC (Hölzel et al., 2007) in meditators compared to non-meditator
controls. Peculiarly, the relation between meditation and activation of the
ACC is not a linear one. Brefczynski-Lewis, Lutz, Schaefer, Levinson, and
Davidson (2007) observed that there is increased ACC activation in practicing meditators, but that the more expertise the practitioner has, the lower the
levels of ACC activation. Brefczynski-Lewis and colleagues interpreted these
findings as evidence that for practiced meditators the maintaining of attention
and the ability to filter out distractions become automatic so that ongoing,
effortful monitoring (based on ACC activity) becomes unnecessary.

One neurophysiological index of conflict monitoring in the ACC is the
N2 component of the event-related potential (ERP). The N2 is a frontocentral negativity elicited between 200 and 400 ms after a stimulus onset (Buss,
Dennis, Brooker, & Sippel, 2011; Dennis & Chen, 2007; Lewis et al., 2008,
Stieben et al., 2007), and N2 amplitude has been shown to vary as a function
of conflict and need for executive control (Bokura, Yamaguchi, & Kobayashi,
2001; Falkenstein, Hoormann, & Hohnsbein, 1999; Forster, Carter, Cohen, &
Cho, 2011). Over the course of development the latency of the N2 component decreases and the amplitude becomes smaller (less negative) suggesting
increases in neural efficiency of top-down executive networks (Espinet, Anderson, & Zelazo, 2012). In studies on self-regulation and executive function, the
N2 component has distinguished between young children (35 to 50 months)
who pass versus fail the Dimensional Change Card Sorting Task (DCCS), a
widely used measure of cognitive flexibility (Espinet et al., 2012), as well as
being associated with performance on the Iowa Gambling Task and the Stroop
task in children between 7 and 16 years of age (Lamm, Zelazo, & Lewis,
2006). Beyond being an index of conflict detection and executive control in

a relatively *cool* environment, the N2 component has also been shown to be a useful index in emotionally *hot* tasks. Stieben et al. (2007) showed that children with self-regulation difficulties showed larger (more negative) N2 amplitudes during negative emotion go/no-go trials compared to healthy controls suggesting they recruited higher levels of executive control, perhaps especially when processing more emotionally charged stimuli. Another study found that children (8–17 years old) with smaller (less negative) N2 amplitudes during no-go trials and greater accuracy overall in the go/no-go task were more likely to have better emotion regulation strategies (Chapman, Woltering, Lamm, & Lewis, 2010). In accordance with the model that mindfulness practice enhances executive attention networks, evidence shows that following *regular* brief mindfulness practice, adult participants showed more negative N2 amplitudes suggestive of enhanced executive control (Moore, Gruber, Derose, & Malinowski, 2012). Furthermore, researchers found that adults with higher levels of dispositional mindfulness showed more negative N1 ERPs to socioemotionally negative stimuli alongside more negative N2 amplitudes (Quaglia, Goodman, & Brown, 2015). Together, these findings suggest that the processing differences associated with mindfulness practice can be seen early in the time course of processing, perhaps indicating a degree of automaticity.

Further support for the suggestion that the attentional effects of mindfulness occur rapidly and in a relatively automatic fashion comes from a study by Ortner, Kilner, and Zelazo (2007). These authors administered the Emotional Interference Task (Buodo et al., 2002) to young adults and then randomly assigned them to a 7-week mindfulness intervention, a 7-week relaxation meditation control condition, or a wait-list control. At pre-test, there was an emotion interference effect: participants showed significantly slower (on the order of 50–100 ms) reaction times following negative pictures than following neutrally valanced images. Following the intervention, participants in the mindfulness group showed a significant reduction in the emotion interference effect when compared to controls. Although this reduction may reflect top-down attentional control, reductions in emotion interference were correlated with reductions in skin conductance responses to the pictures, suggesting that after 7 weeks of practice, participants rapidly processed negative images in way that did not lead to autonomic reactivity and may have obviated the need for more effortful, top-down attentional control. Indeed, these findings are consistent with a core tenet of mindfulness practice, namely that one should notice negative emotions and let them pass by without reacting to them—a gentle interruption.

Emotion regulation and related PFC-amygdala activation shows a paradoxical pattern similar to that seen in ACC activation among practiced meditators. That is, highly experienced meditators show a pattern of *increased* bottom-up processing of negative stimuli and *decreased* top-down control. Hölzel et al. (2011) suggests that it is possible that sufficient expertise in mindfulness changes the meditators' approach to emotional regulation. Whereas beginners at mindfulness rely on top-down inhibition and control of reactions to negative stimuli, practiced meditators are more likely to accept their experience as is and instead observe their emotions as momentary experiences that will pass if left alone.

Neuroscientific evidence drawn from practiced adult mindfulness practitioners as well as amateur meditators supports the suggestion that mindfulness meditation can facilitate top-down attentional control, perhaps in part by reducing interference from more bottom-up processes. Individuals with higher levels of trait mindfulness have been found to show increased activation in PFC (vmPFC, mPFC, vlPFC) along with reduced amygdala activity, as well as stronger pathways between the PFC and amygdala (Creswell, Way, Eisenberger, & Lieberman, 2007). The way mindfulness practice may operate along these pathways is reflected in differential activation in specific brain regions in mindfulness groups and matched control groups. Following 6-week (Allen et al., 2012) or 8-week (Farb et al., 2007) mindfulness interventions, adult participants' dorsolateral PFC, a region strongly associated with EF skills, showed increased activation when compared to an active control group. Further evidence suggests a difference between participants in a traditional 8-week MBSR course and those who attended a 1-month long intensive mindfulness retreat; participants in the MBSR course showed improved ability to orient attention and participants who attended the retreat showed improved receptive attention skills (Jha, Krompinger, & Baime, 2007).

By changing the relationship a student has with their emotions and "turning down the heat" that may interfere with their EF skills, mindfulness may help students to use their EF skills to process academic material and navigate complex social environments of the classroom. Given the neuroscientific evidence, the success of a mindfulness intervention depends on the repeated and supported recruitment of attention skills, the strengthening of neural pathways between the PFC and amygdala involved in emotion regulation, and a gradual shift from more reactive to more reflective responding. Despite the promising findings coming from neuroscience, there remains a need for more rigorous, and controlled studies on the neural correlates of mindfulness meditation, especially in children (see Tang et al., 2015, for a review).

Conceptualizing Mindfulness in Relation to EF Skills

According to one model of self-regulation and its development, the Iterative Reprocessing (IR) model (e.g., Cunningham & Zelazo, 2007; Zelazo, 2015), deliberate self-regulation is the product of a dynamic interaction between more bottom-up (reactive) influences and more top-down (reflective) influences. Top-down influences on self-regulation are made possible by reflection and EF skills. Reflection is the deliberate, sustained consideration (and reconsideration) of something in the context of goal-directed problem solving. With reflection, more details are perceived and integrated into one's representation of one's experience. For example, if a person is experiencing a particular stimulus (e.g., a red rabbit) in the relative absence of reflection, they may only notice a single salient feature, such as its kind. Upon further reflection, however, other aspects of the stimulus, such as the color and the other categories to which it belongs (e.g., pet, animal, etc.), may become integrated into the person's conscious construal.

Reflection provides a necessary foundation for EF skills (cognitive flexibility, working memory, inhibitory control, and hot EF) all of which depend on, and indeed involve, some degree of reflection. In terms of the Iterative Reprocessing model, mindfulness involves sustained reflection on the current object of attention and the current context, and yields a sustained state of purposeful attention or absorption that differs from both the fragmented automaticity associated with multitasking (e.g., Ophir, Nass, & Wagner, 2009), and the mind-wandering that occurs when one's attention is captured by thoughts about the future (e.g., errands to be completed) or the past (e.g., ruminating over an interpersonal conflict; see Smallwood & Schooler, 2006). Conceptualizing mindfulness in terms of the IR model yields predictions regarding the effects of mindfulness meditation on behavior (e.g., increased attentional control) and neural function (e.g., increasingly elaborated hierarchies of activation in prefrontal cortical regions).

From this perspective, mindfulness can be understood to be largely isomorphic with sustained reflection, albeit in a particular context and with a particular attitude. That is, mindfulness as generally practiced corresponds to nonjudgemental reflection in the context of being, as opposed to doing. As Kabat-Zinn (2013) puts it:

> Learning how to stop all your doing and shift over to a "being" mode, learning how to make time for yourself, how to slow down and nurture calmness and self-acceptance in yourself, learning how to observe what your own mind is up to from moment to moment, how to watch your thoughts and how to let go of them without getting so caught up in them and driven by them, how to make room for new ways of seeing old problems and for perceiving the interconnectedness of things, these are some of the lessons of mindfulness.
>
> (p. 20)

Mindfulness may also be practiced in the context of doing, however. Mindful doing involves purposeful reflection on an external situation, including the achievement of a goal, and it is in the context of goal-directed problem solving that mindfulness is most closely aligned with reflection and EF.

Whether in the context of being (e.g., open meditation) or doing (e.g., focused awareness and goal-directed problem solving), mindfulness both supports and depends on EF skills. Consider the example of mindful breathing. The intention to be mindful of breathing must be kept in mind (working memory) and distractions avoided (inhibitory control), and attention will need to be flexibly redirected back to breathing when mind wandering (inevitably) occurs (cognitive flexibility). Improvements in EF, especially the hot EF skills required for controlling attention in emotionally charged situations, may mediate observed mindfulness-induced reductions in stress, social anxiety, depression, and rumination (e.g., Goldin & Gross, 2010). In addition, however, practicing being nonjudgmental may promote calmness and wellbeing, as may focusing on the present moment (e.g., instead of ruminating over a recollected source of anxiety; Kabat-Zinn, 2003). While there are situations in which bottom-up responses are more appropriate than top-down responses (e.g., when a rapid response to a bear in the woods or a snake in the grass is required), one goal of mindfulness meditation is to reduce interference from emotional intrusions. As described earlier, in a study where adult participants were presented with the Emotional Interference task after completing either a 7-week mindfulness training course, 7-week relaxation meditation course, or a wait-list control period, those who practiced mindfulness meditation and relaxation meditation showed attenuated emotional responses as measured by skin conductance responses but only the mindfulness meditation group showed an elimination of the emotional interference effect (Ortner et al., 2007). These findings suggest that mindfulness practice (even after a relatively short period of time) helped participants prevent emotional reactivity from interfering with their performance on a cognitive task.

Two approaches to mindfulness are reviewed in the remainder of this chapter. The first involves the use of mindfulness practices with children, and the second involves the practice of mindfulness by teachers. For each approach, we examine the extent to which mindfulness operates along two main pathways for improving EF skills: the direct practice of reflection (a top-down influence on EF) and the reduction of bottom-up, reactive influences on behavior. As noted, mindfulness practice: (1) encourages an open, nonjudgmental attitude, (2) may reduce anxiety via a focus on the present, and (3) involve activities (such as deep breathing) that directly affect biological markers of stress and anxiety. Moreover, by coordinating the focus of attention in an open way upon present experience, mindfulness may allow for the kind of subjective experience associated with growth and *flow*.

Mindfulness Practices for Use With Children

In adults, mindfulness practices are well illustrated by the activities involved in Mindfulness Based Stress Reduction (MBSR) training (Kabat-Zinn, 1982, 2003). The MBSR program has been widely adopted in clinical settings as a supplemental treatment for a variety of disorders, from chronic pain and cancer to anxiety and depression, and evidence indicates clearly that it is effective. In the typical MBSR program, 8 weeks of group lessons are supplemented by individual practice at home. Mindfulness activities include body scans (i.e., sequentially attending to each part of one's body, from the tip of one's toes to the top of one's head) and breath awareness activities (i.e., noticing the sensations in one's nose, throat, and chest as one breathes). Mindfulness is practiced during sitting meditations as well as during a variety of other activities (e.g., standing, walking, or eating) to encourage the transfer of trained skills to new contexts and the integration of mindfulness into daily life. During MBSR training, individuals are instructed to focus their attention on their moment-to-moment experiences (e.g., noticing the many sensations associated with breathing), and are told that if their attention wanders (e.g., ruminating over an interpersonal conflict), then they should bring it back to the current moment. In this way, one's subjective experiences may be noticed as they occur without triggering an automatic sequence of emotional reactions or evaluations (Grossman, Niemann, Schmidt, & Walach, 2004; Kabat-Zinn, 1982).

Standard adult exercises have been adapted for use with children and adolescents to create developmentally appropriate ways to train the core aspects of mindfulness: the nonjudgmental noticing of one's moment to moment experiences, the monitoring of attention and the redirection of attention when it has wandered, and the nonreactive observation of one's thoughts and feelings. As with adults, mindfulness training with children is typically implemented in small group sessions that include a variety of activities, such as body scans, breathing exercises, and sitting meditations. Small groups of 5–10 children are led through exercises during daily or weekly sessions lasting about 20 minutes for younger (e.g., preschool age) children and longer for older children and adolescents. Each session often involves a series of shorter (e.g., 2 minutes, for the youngest children) goal-directed activities. Having children intentionally attend to their eating, breathing or walking helps transform previously automatic processes into goal-directed actions, providing children with opportunities to engage in goal-directed top-down control of attention. For example, in the MindUP mindfulness curriculum (Hawn Foundation, 2011), children in preschool through 2nd grade will listen to a complicated musical piece that involves many different instrumental parts; after listening to the song once, they split up into small groups and practice listening to a specific instrument (e.g., violin or trumpet). When the groups hear their musical instrument they then engage in a special movement and when the sound disappears they stand still. This goal-directed active listening engages children's mindful awareness to pick out a specific signal within the noise.

Activities may also be illustrated through the use of narratives and/or concrete metaphors. For example, children may be told that thoughts pass through the mind like floats pass by in a parade, and that some of the floats (thoughts) may grab their attention more than others. They are told that just like if they were at a parade, they wouldn't jump onto a float, and instead they can simply observe their thoughts as they occur (Saltzman & Goldin, 2008). Or, children may be asked to fill in an outline figure of their body with emotions they were feeling at the moment. By using abstract drawings and by the creative use of colors, students were able to identify and label their emotions (e.g., Zelazo et al., 2018). Both of these examples demonstrate how mindfulness training can facilitate the noticing and labeling of thoughts, emotions, and feelings. Research with children has shown that labeling relevant features of an object within a task facilitates better top-down regulation of behavior (see Doebel & Zelazo, 2013; Zelazo, 2004). By labeling emotions, thoughts, and feelings during mindful practice children are taught to recognize them and start to approach them nonjudgmentally. In a similar way, the noticing and deliberate attention to emotions and stressors can help reduce their bottom-up influence over goal-directed behavior.

To date, most research on mindfulness training with children has examined interventions that engage children directly, leading them in activities designed to practice the skill of attending mindfully. Often these occur as "pull out" interventions where students are taken out of the classroom for directed practice in specific mindfulness-related activities. In addition, however, some programs, such as MindUP, can be integrated into existing classrooms and are delivered to children by trained teachers.

Challenges in evaluating research on mindfulness in education include inconsistency in program fidelity, uncertainty regarding which outcomes to measure, and a lack of a causal theoretical framework for understanding what it means to engage in mindful activities. These concerns are reflected in the general field of mindfulness research (Davidson & Kaszniak, 2015). For these reasons we have narrowed our discussion to reflect the effects of high-fidelity, research informed practices on theoretically motivated outcome measures related to self-regulation. Specifically, we focus on the effects of mindfulness on children's EF skills and emotional regulation from the perspective of developmental neuroscience and the Iterative Reprocessing model.

Examples of Mindfulness Interventions for Children

An example of a successful mindfulness curriculum for young children is the 12-week mindfulness-based Kindness Curriculum (KC; Flook et al., 2015). The KC curriculum, designed for children ages 4–5 years old, was delivered by trained mindfulness instructors who visited children's classrooms twice a week for 20–30 minutes per week for 12 weeks. The curriculum emphasizes empathy, gratitude, emotion regulation, attention, and mindfulness. Results from an evaluation of this intervention with 99 children aged 4.6 years indicate higher marks on teacher-rated social competence in the group that received KC compared to the wait-list control group (preschool as usual), more generous performance on a sticker sharing task, as well as better end-of year-grades in learning, health, and social/emotional categories. Additionally, this curriculum seemed to benefit particularly those children who had lower baseline functioning prior to the intervention (both social competence and executive function). This pattern of results, which demonstrates that those who start lower see higher gains, is consistent with other EF interventions (Diamond & Lee, 2011), suggesting that interventions such as KC might be preventing a negative spiral of behavior leading to negative cascades of effects that follow students throughout their academic careers. Improving SEL and EF skills might have indirect positive effects on how children interact within their classroom.

The improvements on teacher-rated social competence might also be indicative of improved teacher-student relationships. When looking at academic performance and achievement and the benefits of mindfulness in schools it is important to consider co-relations among teachers, students, and classrooms. It is possible that by improving the SEL and EF skills of the bottom quartile of the class through the KC curriculum, this would lead to improvements on measures of classroom general atmosphere and learning environment. At present, however, there is a paucity of empirical research that examines the effects of mindfulness at the level of the classroom.

A recent randomized study (Zelazo et al., 2018) examined the impact of a Mindfulness + Reflection intervention. This intervention combined traditional mindfulness training (e.g., belly breathing, body scan), which was expected to help children calm down, regulate stress, become aware of moment-to-moment experience, and sustain attention; and reflection training in the context of EF games, which should also help children recognize when they need to "go off autopilot" and instead act deliberately, relying on their EF skills to achieve their goals.

The combined intervention was delivered by trained teachers during 30 daily small-group sessions over 6 weeks in preschool classrooms (average age = 4.8 years). Reflection training occurred in the context of 3 EF-challenging games presented along with reflection protocols designed to encourage explicit consideration of children's own thoughts, emotions, and behavioral tendencies in the context of goal-directed problem solving. For each EF game, reflection protocols were designed to help teachers to scaffold children's performance on the game, adjusting the degree of challenge to maintain engagement, and to encourage children to notice sources of difficulty in the game and acquire strategies for pausing, stepping back, and acting deliberately. A well-established pre-literacy curriculum served as an active control condition, and business as usual (BAU) served as a passive control. All groups showed improvement in EF skills (measured behaviorally) over the 5-month span of the study, which was expected because the preschool period is marked by particularly rapid EF development (Carlson et al., 2013). However, planned contrasts showed that the Mindfulness + Reflection group (only) significantly outperformed the BAU group, with the differences most pronounced at follow-up. This effect was most clearly seen when examining the *rank order* of participants at each time point as a function of group assignment. Children's ranks went up markedly over time for the Mindfulness + Reflection group, whereas they declined for the BAU group and remained stable for the Literacy group.

One key finding that warrants further discussion is the delayed post-test effect finding. These types of delayed effects suggest that some degree of consolidation or continued learning may take place after the intervention is over. Perhaps children benefit from practicing newly learned skills in new situations, increasing the likelihood that these skills will generalize. It is important to note, however, that no studies to date have actually measured the time course of the effects of mindfulness practice using a microgenetic approach and observing children's post-intervention activities (e.g., in the classroom), although the behavioral findings discussed here are consistent with this proposed pattern of change.

Increasing top-down control and strengthening EF skills is only part of the benefits of mindfulness interventions. Studies with adults (e.g., Ortner et al., 2007) suggest that mindfulness meditation can help minimize emotional interference during goal-directed action and improve emotion regulation. For example, adults practiced in mindfulness are more likely to activate brain regions associated with body sensation than regions associated with emotional reactivity (Farb et al., 2007). Body sensation activities and emotion recognition activities in child-focused programs attempt to reframe how emotions are reflected upon and viewed, preventing them from automatically (without awareness) hijacking self-regulation. Although research on the effects of mindfulness on children's emotional regulation are limited, the existing findings are promising. One randomized control study looked at neural correlates of mindfulness or EF training as well as a business as usual (BAU) control group. In this study, 12 hours of mindfulness training for a sample of internationally adopted children was associated with lower post-training anxiety as well as more muted neural responses to experiencing errors (as measured by error-related negativity, ERN) (Esposito, 2015).

In addition to pull-out programs like those studied by Flook et al. (2015) and Zelazo et al. (2018), research has examined more fully integrated curricula like the MindUp Curriculum (Hawn Foundation, 2011). The MindUP curriculum is a comprehensive 15-lesson curriculum with different activities and programs for children ranging from preschool through 8th grade. MindUP draws on findings from contemplative neuroscience as well as research on social and emotional learning (SEL skills). Students learn about their brain, how their brain and emotions influence their behaviors and how to leverage this knowledge to regulate behavior and learn academic material. Critically, MindUP integrates lessons and mindful practices throughout the day for the duration of the year. Across multiple evaluations of MindUP (e.g., Schonert-Reichl & Lawlor, 2010; Schonert-Reichl et al., 2015) researchers found that the curriculum improved student's EF skills and physiological stress reactivity, improved self-reported empathy, emotional control and mindfulness, and resulted in lower self-reported symptoms of depression and increased peer acceptance. The MindUP curriculum demonstrates how an integrated curriculum informed by self-regulation and mindfulness research can have positive effects on students above and beyond business as usual curricula.

Some of the limitations of using a MindUP-style approach to promoting mindfulness are limitations common to other curricula-overhaul interventions like Tools of the Mind (Bodrova & Leong, 2017). These limitations include maintaining teacher fidelity of implementation. When implementing these types of curricula in a controlled environment for a study, fidelity can be measured and controlled for. However, as programs come to scale, they may clash with obstacles in different populations and environments. While it is important to adapt interventions to account for cultural and other differences between groups, it is also important to not deviate too much from what is causing an intervention to work. That being said, more research is needed to distill the "core components" of mindfulness interventions, without which the intervention would fail.

Addressing mindfulness directly, whether in an 8-week pull-out course or as part of an integrated curriculum, may not be appropriate for all settings and populations. One recent intervention studied in our lab, called Ready 4 Routines and designed for families with children aged 3 to 5 years old, integrates lessons and practices from successful EF and mindfulness interventions without explicitly using mindful practices as its core. One mindfulness-informed practice used by Ready 4 Routines is found in the PEER(E) "mantra," a set of guiding principles which structure activities for parents and children: Pause, Engage, Encourage, Reflect and (Extend). The mantra guides parents through a set of processes for supportive engagement with their children. First, a parent must pause, set aside what they were doing previously, take a few breaths, and dedicate their attention to their child. Next, parents engage fully with their child, interacting with them in an autonomy-supportive way in a given game or activity. Throughout the activity, parents encourage their children and guide them through difficult parts of the activity. Once the activity is over, parents and children sit down and reflect upon what they just did and discuss what went well and what could have gone better. Finally, parents are encouraged to extend the lesson of the activity and find new contexts and environments to practice this activity in. Most notably, mindfulness-informed practice comes in during the Pause and Reflect steps where parents are taught how to slow down, take deep breaths and devote their attention to their children and the activity they are about to partake in. Preliminary research on the Ready 4 Routines intervention suggests improvements in children's executive function skills when compared to a control group, as well as a decrease in parenting-related stress. These findings suggest that lessons from mindfulness practice can be applied in non-traditional settings, such as planning daily family routines and during parent-child interactions.

In addition to using mindfulness as a means to improve top-down attention regulation, mindfulness practice can be taught as a way of reframing and lessening the impact of negative emotions and environmental stressors. The *.b* mindfulness program (Mindfulness in Schools Program) is a classroom-based mindfulness curriculum designed for adolescents aged 11–18 years (with a childhood version, *Paws* b for children aged 7–11 years). Research on this 9-lesson intervention suggests that self-reported student wellbeing, stress, and depressive symptoms improved when compared to a control group (Kuyken et al., 2013). However, additional research on the program suggests that positive effects of the intervention might be limited to students who maintain a consistent at-home practice (Huppert & Johnson, 2010). Research into the efficacy of the .b curriculum highlights potential challenges facing at-school mindfulness interventions. A randomized control trial evaluation of the .b curriculum found no significant differences on self-reported anxiety/depression and wellbeing compared to a matched control group (Johnson, Burke, Brinkman, & Wade, 2017). Researchers speculate these findings are due to the test school's significant deviance from the original curriculum, as well as untested practices and increased parental supervision/involvement. Lessons from the .b curriculum advise researchers and administrators who implement mindfulness curricula to be cognizant of how slight changes or alterations to a program may cause unpredictable effects (or lack thereof).

Existing literature suggests that mindfulness-based interventions ranging from short-term pull-out interventions to fully integrated curricula help to promote EF skill and other self-regulation abilities (Zelazo et al., 2018; Flook et al., 2015; Schonert-Reichl et al., 2015). Furthermore, there are promising avenues of research that suggest that mindfulness can help with emotion regulation strategies and even change how participants perceive emotional stimuli (Ortner et al., 2007). Together, these findings help reinforce the importance of reflection in developing self-regulation skills, consistent with the IR model.

Consistent with a developmental systems approach, however, it is important to look beyond just how mindfulness can be used by students to improve academic outcomes and to look to the front of the classroom and consider how mindfulness can be used with teachers. In the next section we will focus on how mindfulness practice has been shown to reduce stress in teachers, improve instruction and classroom quality, and affect learning outcomes for students.

Classroom-level, Teacher-focused Mindfulness Interventions

Many mindfulness programs for schools rely upon outside providers or push-in specialists to deliver content to students, while others provide some training for classroom teachers in order to develop their skills to present curricula to students. Unaddressed in these approaches is the role of the educator in the classroom, in particular the role that the educator plays in creating a safe and supportive learning environment for students. Across the broad spectrum of education research, teachers' attitudes towards, relationships with, and responsiveness to students, are cited as significant factors in student achievement. Despite widespread support within education scholarship, however, the ability of teachers to navigate the complexities of their classrooms and build effective relationships with students is compromised by alarmingly high levels of attrition, job stress, and disengagement. Emerging research suggests that focusing on the teacher through mindfulness-based interventions may have the twin effects of promoting student learning and increasing teacher wellbeing.

Teachers may support child-directed mindfulness activities, for example, commenting on aspects of the environment in a non-evaluative way, or encouraging children to attend more deeply to their experiences, by asking them open-ended questions. They may transform daily experiences into opportunities to promote mindful awareness by probing children to notice what is happening in the current moment in a purposeful and nonreactive way. For example, during meals, children might be challenged to reflect on the food they are eating: Is it hot or cold? Is it hard or soft? Children might also be asked to think about where the food came from and all of the people and events that happened to get that food to their plate: How did it get from the farm to the table? During a sad moment, children might be asked: Where do you feel sad: in your eyes, in your throat, in your chest? Does your sad feeling have a texture? Is it rough or smooth? Light or heavy?

Most likely, however, the success of teachers in supporting children's mindfulness and EF skills depends on teachers' own mindfulness. Illustrating the focus on teachers, Roeser, Skinner, Beers, and Jennings (2012) hypothesized that mindfulness-based interventions may develop teachers' "habits of mind," improving their resiliency and emotional regulation, which in turn would lead to increased wellbeing and reductions in burnout and attrition:

> Why are habits of mind necessary for effective teaching? Human service occupations like teaching, because of their social nature, involve high levels of uncertainty, emotion and attention to others, and thus require habits of mind associated with mental flexibility, emotion regulation, and relationship skills (Helsing, 2007; Shutz & Zembylas, 2009; Zapf, 2002) . . . teachers' work lives are saturated with interactions with students, colleagues, administrators, and parents—interactions that require significant attentional and emotional resources and their effective regulation through habits of mind.
>
> (p. 168)

These improvements to the habits of mind then lead to what the authors deem as "virtuous cycles" such as improved teacher-student relationships, prosocial behaviors, classroom climate and student engagement, potentially effecting positive student outcomes such as increased motivation, belonging, and engagement (see Figure 12.1). The student outcomes are corroborated by research in classroom learning environments (e.g., Raver et al., 2011).

The flow from habits of mind to improved student outcomes, while hypothetical at this stage in the research, is echoed by other scholars who approach the potential connections among teacher reflection and self-care (Shapiro, Rechtschaffen, & de Sousa, 2016), stress and self-efficacy (Flook, Goldberg, Pinger, Bonus, & Davidson, 2013), and coping and resiliency (Skinner & Beers, 2016).

Research on the effects of mindfulness-based interventions on teachers is relatively new, and there is currently limited evidence of a relation between teachers' mindfulness and student outcomes. Scholarship at this point has focused primarily on teacher wellbeing rather than the related effects on student outcomes or teacher practices (Meiklejohn et al., 2012). Recent metaanalyses of mindfulness-based interventions with educators suggest that these interventions show promise for promoting teachers' wellbeing (Emerson et al., 2017; Hwang, Bartlett, Greben, & Hand, 2017; Lomas et al., 2017). Similar

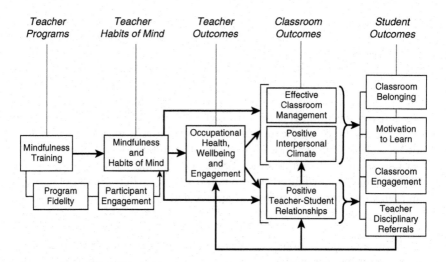

Figure 12.1 A Conceptual Framework for how Mindfulness Training for Teachers Translates Into Outcomes for Teachers, Classrooms, and Students.

Source: From Roeser et al. (2012).

to the limitations in the research on youth described in this chapter, however, studies on educators show the need for increased rigor in research design, diversity of measures utilized to assess wellbeing outcomes of interventions (especially in regards to the use of self-report and mental health measures), greater attention to fidelity reporting, clarity in conceptualization of mindfulness and the intervention content, and additional measures to evaluate the potential outcomes of interventions in classrooms.

Summary and Recommendations for Future Research

The research to date suggests that mindfulness practices can be effective in promoting EF skills and reducing stress in children (Klingbeil et al., 2017; Zenner, Herrnleben-Kurz, & Walach, 2014; Zoogman, Goldberg, Hoyt, & Miller, 2015). Mindfulness also shows promise for promoting the reported wellbeing of educators (Emerson et al., 2017; Hwang et al., 2017; Lomas et al., 2017), which may lead to improved student outcomes. Clearly, however, more rigorous research is needed to demonstrate the link between teacher mindfulness and student outcomes as well as the efficacy of student-focused mindfulness interventions. We conclude with recommendations for future research and a summary of implications for learning and education.

Research on mindfulness is encouraging, but many studies have small sample sizes and inadequate controls. Research is needed that involves random assignment of both trainers and trainees, active control conditions, efforts to equate both student and teacher expectancy effects, and validated behavioral (vs. self- or other-report) measures administered by researchers who are blind to experimental condition. Future research should also investigate translational issues concerning the feasibility of integrating mindfulness training activities into routine school-day activities, move toward standardized interventions, and assess the degree of fidelity and dosage (intervention duration, intensity, and frequency) that is required for mindfulness training to be effective, the influence of classroom and school factors on efficacy, and the time course and duration of any observed effects. Such research has the potential not only to provide important knowledge that may be used in applied settings, but also to provide insight into the causal mechanisms underlying major age-related changes in reflection and EF.

What Has Neuroscience Added to Our Understanding Over and Above Psychology?

Neuroscience adds to our understanding by identifying the mechanisms underlying behavioral changes following mindfulness practice, including the basis of its impact on EF skills, and by pointing toward potential developmental windows of opportunity. The principles of neural plasticity, reciprocal interactions between more top-down (e.g., prefrontal) and more bottom-up (e.g., limbic) influences, and sensitive periods inform efforts to design and optimize interventions to promote the development of EF. While there has been a paucity of neuroimaging research on the effects of mindfulness in children and adolescents to date, the adult literature points to the enhancement of self-regulatory attentional networks as the main mechanism of change following mindfulness practice. This improves top-down attentional control, perhaps in part by reducing interference from more bottom-up processes, particularly with respect to emotion regulation. Research in developmental neuroscience indicates that there are periods of relatively high plasticity when particular parts of the brain and their corresponding functions are especially susceptible to environmental influences. For EF skills, there is a rapid transformation during early childhood from 2 to 6 years of age, so the preschool period may be a window of opportunity for the cultivation of EF skills through techniques such as mindfulness. There is also considerable reorganization of prefrontal systems during the transition to adolescence, suggesting another possible window of opportunity. However, despite the promising findings coming from neuroscience, there remains a need for more rigorous, and controlled studies on the neural correlates of mindfulness meditation, especially in children.

What Are the Concrete Implications of Research and Opportunities for Translation?

Here we consider the implications of research and opportunities of mindfulness. Given the evidence reviewed in this chapter we can recommend several approaches to practicing mindfulness. As reviewed, there are both student-focused and teacher-focused approaches to mindfulness. The student-focused approach can be undertaken through either entire curriculum overhauls (like the MindUP curriculum) or by pull-out mindfulness sessions. Additionally, families may choose to practice mindfulness with their children at home, either through self-guided approaches or commercially available programs.

Alternatively, there are programs that integrate reflective practices and other aspects of mindfulness practice into their repertoire. An intervention such as the Ready4Routines intervention prompts families to pause before starting activities, then reflect on those activities after they're done, and encourages parents and children to engage in breathing-focused activities. Other interventions such as Tools of the Mind also prompt teacher and students to take time to plan and reflect and to allow for a more reflective mindset.

The need for improved research into mindfulness practice and its effects on cognitive functioning remains ever-present. Despite a sharp increase in mindfulness research in the past decade a pattern of methodological issues persists and remains unaddressed by researchers (see Davidson & Kaszniak, 2015, for review). These opportunities for future research rest on a few key principles. The first is that researchers need to take care in specifying what kind of mindfulness practice they are undertaking. As reviewed in this chapter there is a great range of mindfulness-based and mindfulness-informed activities which are employed in the education realm. By documenting the specific mindfulness activities, curricula, and practices being investigated, future researchers can support subsequent replication. The second principle guiding future research is the importance of properly controlled experiments. The possibility of falling into a Hawthorne effect[2] cycle is great and therefore researchers should seek out control conditions that go beyond a business-as-usual (BAU) condition and instead introduce an active but theoretically distinct control condition. For example, the literacy boosting control condition in Zelazo et al. (2018) operates along an orthogonal pathway to the mindfulness + reflection condition, thereby allowing a more robust analysis of existing intervention effects that controls for numerous non-specific factors such as engagement in intentional activities. Finally, the third principle researchers should consider when studying the effects of mindfulness in education is to consider the dynamic, and bidirectional interactions among students, classroom environments, and teachers, and to study these using multiple levels of analysis. As reviewed in this chapter, teachers and students occupy unique roles within the classroom, and by recognizing the demands placed on these roles, one can better understand how and *why* mindfulness may lead to desirable education outcomes.

Further Resources

For more information and additional resources please consider the following:

1. Broderick, P. C., & Frank, J. L. (2014). Learning to BREATHE: An intervention to foster mindfulness in adolescence. *New Directions for Student Leadership, 2014*(142), 31–44.

Table 12.1 List of Available Mindfulness Programs

Program name	Description	Supporting scholarship
Mindful Schools	Short (6-week) online program offerings for educators in developing personal mindfulness practice and bringing mindfulness activities to children. Yearlong teacher certification program offered which combines online cohort learning with an in-person retreat.	Black, D. S., & Fernando, R. (2014). Mindfulness training and classroom behavior among lower-income and ethnic minority elementary school children. *Journal of Child and Family Studies, 23*(7), 1242–1246. Liehr, P., & Diaz, N. (2010). A pilot study examining the effect of mindfulness on depression and anxiety for minority children. *Archives of Psychiatric Nursing.* Galla, B. M. (2016). Within-person changes in mindfulness and self-compassion predict enhanced emotional well-being in healthy, but stressed adolescents. *Journal of Adolescence, 49,* 204–217.
Inward Bound Mindfulness Education (iBme)	Retreat based model that teaches mindfulness through guided practices, reflection, and games and experiential learning activities. Programs are also available for parents, caregivers, and adults in support roles for youth. iBme also offers teacher training for K-12 and higher education instructors interested in bringing mindfulness practices to youth.	
MindUp	15-lesson curriculum designed for grades K-8 with a focus on social-emotional learning (SEL). The program provides support for teachers to integrate into their teaching. The program also provides materials and trained facilitators to help schools implement the program across buildings and districts. The program also offers parent tips to adapt the curriculum for home use.	Maloney, J. E, Lawlor, M. S., Schonert-Reichl, K. A., & Whitehead, J. (2016). A mindfulness-based social and emotional learning curriculum for school-aged children: The MindUP program. In *Handbook of mindfulness in education* (pp. 313–334). New York, NY: Springer. Schonert-Reichl, K. A., Oberle, E., Lawlor, M. S., Abbott, D., Thomson, K., Oberlander, T. F., & Diamond, A. (2015). Enhancing cognitive and social—emotional development through a simple-to-administer mindfulness-based school program for elementary school children: A randomized controlled trial. *Developmental Psychology, 51*(1), 52.

(Continued)

Table 12.1 (Continued)

Program name	Description	Supporting scholarship
Calm Classroom	3-hour online, on-site, and 1-day train the trainer program for educators to deliver classroom activities to their students. One of only a few programs offered in languages other than English.	Moreno, A. J. (2017). A Theoretically and Ethically grounded approach to mindfulness practices in the primary grades. *Childhood Education*, 93(2), 100–108.
Learning to BREATHE	Adolescent-focused program that integrates SEL concepts into mindfulness learning activities. The program emphasizes stress reduction and developing emotional regulation, compassion, and acceptance to navigate the challenges of adolescence. The program offers a 3-day training to prepare educators to deliver the program.	Broderick, P. C., & Frank, J. L. (2014). Learning to BREATHE: An intervention to foster mindfulness in adolescence. *New Directions for Youth Development*, 2014(142), 31–44. Metz, S. M, Frank, J. L., Reibel, D., Cantrell, T, Sanders, R., & Broderick, P. C. (2013). The effectiveness of the learning to BREATHE program on adolescent emotion regulation. *Research in Human Development*, 10(3), 252–272.
Inner Kids Program	Free online program with supporting videos, guided mindfulness practices, and excerpts from texts. Materials are provided for children and guiding adults. Program focuses on social-emotional skills through an exploration of themes such as: appreciation, acceptance, clarity, compassion, joy, and interdependence. At the time of this writing, information regarding training was not available.	Flook, L., Smalley, S.L., Kitil, M.J., Galla, B.M., Kaiser-Greenland, S., Locke, J., Ishijima, E. & Kasari, C. (2010). Effects of mindful awareness practices on executive functions in elementary school children. *Journal of Applied School Psychology*, 26(1), 70–95.
Soles of the Feet	Pull-out intervention targeting aggressive behaviors that consists of 5 sessions lasting 20–30 minutes each. Instruction in practices to identify emotions and de-escalate situations are initially taught to students and then followed by student rehearsal, planning, and gradual application.	Singh N., Wahler R., Adkins A., & Myers R. (2003). Soles of the Feet: A mindfulness-based self-control intervention for aggression by an individual with mild mental retardation and mental illness. *Research in Developmental Disabilities*, 24(3), 158–169. Felver, J.C., Frank, J.L. & McEachern, A.D. (2014). *Mindfulness*, 5(5), 589–597.

Move-Into-Learning	Pull-out elementary school program taught by trained faculty from the Ohio State University's College of Medicine. Includes guided meditations and yoga taught once per week for 8 weeks. Program focuses on stress reduction and social skills.	Klatt, M., Harpster, K., Browne, E., White, S., & Case-Smith, J. (2013). Feasibility and preliminary outcomes for move-into-learning: An arts-based mindfulness classroom intervention. *The Journal of Positive Psychology*, 8(3), 233–241.
Mindfulness in Schools Project (MiSP)	Organization offers both elementary (Paws b) and secondary programs (.b). The elementary program is comprised of six units each delivered in either a one-hour or two half-hour blocks. The secondary program is divided into nine 40 to 60-minute lessons. Schools can introduce staff to MiSP programs through on-site training provided by MiSP trainers or through online coursework. Staff can take 3–4-day trainings to teach MiSP curriculum to students. Training offered for on-site program lead development.	Kuyken, W., Weare, K., Ukoumunne, O.C., Vicary, R., Motton, N., Burnett, R., Cullen, C., Hennelly, S. & Huppert, F (2013). Effectiveness of the Mindfulness in schools programme: Non-randomised controlled feasibility study. *The British Journal of Psychiatry*, 203(2),126–131. Vickery, C. E., & Dorjee, D. (2016). Mindfulness training in primary schools decreases negative affect and increases meta-cognition in children. *Frontiers in Psychology*, 6, 2025.

2. Center on the Developing Child. Retrieved from https://developingchild.harvard.edu/

Center for Healthy Minds at the University of Wisconsin—Madison. Retrieved from https://centerhealthyminds.org/

3. Executive function in education: From theory to practice. Retrieved from www.guilford.com/books/Executive-Function-in-Education/Lynn-Meltzer/9781462534531

4. Hanh, T. N., & Weare, K. (2017). *Happy teachers change the world: A guide for cultivating mindfulness in education.* Berkeley, CA: Parallax Press.

5. Jennings, P. A. (2015). *Mindfulness for teachers: Simple skills for peace and productivity in the classroom (The Norton series on the social neuroscience of education).* New York: W.W. Norton & Co.

6. MindUP school curriculum. Retrieved from https://mindup.org/

7. Meiklejohn, J., Phillips, C., Freedman, M. L., Griffin, M. L., Biegel, G., Roach, A., . . . Isberg, R. (2012). Integrating mindfulness training into K-12 education: Fostering the resilience of teachers and students. *Mindfulness*, 3(4), 291–307.

8. Ready 4 Routines. Retrieved from https://developingchild.harvard.edu/innovation-application/innovation-in-action/ready4routines/

9. Reflection Sciences. Retrieved from https://reflectionsciences.com/

10. Roeser, R. W., Skinner, E., Beers, J., & Jennings, P. A. (2012). Mindfulness training and teachers' professional development: An emerging area of research and practice. *Child Development Perspectives*, 6(2), 167–173.

11. Saltzman, A. (2014). *A still quiet place: A mindfulness program for teaching children and adolescents to ease stress and difficult emotions.* Oakland, CA: New Harbinger Publications.

12. Tools of the Mind. Retrieved from https://toolsofthemind.org/

13. Schonert-Reichl, K. A., & Roeser, R. W. (Eds.). (2016). *Handbook of mindfulness in education: Integrating theory and research into practice.* New York: Springer.

14. University of Minnesota's Earl E Bakken center for spirituality and healing. Retrieved from www.csh.umn.edu/

Notes

1. "When an axon of cell A is near enough to excite B and repeatedly and persistently takes part in firing it, some growth process or metabolic change takes place in one or both cells such that A's efficiency, as one of the cells firing B, is increased." (Hebb, 1949, p. 62)
2. The Hawthorne effect, sometimes referred to as the observer effect, occurs when research participants behave differently when they are being observed or studied. This effect manifests itself in intervention research when the introduction of an intervention per se changes behavior.

References

Allan, N. P., Hume, L. E., Allan, D. M., Farrington, A. L., & Lonigan, C. J. (2014). Relations between inhibitory control and the development of academic skills in preschool and kindergarten: A meta-analysis. *Developmental Psychology, 50*, 2368–2379.

Allen, J. W. P., & Bickhard, M. H. (2018). Stage fright: Internal reflection as a domain general enabling constraint on the emergence of explicit thought. *Cognitive Development, 45*, 77–91.

Allen, M., Dietz, M., Blair, K. S., Van Beek, M., Rees, G., Vestergaard-Poulsen, P., . . . Roepstorff, A. (2012). Cognitive-affective neural plasticity following active-controlled mindfulness intervention. *Journal of Neuroscience, 32*, 15601–15610.

Astle, D. E., Barnes, J., Baker, K., Colclough, G., & Woolrich, M. W. (2015). Cognitive training enhances intrinsic brain connectivity in childhood. *Journal of Neuroscience, 35*(16), 6277–6283.

Badre, D., & D'Esposito, M. (2007). Functional magnetic resonance imaging evidence for a hierarchical organization of the prefrontal cortex. *Journal of Cognitive Neuroscience, 19*, 2082–2099.

Bechara, A., Damasio, A. R., Damasio, H., & Anderson, S. W. (1994). Insensitivity to future consequences following damage to human prefrontal cortex. *Cognition, 50*(1–3), 7–15.

Bengtsson, S. L., Nagy, Z., Skare, S., Forsman, L., Forssberg, H., & Ullén, F. (2005). Extensive piano practicing has regionally specific effects on white matter development. *Nature Neuroscience, 8*(9), 1148–1150. https://doi.org/10.1038/nn1516

Benson, J., Sabbagh, M., Carlson, S. M., & Zelazo, P. D. (2013). Individual differences in executive functioning predict preschoolers' improvement from theory-of-mind training. *Developmental Psychology, 49*, 1615–1627.

Biegel, G. M., Brown, K. W., Shapiro, S. L., & Schubert, C. M. (2009). Mindfulness-based stress reduction for the treatment of adolescent psychiatric outpatients: A randomized clinical trial. *Journal of Consulting and Clinical Psychology, 77*, 855–866.

Bierman, K. L., Domitrovich, C. E., Nix, R. L., Gest, S. D., Welsh, J. A., Greenberg, M. T., . . . Gill, S. (2008). Promoting academic and social-emotional school readiness: The head start REDI program. *Child Development, 79*, 1802–1817.

Bierman, K. L., & Welsh, J. A. (1997). Social relationship deficits. In E. J. Mash & G. Lief (Eds.), *Assessment of childhood disorders* (3rd ed., pp. 328–365). New York: Guilford Press.

Blair, C., Granger, D., Willoughby, M., Mills-Koonce, R., Cox, M., Greenberg, M. T., . . . The FLP Investigators. (2011). Salivary cortisol mediates effects of poverty and parenting on executive functions in early childhood. *Child Development, 82*, 1970–1984.

Bodrova, E., & Leong, D. J. (2017). Tools of the mind: A Vygotskian early childhood curriculum. In M. Fleer & B. van Oers (Eds.), *International handbook of early childhood education*. Dordrecht: Springer.

Bokura, H., Yamaguchi, S., & Kobayashi, S. (2001). Electrophysiological correlates for response inhibition in a Go/NoGo task. *Clinical Neurophysiology, 112*.

Brefczynski-Lewis, J. A., Lutz, A., Schaefer, H. S., Levinson, D. B., & Davidson, R. J. (2007). Neural correlates of attentional expertise in long-term meditation practitioners. *Proceedings of the National Academy of Sciences, 104*(27), 11483–11488. https://doi.org/10.1073/pnas.0606552104

Broderick, P. C., & Metz, S. (2009). Learning to BREATHE: A pilot trial of a mindfulness curriculum for adolescents. *Advances in School Mental Health Promotion, 2*, 35–46.

Brown, K. W., & Ryan, R. M. (2003). The benefits of being present: Mindfulness and its role in psychological well-being. *Journal of Personality and Social Psychology, 84,* 822–848.

Buodo, G., Sarlo, M., & Palomba, D. (2002). Attentional resources measured by reaction times highlight differences within pleasant and unpleasant, high arousing stimuli. *Motivation and Emotion, 26*(2), 123–138. https://doi.org/10.1023/A:1019886501965

Buss, K. A., Dennis, T. A., Brooker, R. J., & Sippel, L. M. (2011). An ERP study of conflict monitoring in 4–8 year old children: Associations with temperament. *Developmental Cognitive Neuroscience, 1,* 131–140.

Butzer, B., Ebert, M., Telles, S., & Khalsa, S. B. S. (2015). School-based yoga programs in the United States: A survey. *Advances in Mind-Body Medicine, 29*(4), 18–26.

Carlson, S. M., Zelazo, P. D., & Faja, S. (2013). Executive function. In P. D. Zelazo (Ed.), *Oxford handbook of developmental psychology* (Vol. 1, pp. 706–743). New York: Oxford University Press.

Carson, J. W., Carson, K. M., Gil, K. M., & Baucom, D. H. (2006). Mindfulness-based relationship enhancement (MBRE) in couples. In R. A. Baer (Ed.), *Mindfulness-based treatment approaches: Clinician's guide to evidence base and applications* (pp. 309–331). San Diego, CA: Elsevier Academic Press.

Chapman, H. A., Woltering, S., Lamm, C., & Lewis, M. D. (2010). Hearts and minds: Coordination of neurocognitive and cardiovascular regulation in children and adolescents. *Biological Psychology, 84,* 296–303.

Chevalier, N., & Blaye, A. (2016). Metacognitive monitoring of executive control engagement during childhood. *Child Development, 87*(4), 1264–1276.

Constantinidis, C., & Klingberg, T. (2016). The neuroscience of working memory capacity and training. *Nature Reviews Neuroscience, 17,* 438–449.

Creswell, J. D., Way, B. M., Eisenberger, N. I., & Lieberman, M. D. (2007). Neural correlates of dispositional mindfulness during affect labeling. *Psychosomatic Medicine, 69*(6), 560–565.

Cunningham, W. A., & Zelazo, P. D. (2007). Attitudes and evaluations: A social cognitive neuroscience perspective. *Trends in Cognitive Sciences, 11,* 97–104.

Davidson, R. J., & Kaszniak, A. W. (2015). Conceptual and methodological issues in research on mindfulness and meditation. *American Psychologist, 70*(7), 581.

Demetriou, A., Makris, N., Spanoudis, G., Kazi, S., Shayer, M., & Kazali, E. (2018). Mapping the dimensions of general intelligence: An integrated differential-developmental theory. *Human Development, 61,* 4–42.

Dennis, T. A., & Chen, C. C. (2007). Neurophysiological mechanisms in the emotional modulation of attention: The interplay between threat sensitivity and attentional control. *Biological Psychology, 76,* 1–10.

Diamond, A. (2013). Executive functions. *Annual Review of Psychology, 64,* 135–168.

Diamond, A., & Lee, K. (2011). Interventions shown to aid executive function development in children 4 to 12 years old. *Science, 333,* 959–964.

Doebel, S., & Zelazo, P. D. (2013). Bottom-up and top-down dynamics in young children's executive function: Labels aid 3-year-olds' performance on the Dimensional Change Card Sort. *Cognitive Development, 28*(3), 222–232. https://doi.org/10.1016/j.cogdev.2012.12.001

Elbert, T., Pantev, C., Wienbruch, C., Rockstroh, B., & Taub, E. (1995). Increased cortical representation of the fingers of the left hand in string players. *Science, 270*(5234), 305–307.

Emerson, L. M., Leyland, A., Hudson, K., Rowse, G., Hanley, P., & Hugh-Jones, S. (2017). Teaching mindfulness to teachers: A systematic review and narrative synthesis. *Mindfulness, 8*(5), 1136–1149.

Espinet, S. D., Anderson, J. E., & Zelazo, P. D. (2012). N2 amplitude as a neural marker of executive function in young children: An ERP study of children who switch versus perseverate on the dimensional change card sort. *Developmental Cognitive Neuroscience, 2*, S49–S58.

Espinet, S. D., Anderson, J. E., & Zelazo, P. D. (2013). Reflection training improves executive function in preschool children: Behavioral and neural effects. *Developmental Cognitive Neuroscience, 4*, 3–15. doi:10.1016/j.dcn.2012.11.009

Esposito, E. A. (2015). Doctoral dissertation, University of Minnesota. Retrieved from conservancy.umn.edu

Evans, G. W., & Schamberg, M. A. (2009). Childhood poverty, chronic stress, and adult working memory. *Proceedings of the National Academy of Sciences, 106*(16), 6545–6549. doi:10.1073/pnas.0811910106

Falkenstein, M., Hoormann, J., & Hohnsbein, J. (1999). ERP components in Go/NoGo tasks and their relation to inhibition. *Acta Psychologica, 101*(2–3), 267–291.

Farb, N. A., Segal, Z. V., Mayberg, H., Bean, J., McKeon, D., Fatima, Z., & Anderson, A. K. (2007). Attending to the present: Mindfulness meditation reveals distinct neural modes of self-reference. *Social Cognitive and Affective Neuroscience, 2*(4), 313–322. doi:10.1093/scan/nsm030

Faul, F., Erdfelder, E., Lang, A. G. et al. (2007). G*Power 3: A flexible statistical power analysis program for the social, behavioral, and biomedical sciences. *Behavior Research Methods, 39*, 175–191. https://doi.org/10.3758/BF03193146

Flook, L., Goldberg, S. B., Pinger, L., Bonus, K., & Davidson, R. J. (2013). Mindfulness for teachers: A pilot study to assess effects on stress, burnout, and teaching efficacy. *Mind, Brain, and Education, 7*(3), 182–195.

Flook, L., Goldberg, S. B., Pinger, L., & Davidson, R. J. (2015). Promoting prosocial behavior and self-regulatory skills in preschool children through a mindfulness-based kindness curriculum. *Developmental Psychology, 51*(1), 44–51. http://doi.org/10.1037/a0038256

Flook, L., Smalley, S. L., Kitil, M. J., Galla, B., Kaiser-Greenland, S., Locke, J., . . . Kasari, C. (2010). Effects of mindful awareness practices on executive functions in elementary school children. *Journal of Applied School Psychology, 26*(1), 70–95.

Forster, S. E., Carter, C. S., Cohen, J. D., & Cho, R. Y. (2011). Parametric manipulation of the conflict signal control-state adaptation. *Journal of Cognitive Neuroscience, 23*, 923–935.

Gibson, E. M., Purger, D., Mount, C. W., Goldstein, A. K., Lin, G. L., Wood, L. S., Inema, I., . . . Monje, M. (2014). Neuronal activity promotes oligodendrogenesis and adaptive myelination in the mammalian brain. *Science, 344*(6183), 1252304–1252304. https://doi.org/10.1126/science.1252304

Giedd, J., Blumenthal, J., Jeffries, N., Castellanos, F. X., Liu, H., Zijdenbos, A., . . . Rapoport, J. L. (1999). Brain development during childhood and adolescence: A longitudinal MRI study. *Nature Neuroscience, 2*, 861–863. doi:10.1038/13158

Goldin, P. R., & Gross, J. J. (2010). Effects of mindfulness-based stress reduction (MBSR) on emotion regulation in social anxiety disorder. *Emotion, 10*, 83–91.

Greenough, W. T., Black, J. E., & Wallace, C. S. (1987). Experience and brain development. *Child Development, 58*(3), 539–559. https://doi.org/10.2307/1130197

Grossman, P., Niemann, L., Schmidt, S., & Walach, H. (2004). Mindfulness-based stress reduction and health benefits: A meta-analysis. *Journal of Psychosomatic Research, 57*, 35–43.

Hajcak, G., & Dennis, T. (2009). Brain potentials during affective picture processing in children. *Biol. Psychol., 80*, 333–338.

Hassinger-Das, B., Jordan, N. C., Glutting, J., Irwin, C., & Dyson, N. (2014). Domain-general mediators of the relation between kindergarten number sense and first-grade mathematics achievement. *Journal of Experimental Child Psychology, 118*, 78–92.

Hawn Foundation. (2011). *The MindUp Curriculum: Brain-focused strategies for learning— and living*. New York: Scholastic Teaching Resources.

Hebb, D. O. (1949). *The organization of behavior*. New York: Wiley.

Hölzel, B. K., Lazar, S. W., Gard, T., Schuman-Olivier, Z., Vago, D. R., & Ott, U. (2011). How does mindfulness meditation work? Proposing mechanisms of action from a conceptual and neural perspective. *Perspectives on Psychological Science, 6*(6), 537–559.

Hölzel, B. K., Ott, U., Hempel, H., Hackl, A., Wolf, K., Stark, R., & Vaitl, D. (2007). Differential engagement of anterior cingulate and adjacent medial frontal cortex in adept meditators and non-meditators. *Neuroscience Letters, 421*(1), 16–21.

Hostinar, C. E., Sullivan, R. M., & Gunnar, M. R. (2014). Psychobiological mechanisms underlying the social buffering of the hypothalamic-pituitary-adrenocortical axis: A review of animal models and human studies across development. *Psychological Bulletin, 140*(1), 256–282.

Huppert, F. A., & Johnson, D. M. (2010). A controlled trial of mindfulness training in schools: The importance of practice for an impact on well-being. *Journal of Positive Psychology, 5*, 264–274. doi:10.1080/17439761003794148

Huttenlocher, P. R. (2002). *Neural plasticity: The effects of environment on the development of the cerebral cortex*. Cambridge, MA: Harvard University Press.

Hwang, Y. S., Bartlett, B., Greben, M., & Hand, K. (2017). A systematic review of mindfulness interventions for in-service teachers: A tool to enhance teacher wellbeing and performance. *Teaching and Teacher Education, 64*, 26–42.

Jacques, S., & Marcovitch, S. (2010). Executive function. In W. Overton (Ed.), *Handbook of lifespan development* (pp. 431–466). New York: Wiley.

Jha, A. J., Krompinger, J., & Baime, M. J. (2007). Mindfulness training modifies subsystems of attention. *Cognitive, Affective, & Behavioral Neuroscience, 7*, 109–119.

Johnson, C., Burke, C., Brinkman, S., & Wade, T. (2017). A randomized controlled evaluation of a secondary school mindfulness program for early adolescents: Do we have the recipe right yet? *Behaviour Research and Therapy, 99*, 37–46.

Kabat-Zinn, J. (1982). An out-patient program in behavioral medicine for chronic pain patients based on the practice of mindfulness meditation: Theoretical considerations and preliminary results. *General Hospital Psychiatry, 4*, 33–47.

Kabat-Zinn, J. (1994). *Where you go there you are: Mindfulness meditation in everyday life*. New York: Hyperion.

Kabat-Zinn, J. (2003). Mindfulness-based interventions in context: Past, present, and future. *Clinical Psychology: Science and Practice, 10*, 144–156.

Kabat-Zinn, J. (2013). *Full catastrophe living* (Revised ed., paperback). New York: Bantam.

Kaiser Greenland, S. (2010). *The mindful child: How to help your kid manage stress and become happier, kinder, and more compassionate*. New York: Free Press.

Kapur, S., Craik, F. I. M., Tulving, E., Wilson, A. A., Houle, S., & Brown, G. M. (1994). Neuroanatomical correlates of encoding in episodic memory: Levels of processing effect. *Proceedings of the National Academy of Sciences, USA, 91*, 2008–2111.

Karbach, J., & Kray, J. (2009). How useful is executive control training? Age differences in near and far transfer of task-switching training. *Developmental Science, 12*(6), 978–990.

Kaunhoven, R. J., & Dorjee, D. (2017). How does mindfulness modulate self-regulation in pre-adolescent children? An integrative neurocognitive review. *Neuroscience and Biobehavioral Reviews, 74*, 163–184.

Keng, S.-L., Robins, C. J., Smoski, M. J., Dagenbach, J., & Leary, M. R. (2013). Reappraisal and mindfulness: A comparison of subjective effects and cognitive costs. *Behaviour Research and Therapy, 51*, 899–904.

Klingbeil, D. A., Renshaw, T. L., Willenbrink, J. B., Copek, R. A., Chan, K. T., Haddock, A., . . . Clifton, J. (2017). Mindfulness-based interventions with youth: A comprehensive meta-analysis of group-design studies. *Journal of School Psychology, 63*, 77–103.

Krech, D., Rosenzweig, M. R., & Bennett, E. L. (1960). Effects of environmental complexity and training on brain chemistry. *Journal of Comparative and Physiological Psychology, 53*(6), 509–519.

Kuyken, W., Weare, K., Ukoumunne, O., Vicary, R., Motton, N., Burnett, R., . . . Huppert, F. (2013). Effectiveness of the mindfulness in schools programme: Non-randomised controlled feasibility study. *British Journal of Psychiatry, 203*(2), 126–131. doi:10.1192/bjp.bp.113.126649

Lamm, C., Zelazo, P. D., & Lewis, M. D. (2006). Neural correlates of cognitive control in childhood and adolescence: Disentangling the contributions of age and executive function. *Neuropsychologia, 44*, 2139–2148.

Lantieri, L. (2008). *Building emotional intelligence: Techniques to cultivate inner strength in children*. Boulder, CO: Sounds True.

Lewis, M. D., Granic, I., Lamm, C., Zelazo, P. D., Stieben, J., Todd, R. M., . . . Pepler, D. (2008). Changes in the neural bases of emotion regulation associated with clinical improvement in children with behavior problems. *Development and Psychopathology, 20*, 913–939.

Lomas, T., Medina, J. C., Ivtzan, I., Rupprecht, S., Hart, R., & Eiroa-Orosa, F. J. (2017). The impact of mindfulness on well-being and performance in the workplace: An inclusive systematic review of the empirical literature. *European Journal of Work and Organizational Psychology, 26*(4), 492–513.

Lutz, A., Dunne, J. D., & Davidson, R. J. (2007). Meditation and the neuroscience of consciousness: An introduction. In P. D. Zelazo, M. Moscovitch & E. Thompson (Eds.), *The Cambridge handbook of consciousness* (pp. 499–551). New York: Cambridge University Press.

Lutz, A., Slagter, H. A., Dunne, J. D., & Davidson, R. J. (2008). Attention regulation and monitoring in meditation. *Trends in Cognitive Sciences, 12*, 163–169.

Lyons, K. E., & Zelazo, P. D. (2011). Monitoring, metacognition, and executive function: Elucidating the role of self-reflection in the development of self-regulation. In J. Benson (Ed.), *Advances in child development and behavior* (Vol. 40, pp. 379–412). Burlington: Academic Press.

Maguire, E. A., Gadian, D. G., Johnsrude, I. S., Good, C. D., Ashburner, J., Frackowiak, R. S. J., & Frith, C. D. (2000). Navigation-related structural change in the hippocampi of taxi drivers. *Proceedings of the National Academy of Sciences USA, 97,* 4398–4403.

Manes, F., Sahakian, B., Clark, L., Rogers, R., Antoun, N., Aitken, M., & Robbins, T. (2002). Decision-making processes following damage to prefrontal cortex. *Brain, 125,* 624–639.

Marcovitch, S., Jacques, S., Boseovski, J. J., & Zelazo, P. D. (2008). Self-reflection and the cognitive control of behavior: Implications for learning. *Mind, Brain, and Education, 2,* 136–141.

Masten, A. S. (2014). *Ordinary magic: Resilience in development.* New York: Guilford.

Masten, A. S., Herbers, J. E., Desjardins, C. D., Cutuli, J. J., McCormick, C. M., Sapienza, J. K., . . . Zelazo, P. D. (2012). Executive function skills and school success in young children experiencing homelessness. *Educational Researcher, 41*(9), 375–384. doi:10.3102/0013189x12459883

McClelland, M. M., Cameron, C. E., Connor, C. M., Farris, C. L., Jewkes, A M., & Morrison, F. J. (2007). Links between behavioral regulation and preschoolers' literacy, vocabulary, and math skills. *Developmental Psychology, 43,* 947–959.

Meiklejohn, J., Phillips, C., Freedman, L., Griffin, M. L., Biegel, G. M., Roach, A. et al. (2012). Integrating mindfulness training into K-12 education: Fostering the resilience of teachers and students. *Mindfulness, 3,* 291–307. doi:10.1007/s12671-012-0094-5

Metis Associates. (2011). *Building inner resilience in teachers and their students: Results of the inner resilience pilot program.* Retrieved March 12, 2012, from http://innerresilience.org/documents/IRP_Pilot_Program_Results_AERA2011_updated_6.9.pdf

Mezzacappa, E. (2004). Alerting, orienting, and executive attention: Developmental properties and sociodemographic correlates in an epidemiological sample of young, urban children. *Child Development, 75*(5), 1373–1386.

Miller, R. C., & Butler, B. (2011). *iRest for kids.* San Rafael, CA: Integrative Restoration Institute. Retrieved from www.irest.us/node/338

Miyake, A., Friedman, N. P., Emerson, M. J., Witzki, A. H., Howerter, A., & Wager, T. D. (2000). The unity and diversity of executive functions and their contributions to complex "Frontal Lobe" tasks: A latent variable analysis. *Cognitive Psychology, 41*(1), 49–100. https://doi.org/10.1006/cogp.1999.0734

Modinos, G., Ormel, J., & Aleman, A. (2010). Individual differences in dispositional mindfulness and brain activity involved in reappraisal of emotion. *Social Cognitive and Affective Neuroscience, 5*(4), 369–377.

Moore, A., Gruber, T., Derose, J., & Malinowski, P. (2012). Regular, brief mindfulness meditation practice improves electrophysiological markers of attentional control. *Frontiers in Human Neuroscience, 6,* 18. doi:10.3389/fnhum.2012.00018

Moriguchi, Y., Sakata, Y., Ishibashi, M., & Ishikawa, Y. (2015). Teaching others rule-use improves executive function and prefrontal activations in young children. *Frontiers in Psychology, 6,* 894. doi:10.3389/fpsyg.2015.00894

Noble, K. G., Norman, M. F., & Farah, M. J. (2005). Neurocognitive correlates of socioeconomic status in kindergarten children. *Developmental Science, 8*(1), 74–87.

Ophir, E., Nass, C., & Wagner, A. D. (2009). Cognitive control in media multitaskers. *Proceedings of the National Academy of Sciences of the United States of America, 106,* 15583–15587.

Ortner, C. N. M., Kilner, S. J., & Zelazo, P. D. (2007). Mindfulness meditation and reduced emotional interference on a cognitive task. *Motivation and Emotion, 31,* 271–283.

Petersen, S., & Posner, M. (2012). The attention system of the human brain: 20 years after. *Annual Review of Neuroscience, 21*, 73–89.

Posner, M. I., & Petersen, S. E. (1990). The attention system of the human brain. *Annual Review of Neuroscience, 13*(1), 25–42.

Posner, M. I., Rothbart, M. K., Sheese, B. E., & Voelker, P. (2014) Developing attention: Behavioral and brain mechanisms. *Advances in Neuroscience, 2014*, 9 pp. https://doi.org/10.1155/2014/405094

Quaglia, J. T., Goodman, R. J., & Brown, K. W. (2015). Trait mindfulness predicts efficient top-down attention to and discrimination of facial expressions. *Journal of Personality, 8*, 393–404.

Raver, C. C., Li-Grining, C., Bub, K., Jones, S. M., Zhai, F., & Pressler, E. (2011). CSRP's impact on low-income preschoolers' preacademic skills: Self-regulation as a mediating mechanism. *Child Development, 82*(1), 362–378.

Roebers, C. M. (2017). Executive function and metacognition: Towards a unifying framework of cognitive self-regulation. *Developmental Review, 45*, 31–51.

Roeser, R. W., Skinner, E., Beers, J., & Jennings, P. A. (2012). Mindfulness training and teachers' professional development: An emerging area of research and practice. *Child Development Perspectives, 6*(2), 167–173.

Rothbart, M. K., Sheese, B. E., Rueda, M. R., & Posner, M. I. (2011). Developing mechanisms of self-regulation in early life. *Emotion Review, 3*, 207–213.

Rueda, M. R., Rothbart, M. K., McCandliss, B. D., Saccomanno, L., & Posner, M. I. (2005). Training, maturation, and genetic influences on the development of executive attention. *Proceedings of the National Academy of Sciences, 102*, 14931–14936.

Saltzman, A., & Goldin, P. (2008). Mindfulness based stress reduction for school-age children. In S. C. Hayes & L. A. Greco (Eds.), *Acceptance and mindfulness interventions for children, adolescents and families* (pp. 139–161). Oakland, CA: Context Press, New Harbinger.

Saltzman, A. (2014). *A still quiet place: A mindfulness program for teaching children and adolescents to ease stress and difficult emotions.* Oakland, CA: New Harbinger.

Schmitt, S. A., McClelland, M. M., Tominey, S. L., & Acock, A. C. (2015). Strengthening school readiness for head start children: Evaluation of a self-regulation intervention. *Early Childhood Research Quarterly, 30*, 20–31.

Scholz, J., Klein, M. C., Behrens, T. E. J., & Johansen-Berg, H. (2009). Training induces changes in white-matter architecture. *Nature Neuroscience, 120*(11), 1367–1368.

Schonert-Reichl, K. A., & Lawlor, M. S. (2010). The effects of a mindfulness-based education program on pre- and early adolescents well-being and social and emotional competence. *Mindfulness, 1*, 137–151.

Schonert-Reichl, K. A., Oberle, E., Lawlor, M. S., Abbott, D., Thomson, K., Oberlander, T. F., & Diamond, A. (2015). Enhancing cognitive and social-emotional development through a simple-to administer mindfulness-based school program for elementary school children: A randomized controlled trial. *Developmental Psychology, 51*, 52–66. http://doi.org/10.1037/a0038454

Shapiro, S. L., & Carlson, L. E. (2009). *The art and science of mindfulness: Integrating mindfulness into psychology and the helping professions.* Washington, DC: American Psychology Press.

Shapiro, S. L., Jazzeri, H., & Golden, P. (2012). Effects of mindfulness training on ethics. *Mindfulness, 2*–12.

Shapiro, S., Rechtschaffen, D., & de Sousa, S. (2016). Mindfulness training for teachers. In K. A. Schonert-Reichl & R. W. Roeser (Eds.). *Handbook of Mindfulness in Education* (pp. 83–97). New York: Springer.

330   *Andrei D. Semenov, Douglas Kennedy, and Philip David Zelazo*

Sheppes, G., & Gross, J. J. (2011). Is timing everything? Temporal considerations in emotion regulation. *Personality and Social Psychology Review, 15*(4), 319–331.

Skinner, E., & Beers, J. (2016). Mindfulness and teachers' coping in the classroom: A developmental model of teacher stress, coping, and everyday resilience. In K. A. Schonert-Reichl & R. W. Roeser (Eds.). *Handbook of Mindfulness in Education* (pp. 99–118). New York: Springer.

Smallwood, J., & Schooler, J. W. (2006). The restless mind. *Psychological Bulletin, 132,* 946–958.

So, K., & Orme-Johnson, D. W. (2001). Three randomized experiments on the longitudinal effects of the transcendental meditation technique on cognition. *Intelligence, 29,* 419–440.

Stieben, J., Lewis, M. D., Granic, I., Zelazo, P. D., Segalowitz, S., & Pepler, D. (2007). Neurophysiological mechanisms of emotion regulation for subtypes of externalizing children. *Developmental Psychopathology, 19,* 455–480.

Takeuchi, H. et al. (2010). Training of working memory impacts structural connectivity. *Journal of Neuroscience, 30,* 3297–3303.

Tan, L., & Martin, G. (2013). Taming the adolescent mind: Preliminary report of a mindfulness-based psychological intervention for adolescents with clinical heterogeneous mental health diagnoses. *Clinical Child Psychology and Psychiatry, 18*(2), 300–312. https://doi.org/10.1177/1359104512455182

Tang, Y. Y., Hölzel, B. K., & Posner, M. I. (2015). The neuroscience of mindfulness meditation. *Nature Reviews Neuroscience, 16*(4), 213.

Tang, Y., Lu, Q., Geng, X., Stein, E. A., Yang, Y., & Posner, M. I. (2010). Short-term meditation induces white matter changes in the anterior cingulate. *Proceedings of the National Academy of Sciences of the United States of America, 107,* 15649–15652.

Tominey, S. L., & McClelland, M. M. (2011). Red light, purple light: Findings from a randomized trial using circle time games to improve behavioral self-regulation in preschool. *Early Education and Development, 22*(3), 489–519.

U.S. Department of Education Office for Civil Rights. (2014, March 21). *Civil rights data collection: Data snapshot (early childhood).* Washington, DC: U.S. Department of Education Office for Civil Rights.

Veen, V. V., & Carter, C. S. (2002). The timing of action-monitoring processes in the anterior cingulate cortex. *Journal of Cognitive Neuroscience, 14*(4), 593–602.

Willard, C. (2010). *Child's mind: Mindfulness practices to help our children be more focused, calm, and relaxed.* Berkeley, CA: Parallax Press.

Zelazo, P. D. (2004). The development of conscious control in childhood. *Trends in Cognitive Sciences, 8,* 12–17.

Zelazo, P. D. (2015). Executive function: Reflection, iterative reprocessing, complexity, and the developing brain. *Developmental Review.* doi:10.1016/j.dr.2015.07.001

Zelazo, P. D., Anderson, J. E., Richler, J., Wallner-Allen, K., Beaumont, J. L., Conway, K. P., . . . Weintraub, S. (2014). NIh toolbox cognition battery (CB): Validation of executive function measures in adults. *Journal of the International Neuropsychological Society, 20*(6), 620–629.

Zelazo, P. D., Blair, C. B., & Willoughby, M. T. (2016). *Executive function: Implications for education.* Washington, DC: National Center for Education Research, Institute of Education Sciences, U.S. Department of Education. Retrieved from ies.ed.gov

Zelazo, P. D., & Cunningham, W. (2007). Executive function: Mechanisms underlying emotion regulation. In J. Gross (Ed.), *Handbook of emotion regulation* (pp. 135–158). New York: Guilford.

Zelazo, P. D., Forston, J. L., Masten, A. S., & Carlson, S. M. (2018). Mindfulness plus reflection training: Effects on executive function in early childhood. *Frontiers in Psychology*, 9(February), 1–12. https://doi.org/10.3389/fpsyg.2018.00208

Zelazo, P. D., & Lyons, K. E. (2012). The potential benefits of mindfulness training in early childhood: A developmental social cognitive neuroscience perspective. *Child Development Perspectives*, 6, 154–160.

Zelazo, P. D., & Müller, U. (2002). The balance beam in the balance: Reflections on rules, relational complexity, and developmental processes. *Journal of Experimental Child Psychology*, 81(4), 458–465.

Zenner, C., Herrnleben-Kurz, S., & Walach, H. (2014). Mindfulness-based interventions in schools—a systematic review and meta-analysis. *Frontiers in Psychology*, 5, 603. doi:10.3389/fpsyg.2014.00603

Zoogman, S., Goldberg, S. B., Hoyt, W. T., & Miller, L. (2015). Mindfulness interventions with youth: A meta-analysis. *Mindfulness*, 6(2), 290–302. doi:10.1007/s12671-013-0260-4

13 The Neuroscience of Sleep and Its Relation to Educational Outcomes

Rachel Sharman, Gaby Illingworth
and Christopher-James Harvey

This chapter will consider the neuroscience of sleep, and how this impacts on educational outcomes with a particular focus on adolescents. First we will outline some of the basic physiology of sleep. We will then consider the broad effects of sleep deprivation on health and well-being and how this might indirectly impact on performance in the classroom before moving on to elucidate the direct effects on cognitive and academic outcomes. Finally we will review the evidence for potential, realistic school-based interventions for targeting academic outcomes via sleep.

What Is Sleep?

Sleep is understood to be '*a reversible behavioural state of perceptual disengagement from, and unresponsiveness to, the environment*' (Carskadon & Dement, 2011, p. 16). In this way, sleep is distinct from coma and anaesthesia: sleep is not an unconscious state. Whilst there is reduced interaction with the external environment you are still able to engage with it. Some stimuli will penetrate the sensory system—think of alarm clocks, for example. Sleep is a highly specialised behaviour, the most dominant single behaviour we engage in as a species. It has myriad functions and involves every aspect of the nervous system and so the effects of sleep deprivation are just as wide reaching.

Sleep has a clear electrophysiological signal within the brain. During sleep we cycle between two states, non-rapid eye movement sleep (NREM) and rapid eye movement sleep (REM). NREM sleep can be further categorised into three stages: N1, N2, and N3. N3 is deep sleep, where the majority of slow wave activity occurs. In healthy adults, we enter sleep through NREM and enter REM about 80 minutes later; we continue cycling in this pattern through the sleep period: every 80 to 120 minutes (Carskadon & Dement, 2011). The exception to this cycling is for infants, under the age of one, where they enter through an active sleep stage (reminiscent of REM) and then follow into a quiet sleep stage (reminiscent of NREM), cycling between these two stages every 50 minutes. In adults, over a typical 8-hour sleep period, we would expect to see around four to five sleep cycles. Structurally, the first third of the night primarily comprises N3 sleep, which is then slowly replaced with elongated REM sleep periods in the later sleep cycles. The proportion of these sleep stages (N1, N2, N3, and REM) across a sleep period are also predictable and change with age. At birth, REM (defined as active sleep in infants) will make up 50% of the infant's sleep, this decreases up to the age of two whereby it reaches around 20–25% and remains at that proportion throughout the lifespan (not withstanding any pathologies that alter REM). Conversely we see a decline in slow wave sleep (N3) as we age (Ohayon, Carskadon, Guilleminault, & Vitiello, 2004).

The most parsimonious explanation of sleep is the two-process model, first proposed by Borbély in 1982. This model posits that there are two systems which drive the timing and depth, or quality, of sleep: the circadian system and the sleep homeostat. The circadian system regulates all of our biological processes and alertness levels through internally generated, approximately 24-hour oscillations in physiology and behaviour. Core body temperature, blood pressure, hormone release and alertness, as examples, all follow a predictable pattern over the day (Monk et al., 1997). These oscillations are driven at a cellular level through clock genes, e.g., PERIOD (PER). These genes result in the generation of various clock proteins which ultimately inhibit their own creation. Once the protein levels drop sufficiently the process begins again: a genetic transcription-translation feedback loop. This whole process occurs over a roughly 24-hour period (Buhr & Takahashi, 2013). Inherited alterations in these clock genes will change the rhythm of the oscillation, speeding up or slowing down the rhythm. An individual with a faster running genetic clock (a shorter oscillation length) will prefer to wake and sleep earlier—designated 'morning types' or 'larks' whereas those with a slower running clock (faster oscillation length) will prefer to wake and sleep later—'late types' or 'owls'. This preference for certain times of day is known as an individual's chronotype (Brown et al., 2008). Almost every cell in our body has this molecular clock machinery that keeps cellular processes to time forming a biological timing network or our body's biological clock.

These cellular clocks located in peripheral sites, such as in the gut or heart, are coordinated by a master clock in the brain, the suprachiasmatic nuclei (SCN): a large grouping of cellular clocks located in the hypothalamus directly above the optic chiasm. The average oscillation time of the molecular SCN is 24.18-hours ±16 minutes and therefore, to keep with external time, we need daily adjustment to maintain a 24-hour rhythm (Czeisler et al., 1999). This adjustment is made via *zeitgebers*, or time-givers, with the most effective being light. Photic entrainment is said to be the key entraining stimuli. Light enters the eye where it interacts with specialised non-vision-producing cells in the retina: photosensitive retinal ganglion cells (pRGC). Owing to the presence of a protein called melanopsin, these cells are intrinsically photosensitive and provide a signal to the SCN, via the retinal-hypothalamic tract (RHT), about the time of day (Do & Yau, 2010; Foster et al., 1991). In terms of impacting the rest/activity cycle, light has a dual effect on the circadian system depending on the time of day that it is experienced: Light in the early morning will advance the clock whereas light in the evening/early night will delay the clock (Czeisler, Richardson, Zimmerman, Moore-Ede, & Weitzman, 1981). Light affects the circadian network in two ways. Firstly, light directly influences the molecular components of the biological clock within the SCN cells by changing the expression of PER within the transcription-translation feedback loop, thus changing the oscillation speed (Yan & Silver, 2004). Secondly, the SCN relays the light/dark signal to the pineal gland regulating the expression of the hormone melatonin. In humans, melatonin levels rise in response to dusk and therefore light in the evening hours will suppress melatonin expression (Brainard, Rollag, & Hanifin, 1997). Melatonin is not a soporific per se, but has receptors in numerous locations around the body and on the SCN itself, so is proposed to act as a synchronising signal between the SCN and the peripheral tissues (Stehle, Von Gall, & Korf, 2003). In the absence of the pRGC or RHT, for example in individuals who have lost their eyes, non-photic stimuli may act as *zeitgebers*. Although providing a weaker adjustment than light, there is evidence that social interaction, food consumption, temperature, exercise, and even the sleep/wake cycle itself can entrain the human circadian rhythm (Mistlberger & Skene, 2005).

Through the plasticity within this pathway, the brain and body respond appropriately to time of day by optimising physiological processes and behaviour in anticipation of environmental changes. However, this temporal optimisation of physiology means our performance on certain tasks will vary across the day. For example, different types of athletic performance have been shown to be better or worse at certain times in the biological day (Thun, Bjorvatn, Flo, Harris, & Pallesen, 2015). There are well-documented circadian variations in alertness, sleepiness, and mood (Monk et al., 1997). The effects of the circadian system are far-reaching: from our hour-to-hour, day-to-day activities right through to impacts on public policy and practice. This will be explored later in this chapter as it relates to adolescents and educational practice.

The second system in Borbély's (1982) two-process model of sleep is the sleep homeostat. The sleep homeostat operates on a simple principle: The longer you are awake, the stronger the pressure for sleep, until it reaches a critical point and sleep is initiated. This system tracks duration of wakefulness via the build-up of various neurochemicals, predominantly adenosine (Donlea, Alam, & Szymusiak, 2017). Adenosine is a by-product of energy metabolism, synthesised from the use of the cellular energy nucleotide, adenosine triophosphate (ATP), by neurons within the brain. Therefore, the longer we are awake, the more energy the neuronal cells have used, and the more adenosine is built up. Adenosine has a dual influence on sleep by inhibiting the wake-promoting neurons (basal forebrain) and stimulating neurons in the sleep-promoting areas of the brain (including the ventrolateral preoptic nucleus in the hypothalamus) (Holst & Landolt, 2015). Adenosine is said to be cleared during deep sleep, specifically during slow wave sleep (to be discussed later), so the longer we are awake the more deep sleep we have/need.

Caffeine is an adenosine antagonist, blocking the adenosine receptors, and stimulating wakefulness.

Good quality sleep occurs when the homeostat and the circadian system are both primed for it: when both systems are in concert. We awaken naturally, without alarms, when sleep pressure is gone. As sleep pressure increases throughout the day, the circadian system drives alertness, working against the increasing homeostatic drive for sleep. We experience fluctuations in our alertness across the day when the circadian system's alerting signal is not strong enough to counter the build-up of sleep pressure, e.g., the postprandial dip which occurs between 1300–1500 hours. If the circadian and homeostat system are not aligned, i.e., if we do not have sufficient sleep in the night to reduce the previous day's sleep pressure, then the alerting effects of the circadian system are not as effective and the natural dips in alertness that happen during the day will be more severe and longer lasting. If we try to sleep when the circadian system is prepared for wake we will experience a poorer quality sleep overall, even if sleep pressure is high. Such is the case for those working night shifts and sleeping in the day for example. This has particular relevance during adolescence.

Changes to Adolescent Sleep

Both of these sleep-driving processes go through a developmental change in adolescence. The circadian clock delays by between 1–3 hours around the onset of puberty (Carskadon et al., 1980). The sleep homeostat becomes less sensitive, so the pressure to sleep builds up more slowly during the day (Carskadon et al., 1980; Jenni, Achermann, & Carskadon, 2005). This means that not only is the adolescent circadian system signalling for sleep later, but the sleep homeostat may not have sufficiently built up enough pressure by the parental desired sleep time to trigger restful sleep. Equally, an early awakening for school may result in waking before sleep pressure has reduced, meaning that the adolescent will feel sleepy at the start of the school day compounding the impact of the delayed circadian rhythm. Additionally, this system also becomes more sensitive to light in early adolescence (Crowley, Acebo, & Carskadon, 2007). This could mean that the effects of artificial light on the system are more pronounced in this population. We do not yet fully understand why or how this delay happens, other than there is potentially an interaction between the SCN and gonadal hormones (Manber, & Armitage, 1999; Hagenauer, Perryman, Lee, & Carskadon, 2009). We do know that these developmental changes are found during the pubertal phase of a number of mammalian species.

Adolescents, due to the delay in the circadian clock, begin to prefer later bedtimes: They drift towards a more evening chronotype, evidenced by a tendency to go to bed later with age (Gradisar, Gardner, & Dohnt, 2011; Sadeh, Raviv, & Gruber, 2000). This preference to head to bed later, coupled with the socially driven demand to be awake early on school days, could be resulting in a progressive shortening of total sleep time as children age (Carskadon, 2011). This is supported by a meta-analysis of quantitative changes in sleep parameters over the lifespan where adolescents reported significantly shorter total sleep times on weekday nights compared to weekend nights during the latter part of puberty (Ohayon et al., 2004). The significant extension of total sleep time on weekend nights demonstrates that adolescents are experiencing partial sleep deprivation during weeknights as the weekend "lie-in" attempts to catch up on lost sleep during the week. This mismatch between week and weekend sleep timing is known as social jet lag and the degree of this discrepancy has been shown to rise rapidly around puberty, peaking at around 19 years for females and 21 years for males (Roenneberg et al., 2004). Internationally, we see that adolescents are not getting the recommended amount of sleep (Ohayon et al., 2004). The National Sleep Foundation (NSF) recommends 8–10 hours' sleep for 14–17 year olds (Hirshkowitz et al., 2015). However, studies in the US (Roberts, Roberts, & Duong, 2009), China (Chen et al., 2014), Australia (Short, Gradisar, Lack, Wright, & Dohnt, 2013) and pilot work in the UK (Sharman et al., 2017) have shown that short sleep is prevalent. Indeed, a review of worldwide sleep patterns has shown that in 53% of samples, teenagers are achieving less than 8 hours' sleep on a weekday night (Gradisar et al., 2011).

Alongside the changes to the sleep homeostat and circadian system, children experience a number of developmental changes in sleep structure over the course of puberty into adulthood. As active sleep decreases in infancy, the proportion of slow wave sleep increases through childhood to puberty and then decreases by around 40% during adolescence (Campbell et al., 2011). Children on the cusp of puberty (tanner stage 1) have around 33% slow wave sleep across the sleep period, whereas at post puberty (tanner stage 5) this reduces to around 22%: a similar proportion to what we would expect in a healthy adult sleeper (Jenni & Carskadon, 2004). Sleep duration also reduces as we age, although from childhood to adolescence this reduction appears to occur mostly on school nights (Ohayon et al., 2004). A reduction in total sleep time would reduce the number of sleep cycles and duration spent in each stage, specifically REM which would be reduced by the curtailing of sleep and loss of the later few sleep cycles where REM dominates.

The potential impact of structural sleep changes will be discussed further on, however, Figure 13.1 outlines the effects of chronic sleep deprivation across various physiological and psychological domains (Wulff, Gatti, Wettstein, & Foster, 2010). In the short term, the effects of sleep deprivation are manageable and reversible: for example, sleepiness, reduced attention span, irritability, increases in impulsive behaviour, poor decision making, increased error rate, changes to appetite, and increased stimulant use. Over the long term, chronic sleep disruption has been associated with an increased risk for obesity, cardiovascular disease, diabetes, cancer, and poor mental health outcomes in later life (Cappuccio, D'Elia, Strazzullo, & Miller, 2010). With the exception of obesity (Must & Strauss, 1999) the extent to which sleep loss in adolescence

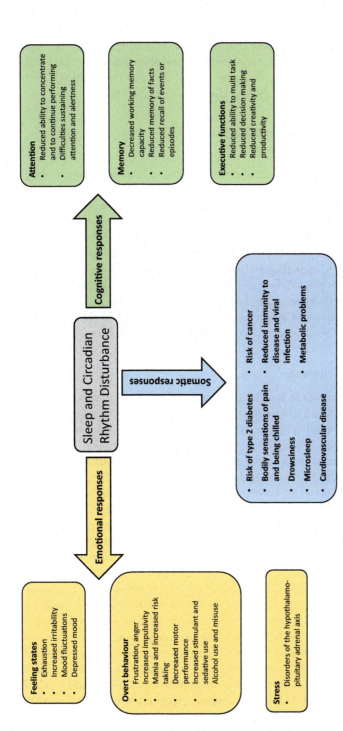

Figure 13.1 The Health Consequences of Shortened or Reduced Sleep and Desynchronized Circadian Rhythms, Classified by Emotional, Cognitive, and Somatic Response, Adapted from Wulff et al., 2010. This demonstrates the potential impact of sleep and circadian rhythm disruption ranging from quite mild consequences of short-term disruption (feeling tired or frustrated) to the consequences of long-term disruption (cancer, metabolic disease).

predicts these more severe health issues is not clear, as most work to date has been with adults. We do know that there are links between different aspects of sleep (duration, reported sleepiness etc.) and short-term outcomes in adolescents (Smaldone, Honig, & Byrne, 2007). This has ramifications on their ability to learn effectively, and also their experience of school.

Sleep and Adolescent Emotional and Behavioural Functioning

There is mounting evidence to show that how well adolescents are sleeping may be associated with their health, emotions, and behaviour. Notably for those working in education, sleep may contribute to psychosocial functioning and emotional/behavioural regulation, and so may influence students' wellbeing, their ability to get on with their peers and teachers, and their behaviour at school. This suggests there is a need for educators to consider sleep and sleep problems as contributory factors to how adolescents function at school as well as potentially challenging classroom behaviours. Sleep-wake patterns (consistency of bedtime and wake time, and the consistency of those patterns across school days and weekends), sleep duration, and levels of sleepiness, have all been investigated as potentially important variables for adolescents.

Emotional Functioning

Sleep plays a key role in how we construct our emotional world. For example, sleep has been shown to increase the speed by which individuals can recognise previously presented (prior to the sleep period) emotional facial expressions (Wagner, Kashyap, Diekelmann, & Born, 2007). Furthermore, sleep appears to favour the retention of emotional versus neutral stimuli in adults (Wagner, Gais, & Born, 2001). The amygdala and the prefrontal cortex (PFC) are two key structures known to be involved in emotional processing, with a function of the PFC being to inhibit the amygdala (Davidson, 2002). Yoo and colleagues (2007), in a functional magnetic resonance imaging study (fMRI) undertaken with young adults, found a 60% increase in amygdala activity in response to an emotional stimulus viewing task when participants were sleep deprived compared to a control group. The authors suggested there was an amplified amygdala response to negative emotional stimuli in individuals who were sleep deprived and a loss of functional connectivity with the medial prefrontal cortex (MPFC), summarised as a failure of top-down, prefrontal control. In short, sleep deprivation may be associated with hyper-connectivity between the amygdala and the rest of the limbic system, notably activation of the autonomic nervous system via the hypothalamus. This has been evidenced in a study by Franzen et al., whereby, compared with controls, individuals who were sleep deprived had greater pupillary response when viewing negatively valenced images compared to neutral or positively valenced images (Franzen, Buysse, Dahl, Thompson, & Siegle, 2009). In addition, the young adults who were sleep deprived showed a faster pupillary response to the negative images, indicating a hyper-responsiveness. This may be particularly salient for adolescents given that the PFC is a brain region which develops slowly and does not reach full maturity until adulthood (Blakemore & Robbins, 2012; Giedd, 2004). Additionally, younger adolescents appear to be less successful at regulating emotional responses to social stimuli (Silvers et al., 2012) and this developmental phenomenon may be compounded by their chronic sleep deprivation.

Studies which have focused on sleep deprivation suggest that sleep is essential for proper emotional regulation (Gregory & Sadeh, 2012). Moodiness, irritability, and a low tolerance for frustration are the symptoms most frequently described in sleep-deprived adolescents (Dahl, 1999) with findings supporting a relationship between sleepiness and impaired mood being considered robust (Fallone, Owens, & Deane, 2002). Sleep may have a general effect on mood lability with adolescents reporting less control over their moods following sleep loss. This can be demonstrated in a variety of ways, so that students may be angrier when faced with a frustrating situation, more likely to cry when upset or sad, and may be sillier in response to a humorous situation (Dahl & Lewin, 2002).

Adolescence is the peak age for the onset of many mental health conditions, such as anxiety (Paus, Keshavan, & Giedd, 2008). Although many other factors can contribute, it appears that healthy sleep plays an important role in maintaining mental health (Short et al., 2013). A wealth of cross-sectional studies have found a concurrent association between short or disturbed sleep and negative psychological outcomes in adolescents, for example depressive symptoms and anxiety (Gregory & Sadeh, 2012; Moore et al., 2009; Pasch, Laska, Lytle, & Moe, 2010; Roberts, Roberts, & Chen, 2001; Wolfson & Carskadon, 1998). It should be noted that a cross-sectional design (which relates to some of the studies mentioned later) limits the ability to attribute causality to sleep and that many of the relationships between sleep and psychological functioning are likely to be bidirectional (Moore et al., 2009).

In a much-cited study, Wolfson and Carskadon (1998) examined sleep patterns and daytime functioning in a large sample (3,120) of students, aged 13 to 19 years. Adolescents reported to have 'short' (<6 hours 45 minutes) school-night sleep time and/or large weekend bedtime delay (>120 minutes) had higher levels of depressed mood and sleep/wake behaviour problems than those who reported 'long' (>8 hours 15 minutes) school-night sleep time with a short weekend bedtime delay (<60 minutes). Therefore, those who had less sleep on school nights, or larger discrepancies between school and weekend bedtimes, or both, were more likely to experience a depressed mood. These findings suggest that there is a relationship between how adolescents sleep and how they feel and behave.

In a more recent study, it was the degree of sleepiness, but not objective estimates or variability in sleep duration, which correlated with adolescents' self-report of symptoms of depression, anxiety, and health (Moore et al., 2009).

The authors proposed that a subjective feeling of sleepiness might result in a general negative mood as well as a reduced ability to regulate emotions. This might then contribute to depressed and anxious feelings and somatic symptoms. However, the converse may also be an explanation, in that more anxious or depressed adolescents, or those with lower perceived health, may feel sleepier.

A systematic review on the functional consequences of inadequate sleep in adolescents, by Shochat, Cohen-Zion, and Tzischinsky (2014) concluded that prospective studies have demonstrated that sleep problems and/or sleep deprivation increase the risk for subsequent mental/emotional dysfunction (e.g., Fredriksen, Rhodes, Reddy, & Way, 2004; Roberts et al., 2009). Fredriksen and colleagues (2004) focused on the role of sleep in predicting psychosocial outcomes using survey data from 11- to 14-year-old students over three consecutive years. The authors reported that while short sleep (sleeping 6 hours or less) on school nights increased the risk of depressive symptoms and lower self-esteem, the latter measures did not predict future short sleep. Sleep seemed to be playing a significant role in predicting depressive symptoms and self-esteem, although it is not possible to confirm a direct causal pathway. Roberts and colleagues examined associations between sleep disturbance and psychosocial outcomes in one baseline study with 11- to 17-year-olds and two prospective investigations from data collected a year later (Roberts, Roberts, & Chen, 2002; Roberts et al., 2009). When looking at psychosocial outcomes, short sleep duration was found to increase the subsequent risk for poor perceived mental health, poor life satisfaction, and problems at school.

As adolescents regularly experience shortened sleep on school nights, experimental studies have been conducted with the aim of better understanding the effects of sleep restriction on adolescents' mood and emotional regulation (Baum et al., 2014; Lo, Ong, Leong, Gooley, & Chee, 2016). Baum et al. (2014) compared sleep restriction (6.5 hours in bed per night for five nights) with an enhanced sleep duration (10 hours in bed per night for five nights) in 50 adolescents, aged 14–17 years, and included questionnaires on mood and mood regulation. They found that adolescents rated themselves as more tense/anxious and angry/hostile during sleep restriction compared with a longer sleep duration. Parents and adolescents also reported greater oppositionality/irritability and poorer emotional regulation during sleep restriction compared with a healthy sleep duration. Importantly, the study demonstrated that after only a few days of shortened sleep, at a level routinely experienced by many adolescents on school nights, adolescents were less able to regulate negative emotions and had worsened mood. However, other studies investigating sleep loss have found a decrease in positive emotions rather than an increase in negative emotions (Lo et al., 2016; Talbot et al., 2010). Lo and colleagues (2016) focused on subjective sleepiness and mood following sleep restriction in 15- to 19-year-old adolescents. During the manipulation period, those experiencing sleep restriction (5 hours in bed per night for a week) demonstrated an increase in subjective sleepiness and a decrease in positive mood whereas negative mood appeared to remain unaffected.

Risk-taking and Health Behaviours

Adolescence has been described as a period of development characterised by making risky decisions (Blakemore & Robbins, 2012). Adolescents appear to be particularly vulnerable to risk-taking behaviour and impulsivity. According to the 'dual systems' hypothesis, there is a developmental mismatch between the earlier maturation of sub-cortical regions (involved in emotional and reward processing) and the later maturation of prefrontal regions (involved in cognitive control) (Casey, Getz, & Galvan, 2008; Steinberg, 2008). Evidence supports a dissociation between the slower, linear development of impulse control and response inhibition versus the nonlinear development of the reward system, which in adolescence is often particularly responsive (Blakemore & Robbins, 2012). Steinberg (2008) suggested that increases in risk-taking were mainly due to increases in sensation-seeking behaviours linked to changes in the dopaminergic system around the time of puberty. Social context is also influential as adolescents are more likely than other age groups to make risky decisions in 'hot' contexts, for example when in the company of their peers. In this instance, peer approval constitutes the potential reward (Blakemore & Robbins, 2012).

Sleep is pertinent as not getting enough sleep may increase the likelihood that students have difficulty coping with everyday tasks and challenges and may subsequently engage in risky behaviours (Pasch et al., 2010). Executive function, which refers to a range of higher-order cognitive processes, can be impaired with insufficient sleep; for example, those reporting high levels of sleepiness have demonstrated detriments in executive functioning (Anderson, Storfer-Isser, Taylor, Rosen, & Redline, 2009). Telzer, Fuligni, Lieberman, and Galván (2013) took (fMRI) scans of 46 adolescents while they completed a cognitive control and risk-taking task. On the basis of their behavioural findings, the authors suggested that adolescents with poorer sleep quality may be more apathetic, less confident, and take less care during decision making. They also suggested that the normative imbalance between affective and cognitive control systems may be exaggerated by poor sleep.

Evidence supports associations between sleep and adolescent risk and health-compromising behaviours (O'Brien & Mindell, 2005; McKnight-Eily et al., 2011; Pasch et al., 2010). However, although these studies provide an insight into relations between sleep and risk behaviours, it is not possible to draw conclusions on the temporality of these associations. O'Brien and Mindell (2005) examined the relationship between adolescents' sleep-wake patterns (including total sleep times, bedtimes, weekend delay, and oversleep) and risk-taking behaviour measured using seven subscales from the Youth Risk Behavior Survey (including safety behaviours, violence behaviours, tobacco, alcohol, marijuana and drug use, and sexual behaviours). Adolescents who reported insufficient sleep also reported increased risk-taking behaviours compared to those who reported more adequate sleep. Students' total sleep time on a school night had a limited relationship to self-reported risk-taking behaviour (i.e., alcohol use). However, the magnitude of the discrepancy between weekday and weekend bedtime did relate to self-reported risk-taking behaviour. This is independent from weekend oversleep where adolescents delay their wake time to 'catch up' on lost sleep.

Pasch and colleagues (2010) also asked adolescents to complete a self-report survey on risk behaviours and sleep measures. Adequate sleep during the school week was associated with lower risk behaviours. It suggested that if students slept less on weekdays, they were more likely to report alcohol use and drunkenness in the past month compared to those who reported longer weekday sleep duration. In addition, some of the variables suggesting inconsistent sleep patterns were significant, with those reporting greater weekend delays and oversleeps more likely to report substance use behaviours and truancy. In a further study focusing on relationships between sleep and risk behaviours, McKnight-Eily and colleagues (2011) investigated associations between insufficient sleep (<8 hours on average school nights) and health-risk behaviours. The authors found that insufficient sleep on an average school night was associated with ten of the 11 health-risk behaviours examined including current cigarette, alcohol, and marijuana use, sexual activity, physical fighting, and seriously considered attempting suicide.

Sleep appears to play a part in adolescent health in other ways. Adequate sleep has been found to positively associate with health-promoting behaviour. Adolescents who obtained adequate sleep (defined in the study as 6–8 hours per night) in a Taiwanese sample were found to have a higher frequency of health-promoting behaviours such as stress management, healthy diet, and exercise, as well as a higher total score of health-promoting behaviour than those who did not obtain adequate sleep (Chen, Wang, & Jeng, 2006). Sleep deprivation has also been found to associate with adolescents' self-report of health-related quality of life and perceived health (Paiva, Gaspar, & Matos, 2015).

In summary, the quantity and quality of sleep experienced by adolescents, (for example, not getting enough sleep, discrepancies between school night and weekend bedtimes, and subjective feelings of sleepiness) may be linked to their psychological and physical wellbeing. This may, in turn, be related to an adolescent's behaviour and their ability to function well at school.

The Direct Impact of Sleep Loss on Education

The Role of Sleep in Memory Consolidation

Learned information (encoded) needs to undergo a process of consolidation to be accessible for retrieval at a later date (memory retention). Jenkins and Dallenbach (1924) were the first researchers to identify that memory retention improves after a period of sleep. Since then, numerous studies have further evaluated and strengthened the importance of sleep in memory processing (for example, see reviews by Diekelmann, Wilhelm, & Born, 2009; Rasch & Born 2013). In their review, Rasch and Born state that sleep is not simply a period of reduced cognitive load where the brain is able to devote energy to memory consolidation but rather sleep affords active memory consolidating processes.

Initially, it was hypothesised that as sleep can be categorised into two distinct states, NREM and REM, so too would these different states have different roles in memory consolidation; this is known as the dual process hypothesis (Stickgold, 2005). This hypothesis states that declarative information (e.g., episodic/events or fact based) is consolidated during NREM sleep, whereas procedural (e.g., riding a bike) information is consolidated during REM sleep. As we know the first third of sleep is predominately NREM sleep, this hypothesis suggests that, in terms of classroom learning, the typical adolescent behaviour of late bedtimes and curtailing sleep would not have a large impact on declarative memory performance. Sleep and memory are independently complex processes; the interaction between the two is still not fully understood (Smith, 2001). Smith concluded that it is the sleep cycles (the repeated cycling between NREM and REM sleep) that result in memory processing. Specifically, memories are selected and processed during the NREM sleep period and are then redistributed and consolidated during the subsequent REM period (Giuditta et al., 1995). Again, in terms of declarative learning in the classroom, it is still NREM sleep whereby newly acquired information is encoded, but it is REM sleep where the information is stored for ease of retrieval at next use. Rasch and Born (2013) suggest therefore that sleep is an active state that is optimised for the consolidation of memories that are encoded during wake, and which are then replayed, consolidated, and reorganised during the different stages of sleep. It is during the deep sleep/slow wave component of NREM sleep that newly learnt information is thought to be replayed, redistributed, and integrated with existing long-term memories. This learnt information/memory is stabilised in a consolidation process during REM (Born & Wilhelm, 2012). Therefore, it is not simply about promoting the initial third of the night, which is predominantly deep sleep, but ensuring that an adolescent has sleep of a sufficient length to achieve a satisfactory number of sleep cycles.

This hypothesis is complemented by the synaptic homeostasis hypothesis which states that during wake we have synaptic potentiation and so during sleep these pathways are reduced to afford greater efficiency of information retrieval and an improved energy balance in the brain. It is suggested that synaptic downscaling occurs in slow wave sleep, and is evidenced through the sleep homeostatic process (from the two-process model), whereby the longer we are awake, the greater the sleep pressure, and the greater the depth of slow wave sleep in the subsequent sleep period (Tononi & Cirelli, 2003, 2006). Therefore, an adolescent who is learning all day and generating new synapses (forming memories) will require a proportionate amount of slow wave sleep during the night to be able to consolidate those memories and efficiently retrieve the newly learnt information later on.

As discussed previously, children have significantly more deep/slow wave sleep than adults. When a small study compared adults' (18–35 years) and children's (8–11 years) abilities to recall a motor sequence following a sleep or wake period, children showed a significantly greater improvement in learning than adults when testing followed a sleep period (Wilhelm et al., 2013). This improvement in learning was associated with the significant difference in slow wave activity in the sleep period after being presented with the sequence to memorise. A review of 15 studies identified measures of sleep, including sleep duration, sleepiness, and poor sleeper status, associated with measures of memory consolidation and working memory in children/adolescents (7–18 years): The poorer the reported sleep measure, the worse the child/adolescent performed on the measure of memory (Kopasz et al., 2010). We know that adolescents have a tendency to curtail sleep on school nights (Ohayon et al., 2004), shortening sleep duration and potentially reducing the number of sleep cycles. Furthermore, adolescents experience a 40% decrease in their slow wave sleep as they move through puberty into adulthood (Campbell et al., 2011). To date, there is very little research evaluating these naturalistic changes in adolescent sleep, specifically the potential impact of the reduction of slow wave sleep, on memory and learning. However, one could theorise that without sufficient NREM sleep or duration of sleep for sufficient sleep cycling, memory encoding and consolidation would be impaired—a salient point for education, considering that it is during adolescence when the majority of students take their final compulsory examinations.

Sleepiness and Learning

Unsurprisingly, research has indicated that older adolescents report higher levels of daytime sleepiness than younger adolescents, an effect potentially driven through the sleep changes at puberty (Sadeh et al., 2000). Additionally, we know that partial sleep deprivation, as indicated by short sleep durations on weeknights, also associates with subjective reports of sleepiness in the classroom (Anderson, Storfer-Isser, Taylor, Rosen, & Redline, 2009; Wolfson & Carskadon, 1998).

Sleepiness, to some degree through fluctuations in our natural daily rhythm, is to be expected in the classroom (Buysse, Monk, Carrier, & Begley, 2005). However, problems can occur, when sleepiness significantly interferes with functioning. Within a study of 236 adolescents, 72 of the students self-reported above-normal levels of daytime sleepiness (Anderson et al., 2009). Compared to the students with normative sleepiness levels, the students reporting higher-than-normal levels of sleepiness had a greater chance of experiencing a night of short sleep (less than 6.5 hours) and greater night-to-night variability in sleep duration. Detriments to parent-reported student executive functioning (metacognition: the ability to track information and monitor actions during daily living activities and behavioural regulation: the ability to self-regulate behaviour) were significantly associated with higher levels of student sleepiness but not with sleep duration. The association found between executive function and sleepiness was driven primarily through changes in metacognition, suggesting that adolescents who feel sleepy in the classroom regardless of the amount they slept the night before may experience an impaired ability to track information and therefore learn efficiently during school.

Potential Resilience to the Direct Impact of Short Term Sleep Loss in Adolescence

There is a distinct lack of evidence supporting objective changes in executive function following sleep loss in adolescents, with some researchers suggesting that adolescents may be more resilient to a forced reduction in sleep duration compared to adults (Carskadon, Harvey, & Dement, 1981a; Carskadon, Harvey, & Dement, 1981b). A preliminary study using fMRI in six sleep-deprived adolescents found that, during a working memory task, adolescents had greater activity than expected in regions specific to attention-based tasks. This may represent a compensatory mechanism which allows performance to remain similar to a well-rested state in the face of compromised sleep (Beebe, DiFrancesco, Tlustos, McNally, & Holland, 2009). In an early study by Carskadon and colleagues (1981a), 12 adolescents were kept awake for 36 hours and, despite increases in both subjective and objective sleepiness, there were no significant effects of sleep deprivation on attention (listening task) in computerised testing, performance (finger tapping speed), and simple addition skills (percentage of correct answers in a numerical task). However, students were found to attempt fewer addition questions in the allotted time when sleep deprived (indicative of reduced processing speed) and had a reduced memory recall ability (paired words). When this group's sleep was reduced to just four hours per night, using the same tasks as the 36-hour sleep restriction study, no changes were identified in processing speed or memory recall ability (Carskadon et al., 1981b), again suggesting that adolescents may be resilient to performance deficits following short-term sleep restriction. A larger study assigned 76 adolescents to one of five sleep conditions ranging from sufficient (9 and 8 hours) to restricted (7, 6, or 5 hours) for four nights (Voderholzer et al., 2011). Restricted sleep was obtained by delaying the bedtime, something which adolescents are known to do and mimicking the adolescent preference for delayed sleep timing. The length of the sleep restriction correlated with an increase in deep sleep (percentage of amount of deep sleep to total sleep time), a shortened time to fall asleep, fewer awakenings, and more efficient sleep. In summary, the shorter sleep resulted in more consolidated sleep. The authors suggested that this response to the short-term sleep restriction afforded adolescents resilience to the immediate impact of sleep loss as, following two nights of recovery sleep, the sleep restricted participants showed no changes in the ability to recall procedural (mirror tracing) or declarative (word pairs) memories.

However, this resilience to shortened sleep seems to occur when only bed times are delayed. Lo and colleagues (2016) restricted (5 hours) or extended (9 hours) sleep for seven nights and tested participants three times each day for deficits in cognitive functioning. Restriction was achieved through delaying bedtimes and earlier rise times. Unsurprisingly, when compared to students in the nine-hour sleep opportunity group, the students under sleep restriction showed deficits in a number of cognitive functions including executive functioning, working memory, and sustained attention. Following sleep restriction, the students in this group had three recovery nights (9 hours per night) and, again, had their cognitive performance tested three times a day. The authors reported that, following two nights of recovery sleep, the students who had been sleep restricted still showed deficits in their processing speed, ability to sustain attention, and alertness levels. These lingering effects of sleep restriction resulted in the students' performance on the cognitive tasks to be lower than at baseline. Similar deficits to working memory were identified by Jiang and colleagues (2011) when 20 adolescents' sleep was restricted to six hours in bed per night for five school nights counterbalanced with five school nights of eight hours' sleep (Jiang et al., 2011). Importantly, the adolescents showed changes in working memory following restricted sleep compared to eight hours of sleep without showing concurrent increases in self-reported sleepiness. This suggests that adolescents may experience impaired cognitive performance in the classroom because of insufficient sleep without reporting subjective complaints of sleep loss. An adolescent may be subjectively unaware of their tiredness.

The Impact of Insufficient Sleep in the Classroom

Many adolescents are thought to suffer from poor sleep quantity and quality which, alongside sleepiness, impacts their ability to learn which in turn affects their academic potential (Curcio, Ferrara, & Gennaro, 2006). Teacher reports have identified that when students (aged 6–12 years) followed a sleep restriction protocol (8 hours for younger students, 6.5 hours for older students), teachers' ratings of academic performance and attention were comparatively lower relative to baseline (Fallone, Acebo, Seifer, & Carskadon, 2005). Fallone and colleagues also attempted to extend the students' sleep (time in bed >10 hours); however, despite increase in teacher-reported attention comparative to baseline, no significant changes in academic performance were reported by the teachers. When slightly older, pre-adolescents (8–12 years), had their sleep restricted or extended by one hour each night for four nights, despite finding no differences in attention between groups, those in the sleep restriction group showed deficits in working memory and a mathematics fluency task comparative to those in the sleep extension group (Vriend et al., 2013). Therefore, this study highlights that even a moderate sleep restriction, if sustained over the week, could have a marked impact on the classroom.

Sixteen adolescents underwent a counterbalanced protocol of school-week sleep extension (10 hours in bed) and sleep restriction (6.5 hours in bed), with a 'washout' period over the weekend when students selected their own bed-times and performance was evaluated in a simulated classroom setting (Beebe, Rose, & Amin, 2010). Following the week of sleep extension/restriction, students went to a simulated classroom on a Saturday morning. This paradigm allowed the researchers to objectively evaluate learning performance (quiz) following a novel learning scenario (a 30-minute educational film) whilst observing classroom behaviour via video recordings and objective measures of sleepiness/alertness using electroencephalography. In the sleep restricted condition, students performed worse in the novel learning quiz, showed more inattentive behaviours in the classroom and had more intrusions of sleep-like activity in the electroencephalogram (increase in theta activity) when com-pared to the sleep extension condition.

The studies just discussed use standard scientific testing platforms to eval-uate cognitive functioning in sleep-deprived adolescents, then apply the changes seen to the classroom environment, which might not provide the most ecologically valid assessment of the true impact of sleep deprivation in the classroom. That said, a small number of studies have attempted to evaluate the direct impact of sleep on academic performance in a classroom setting and have evaluated performance in the classroom using teacher reports or student self-reported academic grades. An early evaluation of 3000 American high school students indicated a relationship between good sleep stability (i.e., fewer awakenings, shorter weekend lie-ins etc.) and academic achievement, with those who had poorer grades reporting shorter sleep durations (Wolf-son & Carskadon, 1998). In another example, a large Swedish survey looked at the sleep of approximately 40,000 adolescents (aged 12–19 years) between 2005 and 2011 (Titova et al., 2015). The authors identified that students who reported any sleep disturbances in the past three months were more likely to fail a subject at school than those who did not report any disturbance. In addition, those who reported significantly insufficient sleep, defined as less than seven hours' sleep on both week and weekend nights, were more likely to fail a subject than those who reported seven hours or more sleep on week and weekend nights.

Both of these studies used subjective reporting of academic performance to elucidate the impact of sleep deprivation on performance in the classroom, a teacher-given grade of their performance in a particular subject (US), and a student report of missed grade target (Sweden). When standard school meas-ures of performance are used (standard examination results), it appears that it is sleep quality that mediates the impact of sleep on academic outcomes as opposed to sleep duration. A small study of 36 Italian adolescents found that although sleep timing (morningness/eveningness) preference correlated with exam results, this relationship was mediated through objective sleep effi-ciency (Tonetti, Fabbri, Filardi, Martoni, & Natale, 2015). Sleep efficiency is a marker of sleep quality encompassing time taken to fall asleep and time awake during the sleep period. Surprisingly, despite the previously mentioned evidence on the impact of short sleep duration on working memory and attention, the study by Tonetti and colleagues did not find any association between subjective or objective sleep duration with final exam results. This finding has been replicated in 75 younger Canadian students (aged approximately 9 years) showing that sleep efficiency, and not sleep duration, associated with academic performance in standard school mathematics, English language, and French as a second language (Gruber et al., 2014).

Sleep plays a vital role in the ability to follow information presented in the classroom and then to encode and consolidate that learned information to memory. Adolescents appear to have some resilience to partial, short-term, sleep restriction but poor sleep quality (lots of awakenings) and poor sleep stability (using the weekend to catch up) has been associated with poorer academic performance. Sleepiness may also impact academic potential, without the student recognising/reporting that they are feeling tired.

What Can Schools Do to Help Improve Adolescent Sleep?

Given that adolescence is a developmental period characterised by significant biological changes and adolescents are known to be a chronically sleep-deprived population, it is important to consider interventions to increase the likelihood that adolescents get enough sleep. As well as the changes in biological processes identified earlier, many other factors have been found to contribute to sleep in this age group. Social and environmental factors, for example, culture (Gradisar et al., 2011) and family environment and structure (Troxel, Lee, Hall, & Matthews, 2014) can influence sleep behaviour. Psychosocial factors with a particular relevance at this age include greater autonomy in setting bedtimes (Carskadon, 2011), an increase in peer influence (Steinberg & Silverberg, 1986), sacrificing sleep in order to fulfil both homework requirements and an increased need for social activities (Wahlstrom et al., 2014), social stresses including anxieties and emotional arousal (Dahl & Lewin, 2002), and use of electronic media before bedtime (Cain & Gradisar, 2010). At an organisational level, schools and educational policy makers are in a unique position to use an understanding of sleep science to address the issue of sleep deprivation. A school is ideally placed to reach the adolescent population. Accordingly, schools have been encouraged to take part in interventions by delaying their start times or implementing sleep education programmes within the classroom.

School Interventions: Start Times

Early school start times could be considered at odds with the biologically driven shift for delayed sleep in adolescence, increasing the likelihood that students will experience insufficient sleep by forcing them to wake at times inappropriate to their biology, and by limiting the window available for sleep during the school week. Later school start times are proposed to benefit students by enabling their circadian rhythms to be synchronised with the school schedule, meaning that they are not required to be in classes before their wake-promoting process is fully engaged (Kirby, Maggi, & D'Angiulli, 2011).

To address the 'epidemic of adolescent sleep loss' (Owens, Drobnich, Baylor, & Lewin, 2014, p. 182), the most high profile and concerted drive for later school start times has occurred in the U.S. Here, the Start School Later organisation has raised public awareness about the relationship between sleep and school hours and campaigned for later start times[1] (www.startschoollater.net). Coupled with this, major health organisations such as the American Academy of Pediatrics (2014), and the American Academy of Sleep Medicine, the professional society dedicated to the promotion of sleep health (Watson et al., 2017), have recommended that start times be no earlier than 8.30 a.m. in middle and high schools. Despite this, according to the Centers for Disease Control and Prevention, most middle and high schools in the US still start before this suggested time, with an average start of 8:03 a.m.

A good deal of research has now provided compelling evidence that delaying school start times leads to an increase in students' sleep duration and a decrease in self-reported sleepiness (Boergers, Gable, & Owens, 2014; Bowers & Moyer, 2017; Minges & Redeker, 2016; Owens, Dearth-Wesley, Herman, Oakes, & Whitaker, 2017). Improvements in other variables such as mood (Owens, Belon, & Moss, 2010), tardiness and disciplinary issues (Thacher & Onyper, 2016) and attendance (Wahlstrom, 2002) have also been reported.

Owens and colleagues (2017) surveyed self-reported sleep duration and daytime sleepiness in 11 secondary and high schools before and after the school start times were delayed by 50 minutes (7:20 to 8:10 a.m.). After the delay, students were found to sleep approximately 30 minutes longer on school nights and reported less daytime sleepiness. A question which has arisen in discussions concerning the validity of delaying start times is whether adolescents will simply go to bed later if they are given the opportunity to sleep later. The schoolnight bedtime in this high school group was only delayed by approximately 7 minutes whereas the wake times were around 38 minutes later. The finding that the bedtime was only marginally delayed is consistent with other studies which have found that bedtimes were mostly unchanged (Boergers et al., 2014; Wahlstrom, 2002).

A meta-analysis conducted by Bowers and Moyer (2017) demonstrated that later school start times were associated with students obtaining more sleep after aggregating data from five longitudinal and 15 cross-sectional studies. In the longitudinal studies included in the analysis, delaying start times was found to increase sleep duration from the first to the second time point by approximately 20 minutes. As well as this extension to sleep, later school start times overall were associated with less daytime sleepiness and a reduction in tardiness, which has implications for increased engagement in learning and improved educational outcomes.

A systematic review by Minges and Redeker (2016) evaluated the effect of delayed start times on sleep, health, and academic parameters in six pre–post studies which satisfied their selection criteria. All six studies reported sleep outcomes; three reported health-related outcomes and five reported academic-related outcomes. Evidence supported delayed start times as an effective method of improving all these outcomes, albeit with caveats. The school delay ranged from 25 to 60 minutes, with a corresponding increase in total sleep time on weekdays observed in all studies, ranging from 25 to 77 minutes per school night, suggesting a dose-response relationship. Improved school-related outcomes included decreased tardiness, less falling asleep in class, fewer students reporting being too tired to do homework, and improved reaction times and attention levels in class. However, the two studies that evaluated academic achievement pre–post delay found no significant difference in self-reported grades of B or higher. While some evidence was found for reduced depression and caffeine use, findings regarding changes in health-related outcomes were mixed and taken from too few studies to make substantive inferences. The authors concluded that future studies were needed using a randomised design with a reporting of consistent outcomes.

Empirical evidence supporting a link between school start times and academic performance is limited to date. Evaluating the potential effect of delayed start times on academic performance is not straightforward. For example, class grading is not standardised and tests which are standardised (e.g., Scholastic Aptitude Test) are not taken by all students. In addition, findings may be compromised by ceiling effects for those students who academically perform very well before any delay is initiated (Wahlstrom, 2002; Wheaton, Chapman, & Croft, 2016). The first longitudinal study of later high school start times was based on findings from seven schools when the Minneapolis Public School District moved start times from 7:15 a.m. to 8:40 a.m. in 1997 (Wahlstrom, 2002). Analysis of class letter grades obtained during the three years before and three years after the change to a later start time faced many obstacles given the difficulty in obtaining 'clean' data (p. 11). Students' letter grades revealed a slight improvement but this was not statistically significant. However, students in schools with the late start were getting an hour's more sleep each school night than their peers whose schools began an hour earlier, and this was still true four years after the change. The authors cautioned that grades were often rather subjective and that when looking at the benefits of later starts, many measures of success, such as student emotional wellbeing, should be used.

Edwards (2012) investigated the impact of school start times on standardised tests (end of grade test scores in maths and reading) in middle school students (grades 6–8) in North Carolina, U.S., from 1999 to 2006. Cross-sectional analysis revealed that later school start times corresponded with higher test scores in both maths and reading, with an average 3 percentile point gain for a one-hour later start time. Longitudinal analysis also revealed a change in the same direction but in this instance a one-hour change corresponded with a 2 percentile point improvement in maths and a 1.5 percentile point improvement in reading. Wheaton and colleagues (2016) reviewed 38 reports encompassing cross-sectional and longitudinal studies of school start times. The authors concluded that some evidence indicated a positive association between later school start times and academic performance. However, this association was not always demonstrated in the findings of these reports and when found, could be relatively weak.

Given the links between sleep and emotional functioning discussed earlier, researchers have also assessed whether later start times might be associated with improved mood. Boergers et al. (2014) found that after a modest 25-minute delay (8 a.m. to 8:25 a.m.) in a private residential high school, students' sleep increased by 29 minutes each school night and their scores decreased on the Depression Mood subscale of the School Sleep Habits Survey (SSHS; Wolfson & Carskadon, 1998), indicating a reduction in depressed mood. This pattern was also found in an independent high school in Rhode Island which delayed from 8:00 a.m. to 8:30 a.m. with a corresponding increase in school-night sleep duration of 45 minutes and a reduction in self-reported depressed mood (Owens et al., 2010). Sleep duration on school nights was negatively correlated with depressive symptoms. There was also a reduction in the percentage of students who reported feeling irritated or annoyed. However, neither of the previously mentioned studies included a control group so positive changes in sleep cannot be attributed solely to delays in start times. In contrast, a Norwegian study did not find a significant difference between an intervention and a control school in positive or negative affect, although the intervention school only implemented the delay on Monday mornings.

School Interventions: Education

School-based sleep education programmes have been proposed as a means to put sleep health on the school agenda and to promote sufficient sleep as an everyday goal for adolescents. Two types of interventions have been identified and implemented: those that aim to change sleep behaviour, and those that aim to disseminate information and improve sleep knowledge (Blunden & Rigney, 2015). Sleep knowledge has generally been found to significantly improve following education (Cain, Gradisar, & Moseley, 2011; Moseley & Gradisar, 2009). Although reviews of the success of sleep education programmes found that increases in sleep knowledge did not necessarily correspond with increased sleep duration or better sleep hygiene practices (Blunden, Chapman, & Rigney, 2012) or sustained sleep behavioural change (Cassoff, Knäuper, Michaelsen, & Gruber, 2013). Adding to this literature, Chan and colleagues (2016) conducted a randomised controlled trial (RCT) with 14 secondary schools in Hong Kong to promote good sleep practices. In agreement with previous studies, sleep knowledge significantly improved in the intervention group compared with the control group. However, this was not translated into an improvement in self-reported sleep duration or pattern. Regarding other outcomes, there was a significant enhancement in students' behavioural health and mental health. The exact reasons for this are unclear and cannot be attributed to improvements in sleep.

An RCT run by Bonnar and colleagues in six Australian high schools has provided promising results (2015). Classes were assigned to one of four conditions: control; sleep education plus parental involvement; sleep education plus bright light therapy; or sleep education plus both parental involvement and bright light therapy. Students' sleep knowledge and sleep (measured by self-report) improved for those who received sleep education relative to the control group. From pre- to post-intervention, sleep onset latency on school nights decreased by 15 minutes and total sleep time on school nights increased by 27 minutes on average for intervention groups. All intervention groups demonstrated similar improvements, which suggested that bright light therapy and parental involvement did not provide additional benefits. Additionally, small improvements were found in depressed mood in each of the intervention groups, whereas only a negligible change occurred for the control group.

From a methodological perspective, study limitations have included small sample size, lack of control group or follow-up measurement. Studies have tended to use a subjective (e.g., sleep diaries, questionnaires) rather than a pseudo-objective measurement (e.g., Actiwatches) of sleep patterns and it has been recommended that the use of standardised tools would facilitate more confidence in data collection and comparability between studies (Blunden & Rigney, 2015).

Concluding Remarks

What Has Neuroscience Added to Our Understanding Over and Above Psychology?

This chapter outlines the important role sleep plays in physical and psychological health, highlighting the direct impact of sleep on brain function and the indirect effect sleep might have via its effect on behaviour and emotion regulation. Whilst many of the outcomes focus on subjective reports of mood and behaviour and so are fundamentally psychological, advances in our understanding of the specific role of sleep stages and how these change in response to development are helping us to fully appreciate the complexity of sleep and its impact on memory and mood. Specific to adolescents, the understanding that the delay in timing is driven at the cellular level is shaping the research in this area. Work investigating delaying the school start time and altering bedtimes is directly driven by this understanding of the basic system. In this way, sleep research very clearly represents the crossroads between biology, psychology, and cognitive neuroscience.

Concrete Implications of Research and Opportunities for Translation

There are very practical implications to much of the research around adolescent sleep and education. Sleep has an impact on behaviour in the classroom and on the ability to learn. Insufficient sleep, poor sleep quality, and sleepiness all impact on a student's academic potential. Furthermore, research suggests that alongside experiencing a resilience to short-term sleep restriction, adolescents do not need to report feeling sleepy for objective sleepiness to have an influence in the classroom. This has since led to researchers trying to identify interventions that can be utilised in schools to address adolescent sleep. As discussed, there is debate around delaying school start times to better suit the adolescent body clock (a neuroscience/biological approach), as well as sleep education interventions (a behavioural/psychological approach) currently being tested and developed which are showing promise. Both have the potential to translate to policy, certainly in the statutory inclusion of healthy sleep education alongside other mandated health and wellbeing topics.

Other avenues for exploration would be the impact of scheduled napping to boost memory consolidation and improve alertness, bright lights in the morning to influence the clock, and the interplay between physical activity and sleep. The question of bright light is particularly interesting, specifically as bright light in the morning is a recognised intervention for advancing the clock. It is not clear why the circadian delay happens in adolescence. Thus, manipulating the clock using light might provide some insight into why the delay happens and its role in development generally, alongside insight into a potential therapeutic tool for adolescents experiencing particularly poor sleep.

With the emerging neuroscience and psychology research, sleepy teenagers in the classroom may no longer need to be the norm.

Further Reading

- Oxford Sparks: What Makes You Tick (including teaching resources)

  www.oxfordsparks.ox.ac.uk/what-makes-you-tick

- BBC Terrific Scientific—What happens when I sleep (including teaching resources)

  www.bbc.co.uk/guides/zx642nb

- National Sleep Foundation—Later School Start Times

  https://sleepfoundation.org/sleep-news/backgrounder-later-school-start-times

- Start School Later coalition

  www.startschoollater.net/why-change.html

- National Sleep Foundation—Teens and Sleep

  https://sleepfoundation.org/sleep-topics/teens-and-sleep

Note

1. www.startschoollater.net

References

American Academy of Pediatrics. (2014). School start times for adolescents. *Pediatrics, 134*(3), 642–649.

Anderson, B., Storfer-Isser, A., Taylor, H. G., Rosen, C. L., & Redline, S. (2009). Associations of executive function with sleepiness and sleep duration in adolescents. *Pediatrics, 123*(4), e701–e707.

Baum, K. T., Desai, A., Field, J., Miller, L. E., Rausch, J., & Beebe, D. W. (2014). Sleep restriction worsens mood and emotion regulation in adolescents. *Journal of Child Psychology and Psychiatry, 55*(2), 180–190.

Beebe, D. W., DiFrancesco, M. W., Tlustos, S. J., McNally, K. A., & Holland, S. K. (2009). Preliminary fMRI findings in experimentally sleep-restricted adolescents engaged in a working memory task. *Behavioral and Brain Functions, 5*(1), 9.

Beebe, D. W., Rose, D., & Amin, R. (2010). Attention, learning, and arousal of experimentally sleep-restricted adolescents in a simulated classroom. *Journal of Adolescent Health, 47*(5), 523–525.

Blakemore, S. J., & Robbins, T. W. (2012). Decision-making in the adolescent brain. *Nature Neuroscience, 15*(9), 1184–1191.

Blunden, S. L., Chapman, J., & Rigney, G. A. (2012). Are education programs successful? The case for improved and consistent efforts. *Sleep Medicine Reviews, 16*(4), 355–370.

Blunden, S. L., & Rigney, G. (2015). Lessons learned from sleep education in schools: A review of dos and don'ts. *Journal of Clinical Sleep Medicine: JCSM: Official Publication of the American Academy of Sleep Medicine, 11*(6), 671.

Boergers, J., Gable, C. J., & Owens, J. A. (2014). Later school start time is associated with improved sleep and daytime functioning in adolescents. *Journal of Developmental & Behavioral Pediatrics, 35*(1), 11–17.

Bonnar, D., Gradisar, M., Moseley, L., Coughlin, A. M., Cain, N., & Short, M. A. (2015). Evaluation of novel school-based interventions for adolescent sleep problems: Does parental involvement and bright light improve outcomes? *Sleep Health, 1*(1), 66–74.

Borbély, A. A. (1982). A two process model of sleep regulation. *Human Neurobiology, 1*(3), 195–204.

Born, J., & Wilhelm, I. (2012). System consolidation of memory during sleep. *Psychological Research, 76*(2), 192–203.

Bowers, J. M., & Moyer, A. (2017). Effects of school start time on students' sleep duration, daytime sleepiness, and attendance: A meta-analysis. *Sleep Health: Journal of the National Sleep Foundation, 3*(6), 423–431.

Brainard, G. C., Rollag, M. D., & Hanifin, J. P. (1997). Photic regulation of melatonin in humans: Ocular and neural signal transduction. *Journal of Biological Rhythms, 12*(6), 537–546.

Brown, S. A., Kunz, D., Dumas, A., Westermark, P. O., Vanselow, K., Tilmann-Wahnschaffe, A., . . . Kramer, A. (2008). Molecular insights into human daily behavior. *Proceedings of the National Academy of Sciences, 105*(5), 1602–1607.

Buhr, E. D., & Takahashi, J. S. (2013). Molecular components of the mammalian circadian clock. In *Circadian clocks* (pp. 3–27). Berlin and Heidelberg: Springer.

Buysse, D. J., Monk, T. H., Carrier, J., & Begley, A. (2005). Circadian patterns of sleep, sleepiness, and performance in older and younger adults. *Sleep, 28*(11), 1365–1376.

Cain, N., & Gradisar, M. (2010). Electronic media use and sleep in school-aged children and adolescents: A review. *Sleep Medicine, 11*(8), 735–742.

Cain, N., Gradisar, M., & Moseley, L. (2011). A motivational school-based intervention for adolescent sleep problems. *Sleep Medicine*, *12*(3), 246–251.

Campbell, I. G., Darchia, N., Higgins, L. M., Dykan, I. V., Davis, N. M., Bie, E. D., & Feinberg, I. (2011). Adolescent changes in homeostatic regulation of EEG activity in the delta and theta frequency bands during NREM sleep. *Sleep*, *34*(1), 83–91.

Cappuccio, F. P., D'Elia, L., Strazzullo, P., & Miller, M. A. (2010). Sleep duration and all-cause mortality: A systematic review and meta-analysis of prospective studies. *Sleep*, *33*(5), 585–592.

Carskadon, M. A. (2011). Sleep in adolescents: The perfect storm. *Pediatric Clinics of North America*, *58*(3), 637–647.

Carskadon, M. A., & Dement, W. C. (2011). Monitoring and staging human sleep. In M. H. Kryger, T. Roth, & W. C. Dement (Eds.), *Principles and practice of sleep medicine* (5th ed., pp. 16–26). St. Louis: Elsevier Saunders.

Carskadon, M. A., Harvey, K., & Dement, W. C. (1981a). Sleep loss in young adolescents. *Sleep*, *4*(3), 299–312.

Carskadon, M. A., Harvey, K., & Dement, W. C. (1981b). Acute restriction of nocturnal sleep in children. *Perceptual and Motor Skills*, *53*(1), 103–112.

Carskadon, M. A., Harvey, K., Duke, P., Anders, T. F., Litt, I. F., & Dement, W. C. (1980). Pubertal changes in daytime sleepiness. *Sleep*, *2*(4), 453–460.

Casey, B. J., Getz, S., & Galvan, A. (2008). The adolescent brain. *Developmental Review*, *28*, 62–77.

Cassoff, J., Knäuper, B., Michaelsen, S., & Gruber, R. (2013). School-based sleep promotion programs: Effectiveness, feasibility and insights for future research. *Sleep Medicine Reviews*, *17*(3), 207–214.

Chan, N. Y., Lam, S. P., Zhang, J., Yu, M. W. M., Li, S. X., Li, A. M., & Wing, Y. K. (2016). Sleep education in Hong Kong. *Sleep and Biological Rhythms*, *14*(1), 21–25.

Chen, M. Y., Wang, E. K., & Jeng, Y. J. (2006). Adequate sleep among adolescents is positively associated with health status and health-related behaviors. *BMC Public Health*, *6*(1), 59.

Chen, T., Wu, Z., Shen, Z., Zhang, J., Shen, X., & Li, S. (2014). Sleep duration in Chinese adolescents: Biological, environmental, and behavioral predictors. *Sleep Medicine*, *15*(11), 1345–1353.

Crowley, S. J., Acebo, C., & Carskadon, M. A. (2007). Sleep, circadian rhythms, and delayed phase in adolescence. *Sleep Medicine*, *8*(6), 602–612.

Curcio, G., Ferrara, M., & De Gennaro, L. (2006). Sleep loss, learning capacity and academic performance. *Sleep Medicine Reviews*, *10*(5), 323–337.

Czeisler, C. A., Duffy, J. F., Shanahan, T. L., Brown, E. N., Mitchell, J. F., Rimmer, D. W., . . . Dijk, D. J. (1999). Stability, precision, and near-24-hour period of the human circadian pacemaker. *Science*, *284*(5423), 2177–2181.

Czeisler, C. A., Richardson, G. S., Zimmerman, J. C., Moore-Ede, M. C., & Weitzman, E. D. (1981). Entrainment of human circadian rhythms by light-dark cycles: A reassessment. *Photochemistry and Photobiology*, *34*(2), 239–247.

Dahl, R. E. (1999). The consequences of insufficient sleep for adolescents: Links between sleep and emotional regulation. *Phi Delta Kappan*, *80*(5), 354.

Dahl, R. E., & Lewin, D. S. (2002). Pathways to adolescent health sleep regulation and behavior. *Journal of Adolescent Health*, *31*(6), 175–184.

Davidson, R. J. (2002). Anxiety and affective style: Role of prefrontal cortex and amygdala. *Biological Psychiatry*, *51*(1), 68–80.

Diekelmann, S., & Born, J. (2010). The memory function of sleep. *Nature Reviews Neuroscience*, 11(2), 114–126.

Diekelmann, S., Wilhelm, I., & Born, J. (2009). The whats and whens of sleep-dependent memory consolidation. *Sleep Medicine Reviews*, 13(5), 309–321.

Do, M. T. H., & Yau, K. W. (2010). Intrinsically photosensitive retinal ganglion cells. *Physiological Reviews*, 90(4), 1547–1581.

Donlea, J. M., Alam, M. N., & Szymusiak, R. (2017). Neuronal substrates of sleep homeostasis; lessons from flies, rats and mice. *Current Opinion in Neurobiology*, 44, 228–235.

Edwards, F. (2012). Early to rise? The effect of daily start times on academic performance. *Economics of Education Review*, 31(6), 970–983.

Fallone, G., Acebo, C., Seifer, R., & Carskadon, M. A. (2005). Experimental restriction of sleep opportunity in children: Effects on teacher ratings. *Sleep*, 28(12), 1561–1567.

Fallone, G., Owens, J. A., & Deane, J. (2002). Sleepiness in children and adolescents: Clinical implications. *Sleep Medicine Reviews*, 6(4), 287–306.

Foster, R. G., Provencio, I., Hudson, D., Fiske, S., De Grip, W., & Menaker, M. (1991). Circadian photoreception in the retinally degenerate mouse (rd/rd). *Journal of Comparative Physiology A*, 169(1), 39–50.

Franzen, P. L., Buysse, D. J., Dahl, R. E., Thompson, W., & Siegle, G. J. (2009). Sleep deprivation alters pupillary reactivity to emotional stimuli in healthy young adults. *Biological Psychology*, 80(3), 300–305.

Fredriksen, K., Rhodes, J., Reddy, R., & Way, N. (2004). Sleepless in Chicago: Tracking the effects of adolescent sleep loss during the middle school years. *Child Development*, 75(1), 84–95.

Giedd, J. N. (2004). Structural magnetic resonance imaging of the adolescent brain. *Annals of the New York Academy of Sciences*, 1021(1), 77–85.

Giuditta, A., Ambrosini, M. V., Montagnese, P., Mandile, P., Cotugno, M., Zucconi, G. G., & Vescia, S. (1995). The sequential hypothesis of the function of sleep. *Behavioural Brain Research*, 69(1), 157–166.

Gradisar, M., Gardner, G., & Dohnt, H. (2011). Recent worldwide sleep patterns and problems during adolescence: A review and meta-analysis of age, region, and sleep. *Sleep Medicine*, 12(2), 110–118.

Gregory, A. M., & Sadeh, A. (2012). Sleep, emotional and behavioral difficulties in children and adolescents. *Sleep Medicine Reviews*, 16(2), 129–136.

Gruber, R., Somerville, G., Enros, P., Paquin, S., Kestler, M., & Gillies-Poitras, E. (2014). Sleep efficiency (but not sleep duration) of healthy school-age children is associated with grades in math and languages. *Sleep Medicine*, 15(12), 1517–1525.

Hagenauer, M. H., Perryman, J. I., Lee, T. M., & Carskadon, M. A. (2009). Adolescent changes in the homeostatic and circadian regulation of sleep. *Developmental Neuroscience*, 31(4), 276–284.

Hirshkowitz, M., Whiton, K., Albert, S. M., Alessi, C., Bruni, O., DonCarlos, L., . . . Neubauer, D. N. (2015). National sleep foundation's sleep time duration recommendations: Methodology and results summary. *Sleep Health*, 1(1), 40–43.

Holst, S. C., & Landolt, H. P. (2015). Sleep homeostasis, metabolism, and adenosine. *Current Sleep Medicine Reports*, 1(1), 27–37.

Jenkins, J. G., & Dallenbach, K. M. (1924). Obliviscence during sleep and waking. *The American Journal of Psychology*, 35(4), 605–612.

Jenni, O. G., Achermann, P., & Carskadon, M. A. (2005). Homeostatic sleep regulation in adolescents. *Sleep*, 28(11), 1446–1454.

Jenni, O. G., & Carskadon, M. A. (2004). Spectral analysis of the sleep electroencephalogram during adolescence. *Sleep, 27*(4), 774–783.

Jiang, F., VanDyke, R. D., Zhang, J., Li, F., Gozal, D., & Shen, X. (2011). Effect of chronic sleep restriction on sleepiness and working memory in adolescents and young adults. *Journal of Clinical and Experimental Neuropsychology, 33*(8), 892–900.

Kirby, M., Maggi, S., & D'Angiulli, A. (2011). School start times and the sleep—wake cycle of adolescents: A review and critical evaluation of available evidence. *Educational Researcher, 40*(2), 56–61.

Kopasz, M., Loessl, B., Hornyak, M., Riemann, D., Nissen, C., Piosczyk, H., & Voderholzer, U. (2010). Sleep and memory in healthy children and adolescents—a critical review. *Sleep Medicine Reviews, 14*(3), 167–177.

Lo, J. C., Ong, J. L., Leong, R. L., Gooley, J. J., & Chee, M. W. (2016). Cognitive performance, sleepiness, and mood in partially sleep deprived adolescents: The need for sleep study. *Sleep, 39*(3), 687–698.

Manber, R., & Armitage, R. (1999). Sex, steroids, and sleep: A review. *Sleep, 22*(5), 540–541.

McKnight-Eily, L. R., Eaton, D. K., Lowry, R., Croft, J. B., Presley-Cantrell, L., & Perry, G. S. (2011). Relationships between hours of sleep and health-risk behaviors in US adolescent students. *Preventive Medicine, 53*(4), 271–273.

Minges, K. E., & Redeker, N. S. (2016). Delayed school start times and adolescent sleep: A systematic review of the experimental evidence. *Sleep Medicine Reviews, 28*, 86–95.

Mistlberger, R. E., & Skene, D. J. (2005). Nonphotic entrainment in humans? *Journal of Biological Rhythms, 20*(4), 339–352.

Moore, M., Kirchner, H. L., Drotar, D., Johnson, N., Rosen, C., Ancoli-Israel, S., & Redline, S. (2009). Relationships among sleepiness, sleep time, and psychological functioning in adolescents. *Journal of Pediatric Psychology, 34*(10), 1175–1183.

Monk, T. H., Buysse, D. J., Reynolds, C. F., Berga, S. L., Jarrett, D. B., Begley, A. E., & Kupfer, D. J. (1997). Circadian rhythms in human performance and mood under constant conditions. *Journal of Sleep Research, 6*(1), 9–18.

Moseley, L., & Gradisar, M. (2009). Evaluation of a school-based intervention for adolescent sleep problems. *Sleep, 32*(3), 334–341.

Must, A., & Strauss, R. S. (1999). Risks and consequences of childhood and adolescent obesity. *International Journal of Obesity, 23*(Suppl 2), S2.

O'Brien, E. M., & Mindell, J. A. (2005). Sleep and risk-taking behavior in adolescents. *Behavioral Sleep Medicine, 3*(3), 113–133.

Ohayon, M. M., Carskadon, M. A., Guilleminault, C., & Vitiello, M. V. (2004). Meta-analysis of quantitative sleep parameters from childhood to old age in healthy individuals: Developing normative sleep values across the human lifespan. *Sleep, 27*(7), 1255–1273.

Owens, J. A., Belon, K., & Moss, P. (2010). Impact of delaying school start time on adolescent sleep, mood, and behavior. *Archives of Pediatrics & Adolescent Medicine, 164*(7), 608–614.

Owens, J. A., Dearth-Wesley, T., Herman, A. N., Oakes, J. M., & Whitaker, R. C. (2017). A quasi-experimental study of the impact of school start time changes on adolescent sleep. *Sleep Health: Journal of the National Sleep Foundation, 3*(6), 437–443.

Owens, J., Drobnich, D., Baylor, A., & Lewin, D. (2014). School start time change: An in-depth examination of school districts in the United States. *Mind, Brain, and Education, 8*(4), 182–213.

Paiva, T., Gaspar, T., & Matos, M. G. (2015). Sleep deprivation in adolescents: Correlations with health complaints and health-related quality of life. *Sleep Medicine, 16*(4), 521–527.

Pasch, K. E., Laska, M. N., Lytle, L. A., & Moe, S. G. (2010). Adolescent sleep, risk behaviors, and depressive symptoms: Are they linked? *American Journal of Health Behavior, 34*(2), 237–248.

Paus, T., Keshavan, M., & Giedd, J. N. (2008). Why do many psychiatric disorders emerge during adolescence? *Nature Reviews Neuroscience, 9*(12), 947–957.

Rasch, B., & Born, J. (2013). About sleep's role in memory. *Physiological Reviews, 93*(2), 681–766.

Roberts, R. E., Roberts, C. R., & Chen, I. G. (2001). Functioning of adolescents with symptoms of disturbed sleep. *Journal of Youth and Adolescence, 30*(1), 1–18.

Roberts, R. E., Roberts, C. R., & Chen, I. G. (2002). Impact of insomnia on future functioning of adolescents. *Journal of Psychosomatic Research, 53*(1), 561–569.

Roberts, R. E., Roberts, C. R., & Duong, H. T. (2009). Sleepless in adolescence: Prospective data on sleep deprivation, health and functioning. *Journal of Adolescence, 32*(5), 1045–1057.

Roenneberg, T., Kuehnle, T., Pramstaller, P. P., Ricken, J., Havel, M., Guth, A., & Merrow, M. (2004). A marker for the end of adolescence. *Current Biology, 14*(24), R1038–R1039.

Sadeh, A., Raviv, A., & Gruber, R. (2000). Sleep patterns and sleep disruptions in school-age children. *Developmental Psychology, 36*(3), 291.

Sharman, R., Illingworth, G., Harvey, C., Jowett, A., Foster, R., & Espie, C. (2017). 0057 A preliminary evaluation of adolescent sleep in the UK—baseline sleeping patterns from the Oxford Teensleep cohort. *Journal of Sleep and Sleep Disorders Research, 40*(Suppl 1), A22.

Shochat, T., Cohen-Zion, M., & Tzischinsky, O. (2014). Functional consequences of inadequate sleep in adolescents: A systematic review. *Sleep Medicine Reviews, 18*(1), 75–87.

Short, M. A., Gradisar, M., Lack, L. C., Wright, H. R., & Dohnt, H. (2013). The sleep patterns and well-being of Australian adolescents. *Journal of Adolescence, 36*(1), 103–110.

Smaldone, A., Honig, J. C., & Byrne, M. W. (2007). Sleepless in America: Inadequate sleep and relationships to health and well-being of our nation's children. *Pediatrics, 119*(Suppl 1), S29–S37.

Smith, C. (2001). Sleep states and memory processes in humans: Procedural versus declarative memory systems. *Sleep Medicine Reviews, 5*(6), 491–506.

Silvers, J. A., McRae, K., Gabrieli, J. D., Gross, J. J., Remy, K. A., & Ochsner, K. N. (2012). Age-related differences in emotional reactivity, regulation, and rejection sensitivity in adolescence. *Emotion, 12*(6), 1235.

Stehle, J. H., Von Gall, C., & Korf, H. W. (2003). Melatonin: A clock-output, a clock-input. *Journal of Neuroendocrinology, 15*(4), 383–389.

Steinberg, L. (2008). A social neuroscience perspective on adolescent risk-taking. *Developmental Review, 28*(1), 78–106.

Steinberg, L., & Silverberg, S. B. (1986). The vicissitudes of autonomy in early adolescence. *Child Development*, 841–851.

Stickgold, R. (2005). Sleep-dependent memory consolidation. *Nature, 437*(7063), 1272–1278.

Talbot, L. S., McGlinchey, E. L., Kaplan, K. A., Dahl, R. E., & Harvey, A. G. (2010). Sleep deprivation in adolescents and adults: Changes in affect. *Emotion, 10*(6), 831.

Telzer, E. H., Fuligni, A. J., Lieberman, M. D., & Galván, A. (2013). The effects of poor quality sleep on brain function and risk taking in adolescence. *Neuroimage, 71*, 275–283.

Thacher, P. V., & Onyper, S. V. (2016). Longitudinal outcomes of start time delay on sleep, behavior, and achievement in high school. *Sleep, 39*(2), 271–281.

Thun, E., Bjorvatn, B., Flo, E., Harris, A., & Pallesen, S. (2015). Sleep, circadian rhythms, and athletic performance. *Sleep Medicine Reviews, 23*, 1–9.

Titova, O. E., Hogenkamp, P. S., Jacobsson, J. A., Feldman, I., Schiöth, H. B., & Benedict, C. (2015). Associations of self-reported sleep disturbance and duration with academic failure in community-dwelling Swedish adolescents: Sleep and academic performance at school. *Sleep Medicine, 16*(1), 87–93.

Tonetti, L., Fabbri, M., Filardi, M., Martoni, M., & Natale, V. (2015). Effects of sleep timing, sleep quality and sleep duration on school achievement in adolescents. *Sleep Medicine, 16*(8), 936–940.

Tononi, G., & Cirelli, C. (2003). Sleep and synaptic homeostasis: A hypothesis. *Brain Research Bulletin, 62*(2), 143–150.

Tononi, G., & Cirelli, C. (2006). Sleep function and synaptic homeostasis. *Sleep Medicine Reviews, 10*(1), 49–62.

Troxel, W. M., Lee, L., Hall, M., & Matthews, K. A. (2014). Single-parent family structure and sleep problems in Black and White adolescents. *Sleep Medicine, 15*(2), 255–261.

Voderholzer, U., Piosczyk, H., Holz, J., Landmann, N., Feige, B., Loessl, B., . . . Nissen, C. (2011). Sleep restriction over several days does not affect long-term recall of declarative and procedural memories in adolescents. *Sleep Medicine, 12*(2), 170–178.

Vriend, J. L., Davidson, F. D., Corkum, P. V., Rusak, B., Chambers, C. T., & McLaughlin, E. N. (2013). Manipulating sleep duration alters emotional functioning and cognitive performance in children. *Journal of Pediatric Psychology, 38*(10), 1058–1069.

Wagner, U., Gais, S., & Born, J. (2001). Emotional memory formation is enhanced across sleep intervals with high amounts of rapid eye movement sleep. *Learning & Memory, 8*(2), 112–119.

Wagner, U., Kashyap, N., Diekelmann, S., & Born, J. (2007). The impact of post-learning sleep vs. wakefulness on recognition memory for faces with different facial expressions. *Neurobiology of Learning and Memory, 87*(4), 679–687.

Wahlstrom, K. (2002). Changing times: Findings from the first longitudinal study of later high school start times. *Nassp Bulletin, 86*(633), 3–21.

Wahlstrom, K., Dretzke, B., Gordon, M., Peterson, K., Edwards, K., & Gdula, J. (2014). Examining the impact of later high school start times on the health and academic performance of high school students: A multi-site study. Retrieved from the University of Minnesota Digital Conservancy, http://hdl.handle.net/11299/162769

Watson, N. F., Martin, J. L., Wise, M. S., Carden, K. A., Kirsch, D. B., Kristo, D. A., . . . Rowley, J. A. (2017). Delaying middle school and high school start times promotes student health and performance: An American academy of sleep medicine position statement. *Journal of Clinical Sleep Medicine: JCSM: Official Publication of the American Academy of Sleep Medicine, 13*(4), 623–625.

Wheaton, A. G., Chapman, D. P., & Croft, J. B. (2016). School start times, sleep, behavioral, health, and academic outcomes: A review of the literature. *Journal of School Health, 86*(5), 363–381.

Wilhelm, I., Rose, M., Imhof, K. I., Rasch, B., Büchel, C., & Born, J. (2013). The sleeping child outplays the adult's capacity to convert implicit into explicit knowledge. *Nature Neuroscience, 16*(4), 391–393.

Wolfson, A. R., & Carskadon, M. A. (1998). Sleep schedules and daytime functioning in adolescents. *Child Development*, 69(4), 875–887.

Wulff, K., Gatti, S., Wettstein, J. G., & Foster, R. G. (2010). Sleep and circadian rhythm disruption in psychiatric and neurodegenerative disease. *Nature Reviews Neuroscience*, 11(8), 589.

Yan, L., & Silver, R. (2004). Resetting the brain clock: Time course and localization of mPER1 and mPER2 protein expression in suprachiasmatic nuclei during phase shifts. *European Journal of Neuroscience*, 19(4), 1105–1109.

Yoo, S. S., Gujar, N., Hu, P., Jolesz, F. A., & Walker, M. P. (2007). The human emotional brain without sleep—a prefrontal amygdala disconnect. *Current Biology*, 17(20), R877–R878.

14 The Effectiveness of Aerobic Exercise for Improving Educational Outcomes

Catherine Wheatley, Thomas Wassenaar, and Heidi Johansen-Berg

Introduction

Since the children of St Ninian's Primary School in Scotland started running a 'Daily Mile' back in 2012, more than 3,000 schools in Britain, Belgium, the Netherlands, and as far afield as Kuwait and Indonesia, have followed their example, with pupils leaving the classroom to spend 15 minutes a day jogging or walking round the playground. Teachers from diverse cultures and socio-economic locations have consistently reported a range of educational improvements, from increased concentration and better classroom behaviour to greater levels of self-efficacy. Fitness is raised; obesity levels are lowered; health benefits accrue.

Without doubt, the Daily Mile is a positive initiative that is delivering benefits to many young people at a critical stage in their development. As a classroom intervention, those involved have described it as a 'no-brainer'. Yet understanding more about how this aerobic exercise is affecting young brains is critically important for the design of successful physical activity interventions and for informing future teaching policy and practice. Would 20 minutes of running be more beneficial than 15? Does it need to be every day? Should pupils run—or would walking or football or yoga be just as effective? Are the benefits immediate—or do they build over time? Scientists at the University of Stirling are starting to shed light on some of these issues by measuring the physical, cognitive and emotional outcomes of running the Daily Mile. Their work is adding to the converging lines of neuroscience, psychology and education research which suggest, on balance, that regular physical activity and improved aerobic fitness have the potential to stimulate positive brain changes, improve cognitive performance and boost academic attainment.

A healthy mind in a healthy body is hardly a new idea. For centuries, philosophers and psychologists have studied the links between body and brain. Among children and adolescents, physical activity is linked to reduced depression and anxiety and improved self-esteem—with potential consequences for classroom behaviour (Biddle & Asare, 2011). Exercise is also thought to affect other behaviours, such as sleep quality and duration, and coping and self-regulation skills, that could themselves impact mental health and, potentially, educational outcomes (Lubans, Richards, Hillman, Faulkner, & Beauchamp, 2016). There is also a long history of studies showing associations between physical activity and cognitive ability in young people. For example, a well-known review of 44 studies (Sibley & Etnier, 2003) found that, overall, physically active groups performed significantly better than inactive groups on tests of cognitive performance that included perceptual skills, verbal and maths assessments, IQ tests and memory. The overall 'effect size' was 0.32, or 'small-to-medium'. The statistician who coined the term described this magnitude of difference as being about the same as the height difference between a 15-year-old girl and a 16-year-old girl (Cohen, 1988). Age was an important moderator: the largest effect size was for middle school pupils aged 8–11, while the smallest was for students in high school, aged 14–17. Although this evidence showed promise, it was inconclusive because many of the studies involved were correlational rather than experimental, and because there were many different methods and outcomes involved, making comparisons difficult. Nevertheless, it paved the way for more research: in a field that initially focused on older adults, and mild cognitive impairment in the aging brain, scientists are now investigating the impact of physical activity on cognitive performance in young people including executive functions such as attention, memory and inhibitory control.

In the lab, neuroscientists are working to establish *how* aerobic exercise might impact the brain and cognitive functioning. Studies using animals have found that, at the molecular level, aerobic exercise increases levels of growth factors responsible for making new connections, especially in the hippocampus, an area responsible for learning and memory (Gomez-Pinilla & Hillman, 2013). At the cellular level, increased growth factor production is thought to promote the development of new blood vessels and neurons, and their integration into existing networks of cells in this region (Cotman, Berchtold, & Christie, 2007). In fact, one of the key reasons for the increasing interest in young people is that childhood and adolescence are periods of sustained brain growth, suggesting that neural systems might be particularly receptive to the benefits of exercise (Foulkes & Blakemore, 2018). We look at these mechanisms in more detail in the section on how aerobic exercise enhances brain plasticity and cognitive function.

In schools, researchers are assessing how prevailing exercise levels are associated with cognitive function and/or attainment, typically measured in terms of maths or verbal reasoning tests. By 2011 a review of 50 studies (Rasberry et al., 2011) concluded that there was a broadly positive relationship, although the authors noted that sometimes no association in either direction was found.

One area of research is assessing how acute, or single, bouts of exercise impact short-term cognitive performance. Understanding more about this could help decide whether to schedule maths, for example, immediately after physical education (PE) lessons when concentration might have improved. We consider the evidence in the third section. Another broad area of study is examining how chronic, or regular, long-term exercise sessions might affect cognitive performance over time. In practical terms, the answer might, for example, suggest whether it is a good idea to timetable a daily aerobics session during break to improve memory during summer exam revision. We evaluate some of this research in the section on effects of chronic aerobic exercise on cognition and the brain.

With association studies it is impossible to disentangle cause and effect—do more active children learn better, or are brighter children more likely to engage in physical activity? To determine whether more physical activity in school leads to improved academic performance requires tests of interventions that increase activity either during PE, during classroom lessons, between periods or after school. A review of eight randomised control trials in schools—in which intervention groups took part in a programme of physical activity while control groups followed an unchanged curriculum—found that exercise had a generally positive effect on both cognition and also academic attainment (Lees & Hopkins, 2013). More recently, a review of intervention studies involving preadolescent children found that single bouts of physical activity had a positive impact on attention, while longer programmes of exercise also boosted executive function and academic attainment (de Greeff, Bosker, Oosterlaan, Visscher, & Hartman, 2017). We look at school-based studies in more detail in the sixth section, What Works? Evidence From Research in Schools.

Taken together, studies in the school setting shed light on *whether* aerobic exercise might improve real-life educational outcomes. Again, firm conclusions are difficult to draw because researchers have measured the impact of different types of exercise on a range of cognitive and academic tests. What's more, conflicting evidence means there are still no clear answers to the question of whether exercise impacts children and adolescents in exactly the same way. For example, one study found that two hours of aerobic PE per week improved the attention and working memory scores of young primary school children (Fisher et al., 2011), while a bout of mid-morning running in school improved adolescents' working memory but made no significant difference to attention (Cooper, Bandelow, Nute, Morris, & Nevill, 2012).

So, while there are positive associations between physical activity, cognition and academic attainment, research findings are inconsistent and the mechanisms that link them are not yet fully understood. Looking ahead, there are grounds for cautious optimism—and certainly a justification for larger randomised controlled trials in schools developed with consultation between academics and educators (Donnelly et al., 2016). In the following sections, we take a critical look at the evidence that aerobic exercise is an effective tool for improving educational outcomes.

Aerobic Exercise, Fitness and the Brain

How exactly we define and measure physical activity becomes important when we start to think about the 'dose-response relationship' between aerobic exercise, cognitive enhancement and educational outcomes. In other words, how often, how hard and how long must pupils exercise to achieve change—and in practical terms, is it possible to deliver the correct frequency, intensity and duration in a school setting? (See the seventh section of this chapter).

In research terms, physical activity is "any body movement produced by skeletal muscles that results in a substantial increase over resting energy expenditure" (Caspersen, Powell, & Christenson, 1985). Moderate-to-vigorous physical activity or MVPA—such as brisk walking, cycling, running or any other aerobic exercise that raises our heart rate and causes us to feel warm and out of breath—is the level of activity important for maintaining physical health. Government guidelines suggest that children and adolescents should complete 60 minutes of MVPA per day (Davies, Burns, Jewell, & McBride, 2011). MVPA, during which the heart and lungs are delivering oxygenated blood to the body, is also thought to be involved in changes to the brain, so interventions to boost aerobic activity of this intensity can potentially deliver double benefits.

Aerobic fitness—a measure of an individual's capacity to supply oxygen to the working muscles—is distinct from other outcomes of regular exercise, such as strength or flexibility. In schools, it is typically measured by the multistage fitness or 'beep' test (Léger, Mercier, Gadoury, & Lambert, 1988). In this assessment, children run between two lines 20 metres apart in time with a pre-recorded soundtrack of 'beeps' which become progressively closer together as the test proceeds. Participants run faster and faster until they can no longer keep in time: the score is the number of laps completed. Some studies ask pupils to wear wrist-based accelerometers, similar to a commercial Fitbit, or heartrate monitors, to provide an objective measure of the intensity and duration of physical activity. Others rely on subjective measures gathered by asking young people to remember what they have been doing over the past week and then fill out a questionnaire. There are pros and cons to both types of measurement: It can be hard to persuade young people to wear a device for extended periods, but can also be difficult for them to accurately recall their physical activity.

The cardiovascular fitness hypothesis (North, McCullagh, & Tran, 1990) argues that regular physical activity *that leads to an improvement in aerobic fitness* is necessary for cognitive benefits. The hypothesis suggests that gains in cardiovascular fitness deliver positive physiological changes to the brain's structure and function. Although a review of 37 mainly adult studies back in 2006 found no conclusive evidence to support a direct connection between fitness and the brain, it remains a useful guide: The review's authors proposed that fitness is in fact just the first step in a cascade of physiological changes that ultimately impact the brain (Etnier, Nowell, Landers, & Sibley, 2006). Since then, more evidence has been developed to suggest that a positive change in aerobic fitness improves young people's cognitive performance. More work is needed, but as a consequence of these findings, many school-based studies examining the impact of *chronic* physical activity on cognitive function and attainment involve regular bouts of MVPA.

A complementary theory suggests that physical activity that also involves motor co-ordination and learning (such as playing tennis, dancing or martial arts) boosts 'motor fitness' (Voelcker-Rehage & Niemann, 2013). This is the type of physical fitness or competence that is measured in terms of flexibility, balance and speed, for example. Motor fitness is in turn linked to executive function (EF), the cognitive processes involved in selecting, coordinating and monitoring goal-directed behaviour. EF includes response inhibition (suppressing an inappropriate response); working memory (holding or manipulating information in mind) and cognitive flexibility (updating strategies in changing contexts). Some researchers have suggested that aerobic activities that include a cognitive component—and especially those involving rhythmic movements and hand-eye co-ordination—pre-activate neural networks and therefore have a bigger impact on children's EF than aerobic exercise alone (Etnier et al., 2006; Voelcker-Rehage & Niemann, 2013).

A third promising area of research, on the bioenergetic effects of exercise, could help explain the impact of *acute* bouts of aerobic exercise on cognitive function. In simple terms, a short-term increase in energy expenditure places the neural system under metabolic stress. This in turn promotes adaptive responses that include the production of proteins involved in the growth and survival of neurons, which promote improved memory and learning (Rothman & Mattson, 2013). In this pathway, the impact of exercise on the brain is not mediated by fitness.

Scientists have also started to explore the impact of short bouts of high-intensity or vigorous exercise on cognition. This type of physical activity, in which participants are working at around 80% of their maximum heart rate for anything from 45 seconds to four minutes, has proven popular because it can deliver equivalent fitness benefits to longer, lower-intensity workouts (Buchheit & Laursen, 2013). Fit to Study, a large-scale randomised controlled trial in British secondary schools, looked at the impact of an intervention to increase vigorous physical activity during school PE academic attainment measured by a maths test (Wassenaar et al., 2019). The trial found no evidence that the intervention led to higher maths scores, but researchers are now looking at whether it led to changes in cognitive function, mental health and brain structure. Meanwhile, a study in Australian high schools found that three sessions of high-intensity training during PE per week, for eight weeks, led to a significant improvement in mood, and a non-significant increase in executive function (Costigan, Eather, Plotnikoff, Hillman, & Lubans, 2016). Another recent intervention study in New Zealand found that a six-week programme of high-intensity training in school led to improvements in cognitive control and working memory compared to a control group (Moreau, Kirk, & Waldie, 2017).

Drawing firm conclusions about whether aerobic exercise—with or without a co-ordination component—can improve cognitive function is difficult based only on evidence from schools. At the moment, it is impossible to prescribe how much, and when, young people should exercise to improve cognitive function and academic attainment. Carefully controlled laboratory studies using brain imaging are helping to shed further light on these questions. The next section explores the immediate impact of a single exercise sessions on cognitive function.

Effects of Acute Aerobic Exercise on Cognition and the Brain

Researchers have been investigating the effects of acute bouts of aerobic exercise on cognitive function for many years, based on the premise that exercise-induced changes in (physiological) arousal alter cognitive functioning (Yerkes & Dodson, 1908).

Technological advances mean that experiments can now be complemented with non-invasive brain research methods, such as magnetic resonance imaging (MRI) or, more often, electroencephalography (EEG). These are used to explore how the brain itself responds and adapts to the short-term increase in energy expenditure brought about by a single aerobic exercise session.

Most of the studies have involved adults—and the results typically show that 20 to 60 minutes of moderate-intensity exercise facilitates subsequent cognitive performance, underpinned by brain changes (Tomporowski, 2003a; Lambourne & Tomporowski, 2010; Chang, Labban, Gapin, & Etnier, 2012; Etnier et al., 1997; Mcmorris & Hale, 2012; Verburgh, Königs, Scherder, & Oosterlaan, 2013).

There is less research looking at the effects of acute exercise on young people's brains and cognitive function, although the studies that do examine these populations have received a good deal of attention. Several reviews (Donnelly et al., 2016; Tomporowski, 2003b; Janssen, Toussaint, van Mechelen, & Verhagen, 2014; Li, O'Connor, O'Dwyer, & Orr, 2017; Brisswalter, Collardeau, & Arcelin, 2002; Best, 2010; Tomporowski, McCullick, Pendleton, & Pesce, 2015) and meta-analyses (de Greeff et al., 2017; Chang et al., 2012; Verburgh et al., 2013; Sibley & Etnier, 2003) have found evidence for positive effects. The benefits seem most apparent for EF, or inhibition, working memory and cognitive flexibility (Verburgh et al., 2013; Best, 2010). But other cognitive domains, such as attention, may also improve with exercise (Janssen et al., 2014; Li et al., 2017), although this could well be because these are the domains most often studied. More research is needed in this area. What's more, the reported effect sizes are often small (remember the height difference between 15- and 16-year-old girls) because of the many factors that can moderate the exercise-cognition relationship, including the type and intensity of exercise, the type and timing of the cognitive assessment, as well as fitness levels of individuals (Chang et al., 2012). In other words, it appears that individual differences may influence the extent to which acute exercise impacts young brains and cognition.

In the lab, studies have shown that acute exercise is particularly beneficial for young people's response inhibition—the ability to suppress inappropriate responses in any given context (Best, 2012; Drollette, Shishido, Pontifex, & Hillman, 2012; Hogan et al., 2013; Soga, Shishido, & Nagatomi, 2015; Vazou & Smiley-Oyen, 2014). In these experiments, participants usually run on a treadmill or cycle for a fixed time, typically at *moderate* intensity (around 60%–70% of maximum heart rate) for between 10 and 30 minutes. Inhibitory control is typically measured using the Flanker task, a computer-based assessment that measures how fast and accurately participants can identify the direction a central symbol is pointing. This task is much easier when the central symbol is congruent with the surrounding symbols like this < < < < < compared to when it is incongruent like this < < > < < for example. The incongruent condition requires response inhibition: the 'left' response that would be elicited by the surrounding left-facing arrows in this example needs to be inhibited in order to produce the correct 'right' response corresponding to the right-facing arrow.

Although heightened inhibitory control is perhaps the most convincing finding in the lab, some experiments have found that acute exercise improves different aspects of EF, or even made no difference at all (Soga et al., 2015; Stroth et al., 2009). For example, some studies have reported improvements in processing speed—the ability to think and respond quickly—which supports more complex cognitive functions (Ellemberg & St-Louis-Deschenes, 2010; Piepmeier et al., 2015). There are mixed results for other cognitive domains including working memory, planning and switching. For instance, separate studies have found that acute bouts of moderate exercise led to no change in working memory (Drollette et al., 2012) and also a decline in memory performance (Soga et al., 2015). By contrast, a single bout of maximal-intensity exercise was found to improve working memory in children and adolescents, but only following a recovery period (Samuel et al., 2017). This study also reported a decline in verbal learning immediately after the activity, which returned to baseline levels after one hour of recovery.

The apparent inconsistencies in the evidence suggests that the beneficial effects of acute exercise on cognition may depend on both the intensity of the activity and the task being used to measure cognitive function (Donnelly et al., 2016). More well-controlled studies are needed to tease apart the effects of these moderating factors.

Scientists are also investigating whether acute exercise is linked to greater activity in the brain areas thought to underpin these cognitive functions. In these studies, young people take part in aerobic activity, and their brain function is compared to a non-active control condition during subsequent cognitive tasks using electroencephalography (EEG) or magnetic resonance imaging (MRI) (Drollette et al., 2014; Pontifex, Saliba, Raine, Picchietti, & Hillman, 2013; Ludyga et al., 2017; Chu et al., 2017; Chen, Zhu, Yan, Yin, & Chen, 2016; Hillman, Pontifex et al., 2009; Stroth et al., 2009). Evidence of higher brain activity in these areas, combined with a better task performance, strengthens the argument that a single exercise session boosts specific types of cognitive function afterwards.

EEG uses electrodes on the surface of the scalp to measure electrical activity that takes place in direct response to a cognitive (or sensory or motor) stimulus. Put simply, the electrodes capture the voltage fluctuations or 'brain waves' caused by the chemical reactions taking place as neurons fire together immediately before, during or after a specific event. These 'event-related potentials' or ERPs can shed light on the psycho-physiological correlates of cognitive function. For instance, the P3 or third peak of the ERP waveform occurs between 300 and 500 milliseconds after the stimulus. It is thought that the *higher* the P3 amplitude, the more *attention* is being paid to the stimulus, where attention might involve being alert to changes in stimuli, being spatially aware of them or being able to detect and resolve conflicting information. The *quicker* the P3 peak occurs, the faster the individual's *processing speed* (Polich, 2007).

Researchers have found that 20 minutes of moderate exercise increases children's P3 amplitude as well as improving their performance on the Flanker task, (Hillman, Buck, Themanson, Pontifex, & Castelli, 2009). In other words, after exercising, children appear to devote more attentional resources during tasks that require greater amounts of response inhibition or focus. There is some evidence that children who struggle to focus, or who have been diagnosed with attention-deficit-hyperactivity disorder, may be especially likely to profit from an exercise session (see box) (Pontifex et al., 2013; Ludyga et al., 2017). Notably, the only study that has so far examined adolescents found no change in P3 amplitudes (measuring attention) after acute activity (Stroth et al., 2019).

EEG is a sensitive measure of changes in brain activity over time, but MRI is the technique that researchers use to capture activity in very specific brain regions. Functional MRI (fMRI) uses a strong magnetic field to measure cerebral blood flow during cognitive tasks (and also at rest) and, by inference, neuronal activity in that area. A small study with just nine participants found that 30 minutes of moderate activity not only improved working memory performance in ten-year-olds, but also led to greater activation of the brain regions that support working memory (Chen et al., 2016).

Effects of Chronic Aerobic Exercise on Cognition and the Brain

What about the impact of repeated acute exercise sessions that, over time, add up to regular training and higher fitness? Interest in the effects of chronic exercise on young people's cognitive function and brains has intensified in recent years, fuelled by growing concern about childhood inactivity, a higher prevalence of diseases like obesity and diabetes in this age group, and, in some places, a shortage of opportunities to be physically active during the school day (Diamond, A. B., 2015; Fedewa & Ahn, 2011; Hillman, Erickson, & Hatfield, 2017). Encouragingly, recent reviews (Donnelly et al., 2016; Li et al., 2017; Khan & Hillman, 2014; Chaddock, Pontifex, Hillman, & Kramer, 2011; Álvarez-Bueno et al., 2017; Biddle & Asare, 2011; Kriemler et al., 2011;

Hsieh et al., 2017; Lind et al., 2017) and meta-analyses (Rasberry et al., 2011; Esteban-Cornejo, Tejero-Gonzalez, Sallis, & Veiga, 2015) highlight beneficial effects of chronic exercise on the brain and show small-to-moderate but significant positive effects of physical activity on cognition in young people. These findings may help justify the need to devote more time to physical activity in school settings.

Studies examining the relationship between physical activity levels and/ or cardiorespiratory fitness and cognition at a single point in time show that higher-fit young people (measured with a beep test in school or a VO2max test in the lab) perform better on working memory, processing speed, response inhibition and attention tasks than lower-fit peers (Donnelly et al., 2016). Meanwhile, trials that investigate the impact of aerobic exercise on intervention and control groups over time can shed light on whether exercise *changes* cognition. Many of these training programmes take place in schools, simply because there is a better chance that young people will stick to them in this setting (Kriemler et al., 2011).

Despite considerable variety in the duration, intensity and type of activity these interventions prescribe, they generally support the findings of observational studies, showing exercise-induced improvements in attention, working memory, cognitive flexibility and inhibitory control (de Greeff et al., 2017; Moreau et al., 2017; Vazou, Pesce, Lakes, & Smiley-Oyen, 2016; Álvarez-Bueno et al., 2017; Hsieh et al., 2017; Lind et al., 2017).

A few of these studies have also used EEG or MRI in an attempt to unpack the fitness-cognition relationships at the level of the brain. Early EEG research suggested that higher-fit children are able to pay more attention in cognitive tasks, as evidenced by a larger P3 amplitude and a better performance on the Flanker task (Hillman, Buck et al., 2009; Pontifex et al., 2011)—these results align with those examining acute physical activity. More recent ERP studies have shown that higher fitness is also associated with an ERP component that reflects more efficient task preparation processes (Stroth et al., 2009; Kamijo & Masaki, 2016).

One puzzling pattern revealed by MRI studies is that, as Flanker inhibition tasks become more challenging, higher-fit children appear to show *lower* activation in brain areas associated with cognitive control compared to less-fit peers as the Voss et al. (2011). Another study found that fitter young people show higher but *decreasing* activation in prefrontal and parietal cortices as the task progressed, while maintaining their accuracy. By contrast, lower-fit children showed no change in brain activation and their accuracy fell over time (Chaddock et al., 2012). One possible interpretation of these findings is that higher aerobic fitness is associated with greater efficiency of these neural networks. To fully understand the mechanisms at work will require further research.

In some studies, researchers use MRI to measure and compare volumes of grey matter (cell bodies, synapses and capillaries) and white matter (the fibres connecting grey matter areas) between higher and lower-fit young people. The hippocampus, involved in memory and learning, and the dorsal striatum, linked to cognitive control and response resolution, are of particular interest. Research has shown that, after a programme of training, higher-fit children and adolescents not only perform better on memory tasks, but also have larger hippocampal volumes (Chaddock et al., 2010a; Herting & Nagel, 2012). As well as achieving higher scores on the Flanker task, fitter children also appear to have larger dorsal striatum volumes (Chaddock et al., 2010a, 2010b; Chaddock, Hillman et al., 2012. Scientists have used a specific type of MRI scan, known as diffusion tensor imaging (DTI), to show that fitness levels also appear to be linked with white matter microstructure that connects different regions of the brain, such as the corpus callosum (Chaddock-Heyman et al., 2014). This in turn is related to more *efficient* cognitive control (Herting & Nagel, 2012; Chaddock-Heyman et al., 2013). White matter microstructure also appears to be improved by exercise—and this in turn has been linked to improved attention (Schaeffer et al., 2014; Krafft et al., 2014).

Higher-fit young people also appear to have higher levels of cerebral blood flow in their hippocampi (Chaddock-Heyman et al., 2016), raising the possibility that fitness-related changes in blood flow may underlie superior cognitive performance. What's more, brain function appears to be influenced by exercise and fitness even when young people are not taking part in cognitive tasks. A few studies have looked at the impact of exercise on resting-state networks: areas of the brain that are active at the same time and which can be thought of as being functionally (rather than structurally) connected. There is initial evidence that exercise may refine, or strengthen, these networks, which may be beneficial for cognitive and behavioural performance.

Overall, what these studies suggest is that chronic exercise is beneficial for cognitive functioning in children and adolescents. They also indicate the changes in brain structure and function that take place over time as fitness improves, which in turn shed light on the potential neural underpinnings of these cognitive improvements. But current research techniques cannot yet reveal the neurobiological mechanisms—the molecular and cellular events—underlying these brain changes. For this, we must turn to animal research.

How Might Aerobic Exercise Enhance Brain Plasticity and Cognitive Function?

In recent years, researchers have started to unravel some of the mechanisms linking exercise and neural *plasticity*—the brain's capacity to reshape and reorganize itself in response to environmental influences and experience. Animal studies, in which researchers can directly examine cellular and molecular brain changes with exercise, have been crucial to this endeavour. Like studies in humans, animal research has consistently shown that exercise enhances rodents' cognitive performance, particularly on tasks that require spatial memory and learning (van Praag, 2008). The hippocampus has been the prime target for research into the mechanisms underlying these cognitive effects

(Leuner & Gould, 2010). Current evidence indicates that many different processes are linked to these cognitive improvements (van Praag, 2008; Cassilhas, Tufik, & De Mello, 2016; Vivar & van Praag, 2017; Basso & Suzuki, 2017; Voss, Vivar, Kramer, & van Praag, 2013; Gomez-Pinilla & Hillman, 2013; Patten et al., 2015). Researchers have suggested that during aerobic exercise there is an increase in blood flow to the brain and an upregulation of the quantity of certain brain chemicals (Vivar & van Praag, 2017; Basso & Suzuki, 2017). But many ways in which exercise-related changes in cerebral blood flow might affect cognitive performance are still uncertain (Ogoh, 2017). We do know that several neurotransmitters are implicated in the exercise-cognition pathway. Animal studies show higher levels of dopamine, serotonin, norepinephrine, epinephrine, glutamate and GABA following a bout of exercise (Basso & Suzuki, 2017). These neurotransmitters are also known to be involved in cognitive processing (Basso & Suzuki, 2017; Mcmorris, 2016), but more work is need to fully understand their role.

Brain-derived neurotrophic factor (BDNF) is thought to be the most important factor upregulated by physical activity, because it supports neural survival, growth, synaptic plasticity (the strengthening and weakening of brain connections) and neurogenesis (the production of new neurons) (Cotman et al., 2007; Lipsky & Marini, 2007; Sleiman & Chao, 2015). It also has an important function in learning and memory (Hall, Thomas, & Everitt, 2000). Animal experiments have shown that acute exercise, and both short (two–seven days) (van Praag, Kempermann, & Gage, 1999; Speisman, Kumar, Rani, Foster, & Ormerod, 2013; Merritt & Rhodes, 2015) and longer exercise programmes (Farmer et al., 2004; Berchtold, Castello, & Cotman, 2010; Molteni, Ying, & Gómez-Pinilla, 2002) can increase BDNF levels in the hippocampus and other brain areas. Crucially, blocking BDNF signalling in animals has been shown to abolish the effects of exercise on learning and memory (Vaynman, Ying, & Gomez-Pinilla, 2004). What's more, BDNF interacts with many other genes and factors that are upregulated with exercise (Voss et al., 2013), supporting its central role in the exercise-cognition pathway.

One factor that interacts with BDNF is insulin-like growth factor (IGF-1). IGF-1 is also known to be involved in synaptic plasticity and neurogenesis (Cassilhas et al., 2016), as well as in learning and memory (Ding, Vaynman, Akhavan, Ying, & Gomez-Pinilla, 2006). What's more, IGF-1 moderates the secretion of other factors such as vascular endothelial growth factor (VEGF), a molecule that plays a role in blood vessel growth. Blocking IGF-1 appears to abolish the secretion of VEGF and reduces the production of new capillaries (Lopez-Lopez, LeRoith, & Torres-Aleman, 2004). Both IGF-1 and VEGF are upregulated with exercise (Tang, Xia, Wagner, & Breen, 2010), and play a role in exercise-induced changes in the brain's network of blood vessels.

Exercise also increases the production of brain blood cells (Lopez-Lopez et al., 2004) and the growth of new blood vessels (Swain et al., 2003) throughout the brain, both of which have been linked to better cognitive performance in animals (Clark, Brzezinska, Puchalski, Krone, & Rhodes, 2009; Rhyu et al., 2010). This improvement in brain blood supply with exercise might facilitate the delivery of nutrients to support synaptic plasticity and neurogenesis. Indeed, an increase in hippocampal neurogenesis is one of the most consistently observed effects of exercise (van Praag, 2008; Triviño-Paredes, Patten, Gil-Mohapel, & Christie, 2016; Ma et al., 2017). In animals, chronic exercise more than doubles the production of new neurons in the hippocampus (van Praag, 2008; van Praag, Christie, Sejnowski, & Gage, 1999; Brown et al., 2003). These neurons link up with others and express properties that facilitate long-term potentiation (LTP)—a physiological process that underlies learning and memory (Schmidt-Hieber, Jonas, & Bischofberger, 2004). Enhanced neurogenesis is also associated with increased synaptic plasticity and better performance on a variety of memory tasks (Farmer et al., 2004; Mustroph et al., 2012; Van der Borght, Havekes, Bos, Eggen, & Van der Zee, 2007; van Praag et al., 1999; Speisman et al., 2013; Merritt & Rhodes, 2015). The causal links between neurogenesis and cognitive performance are hotly debated (Groves et al., 2013), but current evidence suggests that exercise-enhanced neurogenesis may mediate, at least in part, cognitive improvements (Kent, Oomen, Bekinschtein, Bussey, & Saksida, 2015; Yau, Gil-Mohapel, Christie, & So, 2014).

Animal research has helped identify the molecular factors and processes that might underpin effects of exercise on the brain and cognition, but they do not always directly translate to human physiology and behaviour. With advances in neuroimaging techniques (Tardif et al., 2016), researchers can start to bridge the gap between animal and human research. But to understand whether exercise might be an effective tool for improving educational outcomes we need to enter the classroom.

What Works? Evidence From Research in Schools

Studies in schools are crucial from a translational perspective: What 'works' in the lab does not necessarily have the same effect in real-life settings. Scientists from the University of Stirling have shown that The Daily Mile makes primary school children more active, less sedentary and fitter (Chesham et al., 2018). But another research team has cast doubt on whether it also leads, as the movement claims, to greater focus and concentration levels in the classroom. Across 11 schools, it found no evidence significant improvement EF or maths fluency immediately after completing 15 minutes of jogging or walking (Morris et al., 2019). More evidence is needed before firm conclusions can be drawn.

These studies add to the promising—although inconsistent—body of evidence linking physical activity to both cognitive function and academic attainment. Studies involving aerobic exercise during or between lessons have tended to take place in primary schools, where there is flexibility to incorporate such changes. By contrast, secondary schools must balance the requirements of the curriculum, so most physical activity research involving adolescents has typically taken place as part of scheduled PE lessons.

Primary school studies examining the impact of acute exercise on cognitive function have produced conflicting but broadly positive results. For example, 20 minutes of moderate-to-vigorous exercise in school improved planning, but not attention, among children aged 9–10 (Pirrie & Lodewyk, 2012). By contrast, 12 minutes of running around an indoor track at a greater intensity (70%–80% of max heart rate) *boosted* attention, with greater improvements observed in children from lower-income families (Tine & Butler, 2012). Thirty minutes of jogging on a playing field at moderate intensity improved 9–11 year-olds' inhibition, shifting and working memory (Chen, Yan, Yin, Pan, & Chang, 2014).

In secondary schools, the picture is slightly different. Ten minutes of high intensity intermittent running appears to improve adolescents' working memory (Cooper, Bandelow, Nute, Morris, & Nevill, 2015) but not selective attention. A bout of predominantly vigorous exercise led to greater improvements in inhibitory control compared to both light and no exercise (Peruyero, Zapata, Pastor, & Cervelló, 2017).

Some studies have looked at the effect of acute physical activity breaks on cognition. For instance, among children aged 10–11, the biggest gains in selective attention followed a moderate-intensity activity break that involved jogging, passing and dribbling a ball; improvements after vigorous activities and after listening to a story for 15 minutes were smaller. Without any kind of break there was no change in performance on the attention task (Janssen et al., 2014). In another study, although children's executive functions did not improve after a five-, ten- or 15-minute classroom exercise break (or after a sedentary lesson), they did show a moderate improvement on a maths test (Howie, Schatz, & Pate, 2015).

Although the evidence is sometimes contradictory, there are growing indications that complex and cognitively-engaging activities in schools, including dance or martial arts, may be particularly beneficial—especially for attention—when compared with repetitive aerobic exercise such as jogging (Tomporowski et al., 2015; Pesce, 2012). In one study, adolescents who took part in ten minutes of cognitively demanding football drills performed better on attention tests than those who had followed their normal PE lesson (Budde, Voelcker-Rehage, Pietraßyk-Kendziorra, Ribeiro, & Tidow, 2008). Some studies have also found that this type of exercise benefits working memory (Pesce, Crova, Cereatti, Casella, & Bellucci, 2009; Ishihara, Sugasawa, Matsuda, & Mizuno, 2017) and cognitive flexibility (Benzing, Heinks, Eggenberger, & Schmidt, 2016). The evidence in support of inhibition is more mixed (Best, 2012; Jäger, Schmidt, Conzelmann, Roebers, & Anderson, 2014).

What about academic achievement? On balance, current findings suggest that increasing structured physical activity in school—with more activity breaks or after-school sessions, for example—has a positive effect on both maths and reading, with more evidence in favour of maths. Of 14 recent intervention studies, five found positive associations; a further three found links between exercise and some educational outcomes but not others; and six found that attainment was not improved (Donnelly et al., 2016). Interventions designed to boost the frequency, intensity or duration of activity during PE show more mixed results: Only two of six recent studies led to academic gains (Fisher et al., 2011). One possible explanation for this is that the impact of physical activity during PE is associated with additional factors that moderate attainment, such as self-esteem.

There is a small but expanding body of school-based research demonstrating how positive relationships between exercise and educational outcomes in school might be mediated by improved fitness and/or cognition (Reed & Ones, 2006; van der Niet, 2015). But at the moment, although studies show that a particular intervention 'works', we cannot yet confidently say 'how', 'why', or whether the results are replicable. Furthermore, educational outcomes depend on a range of environmental and genetic factors from socio-economic status to developmental disorders. Isolating the impact of aerobic exercise on attainment is not straightforward, and not all studies control for these moderating variables. Recent programmes have used a variety of attainment measures, including maths papers, reading assessments and standard reasoning tests to capture educational outcomes, making comparisons difficult. What's more, most studies do not mention the size of the effect that activity and fitness have on attainment, although there is some evidence that the relationship is not linear: Beyond a certain level of fitness, there are no more advantages to be had in terms of educational outcomes (Hansen, Herrmann, Lambourne, Lee, & Donnelly, 2014).

Crucially, there is no evidence that school-based programmes of physical activity can actually harm academic results by, for example, diverting time or resources away from classroom-based study (Rasberry et al., 2011; Lees & Hopkins, 2013). As financial pressures in the education sector threaten PE classes in the UK, and when American schools routinely cut or even eliminate PE to make way for more teaching in 'core' subjects (SHAPE America—Society of Health and Physical Educators, 2016), the following studies—examples of teaching practices that have 'worked'—make a strong case for physical activity in school.

Physically Active Lessons: The Physical Activity Across the Curriculum study (Donnelly et al., 2009), involving 24 US elementary schools, developed lesson plans that incorporated ten minutes of physical activity into daily lessons, to achieve an extra 90 minutes of moderate-to-vigorous activity per week over three years. For example, a lesson about food groups incorporated running to represent the energy from carbohydrate and bicep curls to represent proteins that build muscles. When compared to pupils in control schools, those in the intervention arm of the study recorded significantly higher reading, maths and spelling scores.

Active Lesson Breaks: A smaller Canadian study (Ma, Le Mare, & Gurd, 2014), which compared 'off-task' behaviour during 50-minute classes with and without activity breaks, found that the same children showed significantly fewer signs of talking, fidgeting or not concentrating during active lessons. In this project, teachers delivered ten-minute classroom-based activity breaks, consisting of 4 minutes of vigorous activity such as squats or jumping jacks, plus time to set up and cool down.

Additional Activity: Latino children in the US took part in a two-year dance programme, involving a video 'exer-game' and aerobic dance moves, completed three times per week (Gao, Hannan, Xiang, Stodden, & Valdez, 2013). All the pupils were from one elementary school, which agreed to combine two 15-minute school breaks to timetable a single exercise session during the school day. Students completing the intervention recorded significantly higher scores on a maths test than those in the comparison group.

Exercise Timing: One elementary school study found that 30 or 40 minutes of walking after noon made significant improvements to the children's performance on a short maths test immediately afterwards, compared with both morning walking and no exercise (McNaughten & Gabbard, 1993).

Physical Education: In Germany, students aged 12–13 spent the first lesson period playing basketball, football, hockey or dancing indoors, three times a week for three months. Sometimes participants arrived at school 45 minutes early to complete the activities: On these days they were not given any homework. These students showed a significant improvement on a maths test compared to control, and no differences were recorded in overall homework time (Spitzer & Hollmann, 2013). In the ten-month Active Smarter Kids trial, Norwegian children aged 10–11 from 30 schools took part in an additional 165 minutes per week of MVPA compared to control, but they showed no change in maths, reading or literacy (Resaland et al., 2016).

Implications for Classroom Practice

For schools considering whether to incorporate more physical activity into the school day, what are the key points to think about?

Notably, schools and teachers have sometimes struggled to fit more physical activity into the school day. A recent review of 39 studies found that classroom-based physical activity interventions improved academic attainment, but that, taken together, they did not lead to a significant increase in actual physical activity because of the time constraints imposed by the syllabus and other learning objectives (Watson, Timperio, Brown, Best, & Hesketh, 2017).

There are no firm answers about the optimum exercise programme, but what we do know suggests that quite a broad range of aerobic activities produces similar positive results, from running and dancing to aerobics and circuit training (Lees & Hopkins, 2013). Typically, the intensity of exercise is moderate-to-vigorous. As little as 45 minutes of additional activity per week has been shown to be effective according to a review (Lees & Hopkins, 2013)—and even less in some individual studies. What's more, there is encouraging evidence that short, vigorous sessions that are relatively easy to incorporate into the school day, have potential to deliver similar cognitive benefits when compared to longer, more moderate-intensity sessions (Moreau et al., 2017; Costigan, Eather, Plotnikoff, Taaffe, & Lubans, 2015). Encouragingly, teachers report that active lessons break up the monotony of a class and actually help with behaviour management and aid concentration rather than opening up the possibility of wild behaviour. These types of lessons also seem to encourage children to be more creative and to retain information, especially spelling (Gibson et al., 2008). On the downside, some teachers have reported struggling to incorporate activity into small classrooms (Gibson et al., 2008). Some pedagogical studies have suggested that redesigning classrooms with standing desks might provide a favourable environment for activity breaks (Lanningham-Foster, Foster, McCrady, & Manohar, 2008).

Trained PE teachers manage physical activity in secondary schools, but there is evidence that more generalist primary school teachers can successfully deliver exercise programmes. The well-known Sports, Play and Active Recreation for Kids (SPARK) programme was implemented in seven elementary schools in an affluent area of California (Sallis et al., 1999). This comprehensive curriculum involves lessons that have a health-fitness activity, such as running and skipping, and a skills-fitness activity, such as playing football or Frisbee. Specialist SPARK teachers and trained elementary school teachers delivered the curriculum three times a week for two years, and their results were compared to control schools teaching PE as usual. Over this period, percentile scores on achievement tests declined in all three conditions, possibly because baseline scores were notably high. More encouragingly, elementary teachers who had received SPARK training produced better academic results on a variety of tests than the specialists.

Teachers should recognise that exercise programmes can also be a potential source of problems, according to a Cochrane Review of school-based projects to promote physical activity and fitness (Dobbins, Husson, Decorby, & LaRocca, 2013). First, they risk drawing attention—and perhaps ridicule—to overweight or unfit pupils, which can be especially damaging during adolescence. Also, as the review points out, for many pupils changing clothes for PE can be a stressful experience. Furthermore, insisting that young people perform vigorous or unfamiliar activities against their will might also affect the quality of their motivation towards exercise: instead of promoting positive perceptions it might in fact have the opposite effect (Standage, Duda, & Ntoumanis, 2003).

But as the children of St Ninian's have demonstrated, spending a few minutes per day taking part in simple activities that certainly improve physical health, that might well be positive for the brain and cognition, and do nothing to damage educational outcomes, is a promising strategy that both primary and secondary teachers would do well to consider in the future.

Box: Aerobic Exercise and Attention Deficit Hyperactivity Disorder (ADHD)

Could exercise and fitness lead to an improvement in the classroom behaviours that typify ADHD? Promising evidence suggests that they might—an exciting prospect given that an estimated 5.9%–7.1% of children and adolescents globally show symptoms of a neurodevelopmental disorder that is associated with poor academic outcomes (Willcutt, 2012). The disorder, characterised by impulsivity, hyperactivity and inattention, is thought to be caused by poor behavioural inhibition—difficulties with preventing inappropriate actions, or stopping them once underway (Barkley, 1997). Put simply, children and adolescents with this type of disorder appear to have smaller regions of the prefrontal cortex associated with executive control and inhibition, areas that also respond to aerobic exercise (Halperin & Healey, 2011). Research has started to test whether exercise programmes might improve performance on tasks that measure inhibition. For example, an eight-week programme of swimming and motor-skill games in the water improved participants' scores on one such task, relative to control (Chang, Hung, Huang, Hatfield, & Hung, 2014). There are also suggestions that acute exercise might be beneficial: 30 minutes of moderate-intensity cycling improved inhibitory control, compared to a group watching a TV documentary (Piepmeier et al., 2015). Similar effects have been found with shorter, higher-intensity exercise too. In a randomised control trial, five minutes of vigorous trampolining boosted inhibitory control (Gawrilow, Stadler, Langguth, Naumann, & Boeck, 2016). Whatever the mechanisms involved, a recent review of 30 such studies (Ng, Ho, Chan, Yong, & Yeo, 2017) found that moderate-to-vigorous activity did appear to alleviate the cognitive, behavioural and physical *symptoms* of ADHD—encouraging news for these children and their teachers.

Recommendations

What Neuroscience Has Added to Our Understanding Over and Above Psychology

Evidence from psychology suggests that physical activity can enhance mental health, wellbeing and self-esteem, and that these can in turn improve aspects of *behaviour* to deliver improved educational outcomes. But neuroscience proposes a pathway in which physical activity impacts aspects of *neurobiology*, including the growth of, and connections between, brain cells to improve cognition and, potentially, academic attainment. More research is needed, but on balance the evidence so far suggests that young people's executive functions—their response inhibition, their cognitive flexibility and their ability to use working memory—could all be improved by physical activity. Firm conclusions are hard to draw, based on current findings, but it may be that primary-age children stand to benefit most: The weight of evidence is in their favour for now. What's more, they are typically less self-conscious about school-based exercise than adolescents and therefore more likely to comply with a programme of exercise. Also, strong executive functioning during the early years can underpin and support academic and also behavioural development into adolescence. Children from low socio-economic backgrounds may also benefit disproportionately.

Concrete Implications of Research and Opportunities for Translation

Increasing aerobic exercise in school will almost certainly improve or maintain students' physical and mental health, and there are signs that it might also improve behaviour, concentration and academic attainment, especially in maths. Critically, there is no evidence that diverting classroom time away from desk-based study and towards more physical activity will harm educational outcomes. A growing number of schools, particularly at the primary stage, are not only implementing exercise interventions but also reporting positive results. Overall, incorporating more physical activity into the school day can be relatively straightforward and inexpensive: Activity breaks within lessons, or a timetabled daily run, are practical choices for increasing fitness in primary school, while introducing structured fitness activities during PE is an option in secondary settings.

Further Resources for the Reader to Learn More About the Topic

* For more information on the Take10! lesson plans used in the Physical Activity Across the Curriculum study. Retrieved from www.take10.net
* For more information on the SPARK PE programme. Retrieved from www.sparkpe.org
* For more information about the physical activity guidelines for children. Retrieved from www.nhs.uk/Livewell/fitness/Pages/physical-activity-guidelines-for-children.aspx
* For more information about the exercise- cognition relationship: McMorris, T., Tomporowski, P., & Audiffren, M. (2014). *Exercise and cognitive function*. Chichester: John Wiley & Sons.

References

Álvarez-Bueno, C., Pesce, C., Cavero-Redondo, I., Sánchez-López, M., Martínez-Hortelano, J. A., & Martínez-Vizcaíno, V. (2017). The effect of physical activity interventions on children's cognition and metacognition: A systematic review and meta-analysis. *J. Am. Acad. Child Adolesc. Psychiatry*, 56(9), 729–738.

Barkley, R. A. (1997). Behavioral inhibition, sustained attention, and executive functions: Constructing a unifying theory of ADHD. Behavioral inhibition, sustained attention, and executive functions: Constructing a unifying theory of ADHD. *Psychol. Bull.*, 121(1), 65–94.

Basso, J. C., & Suzuki, W. A. (2017). The effects of acute exercise on mood, cognition, neurophysiology, and neurochemical pathways: A review. *Brain Plast.*, 2, 127–152.

Benzing, V., Heinks, T., Eggenberger, N., & Schmidt, M. (2016). Acute cognitively engaging exergame-based physical activity enhances executive functions in adolescents. *PLoS One*, 11(12), 1–15.

Berchtold, N. C., Castello, N., & Cotman, C. W. (2010). Exercise and time-dependent benefits to learning and memory. *Neuroscience*, 167(3), 588–597.

Berchtold, N. C., Chinn, G., Chou, M., Kesslak, J. P., & Cotman, C. W. (2005). Exercise primes a molecular memory for brain-derived neurotrophic factor protein induction in the rat hippocampus. *Neuroscience*, 133(3), 853–861.

Best, J. R. (2010). Effects of physical activity on children's executive function: Contributions of experimental research on aerobic exercise. *Dev. Rev.*, 30(4), 331–351.

Best, J. R. (2012). Exergaming immediately enhances children's executive function. *Developmental Psychology*, 48, 5. St. Louis, MO: American Psychological Association, Washington University School of Medicine, Department of Psychiatry, pp. 1501–1510. Retrieved from bestj@psychiatry.wustl.edu

Biddle, S. J. H., & Asare, M. (2011). Physical activity and mental health in children and adolescents: A review of reviews. *Br. J. Sports Med.*, 45(11), 886–895. doi:10.1136/bjsports-2011-090185

Brisswalter, J., Collardeau, M., & Arcelin, R. (2002). Effects of acute physical exercise characteristics on cognitive performance. *Sport. Med.*, 32(9), 555–566.

Brown, J. et al. (2003). Enriched environment and physical activity stimulate hippocampal but not olfactory bulb neurogenesis. *Eur. J. Neurosci.*, 17(10), 2042–2046.

Buchheit, M., & Laursen, P. B. (2013). High-intensity interval training, solutions to the programming puzzle: Part I: Cardiopulmonary emphasis. *Sport. Med.*, 43(5), 313–338.

Budde, H., Voelcker-Rehage, C., Pietraßyk-Kendziorra, S., Ribeiro, P., & Tidow, G. (2008). Acute coordinative exercise improves attentional performance in adolescents. *Neurosci. Lett.*, 441(2), 219–223.

Caspersen, C. J., Powell, K. E., & Christenson, G. M. (1985). Physical activity, exercise, and physical fitness: Definitions and distinctions for health-related research. *Public Health Rep.*, 100(2), 126.

Cassilhas, R. C., Tufik, S., & De Mello, M. T. (2016). Physical exercise, neuroplasticity, spatial learning and memory. *Cell. Mol. Life Sci.*, 73(5), 975–983.

Chaddock, L., Hillman, C. H., Pontifex, M. B., Johnson, C. R., Raine, L. B., & Kramer, A. F. (2012). Childhood aerobic fitness predicts cognitive performance one year later. *J. Sports Sci.*, 30(5), 421–430.

Chaddock, L., Pontifex, M. B., Hillman, C. H., & Kramer, A. F. (2011). A review of the relation of aerobic fitness and physical activity to brain structure and function in children. *J. Int. Neuropsychol. Soc.*, 17(6), 975–985.

Chaddock, L. et al. (2010a). A neuroimaging investigation of the association between aerobic fitness, hippocampal volume, and memory performance in preadolescent children. *Brain Res.*, 1358, 172–183.

Chaddock, L. et al. (2010b). Basal ganglia volume is associated with aerobic fitness in preadolescent children. *Dev. Neurosci., 32*(3), 249–256.

Chaddock, L. et al. (2012). A functional MRI investigation of the association between childhood aerobic fitness and neurocognitive control. *Biol. Psychol., 89*(1), 260–268.

Chaddock-Heyman, L. et al. (2013). White matter microstructure is associated with cognitive control in children. *Biol. Psychol., 94*(1), 109–115.

Chaddock-Heyman, L. et al. (2014). Aerobic fitness is associated with greater white matter integrity in children. *Front. Hum. Neurosci., 8*, 1–7.

Chaddock-Heyman, L. et al. (2016). Aerobic fitness is associated with greater hippocampal cerebral blood flow in children. *Dev. Cogn. Neurosci., 20*, 52–58.

Chang, Y.-K., Hung, C.-L., Huang, C.-J., Hatfield, B. D., & Hung, T.-M. (2014). Effects of an aquatic exercise program on inhibitory control in children with ADHD: A preliminary study. *Arch. Clin. Neuropsychol., 29*(3), 217–223.

Chang, Y.-K., Labban, J. D., Gapin, J. I., & Etnier, J. L. (2012). The effects of acute exercise on cognitive performance: A meta-analysis. *Brain Res., 1453*(250), 87–101.

Chen, A.-G., Yan, J., Yin, H.-C., Pan, C.-Y., & Chang, Y.-K. (2014). Effects of acute aerobic exercise on multiple aspects of executive function in preadolescent children. *Psychol. Sport Exerc., 15*(6), 627–636.

Chen, A.-G., Zhu, L., Yan, J., Yin, H., & Chen, A. (2016, November). Neural basis of working memory enhancement after acute aerobic exercise: fMRI study of preadolescent children. *Front. Psychol., 7*, 1–9.

Chesham, R. A., Booth, J. N., Sweeney, E. L., Ryde, G. C., Gorely, T., Brooks, N. E., & Moran, C. N. (2018). The Daily Mile makes primary school children more active, less sedentary and improves their fitness and body composition: A quasi-experimental pilot study. *BMC Medicine, 16*(1), 64.

Chu, C., Kramer, A. F., Song, T., Wu, C., Hung, T., & Chang, Y. (2017). Acute exercise and neurocognitive development in preadolescents and young adults: An ERP study. *Neural Plast.*, 14–16.

Clark, P. J., Brzezinska, W. J., Puchalski, E. K., Krone, D. A., & Rhodes, J. S. (2009). Functional analysis of neurovascular adaptations to exercise in the dentate gyrus of young adult mice associated with cognitive gain. *Hippocampus, 19*(10), 937–950.

Cohen, J. (1988). *Statistical power analysis for the behavioral sciences* (2nd ed.). Hillsdale: Lawrence Erlbaum Associates.

Cooper, S. B., Bandelow, S., Nute, M. L., Morris, J. G., & Nevill, M. E. (2012). The effects of a mid-morning bout of exercise on adolescents' cognitive function. *Ment. Health Phys. Act., 5*(2), 183–190.

Cooper, S. B., Bandelow, S., Nute, M. L., Morris, J. G., & Nevill, M. E. (2015). Breakfast glycaemic index and exercise: Combined effects on adolescents' cognition. *Physiol. Behav., 139*, 104–111.

Costigan, S. A., Eather, N., Plotnikoff, R. C., Hillman, C. H., & Lubans, D. R. (2016). High-intensity interval training for cognitive and mental health in adolescents. *Med. Sci. Sports Exerc., 48*(10), 1985–1993.

Costigan, S. A., Eather, N., Plotnikoff, R. C., Taaffe, D. R., & Lubans, D. R. (2015). High-intensity interval training for improving health-related fitness in adolescents: A systematic review and meta-analysis. *Br. J. Sports Med.*, doi:10.1136/bjsports-2014-094490

Cotman, C. W., Berchtold, N. C., & Christie, L.-A. (2007). Exercise builds brain health: Key roles of growth factor cascades and inflammation. *Trends Neurosci., 30*(9), 464–472.

Davies, S., Burns, H., Jewell, T., & McBride, M. (2011). *Start active, stay active: A report on physical activity from the four home countries' chief medical officers department*, p. 1e61.

de Greeff, J. W., Bosker, R. J., Oosterlaan, J., Visscher, C., & Hartman, E. (2017). Effects of physical activity on executive functions, attention and academic performance in preadolescent children: A meta-analysis. *J. Sci. Med. Sport, 21*(5), 501–507.

Diamond, A. (2015). Effects of physical exercise on executive functions: Going beyond simply moving to moving with thought. *Ann. Sport. Med. Res., 2*(1), 1011.

Diamond, A. B. (2015). The cognitive benefits of exercise in youth. *Curr. Sports Med. Rep., 14*(4), 320–326.

Ding, Q., Vaynman, S., Akhavan, M., Ying, Z., & Gomez-Pinilla, F. (2006). Insulin-like growth factor I interfaces with brain-derived neurotrophic factor-mediated synaptic plasticity to modulate aspects of exercise-induced cognitive function. *Neuroscience, 140*(3), 823–833.

Dobbins, M., Husson, H., Decorby, K., & LaRocca, R. L. (2013). School-based physical activity programs for promoting physical activity and fitness in children and adolescents aged 6 to 18 (review). *Cochrane Database Syst. Rev., 18*(2).

Donnelly, J. E. et al. (2009). Physical activity across the curriculum (PAAC): A randomized controlled trial to promote physical activity and diminish overweight and obesity in elementary school children. *Prev. Med. (Baltim)., 49*(4), 336–341.

Donnelly, J. E. et al. (2016). Physical activity, fitness, cognitive function, and academic achievement in children: A systematic review. *Med. Sci. Sports Exerc., 48*(6), 1197.

Drollette, E. S., Shishido, T., Pontifex, M. B., & Hillman, C. H. (2012). Maintenance of cognitive control during and after walking in preadolescent children. *Med. Sci. Sports Exerc., 44*(10), 2017–2024.

Drollette, E. S. et al. (2014). Acute exercise facilitates brain function and cognition in children who need it most: An ERP study of individual differences in inhibitory control capacity. *Dev. Cogn. Neurosci., 7*, 53–64.

Ellemberg, D., & St-Louis-Deschenes, M. (2010). The effect of acute physical exercise on cognitive function during development. *Psychol. Sport Exerc., 11*, 122–126.

Esteban-Cornejo, I., Tejero-Gonzalez, C. M., Sallis, J. F., & Veiga, O. L. (2015). Physical activity and cognition in adolescents: A systematic review. *J. Sci. Med. Sport, 18*(5), 534–539.

Etnier, J. L., Nowell, P. M., Landers, D. M., & Sibley, B. A. (2006). A meta-regression to examine the relationship between aerobic fitness and cognitive performance. *Brain Res. Rev., 52*(1), 119–130.

Etnier, J. L., Salazar, W., Landers, D. M., Petruzzello, S. J., Han, M., & Nowell, P. (1997). The influence of physical fitness and exercise upon cognitive functioning: A meta-analysis. *J. Sport Exerc. Psychol., 19*, 249–277.

Farmer, J., Zhao, X., van Praag, H., Wodtke, K., Gage, F. H., & Christie, B. R. (2004). Effects of voluntary exercise on synaptic plasticity and gene expression in the dentate gyrus of adult male sprague-dawley rats in vivo. *Neuroscience, 124*(1), 71–79.

Fedewa, A. L., & Ahn, S. (2011). The effects of physical activity and physical fitness on children's achievement and cognitive outcomes: A meta-analysis. *Res. Q. Exerc. Sport, 82*(3), 521–535.

Fisher, A. et al. (2011). Effects of a physical education intervention on cognitive function in young children: Randomized controlled pilot study. *BMC Pediatr., 11*(1), 97.

Foulkes, L., & Blakemore, S.-J. (2018). Studying individual differences in human adolescent brain development. *Nat. Neurosci., 1*.

Gao, Z., Hannan, P., Xiang, P., Stodden, D. F., & Valdez, V. E. (2013). Video game-based exercise, Latino children's physical health, and academic achievement. *Am. J. Prev. Med.*, *44*(Suppl. 3), S240–S246.

Gawrilow, C., Stadler, G., Langguth, N., Naumann, A., & Boeck, A. (2016). Physical activity, affect, and cognition in children with symptoms of ADHD. *J. Atten. Disord.*, *20*(2), 151–162.

Gibson, C. A. et al. (2008). Physical activity, overweight and central adiposity in Swedish children and adolescents: The European youth heart study. *Int. J. Behav. Nutr. Phys. Act.*, *5*, 36.

Gomez-Pinilla, F., & Hillman, C. (2013). The influence of exercise on cognitive abilities. *Compr. Physiol.*, *3*(1), 403–428.

Groves, J. O. et al. (2013). Ablating adult neurogenesis in the rat has no effect on spatial processing: Evidence from a novel pharmacogenetic model. *PLoS Genet.*, *9*(9), e1003718.

Hall, J., Thomas, K. L., & Everitt, B. J. (2000). Rapid and selective induction of BDNF expression in the hippocampus during contextual learning. *Nat. Neurosci.*, *3*(6), 533–535.

Halperin, D., & Healey, J. M. (2011). The influences of environmental enrichment, cognitive enhancement, and physical exercise on brain development: Can we alter the developmental trajectory of ADHD? *Neurosci. Biobehav. Rev.*, *35*(3), 621–634.

Hansen, D. M., Herrmann, S. D., Lambourne, K., Lee, J., & Donnelly, J. E. (2014). Linear/nonlinear relations of activity and fitness with children's academic achievement. *Med. Sci. Sports Exerc.*, *46*(12), 2279.

Herting, M. M., & Nagel, B. J. (2012). Aerobic fitness relates to learning on a virtual Morris water task and hippocampal volume in adolescents. *Behav. Brain Res.*, *233*(2), 517–525.

Hillman, C. H., Buck, S. M., Themanson, J. R., Pontifex, M. B., & Castelli, D. M. (2009). Aerobic fitness and cognitive development: Event-related brain potential and task performance indices of executive control in preadolescent children. *Dev. Psychol.*, *45*(1), 114–129.

Hillman, C. H., Erickson, K. I., & Hatfield, B. D. (2017). Run for your life! Childhood physical activity effects on brain and cognition. *Kinesiol. Rev.*, *6*(1), 12–21.

Hillman, C., Kamijo, K., & Scudder, M. (2011). A review of chronic and acute physical activity participation on neuroelectric measures of brain health and cognition during childhood. *Prev. Med.*, S21–S28.

Hillman, C. H., Pontifex, M. B., Raine, L. B., Castelli, D. M., Hall, E. E., & Kramer, A. F. (2009). The effect of acute treadmill walking on cognitive control and academic achievement in preadolescent children. *Neuroscience*, *159*(3), 1044–1054.

Hogan, M., Kiefer, M., Kubesch, S., Collins, P., Kilmartin, L., & Brosnan, M. (2013). The interactive effects of physical fitness and acute aerobic exercise on electrophysiological coherence and cognitive performance in adolescents. *Exp. Brain Res.*, *229*, 85–96.

Howie, E. K., Schatz, J., & Pate, R. R. (2015). Acute effects of classroom exercise breaks on executive function and math performance: A dose—response study. *Res. Q. Exerc. Sport*, *86*(3), 217–224.

Hsieh, S. et al. (2017). Effects of childhood gymnastics program on spatial working memory. *Med. Sci. Sports Exerc.*, *49*, 2537–2347.

Ishihara, T., Sugasawa, S., Matsuda, Y., & Mizuno, M. (2017). The beneficial effects of game-based exercise using age-appropriate tennis lessons on the executive functions of 6–12-year-old children. *Neurosci. Lett.*, *642*, 97–101.

Jäger, K., Schmidt, M., Conzelmann, A., Roebers, C. M., & Anderson, P. J. (2014, December). Cognitive and physiological effects of an acute physical activity intervention in elementary school children. *Front. Psychol.*, 5, 1–11.

Janssen, M., Chinapaw, M. J. M., Rauh, S. P., Toussaint, H. M., Van Mechelen, W., & Verhagen, E. (2014). A short physical activity break from cognitive tasks increases selective attention in primary school children aged 10–11. *Ment. Health Phys. Act.*, 7(3), 129–134.

Janssen, M., Toussaint, H. M., van Mechelen, W., & Verhagen, E. A. (2014). Effects of acute bouts of physical activity on children's attention: A systematic review of the literature. *Springerplus*, 3, 410.

Kamijo, K., & Masaki, H. (2016, August). Fitness and ERP indices of cognitive control mode during task preparation in preadolescent children. *Front. Hum. Neurosci.*, 10, 1–10.

Kent, B. A., Oomen, C. A., Bekinschtein, P., Bussey, T. J., & Saksida, L. M. (2015). Cognitive enhancing effects of voluntary exercise, caloric restriction and environmental enrichment: A role for adult hippocampal neurogenesis and pattern separation? *Curr. Opin. Behav. Sci.*, 4, 179–185.

Khan, N. A., & Hillman, C. H. (2014). The relation of childhood physical activity and aerobic fitness to brain function and cognition: A review. *Pediatr. Exerc. Sci.*, 26(2), 138–146.

Krafft, C. E. et al. (2014). Improved frontoparietal white matter integrity in overweight children is associated with attendance at an after-school exercise program. *Dev. Neurosci.*, 36(1), 1–9.

Kriemler, S., Meyer, U., Martin, E., van Sluijs, E. M. F., Andersen, L. B., & Martin, B. W. (2011). Effect of school-based interventions on physical activity and fitness in children and adolescents: A review of reviews and systematic update. *Br. J. Sports Med.*, 45(11), 923–930.

Lambourne, K., & Tomporowski, P. (2010). The effect of exercise-induced arousal on cognitive task performance: A meta-regression analysis. *Brain Res.*, 1341, 12–24.

Lanningham-Foster, L., Foster, R., McCrady, S., & Manohar, C. (2008). Changing the school environment to increase physical activity in children. *Obesity*, 16(8), 1849–1853.

Lees, C., & Hopkins, J. (2013). Effect of aerobic exercise on cognition, academic achievement, and psychosocial function in children: A systematic review of randomized control trials. *Prev. Chronic Dis.*, 10(10), doi: 10.5888/pcd10.130010

Léger, L. A., Mercier, D., Gadoury, C., & Lambert, J. (1988). The multistage 20 metre shuttle run test for aerobic fitness. *J. Sports Sci.*, 6(2), 93–101.

Leuner, B., & Gould, E. (2010). Structural plasticity and hippocampal function. *Annu. Rev. Psychol.*, 61(1), 111–140.

Li, J. W., O'Connor, H., O'Dwyer, N., & Orr, R. (2017). The effect of acute and chronic exercise on cognitive function and academic performance in adolescents: A systematic review. *J. Sci. Med. Sport*, 20(9), 841–848.

Lind, R. R. et al. (2017). Improved cognitive performance in preadolescent Danish children after the school-based physical activity programme "FIFA 11 for health" for Europe—A cluster-randomised controlled trial. *Eur. J. Sport Sci.*, 18(1), 130–139.

Lipsky, R. H., & Marini, A. M. (2007). Brain-derived neurotrophic factor in neuronal survival and behavior-related plasticity. *Ann. N. Y. Acad. Sci.*, 1122, 130–143.

Lopez-Lopez, C., LeRoith, D., & Torres-Aleman, I. (2004). Insulin-like growth factor I is required for vessel remodeling in the adult brain. *Proc. Natl. Acad. Sci. U. S. A.*, 101(26), 9833–9838.

Lubans, D., Richards, J., Hillman, C., Faulkner, G., & Beauchamp, M. (2016). Physical activity for cognitive and mental health in youth: A systematic review of mechanisms. *Pediatrics, 138*(3).

Ludyga, S. et al. (2017, October). Developmental cognitive neuroscience an event-related potential investigation of the acute effects of aerobic and coordinative exercise on inhibitory control in children with ADHD. *Dev. Cogn. Neurosci., 28*, 21–28.

Ma, C. L., Ma, X. T., Wang, J. J., Liu, H., Chen, Y. F., & Yang, Y. (2017). Physical exercise induces hippocampal neurogenesis and prevents cognitive decline. *Behav. Brain Res., 317*, 332–339.

Ma, J. K., Le Mare, L., & Gurd, B. J. (2014). Classroom-based high-intensity interval activity improves off-task behaviour in primary school students. *Appl. Physiol. Nutr. Metab., 39*(12), 1332–1337.

Mcmorris, T. (2016). Developing the catecholamines hypothesis for the acute exercise-cognition interaction in humans: Lessons from animal studies. *Physiol. Behav., 165*, 291–299.

Mcmorris, T., & Hale, B. J. (2012). Brain and cognition differential effects of differing intensities of acute exercise on speed and accuracy of cognition: A meta-analytical investigation. *Brain Cogn., 80*(3), 338–351.

McNaughten, D., & Gabbard, C. (1993). Physical exertion and immediate mental performance of sixth-grade children. *Percept. Mot. Skills, 77*(Suppl. 3), 1155–1159.

Merritt, J. R., & Rhodes, J. S. (2015). Mouse genetic differences in voluntary wheel running, adult hippocampal neurogenesis and learning on the multi-strain-adapted plus water maze. *Behav. Brain Res., 280*, 62–71.

Molteni, R., Ying, Z., & Gómez-Pinilla, F. (2002). Differential effects of acute and chronic exercise on plasticity-related genes in the rat hippocampus revealed by microarray. *Eur. J. Neurosci., 16*(6), 1107–1116.

Moreau, D., Kirk, I. J., & Waldie, K. E. (2017). High-intensity training enhances executive function in children in a randomized, placebo-controlled trial. *Elife, 6*.

Morris, J. L., Daly-Smith, A., Archbold, V. S., Wilkins, E. L., & McKenna, J. (2019). The Daily Mile™ initiative: Exploring physical activity and the acute effects on executive function and academic performance in primary school children. *Psychology of Sport and Exercise, 45*, 101583.

Mustroph, M. L., Chen, S., Desai, S. C., Cay, E. B., DeYoung, E. K., & Rhodes, J. S. (2012). Aerobic exercise is the critical variable in an enriched environment that increases hippocampal neurogenesis and water maze learning in male C57BL/6J mice. *Neuroscience, 219*, 62–71.

Neeper, S. A., Gomez-Pinilla, F., Choi, J., & Cotman, C. (1995). Exercise and brain neurotrophins. *Nature, 373*, 109.

Neeper, S. A., Gómez-Pinilla, F., Choi, J., & Cotman, C. W. (1996). Physical activity increases mRNA for brain-derived neurotrophic factor and nerve growth factor in rat brain. *Brain Res., 726*(1–2), 49–56.

Ng, Q. X., Ho, C. Y. X., Chan, H. W., Yong, B. Z. J., & Yeo, W. S. (2017, November). Managing childhood and adolescent attention-deficit/hyperactivity disorder (ADHD) with exercise: A systematic review. *Complement. Ther. Med., 34*, 123–128.

North, C. T., McCullagh, P., & Tran, Z. V. (1990). Effect of exercise on depression. *Exerc. Sport Sci. Rev., 18*(1), 379–416.

Ogoh, S. (2017). Relationship between cognitive function and regulation of cerebral blood flow. *J. Physiol. Sci., 67*(3), 345–351.

Patten, A. R., Yau, S. Y., Fontaine, C. J., Meconi, A., Wortman, R. C., & Christie, B. R. (2015). The benefits of exercise on structural and functional plasticity in the rodent hippocampus of different disease models. *Brain Plast.*, *1*, 97–127.

Peruyero, F., Zapata, J., Pastor, D., & Cervelló, E. (2017). The acute effects of exercise intensity on inhibitory cognitive control in adolescents. *Front. Psychol.*, 8(921), 1–7.

Pesce, C. (2012). Shifting the focus from quantitative to qualitative exercise characteristics in exercise and cognition research. *J. Sport Exerc. Psychol.*, *34*(6), 766–786.

Pesce, C., Crova, C., Cereatti, L., Casella, R., & Bellucci, M. (2009). Physical activity and mental performance in preadolescents: Effects of acute exercise on free-recall memory. *Ment. Health Phys. Act.*, *2*(1), 16–22.

Piepmeier, A. T. et al. (2015). The effect of acute exercise on cognitive performance in children with and without ADHD. *J. Sport Heal. Sci.*, *4*(1), 97–104.

Pirrie, A. M., & Lodewyk, K. R. (2012). Investigating links between moderate-to-vigorous physical activity and cognitive performance in elementary school students. *Ment. Health Phys. Act.*, *5*(1), 93–98.

Polich, J. (2007). Updating P300: An integrative theory of P3a and P3b. *Clin. Neurophysiol.*, *118*(10), 2128–2148.

Pontifex, M. B., Saliba, B. J., Raine, L. B., Picchietti, D. L., & Hillman, C. H. (2013). Exercise improves behavioral, neurocognitive, and scholastic performance in children with attention-deficit/hyperactivity disorder. *J. Pediatr.*, *162*(3), 543–551.

Pontifex, M. B. et al. (2011). Cardiorespiratory fitness and the flexible modulation of cognitive control in preadolescent children. *J. Cogn. Neurosci.*, *23*(6), 1332–1345.

Rasberry, C. N. et al. (2011). The association between school-based physical activity, including physical education, and academic performance: A systematic review of the literature. *Prev. Med. (Baltim).*, *52*(Suppl.), S10–S20.

Reed, J., & Ones, D. S. (2006). The effect of acute aerobic exercise on positive activated affect: A meta-analysis. *Psychol. Sport Exerc.*, *7*(5), 477–514.

Resaland, G. K. et al. (2016). Effects of physical activity on schoolchildren's academic performance: The active smarter kids (ASK) cluster-randomized controlled trial. *Prev. Med. (Baltim).*, *91*, 322–328.

Rhyu, I. J. et al. (2010). Effects of aerobic exercise training on cognitive function and cortical vascularity in monkeys. *Neuroscience*, *167*(4), 1239–1248.

Rothman, S. M., & Mattson, M. P. (2013). Activity-dependent, stress-responsive BDNF signaling and the quest for optimal brain health and resilience throughout the lifespan. *Neuroscience*, *239*, 228–240.

Sallis, J. F., McKenzie, T. L., Kolody, B., Lewis, M., Marshall, S., & Rosengard, P. (1999). Effects of health-related physical education on academic achievement: Project SPARK. *Res. Q. Exerc. Sport*, *70*(2), 127–134.

Samuel, R. D., Zavdy, O., Levav, M., Reuveny, R., Katz, U., & Dubnov-Raz, G. (2017). The effects of maximal intensity exercise on cognitive performance in children by. *J. Hum. Kinet.*, *57*, 85–96.

Schaeffer, D. J. et al. (2014). An 8-month exercise intervention alters frontotemporal White matter integrity in overweight children. *Psychophysiology*, *51*(8), 728–733.

Schmidt-Hieber, C., Jonas, P., & Bischofberger, J. (2004). Enhanced synaptic plasticity in newly generated granule cells of the adult hippocampus. *Nature*, *429*(6988), 184–187.

SHAPE America—Society of Health and Physical Educators. (2016). *Shape of the nation 2016: Status of physical education in the USA*. Report.

Sibley, B. A., & Etnier, J. L. (2003). The relationship between physical activity and cognition in children: A meta-analysis. *Pediatr. Exerc. Sci.*, *15*, 243–256.

Sleiman, S. F., & Chao, M. V. (2015). Downstream consequences of exercise through the action of BDNF. *Brain Plast.*, *1*(1), 143–148.

Soga, K., Shishido, T., & Nagatomi, R. (2015). Executive function during and after acute moderate aerobic exercise in adolescents. *Psychol. Sport Exerc.*, *16*, 7–17.

Speisman, R. B., Kumar, A., Rani, A., Foster, T. C., & Ormerod, B. K. (2013). Daily exercise improves memory, stimulates hippocampal neurogenesis and modulates immune and neuroimmune cytokines in aging rats. *Brain. Behav. Immun.*, *28*, 25–43.

Spitzer, U. S., & Hollmann, W. (2013). Experimental observations of the effects of physical exercise on attention, academic and prosocial performance in school settings. *Trends Neurosci. Educ.*, *2*(1), 1–6.

Standage, M., Duda, J. L., & Ntoumanis, N. (2003). A model of contextual motivation in physical education: Using constructs from self-determination and achievement goal theories to predict physical activity intentions. *J. Educ. Psychol.*, *95*(1), 97–110.

Stroth, S., Kubesch, S., Dieterle, K., Ruchsow, M., Heim, R., & Kiefer, M. (2009). Physical fitness, but not acute exercise modulates event-related potential indices for executive control in healthy adolescents. *Brain Res.*, *1269*, 114–124.

Swain, R. A. et al. (2003). Prolonged exercise induces angiogenesis and increases cerebral blood volume in primary motor cortex of the rat. *Neuroscience*, *117*(4), 1037–1046.

Tandon, P. S. et al. (2016). The relationship between physical activity and diet and young children's cognitive development: A systematic review. *Prev. Med. Reports*, *3*, 379–390.

Tang, K., Xia, F. C., Wagner, P. D., & Breen, E. C. (2010). Exercise-induced VEGF transcriptional activation in brain, lung and skeletal muscle. *Respir. Physiol. Neurobiol.*, *170*(1), 16–22.

Tardif, C. L. et al. (2016). Advanced MRI techniques to improve our understanding of experience-induced neuroplasticity. *Neuroimage*, *131*, 55–72.

Tine, M. T., & Butler, A. G. (2012). Acute aerobic exercise impacts selective attention: An exceptional boost in lower-income children. *Educ. Psychol.*, *32*(7), 821–834.

Tomporowski, P. D. (2003a). Effects of acute bouts of exercise on cognition. *Acta Psychol. (Amst).*, *112*, 297–324.

Tomporowski, P. D. (2003b). Cognitive and behavioral responses to acute exercise in youths: A review. *Pediatr. Exerc. Sci.*, *15*(4), 348–359.

Tomporowski, P. D., McCullick, B., Pendleton, D. M., & Pesce, C. (2015). Exercise and children's cognition: The role of exercise characteristics and a place for metacognition. *J. Sport Heal. Sci.*, *4*(1), 47–55.

Triviño-Paredes, J., Patten, A. R., Gil-Mohapel, J., & Christie, B. R. (2016). The effects of hormones and physical exercise on hippocampal structural plasticity. *Front. Neuroendocrinol.*, *41*, 23–43.

Van der Borght, K., Havekes, R., Bos, T., Eggen, B. J. L., & Van der Zee, E. A. (2007). Exercise improves memory acquisition and retrieval in the Y-maze task: Relationship with hippocampal neurogenesis. *Behav. Neurosci.*, *121*(2), 324–334.

van der Niet, A. G., Smith, J., Scherder, E. J. A., Oosterlaan, J., Hartman, E., & Visscher, C. (2015). Associations between daily physical activity and executive functioning in primary school-aged children. *J. Sci. Med. Sport*, *18*(6), 673–677.

van Praag, H. (2008). Neurogenesis and exercise: Past and future directions. *NeuroMolecular Med.*, *10*(2), 128–140.

van Praag, H., Christie, B. R., Sejnowski, T. J., & Gage, F. H. (1999). Running enhances neurogenesis, learning, and long-term potentiation in mice. *Proc. Natl. Acad. Sci.*, 96(23), 13427–13431.

van Praag, H., Kempermann, G., & Gage, F. H. (1999). Running increases cell proliferation and neurogenesis in the adult mouse dentate gyrus. *Nat Neurosci*, 2(3), 266–270.

Vaynman, S., Ying, Z., & Gomez-Pinilla, F. (2004). Hippocampal BDNF mediates the efficacy of exercise on synaptic plasticity and cognition. *Eur. J. Neurosci.*, 20(10), 2580–2590.

Vazou, S., Pesce, C., Lakes, K., & Smiley-Oyen, A. (2016). More than one road leads to Rome: A narrative review and meta-analysis of physical activity intervention effects on cognition in youth. *Int. J. Sport Exerc. Psychol.*, 1–26.

Vazou, S., & Smiley-Oyen, A. (2014). Moving and academic learning are not antagonists: Acute effects on executive function and enjoyment. *J. Sport Exerc. Psychol.*, 36, 474–485.

Verburgh, L., Königs, M., Scherder, E. J. A., & Oosterlaan, J. (2013). Physical exercise and executive functions in preadolescent children, adolescents and young adults: A meta-analysis. *Br. J. Sports Med.*, 1–8.

Vivar, C., & van Praag, H. (2017). Running changes the brain: The long and the short of it. *Physiology*, 32(6), 410–424.

Voelcker-Rehage, C., & Niemann, C. (2013). Structural and functional brain changes related to different types of physical activity across the life span. *Neurosci. Biobehav. Rev.*, 37(9), 2268–2295.

Voss, M. W., Vivar, C., Kramer, A. F., & van Praag, H. (2013). Bridging animal and human models of exercise-induced brain plasticity. *Trends Cogn. Sci.*, 17(10), 525–544.

Voss, M. W. et al. (2011). Aerobic fitness is associated with greater efficiency of the network underlying cognitive control in. *Neuroscience*, 199, 166–176.

Wassenaar, T. M., Wheatley, C. M., Beale, N., Salvan, P., Meaney, A., Possee, J. B., . . . & Johansen-Berg, H. (2019). Effects of a programme of vigorous physical activity during secondary school physical education on academic performance, fitness, cognition, mental health and the brain of adolescents (Fit to Study): Study protocol for a cluster-randomised trial. *Trials*, 20(1), 189.

Watson, A., Timperio, A., Brown, H., Best, K., & Hesketh, K. D. (2017). Effect of classroom-based physical activity interventions on academic and physical activity outcomes: A systematic review and meta-analysis. *Int. J. Behav. Nutr. Phys. Act.*, 14(1), 114.

Willcutt, E. G. (2012). The prevalence of DSM-IV attention-deficit/hyperactivity disorder: A meta-analytic review. *Neurotherapeutics*, 9(3), 490–499.

Yau, S., Gil-Mohapel, J., Christie, B., & So, K. (2014). Physical exercise-induced adult neurogenesis: A good strategy to prevent cognitive decline in neurodegenerative diseases? *BioMed Res. . . . .*, Figure 1.

Yerkes, R. M., & Dodson, J. D. (1908). The relation of strength of stimulus to rapidity of habit-formation. *J. Comp. Neurol. Psychol.*, 18, 459–482.

15 The Cognitive Benefits and Disadvantages of Bilingualism Across the Lifespan and Implications for Education

Jacqueline Phelps and Roberto Filippi

Acknowledgements

This work was supported by the Leverhulme Trust UK [RPG-2015–024] and the British Academy [SG162171]. A special thought goes to Prof. Annette Karmiloff-Smith who inspired our research.

A Multilingual World

Bilingualism is becoming the rule rather than the exception in our increasingly interconnected world: Data suggest that there are many more bilinguals or multilinguals in the world than there are monolinguals. A decade ago, it was estimated that for every native speaker of English, there were three or four non-native speakers (Crystal, 2008). More recently, a study for the European Commission (2012) of 26,751 respondents across 27 member states reported that just over half (54%) of Europeans were able to hold a conversation in at least one additional language; a quarter were able to speak at least two additional languages, and one in ten were conversant in at least three. Additionally, global migration results in the phenomenon of many more children worldwide who are formally educated (partly or wholly) through a second language than there are children educated exclusively via their first language (Tucker, 2001). Thus the topic of multilingualism and its impact on children's cognitive development is of particular current concern to policy makers, researchers and educationalists.

For some, *bilingualism* + *education* = *success*, especially in achieving extra qualifications in foreign languages for a minimum of effort. The benefits of a bilingual upbringing, however, go beyond language examinations. There are the social benefits of interacting with different groups of friends in different countries/cultures; a broader outlook on life; enhanced overall communication skills; and an additional linguistic skill for life that will ultimately benefit prospects.

However, the *bilingualism* + *education* equation is not necessarily as straightforward for all. The question whether acquiring more than one language can be detrimental to cognitive development has always concerned parents and educators. In the modern U.K. school system, children raised in a multilingual environment are labelled as "English as an additional language" (EAL), vaguely implying that they might require some sort of special learning needs support. What is more, recent U.K. data (Strand, Malmberg, & Hall, 2015) showed reception-age EAL children lagging behind their peers in mathematics and literacy (44% of dual learner pupils achieved the expected level of mathematics and literacy, compared to 54% of their monolingual peers). Consequently, there are cases in which educators suggest parents of multilingual/multicultural families to stick to one language, arguing that adding a second or a third language may "confuse" their children (Festman, Poarch, & Dawaele, 2017).

Such a reaction may be instinctive, but is it supported by research-based evidence? In this chapter, we first set out to review the research field on bilingualism and its purported effects on cognition, both for children and across the lifespan. We explore some of the factors behind the conflicting and often contradictory results and interpretations. We then highlight the contributions of neuroscience to the debate thus far and identify future opportunities in the field of research. We conclude with implications for education and recommendations of further resources.

Research Into Bilingualism and Its Cognitive Effects: A Brief History

Early studies of bilingualism in childhood concluded that the management of two or more languages led to cognitive overload and "mental confusion" and was detrimental to children's intellectual development (e.g., Saer, 1923). According to several early studies, bilingual children performed significantly worse than their monolingual peers in IQ tests (Graham, 1925; Jones & Stewart, 1951; Lewis, 1959; Wang, 1926), arithmetic and reading (Macnamara, 1966; Manuel, 1935) and verbal intelligence (Darcy, 1953).

These results have since been criticised as misleading, however, for a number of reasons. First, early studies of bilingual children did not control for socio-economic status (SES). SES (often measured by maternal level of education and/or family income) is a compound of social background, income and occupational prestige and a well-documented environmental influence on cognitive development (Espy, Molfese, & DiLalla 2001; Hoff, 2003; Walker, Greenwood, Hart, & Carta, 1994; Mezzacappa, 2004) and thus recruitment of a bilingual sample from a lower SES than the monolingual children may have confounded early results. Secondly, studies such as Macnamara's (1966) put bilingual participants at a disadvantage by testing them in their weaker language.

Similarly, academic assessments demonstrating a shortfall in bilingual children's progress have often been based on standardised tests (e.g., vocabulary size); or not appropriately comparative separate measures (see Hakuta, 1986, for a review).

There have been objections to the drawing of conclusions about a child's cognitive ability from performance in one (usually weaker) language. Success in school depends upon the child's mastery of *academic* language, which is often very different from the language used at home (Tucker, 2001). Put succinctly, "A bilingual child is cognitively more able than his single-language skills reflect" (Hoff et al., 2012, p. 24). Total vocabulary across a bilingual child's languages has been shown to be equivalent to a monolingual child's in their one language (Hoff et al., 2012; Pearson, Fernández, & Oller, 1993). In addition, the development of academic language requires typically five to seven years of formal instruction (Cummins, 1984), which may explain (temporary) poorer academic outcomes. McLeod, Harrison, Whiteford, and Walker's (2015) study of schoolchildren found that any areas where the multilingual children lagged behind monolingual children at age 4–5 had closed by ages 6–7 and 8–9. Similarly, the report on English as an Additional Language and Educational achievement in the U.K. (Strand et al., 2015) concluded that any association between bilingualism and underachievement decreased significantly with age until there was virtually no attainment gap at age 16. Poor academic performance was a function of language skills, not cognition.

Indeed, the belief that bilingualism was somehow detrimental to cognition began to be overturned after a landmark study by Peal and Lambert (1962), which proposed that bilingual children, rather than being at a cognitive disadvantage, demonstrated an enhanced cognitive ability after performing better than their monolingual peers on a battery of verbal and nonverbal IQ tests. These tests controlled for the confounds of prior studies (SES, quality of schooling). This finding was among the first to suggest that the bilingual experience enhanced rather than detracted from cognitive ability. This triggered a stream of research, which proposed a variety of cognitive benefits of bilingual experience; Barac, Bialystok, Castro, and Sanchez (2014) reviewed no fewer than 102 studies claiming a cognitive effect of bilingualism on children. Some studies spanned age groups: even pre-verbal infants have been attributed enhanced cognitive functions due to the early processing of bilingual speech (studies include: Bosch & Sebastián-Gallés, 1997; Byers-Heinlein, Burns, & Werker, 2010; Ibanez-Lillo, Pons, Costa, & Sebastián-Gallés, 2010; Kovács & Mehler, 2009a, 2009b; Kuhl et al., 2006).

Other studies of bilingualism ranged across areas of cognition. A nonexhaustive list includes a bilingual advantage in: symbol-reorganisation tasks (Peal & Lambert, 1962), sensitivity to facial expressions (Bain, 1975), recognising feedback cues (Ben-Zeev, 1977), science problems (Kessler & Quinn, 1980), numeric symbols (Saxe, 1988), geometric design problems (Ricciardelli, 1992), and creative thinking (Hommel, Colzato, Fischer, & Christoffels, 2011).

Bialystok (2001) comprehensively reviewed studies of children's cognitive processes affected by bilingualism up to that point, and concluded that the most consistent finding was an advantage in selective attention and inhibition. She proposed that the experience of processing and producing two languages (L1 and L2) significantly accelerated bilingual children's ability to attend selectively to relevant information and control interference (inhibit attention to misleading information or competing responses), through the management of multiple active languages. She hypothesised that regular, long-term "exercise" of this enhanced control generalised beyond language control into an enhancement of executive control, demonstrated in non-verbal tasks.

This enhanced control of selective attention due to bilingualism has been coined the "bilingual advantage". On the one hand, it has been supported by theoretical models and behavioural evidence (by performance in non-verbal tasks). On the other, it has been contested by researchers using similar paradigms. Let us examine the evidence on both sides.

Theoretical Models Underpinning the "Bilingual Advantage"

Theoretical models supporting the notion of a bilingual advantage are predicated on the notion of "executive control" or "executive functions" (EF), the set of higher-order cognitive processes involved in the control of attention, thought and action. These are either presented as a unified function of a central executive (e.g., Baddeley's unitary construct, 1996); connected but disassociable functions (as in Miyake et al.'s unity/diversity framework, 2000); or up to 15 separate executive functions (Best, Miller, & Jones, 2009). In all models, they are responsible for sustaining attention in the presence of distracting information and switching attention between two or more tasks or stimuli.

Green (1998) proposed that bilinguals recruit these domain-general (i.e., not language specific) inhibitory control mechanisms in order to inhibit nontarget lexical representations during language production. This influential model of inhibitory control (ICM) led to Green and Abutalebi's (2013) Adaptive Control Hypothesis, a detailed framework for the mechanisms underlying bilingual control of attention. They identified eight control processes employed in bilingual interactional contexts, one of which was interference control (conflict monitoring and interference suppression), and predicted bilingual advantages in the control of non-verbal tasks as a result, a prediction that formed the basis of multiple studies.

Behavioural Evidence for the Bilingual Advantage: Performance in Non-verbal Tests

Studies investigating the bilingual advantage can be broadly divided into two areas. The first is behavioural studies, where bilingual and monolingual participants' performance across a number of cognitive tasks is measured and compared. The second is neuroimaging studies (structural and functional). Let us examine the behavioural evidence first.

A number of non-verbal tasks have been used to investigate Bialystok's (2001) and Green and Abutalebi's (2013) prediction that bilinguals would outperform monolinguals on tests involving attentional control and inhibition. Most of the tasks used have focused on interference in the *visual* domain and have included the Dimensional Change Card Sort (DCCS) task (e.g., Bialystok, 1999), the Stroop task (e.g., Poulin-Dubois, Blaye, Coutya, & Bialystok, 2011), the flanker task (e.g., Calvo & Bialystok, 2014), the Attentional Network Task (ANT) (e.g., Carlson & Meltzoff, 2008) and the Simon task (e.g., Poarch & van Hell, 2012). These all follow a similar logic to manipulate switching between rules, inhibiting irrelevant messages and updating information: In the DCCS task, participants are asked to remember and apply a rule for sorting cards (e.g., by colour), then suppress the first rule in favour of a second different rule (e.g., sort by shape). In the flanker task, the participant presses a button on the right/left in response to the direction in which a distinctive arrow is pointing. These central arrows are flanked by other arrows either pointing in the same direction (congruent), or the opposite direction (incongruent).

The ANT is a version of the flanker task with additional visual cues. Trials are preceded by a fixation cross, an alerting cue to indicate a trial is about to begin, or an orienting cue to indicate if the arrows will appear above or below the fixation cross. A variation for children (as used by Carlson & Meltzoff, 2008) is a computerised game featuring *hungry fish*. Children are instructed to feed the fish as soon as they appear on screen, by clicking the left button (for fish facing left) and right button (for fish facing right). On no-flanker trials, one fish appears on its own on the screen. In flanker trials, the target fish is always in the centre of a row of five fish. Congruent trials show all fish facing in the same direction; incongruent trials show the central fish facing in a different direction from the four fish surrounding it (creating attentional conflict).

The most widely used task for assessing attentional control has been the Simon task (Simon, 1967). In the standard computerised version of the Simon task, one of two stimuli (a blue or red shape) appears on either the left or the right side of a computer screen. Participants are required to respond as quickly and accurately as possible by pressing a left or right button (each of which is associated with one of the two colours). This button/colour mapping allows manipulation of trials such that some are congruent (i.e., the correct response is on the same side as the stimulus, left/left or right/right) and some are incongruent (i.e., the correct response on the opposite side to the stimulus, left/right or right/left). According to Lu and Proctor (1995), the Simon effect—a longer reaction time for incongruent spatial stimuli—is a widespread and persistent phenomenon that can be attributed to response selection processes.

Many of the studies have proposed an advantage of bilingual experience on children's performance in these visual tasks. Two-year-olds have demonstrated a bilingual advantage on the Stroop task (Poulin-Dubois et al., 2011), 3–4 year olds on the DCCS task (Bialystok, 1999; Bialystok & Martin, 2004), and 5–8 year olds on the Simon task (Poarch & van Hell, 2012).

Additional tests on children in the visual domain have included Bialystok's (1992) Embedded Figures task, in which bilingual 7–9-year-olds were more successful at finding a simple pattern concealed in a more complex picture. Similar results were found in 6-year-old children's performance on the ambiguous figures task, a task that asked participants to identify the alternative image in a reversible figure (Bialystok & Shapero, 2005).

For both children and adults, there have been far fewer studies of attentional control in the *auditory* domain. This is surprising given that bilinguals hear and suppress conflicting auditory information in different languages on a regular basis. A bilingual advantage has been reported in studies ranging from the presentation of single syllables in different ears (e.g., Soveri, Laine, Hämäläinen, & Hugdahl, 2011) to whole sentence comprehension (e.g., Filippi, Leech, Thomas, Green, & Dick, 2012; Filippi et al., 2015) under conditions of auditory verbal interference. These studies compared bilingual and monolingual groups' comprehension of simple (e.g., canonical: Subject-Verb-Object) and complex (e.g., non-canonical: Object-Verb-Subject) sentences with and without verbal interference. For adults, Filippi et al. (2012) found that the bilingual group significantly outperformed their Italian monolingual peers, especially in the comprehension of non-canonical sentences, in the condition of auditory interference. For children aged 7–10, (Filippi et al., 2015) the bilingual group showed an advantage in controlling interference in complex (non-canonical) sentences when the interference was in an unknown language (Greek, in this study). In addition, bilingual children exhibited significantly improved comprehension of non-canonical sentences in the presence of both types of linguistic interference (English and Greek) with increasing age. This suggested that the bilingual advantage in controlling auditory verbal interference improved throughout development.

So far the evidence seems to be building that there is a discernible "bilingual advantage" across visual nonverbal and auditory verbal tasks.

The Case for the Opposition

However, evidence for the bilingual advantage has not always been straightforward. There have been inconsistent results, which have raised doubts. For example, tests using the Simon task on both middle-aged (age 30–54) and older adults (age 60–88) have indicated bilingual advantage across both age groups (Bialystok, Craik, Klein, & Viswanathan, 2004); but the same tests on young adults revealed no difference between the bilingual and monolingual groups (Bialystok et al., 2004.). Similarly, the field has continued to be plagued with criticism over the confound of SES. Attempts to counter the low SES of bilinguals (which would drag down the results, as discussed earlier in the summary of early studies) have included adjusting the (comparable) raw scores between bilingual and monolingual kindergarten children and statistically control for the bilingual group's lower SES and verbal scores (Carlson & Meltzoff, 2008). The final result in this study was a statistically significant advantage for the bilingual children in tasks managing conflicting attentional demands, including the Advanced DCCS and a modified ANT task. This method, however, has been criticised as deliberately skewing the results in another direction.

The opposite SES criticism has also been levied at bilingual advantage researchers—that is, that studies often recruit bilinguals from *higher* SES back-grounds than their monolingual samples and that this recruitment puts the bilinguals at a considerable advantage. Morton and Harper (2007) replicated a study using the Simon task and claimed that any "bilingual advantage" could in fact be attributed to the higher SES of the bilingual sample.[1]

Some arguments have claimed that cognitive abilities other than bilin-gualism enhanced performance on controlled attention tasks (e.g., working memory, Namazi & Thordardottir, 2010). By far the most damaging, though, have been the studies which have aimed to replicate the Simon, flanker, ANT and Stroop tasks with large bilingual and monolingual samples and found no difference at all. No bilingual advantage was found for groups of young adults in the flanker and Simon tasks in separate studies (Humphrey & Val-ian, 2012; Paap & Greenberg, 2013); no bilingual advantage for a large sample of Welsh children and adults tested in the DCCS (n = 650) and Simon (n =557) (Gathercole et al., 2014); no bilingual advantage for the ANT task in a large sample of 180 bilingual and 180 monolingual children aged 7–12 (Antón et al., 2014); and finally no significant bilingual advantage in an even larger sample of 252 monolingual and 252 bilingual children aged 8–13 on a verbal and numerical Stroop task (Duñabeitia et al., 2014).

As detailed here, researchers on both sides of the bilingual advantage debate claim they have decisive evidence supporting their side of the argument. The field has become increasingly antagonistic. Paap, Johnson, and Sawi (2015) have even asserted that most studies resulting in significant bilingual advan-tage are the product of confirmation and publication bias, "questionable use of data" (p. 265), small sample sizes, and deliberate misinterpretation of results. Paap, Johnson, and Sawi (2016) have also claimed a crisis of confidence in the bilingual advantage field because results have failed to match political and societal expectations biased towards multiculturalism. In response, sup-porters of the bilingual advantage have accused their opponents of categorical hypothesising (in which support of one position invalidates the other, Kroll & Bialystok, 2013), "claiming evidence from non-evidence" (Bialystok, 2009, p. 499) and misrepresenting the body of positive research (Bialystok, 2016).

Can Neuroscience Illuminate a Path?

There has been hope that neuroscience can weigh in decisively on either side. One area to benefit from neuroscientific evidence is the study of the cogni-tive effects of a lifetime of bilingual experience in older adults. It has been proposed that lifelong bilingualism confers neuroprotective effects, through slower cognitive ageing (Bialystok, Craik, & Luk, 2008) and a later onset of dementia (Alladi, Shailaja, Santhoshi, Nigam, & Kaul, 2011; Bialystok, Craik, & Freedman, 2007). Alladi and colleagues (2015) and Wood (2016) found that bilingualism was independently associated with substantially reduced poststroke impairment, in non-linguistic areas of cognition (40.5% of the bilingual sample exhibited normal cognition after suffering a stroke versus 19.6% of the monolinguals). Alladi et al.'s (2015) conclusion was that a lifetime of negotiating two or more languages concurrently had increased the bilingual patients' *cognitive reserve*, that is, the ability to maintain cognitive functions despite neural damage or brain pathology (Stern, 2009).

There is also neuroanatomical evidence that long-term bilingualism has neuroprotective benefits. Cognitive impairment and early stages of dementia are associated with grey matter loss, disruption of white matter and deterioration of the temporal poles and orbitofrontal cortex (Abutalebi & Green, 2016). In a review of neuroimaging studies investigating bilingualism, Abutalebi and Green (2016) reported that bilinguals displayed more grey matter density in the dorsal anterior cingulate cortex and pre-supplementary motor area compared to monolinguals. They also showed more grey matter density in the temporal, inferior parietal lobule (where reduced grey matter is observable in the early stages of dementia) and greater myelination (protection) of white matter in the frontal lobes and corpus callosum (demyelination is associated with neurodegenerative conditions).

The claim of neuroplastic change as a result of bilingualism[2] is not limited to studies of old age and cognitive reserve. There is a growing body of researchers (Baum & Titone, 2014; Del Maschio & Abutalebi, 2018; Li, Legault, & Litcofsky, 2014) who believe that "the quantity and quality of second-language experience affects brain structure" (Del Maschio & Abutalebi, 2018, p. 325). This belief is based on several neuroimaging studies. The first of these studies to claim that second language acquisition could change brain structure was by Mechelli et al. (2004). They found changes in grey matter density in the left inferior parietal cortex and attributed it to proficiency and age of acquisition in bilingual adult speakers. Other studies have proposed additional differences in frontal lobe neuroanatomy as a result of bilingualism. Examples include differences in the cortical thickness in the left and right inferior frontal gyrus (IFG) for monolinguals and sequential bilinguals (Klein, Mok, Chen, & Watkins, 2014); enhanced white matter integrity in the brains of bilinguals versus monolinguals (Cummine & Boliek, 2013; Mohades et al., 2012); and even differences in white matter connectivity between multilingual experts (phoneticians) versus standard multilinguals (Vandermosten, Price, & Golestani, 2016).

However appealing it is to conclude cognitive effects from these neuroanatomical changes (for example, decreased grey matter density is associated with cognitive decline [Tisserand et al., 2004], so reverse inference is tempting), it is still not clear whether the multilingual brain can be described as "superior" to a monolingual one in terms of cognitive functioning across the lifespan.

Neuroscience has also helped to identify the regions of the brain associated with both the language representation and other non-linguistic cognitive activity in bilinguals. Prior to modern functional brain imaging techniques, clinical observations of bilinguals with language impairments or undergoing neurosurgery led many to believe that bilinguals processed their languages in different areas of the brain (e.g., Aglioti & Fabbro, 1993). Recent findings have indicated that multiple overlapping brain regions, e.g., the regions of the dorsal audio-motor interface, are activated during the processing of two languages (see review by Golestani, 2016). More importantly, though, for the bilingual advantage hypothesis, are the findings of additional brain activity in areas not specifically associated with language processing, but usually related to executive control, such as the anterior cingulate cortex (ACC), the prefrontal areas, the inferior parietal lobules, and subcortical structures (Abutalebi & Green, 2016).

These areas were also identified in a review of neural studies (Roberts & Hall, 2008) investigating the Stroop, Simon and flanker selective attention tasks commonly used in behavioural studies. They proposed that the neural location of conflict processing was reliably associated with the fronto-parietal network: specifically, activation in the anterior cingulate cortex (ACC), and bilaterally in the inferior frontal gyrus (IFG), anterior insula, and the parietal lobe. They then analysed MRI data from both visual and auditory Stroop tasks (monolingual participants only) and found that there was significant interaction between the type of conflict (visual or auditory) and the location of conflict-related activation. The visual peak of activation was in the superior parietal lobe (SPL) and the auditory peak in the inferior parietal lobe (IPL). This suggested different brain regions were used for the processing of interference in different domains.

In summary, neural studies have corroborated changes in neuroanatomy as a result of bilingualism (e.g., Li et al., 2014). They have also helped identify the loci for the processing of multiple languages and for visual and auditory selective attention tasks. However, this does not resolve the debate of whether bilingualism creates a cognitive advantage in such tasks. Has such evidence been found?

Some neural studies specifically investigating the bilingual advantage have indeed identified neural activity correlating with performance in nonverbal tasks. For example, bilinguals who exhibited a reduced switching cost in a visual task also activated different areas of the frontal cortex (Garbin et al., 2010). A study combining functional and structural imaging found that not only did bilinguals outperform monolinguals behaviourally on conflict control tasks, but bilinguals showed both less activity (interpreted as showing more automated processing) and greater grey matter density in the dorsal ACC (Abutalebi et al., 2011).

Greater grey matter density was also found in an area of the posterior paravermis of the right cerebellum for participants who were better at controlling verbal interference during an auditory selective attention task, from analysis of both MRI images (Filippi et al., 2011) and PET scans (Crinion et al., 2006). Another method, the EEG (electroencephalogram, a measure of brain activity), was used to compare monolingual and bilingual adolescents' encoding of a speech syllable (Krizman, Marian, Shook, Skoe, & Kraus,

2012). They found that bilinguals showed enhanced encoding of the fundamental frequency of the syllable when presented in a noisy background, suggesting that bilinguals exhibited greater selective attention and better auditory processing efficiency, especially under the condition of multitalker babble.

However, neuroscientific evidence so far has not been decisive in the bilingual advantage debate, due to inconsistencies in methodology and contradictory interpretations. From the preceding cases, increased neural activity in some studies has been viewed as "better" or "faster" cognitive processing; reduced neural activity in others has been interpreted as evidence of more automated processing. A comprehensive review exploring inconsistencies in the neuroanatomical research on bilingualism to date, with particular focus on sample selection and methodological issues (García-Pentón et al., 2016a, "The neuroanatomy of bilingualism: how to turn a hazy view into the full picture"), provoked six commentaries from researchers in the bilingual advantage field, each with a different point of view. The conclusions were deemed in turn overly optimistic (Paap, 2016) and unnecessarily pessimistic (Bialystok, 2016). Suggestions were made to develop more theoretical models and seek more behavioural data as validation of neural interpretations (de Bruin & Della Sala, 2016) and extend collaboration between different researchers (Luk & Pliatsikas, 2016). There were objections to the negative connotations of the word "hazy" (Kroll & Chiarello, 2016) and a justification for the inconsistencies (on the grounds of gender and age). In contrast, there was also the view that the studies reviewed were in fact more consistent than suggested (Abutalebi & Green, 2016).

Finally, García-Pentón et al.'s (2016b) response to the commentaries acknowledged the need to link behaviour with neural structure and reiterated the need for methodological uniformity.

The preceding demonstrates the breadth of opinion around the neuroscientific evidence for a bilingual advantage. The same information is interpreted in six different ways; some of the opinions are diametrically opposed; some request more behavioural data, some more neural data; Abutalebi and Green argue that there is less inconsistency than claimed.

Before we write off the whole debate, however, as an intractable mess, let us try to unravel some of the complications.

Why There Is No Simple Answer

As demonstrated, the bilingual advantage debate is currently extremely polarised. Some have proposed a compromise position—i.e., admit that a bilingual advantage is sometimes present, but sometimes not because other variables have confounded the result. Critics such as Paap et al. (2015) have begrudged these as "very specific and undetermined circumstances"; Kroll and Bialystok (2013) defended them as an inevitable consequence of testing on participants with complex linguistic backgrounds. In fact, there are many variables that can confound both sides of the argument. For example, Bialystok et al.

(2004) found that prolonged practice for monolinguals affected performance on the Simon task so much that any bilingual advantage disappeared. Paap and Greenberg's (2013) procedure included an extensive (20 trials) practice of the Simon test, which may have caused the null result. There are many more variables, which could affect results on both sides of the debate. Reviews of the literature (e.g., Costa, Hernández, Costa-Faidella, & Sebastián-Gallés, 2009; Hilchey & Klein, 2011; Kroll & Bialystok, 2013; Valian, 2015a) reveal three main sources of inconsistencies in the results.

Inconsistency 1: Age

The first inconsistency is across age groups. It has been well documented that there is no discernible bilingual advantage in studies with samples of young adults (Humphrey & Valian, 2012; Kousaie & Phillips, 2012a; Paap & Greenberg, 2013). This is especially true of the Simon task, even when the same study did find a bilingual advantage in groups of bilingual and monolingual children, middle adults and older adults (Bialystok, Martin, & Viswanathan, 2005).

There are several explanations offered for this anomaly. Barac et al. (2014) advised there are limits to the effect of a bilingual improvement in cognitive functioning. It has been hypothesised that young adults' baseline cognition is much higher and so the effect of bilingualism is limited. The first explanation for this "cognitive ceiling" is that young adults have developed peak cognitive ability (as suggested by Bialystok et al., 2005). The other (as proposed by Valian, 2015a) is young adults' disproportionately stimulating environment relative to other life stages. She suggested that bilingualism was just one of many cognitively enriching activities that can stimulate non-verbal performance and that these activities are at a peak in young adulthood—such as music training (shown to have the same effect as bilingualism on the Simon task, Bialystok & DePape, 2009), computers (Bialystok et al., 2005) or video games (Bialystok, 2006; Bavelier, Achtman, Mani, & Föcker, 2012).

According to Valian (2015a), young adults exist in an environment of peak stimulation, which raises overall functioning, and diminishes the impact of bilingualism.

Inconsistency 2: The Inherent Variability of the Bilingual Experience

The second broad area is the variability of bilingualism itself. Bilingualism is not a categorical variable (Bialystok, Craik, Green, & Gollan, 2009; Carlson & Meltzoff, 2008), and requires detangling of various complex elements for research to progress (Kaushanskaya & Prior, 2015). These elements are both numerous and contradictory. For example, age of acquisition has been variously proposed to have a linear association with cognitive control (Luk, De Sa, & Bialystok, 2011); to make no difference (Pelham & Abrams, 2014); and for late L2 acquisition to present a disadvantage relative to monolinguals in tests of auditory interference (Mayo, Florentine, & Buus, 1997; Shi, 2010). The impact of age of acquisition on neuroanatomical outcomes has also varied between studies. A study whose focus was cortical thickness in bilinguals (Klein et al., 2014) found equivalent thickness in monolinguals and simultaneous bilinguals (L2 learners at the age of 0–3) in all areas, but sequential learners showed greater cortical thickness in the left inferior frontal gyrus (IFG) and thinner cortex in the right IFG. These differences correlated significantly with the age of acquisition. They concluded that learning a second language later than the first modified the brain structure in an age-dependent manner; but acquiring both languages simultaneously had no additional effect on brain development.

Conversely, grey matter (GM) density was found to be greater for bilinguals than monolinguals in the left inferior parietal lobule (IPL), and the effect was greater in the early bilinguals than in the late bilinguals (Mechelli et al., 2004).

L2 proficiency, another variable, has also been associated with GM density increases (Del Maschio & Abutalebi, 2018). In behavioural tests, proficiency has been proposed to have an effect on the extent of bilingual advantage (Luk, 2008); others (Linck, Hoshino, & Kroll, 2008) suggested a bilingual advantage was conferred by minimal exposure to a second language. They compared bilinguals of different levels with monolinguals and found the most inexperienced bilinguals showed the greatest bilingual advantage in the Simon task.

There is also the question of similarity between L1 and L2, which has been argued to reduce bilingual advantage (Bialystok et al., 2009), versus the claim that minimal typological difference between languages is sufficient to confer bilingual advantages in executive control tasks, including the Simon task (Antoniou, Grohmann, Kambanaros, & Katsos, 2016).

Finally, another influential variable within bilingualism is the interactional language context. According to Green and Abutalebi's (2013) Adaptive Control Hypothesis, the language context in which interference suppression and conflict monitoring are highest is the dual-language context. This is a context in which both languages are used but with different speakers. This theory was also supported by Costa et al. (2009), who claimed that bilingual speakers in diglossic environments (where the two languages are used in different contexts) have less need of linguistic attentional control and so may not show an advantage. Indeed, the uneven manifestation of a bilingual advantage has been attributed solely to the variability of language switching (Prior & Gollan, 2011).

Inconsistency 3: The Results Are Only as Good as the Tasks Used

The third source of inconsistencies in the study of a bilingual advantage is ambiguity about whether the tests truly measure the executive functions they target. As discussed by Paap et al. (2015) and Valian (2015a), many studies compare slightly different tasks that supposedly measure the same functions.

This issue of task equivalence is most evident in the review of the tasks in the visual domain—namely the Simon, flanker, ANT and Stroop tasks, all cited as tests under the umbrella of controlled attention. However, different tasks within the same study often have contradictory results. Yang and Lust (2004) found no difference between monolingual and bilingual children's performance on the Dimensional Card Change Sorting (DCCS) task but an advantage of bilinguals in an ANT test. Martin-Rhee and Bialystok (2008) conducted three studies on children aged 4 and 8 and found a consistent advantage for bilingual children in all three presentations of the Simon task but not in a modified version of the Stroop task. This could be interpreted as a lack of true bilingual advantage, or evidence that the tasks do not tap into the same cognitive functions (in that age group), so produce different results.

Conversely, the same tasks have also been used to measure different processes. For example, Bialystok et al. (2008) considered the Simon task to be a test of interference suppression, whereas Yudes, Macizo, and Bajo (2011) considered the Simon task to be an index of inhibition. Valian (2015b) cited that the Stroop task has variously been claimed to measure interference, processing speed, automatic response inhibition, and (dependent on working memory capacity) ability to maintain goals and resolve conflicts.

In fact, although Green and Abutalebi (2013) defined eight distinct control processes, contributing in varying degrees to overall adaptive control, researchers have not succeeded in isolating each control process with a separate task. This has led to testing the same functions with different tasks, or different functions with the same tasks, with inconsistent results. Valian (2015b) stressed the need for more tests that are specific for aspects of executive functioning but was not confident that such specific tests could be devised.

Similarly, various neuroimaging studies have found different regions or patterns of activation for these tasks supposedly measuring the same function. Ali, Green, Kherif, Devlin, and Price (2010) found that different areas of the brain were activated for the Stroop and Simon task according to analysis of fMRI data (the left head of caudate identified as significant for inhibiting a response on the Stroop task but not for the Simon task). Kousaie and Phillips' (2012a) study using ERP measures not only revealed differences in neural activity between the groups (monolinguals and bilinguals); but between the tasks (e.g., greater N2 and ERN amplitude for monolinguals in the Stroop task, indicating more effortful conflict resolution and greater post-response conflict). These results suggested that different functions and strategies were used to process the Simon, Stroop and flanker tasks.

One interpretation is that, although all the aforementioned tasks are cited as demonstrating attentional control and inhibition, there are subtle variations between tests, meaning that they are processed differently (as shown earlier), and measure different but related mechanisms (e.g., response inhibition or interference suppression).

Interestingly, neural studies have also highlighted bilingual processing differences that were not apparent from behavioural tests: Bialystok et al. (2005)

used magneto-encephalography (MEG) to observe neural differences while groups of bilinguals and monolinguals were processing the Simon task. The behavioural results of the Simon test showed no consistent bilingual advantage, and analyses of the MEG data showed activity in the left and medial prefrontal areas for all three groups. However, the two bilingual groups showed activity in selected left hemisphere regions, whereas the monolingual group showed activity in the middle frontal regions. This finding was replicated in other tasks in the visual domain: Luk, Anderson, Craik, Grady, and Bialystok (2010) analysed fMRI data from participants performing a flanker task. Although there was no significant difference between the language groups' response times, different brain regions were activated by each of the groups in the same tasks (e.g., in incongruent trials, monolinguals activated the left temporal pole and left superior parietal regions; the bilinguals activated an extensive network including bilateral frontal, temporal and subcortical regions). Kousaie and Phillips (2012a, 2012b) found no bilingual advantage in groups of young adults in the Stroop, flanker and Simon tasks and no difference in groups of young and older adults in the Stroop task, but ERP data (2012a) revealed different patterns of activation for monolinguals and bilinguals in the tasks. These results do not imply cognitive differences in themselves (behavioural data was equivalent after all) but indicate that bilinguals and monolinguals may take a slightly different neural path to get to the same destination.

Time for a New Approach?

Numerous studies, both behavioural and neuroimaging, have yielded at best inconsistent and at worst contradictory results. The reasons for some of these inconsistent results have been explained already. Clearly the debate is far from being resolved, and conducting the same tests with the same (inconsistent) results will have diminishing returns. What research so far has revealed is that the study of a bilingual advantage is much more nuanced than previously supposed and the results of studies on both sides of the debate are only as good as the tasks and samples included. Put succinctly, "If one asks a simple question about a complex phenomenon, one is likely to get a simple (and unsatisfying) answer" (Baum & Titone, 2014, p. 881).

Perhaps it is time to recognise that the antagonistic yes/no debate surrounding a purported bilingual advantage is counterproductive and even risks discrediting the field. The limitations of using simple group comparisons with the same (perhaps ineffective, as discussed) tasks have resulted in a research stalemate. The field now needs new approaches that will garner more insights.

One suggestion is to encourage a broader approach that seeks to understand the multi-dimensional dynamics of multilanguage development by integrating research from various levels of analysis (e.g., genes, brain, cognition, behaviour, social context) across the lifespan (D'Souza & Filippi, 2017; Filippi, D'Souza, & Bright, 2018).

A developmental approach to bilingual research is especially relevant to education—after all, models of bilingual language processing in the bilingual brain such as the one proposed by Green and Abutalebi (2008, 2013) provide useful frameworks for understanding neurocognitive adaptation to the demands of bilingual communication but they are not developmental accounts; they describe how processing may occur in the *adult* brain. A critical but unresolved issue, therefore, is how multi-linguistic experience impacts on crucial cognitive processes across the lifespan, from infancy to old age.

New cognitive abilities are claimed to arise from context-dependent interactions that occur both within the child (e.g., between neural systems) and between the child and the environment (e.g., when the child selects a new object to explore). Moreover, because contexts change over time, it is vital to understand cognitive development by tracing higher-level cognitive functions back to their low-level roots in early childhood (Karmiloff-Smith, 1998). This is an important research strategy because changes in neural structures early in development are likely to constrain the emergence of later developing neural structures. For instance, if a group of neurons are recruited to process a child's first language, and the response properties of the neurons become increasingly selective to processing stimuli from that first language (a developmental process called 'specialisation', Johnson, 2011), then the ability of that coalition of neurons to process a second language will decrease over developmental time. This is due to 'neural commitment' (Kuhl et al., 2006). As an analogy, a radio tuned to receive a particular signal has a reduced chance of picking up any other signal. Likewise, if a population of neurons becomes specialised for responding to a particular set of stimuli early in development (e.g., spoken English), then this will alter their ability to respond to a different set of stimuli later in development (e.g., spoken Italian). Therefore, it is imperative to investigate multiple cognitive and non-cognitive domains so that researchers can work towards a comprehensive understanding of the complexities of language development—which is both constrained and underpinned by interdependencies among dynamically evolving internal (e.g., attention, memory) and external (e.g., social interaction) factors (see Filippi et al., 2018, for further discussion).

What happens early in development may affect what can occur later in development (see D'Souza & Karmiloff-Smith, 2016), and for this reason, any broad theoretical consideration of the bilingual advantage will most likely be inadequate unless it incorporates a developmental perspective. A developmental approach is therefore critical for moving away from the *advantage/disadvantage* debate and reinvigorating research in this field with theoretical progress.

As discussed earlier, current models such as the Inhibitory Control Model (ICM) are based on the adult brain and to date the theoretical frameworks have not incorporated early development. As an example, according to the ICM, the bilingual advantage arises because managing two languages during language production draws upon, and thus strengthens, inhibitory control mechanisms. However, this prediction does not account for evidence showing that preverbal infants raised in a multilingual environment may have better executive control than infants raised monolingually (e.g., Kóvacs & Mehler, 2009a, 2009b). Theoretical revision is therefore needed.

By employing a developmental approach to bilingual research it will be possible to build and compare developmental trajectories. That is, one set of developmental constraints may operate in bilinguals, while a different set may operate in monolinguals. These developmental constraints may lead to an inhibitory control advantage in bilinguals at one time point but not at another time point. Indeed, Donnelly, Brooks, and Homer (2015) found that, whereas bilingual adults show an inhibitory control advantage, bilingual children instead show a more general executive control advantage.

Conclusions and Recommendations

What Has Neuroscience Added to Our Understanding Over and Above Psychology?

One of the questions we were asked to consider when writing this chapter was the contribution of neuroscience over and above psychology. As discussed, the debate in response to behavioural evidence has been demystified somewhat by some neuroscientific findings but even these are subject to differing interpretations. In summary, the contribution of neuroscience to the research on the cognitive effects of bilingualism has been proposed on the following levels:

1. More clarity over the areas of the brain used during bilingual language processing (as summarised by Del Maschio & Abutalebi, 2018) and performance in nonverbal tasks (as summarised by Roberts & Hall, 2008).
2. Validation of behavioural data (e.g., the studies by Filippi et al., 2011, 2012, 2015; Krizman et al., 2012) demonstrating a bilingual advantage in selected verbal and nonverbal tasks.
3. Evidence that bilingual experience can be an agent for neuroplastic change (e.g., review by Li et al., 2014).
4. Unexpectedly, suggesting differences in cognitive architecture that behavioural tests alone did not discern, through:

    a. Identification of different neural areas for nonverbal tasks that supposedly measure the same function (Ali et al., 2010; Kousaie & Phillips, 2012a); and
    b. demonstration of a difference in neural activity across groups when behavioural results are the same (Bialystok et al., 2005; Luk et al., 2010).

These last findings perhaps indicate that, even when performance is comparable, bilinguals and monolinguals recruit their mental resources differently; a finding that takes the research into the cognitive effects of bilingualism well beyond a simple yes/no debate about advantage, to one about *differences* and how to best capitalise on them. In fact, Baum and Titone (2014) suggest that the debate should move beyond a simple yes/no bilingual advantage and address questions such as: are there certain things that bilinguals do that have no parallel with monolinguals? Developmental studies exploring differences across the lifespan, rather than validating performance data from tasks, would help move the debate on to another level.

What Are the Concrete Implications of Research and Opportunities for Translation?

The research literature is all very well, but can feel far removed from the reality of bringing up a bilingual child or providing for EAL (English as an additional language) students in the classroom. As discussed, bilingualism in the education sector in the U.K. is not insignificant: the percentage of pupils in English schools aged 5–16 recorded as EAL more than doubled between 1997 and 2013 from 7.6% to 16.2% (Strand et al., 2015) and is still rising. What clear messages can be discerned from the (often confusing) research literature?

The first is that bilingualism in itself is not a negative influence on children's cognitive abilities, as historically supposed. As previously discussed, independent studies (McLeod et al., 2015; Strand et al., 2015) have concluded that any gap in achievement at reception age (4–5) between bilinguals and monolinguals has usually diminished by age 8–9 and virtually disappeared by age 16.

Beyond academic performance, any fears of "mental overload" induced by bilingualism have been refuted. A practitioner review of multilingualism and neurodevelopmental disorders (Uljarević, Katsos, Hudry, & Gibson, 2016) stated categorically that multilingualism consistently showed no adverse effects on various aspects of functioning across a range of conditions, including Autistic Spectrum Disorder (ASD), Attention Deficit Hyperactivity Disorder and Communication Disorders.

The same review (Uljarević et al., 2016) advised that detection of an "atypical" language profile for an EAL child was not necessarily in itself cause for concern. This is of interest to practitioners who diagnose and manage Developmental Language Disorder (DLD), who may assume that some atypical language patterns produced by second language learners are manifestations of DLD. A new field of research, the study of bilingual children with DLD (BIDLD), aims to disentangle the effects of bilingualism from those of DLD, making use of both models of bilingualism and models of language impairment (see further resources at end of chapter for details) to improve language assessment for bilingual children and avoid incorrect diagnoses.

The implications of bilingualism in education also extend beyond EAL. There is also the question of when best to introduce the acquisition of additional languages. Evidence concurs that the best time to learn a second language is as early as possible, based on studies measuring English proficiency of non-native speakers in the U.S. (e.g., Johnson & Newport, 1989; DeKeyser,

2000; Hakuta, Bialystok, & Wiley, 2003). These found that ability either decreased sharply or gradually if acquired after puberty and was at its peak for those who acquired L2 in early childhood. Evidence for a critical window (i.e., that language can only be acquired before a certain point in development) is not as well established for L2 as it is for L1, given that many individuals learn a second language successfully (and even to advanced level) after puberty. Nevertheless, be it previous language experience, age-related plasticity or a sensitive period that inhibits the learning of new sounds and grammar systems (as discussed in Del Maschio & Abutalebi, 2018), proficiency appears to be negatively correlated with age of acquisition.

As well as the obvious communicative advantage of acquiring an additional language, bilingualism has been proposed to confer cognitive benefits, either in the form of cognitive reserve in later life, or a cognitive boost during childhood. The benefits are either claimed as superior executive functioning in the area of selective attention, unique to bilingualism ("bilingual advantage"); or higher cognitive functioning as also enhanced by music training, video game playing or other cognitively stimulating activities (Valian, 2015a). Either way, we can conclude that bilingual children are most definitely not disadvantaged cognitively by their multiple languages and may indeed find cognitively demanding tasks easier as a result. One of the consequent implications for the classroom therefore is that, if bilingualism is fast becoming the new normal, what steps can be taken to ensure that monolingual children keep up cognitively? Luckily, bilingualism is but one of many levers to enhance cognition so the future is not bleak for monolinguals. We hope that a consequence of this review, however, is a reconsideration of the term "English as an Additional Language"—which currently still has a vaguely negative connotation and focus on the benefits of experience of multiple languages, both within the classroom and in the wider (global) community.

Further Resources

Following are some links which may help those wanting more practical guidance on educating bilingual children and staying up to date with latest research developments in the field of bilingualism:

- The Multilanguage & Cognition Lab (MULTAC) at University College London, Institute of Education. Here you can contact active researchers for advice and take part in scientific studies: www.ucl.ac.uk/ioe/departments-centres/centres/centre-for-language-literacy-and-numeracy/multilanguage-and-cognition-lab
- Resources about bilingualism and raising bilingual families can be found on this European Commission-funded website. www.multilingual-families.eu
- *Life as a Bilingual* is a blog by eminent linguist François Grosjean, author of *Bilingual: Life and Reality*. The website also contains interviews, articles and links to books: www.psychologytoday.com/blog/life-bilingual

- *Bilingualism Matters* is an international network of researchers who promote bilingualism. Their branches and partners include

Internationally: www.bilingualism-matters.ppls.ed.ac.uk/branch-network/
In the U.K.:

London	www.ucl.ac.uk/bi-multilingualism/
Edinburgh	www.bilingualism-matters.ppls.ed.ac.uk
Reading	www.reading.ac.uk/celm/bilingualism-matters/
Belfast	www.ulster.ac.uk/research/institutes/social-sciences/research/research-groups/ucom
Cambridge	https://sites.google.com/site/cambiling/

The Cambridge team have also produced a short film, designed to be used in schools and communities as a springboard to discussions about multilingualism. Access the film with an accompanying transcript and letter here:

https://sites.google.com/site/cambiling/your-languages-your-future

- For teachers and practitioners with specific EAL concerns:

  - The National Association for Language Development In the Curriculum (NALDIC) is the UK subject association for English as an additional language (EAL) and provides advice and resources. https://naldic.org.uk
  - The Bell Foundation is a charity that promotes intercultural understanding through language education. www.bell-foundation.org.uk
  - From their website, there is a free download of the EAL assessment framework: www.bell-foundation.org.uk/eal-programme/teaching-resources/eal-assessment-framework/
  - Another assessment tool has been developed for bilingual toddlers, to evaluate their word development at 24 months: www.psy.plymouth.ac.uk/UKBTAT/
  - Advice on bilingualism and Developmental Language Disorder (previously called Specific Language Impairment) can be found at www.bi-sli.org
  - *Bilingualism* offers professional advice by speech and language therapists. www.bilingualism.co.uk/.

- Finally, for more general language development, www.lucid.ac.uk is an ERSC international centre for language and communicative development, with many resources for parents, practitioners and researchers.

Notes

1. In a subsequent attempt to disentangle SES from performance, Calvo and Bialystok (2014) tested 175 children aged 6 from different socioeconomic backgrounds and

proposed that bilingualism had a separate effect from SES on the performance of the Flanker task (bilinguals were significantly more accurate). Indeed, Engel de Abreu, Cruz-Santos, Tourinho, Martin, and Bialystok (2012) found that bilingual children from a disadvantaged background had a unique advantage in the Flanker task—contrasting with initial studies, which seemingly indicated the opposite effect.

2. Proposed change to neuroanatomy as a result of cognitive "exercise" is not unique to bilingualism. One of the most cited studies into neuroplasticity is that of Maguire and colleagues (2000), whose work showed that London taxi drivers had enlarged regions of the hippocampus responsible for spatial navigation as the result of their extensive experience in route-finding.

References

Abutalebi, J., Della Rosa, P. A., Green, D. W., Hernandez, M., Scifo, P., Keim, R., . . . Costa, A. (2011). Bilingualism tunes the anterior cingulate cortex for conflict monitoring. *Cerebral Cortex, 22*(9), 2076–2086.

Abutalebi, J., & Green, D. W. (2016). Neuroimaging of language control in bilinguals: Neural adaptation and reserve. *Bilingualism: Language and Cognition, 19*(4), 689–698.

Aglioti, S., & Fabbro, F. (1993). Paradoxical selective recovery in a bilingual aphasic following subcortical lesions. *Neuroreport: An International Journal for the Rapid Communication of Research in Neuroscience, 4*(12), 1359–1362.

Ali, N., Green, D. W., Kherif, F., Devlin, J. T., & Price, C. J. (2010). The role of the left head of caudate in suppressing irrelevant words. *Journal of Cognitive Neuroscience, 22*(10), 2369–2386.

Alladi, S., Bak, T. H., Mekala, S., Rajan, A., Chaudhuri, J. R., Mioshi, E., . . . Kaul, S. (2015). Impact of bilingualism on cognitive outcome after stroke. *Stroke.* doi:10.1161/STROKEAHA.115.010418

Alladi, S., Shailaja, M., Santhoshi, C., Nigam, R., & Kaul, S. (2011). Age of dementia onset delayed by bilingualism, but advanced by stroke. *Alzheimer's & Dementia, 7*(4), e21.

Antón, E., Duñabeitia, J. A., Estévez, A., Hernández, J. A., Castillo, A., Fuentes, L. J., . . . Carreiras, M. (2014). Is there a bilingual advantage in the ANT task? Evidence from children. *Frontiers in Psychology, 5.*

Antoniou, K., Grohmann, K. K., Kambanaros, M., & Katsos, N. (2016). The effect of childhood bilectalism and multilingualism on executive control. *Cognition, 149,* 18–30.

Baddeley, A. (1996). Exploring the central executive. *The Quarterly Journal of Experimental Psychology: Section A, 49*(1), 5–28.

Bain, B. (1975). Toward an integration of Piaget and Vygotsky: Bilingual considerations. *Linguistics, 13*(160), 5–20.

Barac, R., Bialystok, E., Castro, D., & Sanchez, M. (2014). The cognitive development of young dual language learners: A critical review. *Early Childhood Research Quarterly, 29,* 699–714.

Baum, S., & Titone, D. (2014). Moving toward a neuroplasticity view of bilingualism, executive control, and aging. *Applied Psycholinguistics, 35*(5), 857–894.

Bavelier, D., Achtman, R. L., Mani, M., & Föcker, J. (2012). Neural bases of selective attention in action video game players. *Vision Research, 61,* 132–143.

Ben-Zeev, S. (1977). The influence of bilingualism on cognitive strategy and cognitive development. *Child Development,* 1009–1018.

Best, J. R., Miller, P. H., & Jones, L. L. (2009). Executive functions after age 5: Changes and correlates. *Developmental Review, 29*(3), 180–200.

Bialystok, E. (1992). Attentional control in children's metalinguistic performance and measures of field independence. *Developmental Psychology, 28*(4), 654.

Bialystok, E. (1999). Cognitive complexity and attentional control in the bilingual mind. *Child Development, 70*(3), 636–644.

Bialystok, E. (2001). *Bilingualism in development: Language, literacy, and cognition.* New York: Cambridge University Press.

Bialystok, E. (2006). Effect of bilingualism and computer video game experience on the Simon task. *Canadian Journal of Experimental Psychology, 60*(1), 68.

Bialystok, E. (2009). Claiming evidence from non-evidence: A reply to Morton and Harper. *Developmental Science, 12*(4), 499–501.

Bialystok, E. (2016). How hazy views become full pictures. *Language, Cognition and Neuroscience, 31*(3), 328–330.

Bialystok, E., Craik, F. I., & Freedman, M. (2007). Bilingualism as a protection against the onset of symptoms of dementia. *Neuropsychologia, 45*(2), 459–464.

Bialystok, E., Craik, F. I., Grady, C., Chau, W., Ishii, R., Gunji, A., & Pantev, C. (2005). Effect of bilingualism on cognitive control in the Simon task: Evidence from MEG. *Neuroimage, 24*(1), 40–49.

Bialystok, E., Craik, F. I., Green, D. W., & Gollan, T. H. (2009). Bilingual minds. *Psychological Science in the Public Interest, 10*(3), 89–129.

Bialystok, E., Craik, F. I., Klein, R., & Viswanathan, M. (2004). Bilingualism, aging, and cognitive control: Evidence from the Simon task. *Psychology and Aging, 19*(2), 290.

Bialystok, E., Craik, F., & Luk, G. (2008). Cognitive control and lexical access in younger and older bilinguals. *Journal of Experimental Psychology: Learning, Memory, and Cognition, 34*(4), 859.

Bialystok, E., & DePape, A. M. (2009). Musical expertise, bilingualism, and executive functioning. *Journal of Experimental Psychology: Human Perception and Performance, 35*(2), 565.

Bialystok, E., & Martin, M. M. (2004). Attention and inhibition in bilingual children: Evidence from the dimensional change card sort task. *Developmental Science, 7*(3), 325–339.

Bialystok, E., Martin, M. M., & Viswanathan, M. (2005). Bilingualism across the lifespan: The rise and fall of inhibitory control. *International Journal of Bilingualism, 9*(1), 103–119.

Bialystok, E., & Shapero, D. (2005). Ambiguous benefits: The effect of bilingualism on reversing ambiguous figures. *Developmental Science, 8*(6), 595–604.

Bosch, L., & Sebastián-Gallés, N. (1997). Native-language recognition abilities in 4-month-old infants from monolingual and bilingual environments. *Cognition, 65*(1), 33–69.

Byers-Heinlein, K., Burns, T. C., & Werker, J. F. (2010). The roots of bilingualism in newborns. *Psychological Science, 21*(3), 343–348.

Calvo, A., & Bialystok, E. (2014). Independent effects of bilingualism and socioeconomic status on language ability and executive functioning. *Cognition, 130*(3), 278–288.

Carlson, S. M., & Meltzoff, A. N. (2008). Bilingual experience and executive functioning in young children. *Developmental Science, 11*(2), 282–298.

Costa, A., Hernández, M., Costa-Faidella, J., & Sebastián-Gallés, N. (2009). On the bilingual advantage in conflict processing: Now you see it, now you don't. *Cognition, 113*(2), 135–149.

Crinion, J., Turner, R., Grogan, A., Hanakawa, T., Noppeney, U., Devlin, J. T., . . . Usui, K. (2006). Language control in the bilingual brain. *Science, 312*(5779), 1537–1540.

Crystal, D. (2008). Two thousand million? *English Today, 24*(1), 3–6.

Cummine, J., & Boliek, C. A. (2013). Understanding white matter integrity stability for bilinguals on language status and reading performance. *Brain Structure and Function, 218*(2), 595–601.

Cummins, J. (1984). Minority students and learning difficulties: Issues in assessment and placement. In *Early bilingualism and child development*. Amsterdam: Swets Publishing Service. Reprinted in Cummins, J., & Swain, M. (Eds.). (1986). *Bilingualism in education*. London: Longman.

Darcy, N. T. (1953). A review of the literature on the effects of bilingualism upon the measurement of intelligence. *The Pedagogical Seminary and Journal of Genetic Psychology, 82*(1), 21–57.

de Bruin, A., & Della Sala, S. (2016). The importance of language use when studying the neuroanatomical basis of bilingualism. *Language, Cognition and Neuroscience, 31*(3), 335–339.

DeKeyser, R. M. (2000). The robustness of critical period effects in second language acquisition. *Studies in Second Language Acquisition, 22*(4), 499–533.

Del Maschio, N., & Abutalebi, J. (2018). Neurobiology of bilingualism. *Bilingual Cognition and Language: The State of the Science Across Its Subfields, 54*, 325.

Donnelly, S., Brooks, P. J., & Homer, B. D. (2015). Examining the bilingual advantage on conflict resolution tasks: A meta-analysis. *CogSci*.

D'Souza, D., & Filippi, R. (2017). Progressive modularization: Reframing our understanding of typical and atypical language development. *First Language, 37*(5), 518–529.

D'Souza, D., & Karmiloff-Smith, A. (2016). Why a developmental perspective is critical for understanding human cognition. *Behavioral and Brain Sciences, 39*, e122.

Duñabeitia, J. A., Hernández, J. A., Antón, E., Macizo, P., Estévez, A., Fuentes, L. J., & Carreiras, M. (2014). The inhibitory advantage in bilingual children revisited. *Experimental Psychology, 61*(3), 234–251.

Engel de Abreu, P. M., Cruz-Santos, A., Tourinho, C. J., Martin, R., & Bialystok, E. (2012). Bilingualism enriches the poor: Enhanced cognitive control in low-income minority children. *Psychological Science, 23*(11), 1364–1371.

Espy, K. A., Molfese, V. J., & DiLalla, L. F. (2001). Effects of environmental measures on intelligence in young children: Growth curve modeling of longitudinal data. *Merrill-Palmer Quarterly, 47*(1), 42–73.

Festman, J., Poarch, G. J., & Dewaele, J. M. (2017). *Raising multilingual children*. Bristol: Multilingual Matters.

Filippi, R., D'Souza, D., & Bright, P. (2018). A developmental approach to bilingual research: The effects of multi-language experience from early infancy to old age. *International Journal of Bilingualism*.

Filippi, R., Leech, R., Thomas, M. S., Green, D. W., & Dick, F. (2012). A bilingual advantage in controlling language interference during sentence comprehension. *Bilingualism: Language and Cognition, 15*(4), 858–872.

Filippi, R., Morris, J., Richardson, F. M., Bright, P., Thomas, M. S., Karmiloff-Smith, A., & Marian, V. (2015). Bilingual children show an advantage in controlling verbal interference during spoken language comprehension. *Bilingualism: Language and Cognition, 18*(3), 490–501.

Filippi, R., Richardson, F. M., Dick, F., Leech, R., Green, D. W., Thomas, M. S., & Price, C. J. (2011). The right posterior paravermis and the control of language interference. *Journal of Neuroscience, 31*(29), 10732–10740.

Garbin, G., Sanjuan, A., Forn, C., Bustamante, J. C., Rodríguez-Pujadas, A., Belloch, V., . . . Ávila, C. (2010). Bridging language and attention: Brain basis of the impact of bilingualism on cognitive control. *Neuroimage*, 53(4), 1272–1278.

García-Pentón, L., Fernández García, Y., Costello, B., Duñabeitia, J. A., & Carreiras, M. (2016a). The neuroanatomy of bilingualism: How to turn a hazy view into the full picture. *Language, Cognition and Neuroscience*, 31(3), 303–327.

García-Pentón, L., Fernández García, Y., Costello, B., Duñabeitia, J. A., & Carreiras, M. (2016b). "Hazy" or "jumbled"? Putting together the pieces of the bilingual puzzle. *Language, Cognition and Neuroscience*, 31(3), 353–360.

Gathercole, V. C. M., Thomas, E. M., Kennedy, I., Prys, C., Young, N., Guasch, N. V., . . . Jones, L. (2014). Does language dominance affect cognitive performance in bilinguals? Lifespan evidence from preschoolers through older adults on card sorting, Simon, and metalinguistic tasks. *Frontiers in Psychology*, 5.

Golestani, N. (2016). Neuroimaging of phonetic perception in bilinguals. *Bilingualism: Language and Cognition*, 19(4), 674–682.

Graham, V. T. (1925). The intelligence of Jewish and Italian children in the habit clinics of the Massachusetts division of mental hygiene. *J. Abn. & Soc. Psychol.*, 9, 338–397.

Green, D. W. (1998). Mental control of the bilingual lexico-semantic system. *Bilingualism: Language and Cognition*, 1(2), 67–81.

Green, D. W., & Abutalebi, J. (2008). Understanding the link between bilingual aphasia and language control. *Journal of Neurolinguistics*, 21(6), 558–576.

Green, D. W., & Abutalebi, J. (2013). Language control in bilinguals: The adaptive control hypothesis. *Journal of Cognitive Psychology*, 25(5), 515–530.

Hakuta, K. (1986). *Mirror of language: The debate on bilingualism*. New York, NY: Basic Books.

Hakuta, K., Bialystok, E., & Wiley, E. (2003). Critical evidence: A test of the critical-period hypothesis for second-language acquisition. *Psychological Science*, 14(1), 31–38.

Hilchey, M. D., & Klein, R. M. (2011). Are there bilingual advantages on nonlinguistic interference tasks? Implications for the plasticity of executive control processes. *Psychonomic Bulletin & Review*, 18(4), 625–658.

Hoff, E. (2003). Causes and consequences of SES-related differences in parent-to-child speech. In M. H. Bornstein & R. H. Bradley (Eds.), *Monographs in parenting series. Socioeconomic status, parenting, and child development* (pp. 147–160). Mahwah, NJ: Lawrence Erlbaum Associates.

Hoff, E., Core, C., Place, S., Rumiche, R., Señor, M., & Parra, M. (2012). Dual language exposure and early bilingual development. *Journal of Child Language*, 39(1), 1–27.

Hommel, B., Colzato, L. S., Fischer, R., & Christoffels, I. K. (2011). Bilingualism and creativity: Benefits in convergent thinking come with losses in divergent thinking. *Frontiers in Psychology*, 2.

Humphrey, A. D., & Valian, V. V. (2012, November). *Multilingualism and cognitive control: Simon and flanker task performance in monolingual and multilingual young adults.* 53rd Annual meeting of the psychonomic society, Minneapolis, MN.

Ibanez-Lillo, A., Pons, F., Costa, A., & Sebastián-Gallés, N. (2010). *Inhibitory control in 8-month-old monolingual and bilingual infants: Evidence from an anticipatory eye movement task.* Poster presented at the 22nd Biennial International Conference on Infant Studies, Baltimore, MD.

Johnson, J. S., & Newport, E. L. (1989). Critical period effects in second language learning: The influence of maturational state on the acquisition of English as a second language. *Cognitive Psychology*, 21(1), 60–99.

Johnson, M. H. (2011). Interactive specialization: A domain-general framework for human functional brain development? *Developmental Cognitive Neuroscience, 1*(1), 7–21.

Jones, W. R., & Stewart, W. A. C. (1951). Bilingualism and verbal intelligence. *British Journal of Mathematical and Statistical Psychology, 4*(1), 3–8.

Karmiloff-Smith, A. (1998). Development itself is the key to understanding developmental disorders. *Trends in Cognitive Sciences, 2*(10), 389–398.

Kaushanskaya, M., & Prior, A. (2015). Variability in the effects of bilingualism on cognition: It is not just about cognition, it is also about bilingualism. *Bilingualism: Language and Cognition, 18*(1), 27–28.

Kessler, C., & Quinn, M. E. (1980). Positive effects of bilingualism on science problem-solving abilities. In *Current issues in bilingual education: Proceedings of the Georgetown University roundtable on languages and linguistics*, Washington, DC (pp. 295–308).

Klein, D., Mok, K., Chen, J. K., & Watkins, K. E. (2014). Age of language learning shapes brain structure: A cortical thickness study of bilingual and monolingual individuals. *Brain and Language, 131*, 20–24.

Kousaie, S., & Phillips, N. A. (2012a). Conflict monitoring and resolution: Are two languages better than one? Evidence from reaction time and event-related brain potentials. *Brain Research, 1446*, 71–90.

Kousaie, S., & Phillips, N. A. (2012b). Ageing and bilingualism: Absence of a "bilingual advantage" in stroop interference in a nonimmigrant sample. *The Quarterly Journal of Experimental Psychology, 65*(2), 356–369.

Kovács, Á. M., & Mehler, J. (2009a). Cognitive gains in 7-month-old bilingual infants. *Proceedings of the National Academy of Sciences, 106*(16), 6556–6560.

Kovács, Á. M., & Mehler, J. (2009b). Flexible learning of multiple speech structures in bilingual infants. *Science, 325*(5940), 611–612.

Krizman, J., Marian, V., Shook, A., Skoe, E., & Kraus, N. (2012). Subcortical encoding of sound is enhanced in bilinguals and relates to executive function advantages. *Proceedings of the National Academy of Sciences, 109*(20), 7877–7881.

Kroll, J. F., & Bialystok, E. (2013). Understanding the consequences of bilingualism for language processing and cognition. *Journal of Cognitive Psychology, 25*(5), 497–514.

Kroll, J. F., & Chiarello, C. (2016). Language experience and the brain: Variability, neuroplasticity, and bilingualism. *Language, Cognition and Neuroscience, 31*(3), 345–348.

Kuhl, P. K., Stevens, E., Hayashi, A., Deguchi, T., Kiritani, S., & Iverson, P. (2006). Infants show a facilitation effect for native language phonetic perception between 6 and 12 months. *Developmental Science, 9*(2), F13–F21.

Lewis, D. G. (1959). Bilingualism and non-verbal intelligence: A further study of test results. *British Journal of Educational Psychology, 29*(1), 17–22.

Li, P., Legault, J., & Litcofsky, K. A. (2014). Neuroplasticity as a function of second language learning: Anatomical changes in the human brain. *Cortex, 58*, 301–324.

Linck, J. A., Hoshino, N., & Kroll, J. F. (2008). Cross-language lexical processes and inhibitory control. *The Mental Lexicon, 3*(3), 349–374.

Lu, C. H., & Proctor, R. W. (1995). The influence of irrelevant location information on performance: A review of the Simon and spatial stroop effects. *Psychonomic Bulletin & Review, 2*(2), 174–207.

Luk, G. C. (2008). *The anatomy of the bilingual influence on cognition: Levels of functional use and proficiency of language* (Unpublished dissertation), ProQuest.

Luk, G., Anderson, J. A., Craik, F. I., Grady, C., & Bialystok, E. (2010). Distinct neural correlates for two types of inhibition in bilinguals: Response inhibition versus interference suppression. *Brain and Cognition, 74*(3), 347–357.

Luk, G., De Sa, E., & Bialystok, E. (2011). Is there a relation between onset age of bilingualism and enhancement of cognitive control? *Bilingualism: Language and Cognition, 14*(4), 588–595.

Luk, G., & Pliatsikas, C. (2016). Converging diversity to unity: Commentary on the neuroanatomy of bilingualism. *Language, Cognition and Neuroscience, 31*(3), 349–352.

Macnamara, J. (1966). *Bilingualism and primary education: A study of Irish experience.* Edinburgh, Scotland: Edinburgh University Press.

Maguire, E. A., Gadian, D. G., Johnsrude, I. S., Good, C. D., Ashburner, J., Frackowiak, R. S., & Frith, C. D. (2000). Navigation-related structural change in the hippocampi of taxi drivers. *Proceedings of the National Academy of Sciences, 97*(8), 4398–4403.

Manuel, H. T. (1935). A comparison of Spanish-speaking and English-speaking children in reading and arithmetic. *Journal of Applied Psychology, 19*(2), 189.

Martin-Rhee, M. M., & Bialystok, E. (2008). The development of two types of inhibitory control in monolingual and bilingual children. *Bilingualism: Language and Cognition, 11*(1), 81–93.

Mayo, L. H., Florentine, M., & Buus, S. (1997). Age of second-language acquisition and perception of speech in noise. *Journal of Speech, Language, and Hearing Research, 40*(3), 686–693.

McLeod, S., Harrison, L., Whiteford, C., & Walker, S. (2015). Multilingualism and speech-language competence in early childhood: Impact on academic and social-emotional outcomes at school. *Early Childhood Research Quarterly, 34,* 53–66.

Mechelli, A., Crinion, J. T., Noppeney, U., O'Doherty, J., Ashburner, J., Frackowiak, R. S., & Price, C. J. (2004). Neurolinguistics: Structural plasticity in the bilingual brain. *Nature, 431*(7010), 757–757.

Mezzacappa, E. (2004). Alerting, orienting, and executive attention: Developmental properties and sociodemographic correlates in an epidemiological sample of young, urban children. *Child Development, 75*(5), 1373–1386.

Miyake, A., Friedman, N. P., Emerson, M. J., Witzki, A. H., Howerter, A., & Wager, T. D. (2000). The unity and diversity of executive functions and their contributions to complex "frontal lobe" tasks: A latent variable analysis. *Cognitive Psychology, 41*(1), 49–100.

Mohades, S. G., Struys, E., Van Schuerbeek, P., Mondt, K., Van De Craen, P., & Luypaert, R. (2012). DTI reveals structural differences in white matter tracts between bilingual and monolingual children. *Brain Research, 1435,* 72–80.

Morton, J. B., & Harper, S. N. (2007). What did Simon say? Revisiting the bilingual advantage. *Developmental Science, 10*(6), 719–726.

Namazi, M., & Thordardottir, E. (2010). A working memory, not bilingual advantage, in controlled attention. *International Journal of Bilingual Education and Bilingualism, 13*(5), 597–616.

Paap, K. R. (2016). The neuroanatomy of bilingualism: Will winds of change lift the fog? *Language, Cognition and Neuroscience, 31*(3), 331–334.

Paap, K. R., & Greenberg, Z. I. (2013). There is no coherent evidence for a bilingual advantage in executive processing. *Cognitive Psychology, 66*(2), 232–258.

Paap, K. R., Johnson, H. A., & Sawi, O. (2015). Bilingual advantages in executive functioning either do not exist or are restricted to very specific and undetermined circumstances. *Cortex, 69,* 265–278.

Paap, K. R., Johnson, H. A., & Sawi, O. (2016). Should the search for bilingual advantages in executive functioning continue? *Cortex, 74*(4), 305–314.

Peal, E., & Lambert, W. E. (1962). The relation of bilingualism to intelligence. *Psychological Monographs: General and Applied, 76*(27), 1–23.

Pearson, B. Z., Fernández, S. C., & Oller, D. K. (1993). Lexical development in bilingual infants and toddlers: Comparison to monolingual norms. *Language Learning, 43*(1), 93–120.

Pelham, S. D., & Abrams, L. (2014). Cognitive advantages and disadvantages in early and late bilinguals. *Journal of Experimental Psychology: Learning, Memory, and Cognition, 40*(2), 313.

Poarch, G. J., & van Hell, J. G. (2012). Executive functions and inhibitory control in multilingual children: Evidence from second-language learners, bilinguals, and trilinguals. *Journal of Experimental Child Psychology, 113*(4), 535–551.

Poulin-Dubois, D., Blaye, A., Coutya, J., & Bialystok, E. (2011). The effects of bilingualism on toddlers' executive functioning. *Journal of Experimental Child Psychology, 108*(3), 567–579.

Prior, A., & Gollan, T. H. (2011). Good language-switchers are good task-switchers: Evidence from Spanish—English and Mandarin—English bilinguals. *Journal of the International Neuropsychological Society, 17*(4), 682–691.

Ricciardelli, L. A. (1992). Bilingualism and cognitive development in relation to threshold theory. *Journal of Psycholinguistic Research, 21*(4), 301–316.

Roberts, K. L., & Hall, D. A. (2008). Examining a supramodal network for conflict processing: A systematic review and novel functional magnetic resonance imaging data for related visual and auditory stroop tasks. *Journal of Cognitive Neuroscience, 20*(6), 1063–1078.

Saer, D. J. (1923). The effect of bilingualism on intelligence. *British Journal of Psychology, 14*(1), 25–38.

Saxe, G. (1988). Linking language with mathematics achievement: Problems and prospects. In R. R. Cocking & J. P. Mestre (Eds.). *Linguistic and cultural influences on learning mathematics* (pp. 47–62). Hillsdale, NJ: Lawrence Erlbaum Associates.

Shi, L. F. (2010). Perception of acoustically degraded sentences in bilingual listeners who differ in age of English acquisition. *Journal of Speech, Language, and Hearing Research, 53*(4), 821–835.

Simon, H. A. (1967). Motivational and emotional controls of cognition. *Psychological Review, 74*(1), 29.

Soveri, A., Laine, M., Hämäläinen, H., & Hugdahl, K. (2011). Bilingual advantage in attentional control: Evidence from the forced-attention dichotic listening paradigm. *Bilingualism: Language and Cognition, 14*(3), 371–378.

Stern, Y. (2009). Cognitive reserve. *Neuropsychologia, 47*(10), 2015–2028.

Strand, S., Malmberg, L., & Hall, J. (2015). *English as an additional language (EAL) and educational achievement in England: An analysis of the national pupil database.* London: EEF [online].

Tisserand, D. J., Van Boxtel, M. P., Pruessner, J. C., Hofman, P., Evans, A. C., & Jolles, J. (2004). A voxel-based morphometric study to determine individual differences in gray matter density associated with age and cognitive change over time. *Cerebral Cortex, 14*(9), 966–973.

Tucker, G. R. (2001). *A global perspective on bilingualism and bilingual education.* Georgetown University Round Table on Languages and Linguistics 1999, 332.

Uljarević, M., Katsos, N., Hudry, K., & Gibson, J. L. (2016). Practitioner review: Multilingualism and neurodevelopmental disorders—an overview of recent research and discussion of clinical implications. *Journal of Child Psychology and Psychiatry, 57*(11), 1205–1217.

Vandermosten, M., Price, C. J., & Golestani, N. (2016). Plasticity of white matter connectivity in phonetics experts. *Brain Structure and Function, 221*(7), 3825–3833.

Valian, V. (2015a). Bilingualism and cognition. *Bilingualism: Language and Cognition, 18*(1), 3–24.

Valian, V. (2015b). Bilingualism and cognition: A focus on mechanisms. *Bilingualism: Language and Cognition, 18*(1), 47–50.

Walker, D., Greenwood, C., Hart, B., & Carta, J. (1994). Prediction of school outcomes based on early language production and socioeconomic factors. *Child development, 65*(2), 606–621.

Wang, S. L. (1926). A demonstration of the language difficulty involved in comparing racial groups by means of verbal intelligence tests. *Journal of Applied Psychology, 10*(1), 102.

Wood, H. (2016). Stroke: Bilingualism is associated with better cognitive outcomes after stroke. *Nature Reviews Neurology, 12*(1), 4–4.

Yang, S., & Lust, B. (2004, November). *Testing effects of bilingualism on executive attention: Comparison of cognitive performance on two non-verbal tests*. Boston University Conference on Language Development, 5–7.

Yudes, C., Macizo, P., & Bajo, T. (2011). The influence of expertise in simultaneous interpreting on non-verbal executive processes. *Frontiers in Psychology, 2*, 309.

16 Music Training, Individual Differences, and Plasticity

E. Glenn Schellenberg

Funded by the Natural Sciences and Engineering Research Council of Canada.

An exciting and relatively recent avenue of scientific investigation focuses on *plasticity*, which refers to a living organism's capacity to change due to experience. *Neuroplasticity* refers more specifically to changes in brain structure and/ or function. This phenomenon became popularized after the publication of *The Brain That Changes Itself* (Doidge, 2007). Although the book was written for a general audience, it was well received, garnering positive reviews from the popular press (e.g., *The Guardian, The New York Times*), neuroscientists (e.g., Michael M. Merzenich, Vilayanur S. Ramachandran), and intellectuals and artists (e.g., Yoko Ono, Jeanette Winterson). It provided an accessible review of research, documenting primarily how the brain works to heal and reorganize itself in the face of trauma or atypical development, sometimes in response to specific interventions, but sometimes more or less on its own.

Because neuroplasticity has profound implications for health in general and rehabilitation in particular, it remains a focus of much neuroscientific research. Most of the available literature includes typically developing individuals as participants, however, which raises a different question: do the neuroplastic consequences that are observed after brain trauma extend to typical brains? For example, it is one thing to document how the brain reorganizes itself after left hemisphere damage, such that language use becomes more of a right hemisphere function. It is quite another thing to speculate that individual differences in experience and learning, such as differences in amount of music training, influence brain structure and function in a systematic way among typically developing individuals.

The word *systematic* is crucial. From a personal perspective, I have no doubt that my development, behavior, and brain structure were affected by waking up early before school as a child to practice the piano, on a daily basis, from the age of 5 until I was 16. It is much less clear, however, that a similar history of childhood experience would engender similar effects for another person. After all, development is the result of an interaction between genes and the environment, such that the consequences of years of piano training would almost certainly be influenced by preexisting traits and behaviors (e.g., Ullén, Hambrick, & Mosing, 2016).

The focus of the present chapter is on music training, and whether it has systematic consequences that extend beyond musical knowledge and ability, which are obvious outcomes, to nonmusical cognitive abilities, which are far less obvious. The overarching thesis is that a focus on plasticity, particularly by neuroscientists, has led to an imbalance between the relative emphasis placed on nature and nurture—a kind of radical environmentalism. I use the term "radical" to describe a tendency to interpret correlational findings as evidence of causation, specifically that music training causes systematic effects on brain development, which then extend to behavior. This interpretation, which ignores the role of preexisting individual differences, is further belied by (1) an apparent obliviousness about the genetic contribution to most human behaviors and traits, and (2) centuries of evidence that near-transfer effects tend to be relatively small, whereas far transfer is virtually nonexistent.

Genetics

In this section, I argue that musicians are as much born as they are made. Claims that music training represents a good or an ideal model for the study of plasticity (e.g., Herholz & Zatorre, 2012; Hyde et al., 2009; Jäncke, 2009; Münte, Altenmüller, & Jäncke, 2002; Schlaug, 2001; Strait & Kraus, 2014) rest on the assumption that musically trained and untrained individuals differ *only* in music training, which is untrue. Rather, music training is at least partly confounded with other variables, including cognitive abilities, personality, and demographics (Corrigall, Schellenberg, & Misura, 2013). In other words, whether one becomes a musician is not akin to random assignment. Consequently, comparisons of musically trained and untrained individuals cannot lead to clear interpretations of a causal role for the training, unless researchers (1) assign individuals randomly to music training and appropriate control conditions for many years, which is unadvisable because of attrition and artificiality, or (2) measure all possible confounding variables with perfect accuracy, hold them constant in the statistical analyses, and argue persuasively that the reverse causal direction is implausible. Some scholars claim that evidence of an association between "dose" (years of music training) and "response" (performance on a nonmusical variable, size of a brain region) allows for inferences of causation. This is also untrue because confounding variables have a similar dose-response association with music training (Corrigall et al., 2013).

General cognitive ability, which is typically measured with tests of IQ, has a strong genetic component (Deary et al., 2012; Mackintosh, 2011; Plomin & von Stumm, 2018). Contrary to what one might expect, the genetic contribution increases as individuals age, with heritability reaching over 60% by old age (Deary et al., 2012; McClearn et al., 1997). This increase—or genetic *amplification* (Plomin & DeFries, 1985)—is thought to be due to the fact that as individuals age, they are more likely to be found in environments that match their genetic potential (i.e., a gene-environment correlation; Scarr & McCartney, 1983). In other words, as we get older, genes increasingly determine the environments we are in, which in turn magnify our genetic predispositions.

Music training is likely to work similarly, with predispositions (re: general cognitive ability, personality, and music aptitude) influencing who takes music lessons, which then, potentially, magnify these predispositions. Socioeconomic status (SES) also plays a role, because music lessons cost money, and parents need to be supportive and cooperative. Although SES seems likes a prime example of an environmental influence, IQ predicts many markers of SES, such as years of education, income, occupational status, and lifetime achievement (for review see Mackintosh, 2011; Wai, Worrell, & Chabris, 2017). In short, because SES co-varies with IQ, it is a variable that incorporates influences of genes *and* the environment.

Another variable that co-varies with music training is personality, particularly the trait called *openness-to-experience*. Openness refers to intellectual curiosity, or an interest in new ideas, novelty in general, and aesthetics and the arts. The genetic contribution to openness is substantial, although slightly smaller than it is for general cognitive ability (Bouchard & McGue, 2003; Power & Pluess, 2015; Vernon, Martin, Schermer, & Mackie, 2008). Moreover, twin studies confirm that the association between openness and cumulative duration of music practice is higher among monozygotic than dizygotic twins (Butkovic, Ullén, & Mosing, 2015). Finally, and perhaps most importantly, music aptitude is a marker of general intelligence (Swaminathan & Schellenberg, 2018a; Swaminathan, Schellenberg, & Khalil, 2017; Swaminathan, Schellenberg, & Venkatesan, 2018). This correlation appears to be explained by genetics but not by shared or nonshared environment (Mosing, Pedersen, Madison, & Ullén, 2014). A different genetic component provides additional but independent explanatory power of associations among different tests of aptitude, specifically those that measure the discrimination of tone sequences based on rhythm, melody, or pitch (Mosing, Pedersen et al., 2014). Heritability estimates for these tests range between 12% and 59%, with shared-environment effects evident only on the pitch task, and only for males (Ullén, Mosing, Holm, Eriksson, & Madison, 2014). In short, unless we assume that music aptitude is unrelated to music training, which is nonsensical, taking music lessons has at least two genetic components: one related to general intelligence, the other to music-specific listening skills.

The contribution of genetics to music training is further documented by findings showing that musical skill and achievement are much more than just practice (Hambrick & Tucker-Drob, 2015; Macnamara, Hambrick, & Oswald, 2014), as some scholars used to claim (Ericsson, Krampe, & Tesch-Römer, 1993; Howe, Davidson, & Sloboda, 1998). Notably, twin studies reveal that the link between practicing music and musical ability is stronger among monozygotic than among dizygotic twins (Mosing, Madison, Pedersen, Kuja-Halkola, & Ullén, 2014). In fact, individual differences in practicing music— typically considered to represent an environment influence—are actually heritable to a substantial degree (i.e., 40%–70%; Hambrick & Tucker-Drob, 2015; Mosing, Madison et al., 2014). Moreover, when differences between monozygotic twins are analyzed on their own (thereby ruling out a role for genetics), practice is unrelated to musical ability as measured by an aptitude test (Mosing, Madison et al., 2014). Nevertheless, for individuals who have the genetic potential, practice is essential to becoming musically accomplished (Hambrick & Tucker-Drob, 2015).

Other findings from twin studies suggest that the link between amount of music training and fluid intelligence "is mostly due to shared genetic influences" (Mosing, Madison, Pedersen, & Ullén, 2016, p. 504). This result raises doubts about the proposal that music training causes increases in general cognitive ability. Rather, higher-functioning individuals may be more likely than other individuals to take music lessons and practice music, particularly for long durations of time. Recent results reveal, moreover, that identical twins are more likely than fraternal twins to play the same instrument and the same genre of music (Mosing & Ullén, 2018). In other words, genetics appears to play a role in the instrument one plays, and the genre of music one chooses to play.

Transfer

Transfer refers to situations in which learning and knowledge in one domain lead to faster learning or better performance in a different domain. Near transfer occurs between domains that are closely related, such as if learning and improvement on one test of working memory (e.g., n-back) lead to better performance on a different test of working memory (e.g., counting span). Far transfer, by contrast, occurs between two domains that differ substantially, such as if working memory training leads to better performance on a test of fluid intelligence. Claims that music training leads to benefits in nonmusical cognitive domains are claims of far transfer.

The concept of far transfer is central to the belief in a liberal-arts education. Most people in the developed world think that completing a university degree has cognitive benefits that extend beyond the actual courses one takes. For more than 100 years, however, results from laboratory studies indicate that far transfer is much less likely than near transfer, and that transfer is most likely when the learning and transfer domains have considerable overlap (Thorndike & Woodworth, 1901). In applied contexts, interventions such as *Head Start* are based on the idea that far transfer can ameliorate poor cognitive abilities that are often evident in young children from poor families. Nevertheless, these sorts of interventions have only modest success at best, and there is almost no evidence of long-term cognitive benefits (Love, Chazan-Cohen, Raikes, & Brookes-Gunn, 2013; U.S. Department of Health and Human Services & Administration for Children and Families, 2010).

In the present climate of enthusiasm for plasticity, commercial software developers and scholars have resurrected interest in the possibility of far-transfer effects and stimulated much scholarly debate. An overview of publicly available "brain-training" programs (e.g., *CogMed*, *Lumosity*) came to a conclusion, however, that closely matched the one reached by Thorndike and Woodworth 115 years earlier (Simons et al., 2016). Training clearly improved performance on the actual task that was trained, but the effects were much weaker for closely related transfer tasks, and virtually nonexistent for distantly related tasks.

Basic research on far transfer has focused on working memory training in the laboratory. In a recent meta-analytic review (Melby-Lervåg, Redick, & Hulme, 2016), working memory training led to improvements on non-trained tests of working memory, but these were short lived. There was no evidence of far-transfer effects, however, particularly for studies that had *active* control groups. (With *passive* control groups, observed effects could be due to other aspects of the training program.) Finally, the magnitude of improvements in working memory was not related to the magnitude of far-transfer effects, which undermines the possibility that far transfer actually occurred.

Some findings suggest that positive results from working memory training are evident with particular learning protocols (Jaeggi, Buschkuehl, Jonides, & Perrig, 2008; Jaeggi, Buschkuehl, Jonides, & Shah, 2011). For example, one meta-analysis concluded that n-back tasks lead to improvements in fluid intelligence (Au et al., 2015). A more detailed follow-up meta-analysis, which included a larger number of original studies, reached a different conclusion. N-back training led to improvements on novel n-back tasks, but transfer effects to other working memory tasks and to fluid intelligence were minimal and independent of the amount of training (Soveri, Antfolk, Karlsson, Salo, & Laine, 2017). In a meta-analysis of studies with typically developing children from 3–16 years of age, working memory training transferred to other tests of working memory, but far-transfer effects to fluid intelligence and academic skills were very small (Sala & Gobet, 2017c). The authors concluded, therefore, that "far transfer rarely occurs and its effects are minimal" (p. 671). This result is germane to the present chapter because music lessons are usually taken by typically developing children.

One might wonder about the applied relevance of transfer effects. Perhaps working memory training is more effective in this regard among people who need it the most. If this were the case, targeted interventions could be important for ameliorating cognitive deficits, even if they are less important more generally. Although this is a reasonable hypothesis, the evidence actually suggests otherwise. For example, in a study that included 23 training sessions, adult participants who began the training with good working memory abilities actually improved the most, and there was no evidence of far transfer to different tasks (Foster et al., 2017).

In short, although tests of fluid intelligence (e.g., Raven's matrices) place demands on working memory, actual training in working memory does not seem to influence performance reliably. Even near-transfer effects to other tests of working memory are transient. Learning and performing music also place demands on working memory, but the training process is much less focused. If intensive laboratory-based procedures fail to produce far transfer, one has to question why music training would lead to particularly *distant* transfer effects. Perhaps the long timescale (i.e., year of lessons compared to weeks of lab-based training) is implicated, or the fact that much of nonmusical learning (re: working memory and other executive functions) is implicit rather than explicit. Music training also involves sensory-motor integration and goal-oriented decision making, which could improve performance on tests of fluid intelligence. In any event, causal evidence regarding these hypotheses is difficult to obtain.

Music Training and Nonmusical Cognitive Abilities

Music training is associated positively with performance on a wide variety of nonmusical tasks. Consequently, positive findings are plentiful and research in this area has been rambunctious for several years. For example, a search of *PsycINFO* (29 May 2018) with keywords "music training" or "music lessons" revealed 455 sources published since the year 2000. My colleagues and I have previously provided detailed reviews of the documented associations (Schellenberg, 2016; Schellenberg & Weiss, 2013; Swaminathan & Schellenberg, 2016, 2018b). In each case, we concluded that music training had moderate positive associations with performance on tests of general cognitive ability (e.g., IQ, working memory), language ability (speech perception, vocabulary), and visuospatial skills (visual search, mental rotation).

We also concluded that the evidence for a causal role for music training is very weak. Recent reviews from other research teams reached similar conclusions (Benz, Sellaro, Hommel, & Colzato, 2016; Dumont, Syurina, Feron, & van Hooren, 2017), specifically that there is suggestive evidence that music training improves cognitive abilities, but that the jury is still out regarding the causal role of music training and the underlying mechanisms. By contrast, Costa-Giomi (2012, 2015) considers the evidence showing that music training confers intellectual benefits to be *convincing* in the short-term (after 1 or 2 years of lessons), but she also notes that nonmusical individual differences complicate the issue of longer-term effects by influencing who takes music lessons and practices for years on end. A notable exception is that music training, particularly when it focuses on rhythm perception, appears to improve listening skills that are required for perceiving and isolating the sounds of speech (i.e., phonological awareness), at least for some populations (e.g., young children, children with dyslexia).

In the review of the literature that follows, I focus on evidence from longitudinal studies published since 2000. Before I begin, let me summarize the issues that inform my critique. Some scholars argue that longitudinal research allows for inferences of causation even when participants are not assigned randomly to the music training and control conditions (e.g., Hyde et al., 2009; Tierney, Krizman, & Kraus, 2015). Their point is that if group differences are absent before the intervention begins, any differences that are evident afterward must be due to the different experiences. This view ignores the possibility of genetic *innovation*, specifically that some genetically determined behaviors emerge later in development (Plomin, DeFries, Knopik, & Neiderhiser, 2016). For example, gene-influenced individual differences in a nonmusical ability might be evident at 6 years of age but not at 5 years. Moreover, other environmental effects that are correlated with music training, such as SES, could affect phenotypical behavior differently at different points in time. Affluence, for example, could have little to no effect on a toddler's personality but a large effect for a teenager. In short, it is cavalier to assume that children and their families who opt to take music lessons are identical to other families, except for the decision to enroll in music training.

A related complication when self-selection is involved concerns the way group equivalence is determined before the intervention. Simply documenting that groups do not differ significantly (with $p > .05$) on some variables is not the same thing as "matching" groups. This is a problem in longitudinal designs (e.g., Norton et al., 2005; Habibi et al., 2014), but even more so for cross-sectional designs when potential confounding variables are not held constant in the analysis (e.g., Mongelli et al., 2017).

A separate issue concerns how participants are assigned to the intervention and control groups. Rather than assigning children randomly and individually (e.g., Schellenberg, 2004), it is often more convenient or practical to provide an intervention to preexisting *groups* of children (e.g., some kindergarten classes), while assigning other groups (other kindergarten classes) to the control condition (e.g., Gromko, 2005; Jaschke, Honing, & Scherder, 2018; Portowitz, Lichtenstein, Egorova, & Brand, 2009; Rauscher & Zupan, 2000). Even though these groups may be assigned randomly to the conditions, the design is sub-optimal because other factors that distinguish the groups (e.g., teaching quality, intragroup dynamics) could influence whether an intervention is successful. Thus, studies with group assignment designs are not considered further.

Another complicating factor is the choice of an appropriate control condition. Often, the control group does nothing in place of the music training intervention. Such *passive* control groups preclude the possibility of a clear interpretation of subsequent group differences, which could have stemmed from nonmusical aspects of the experience (e.g., more contact with an adult, more time spent in a structured learning environment). Ideally, the control group should be involved in some nonmusical training that is as similar as possible to music lessons, but without the music. For example, an *active* control group could involve painting training, drama lessons, or instruction in a foreign language, taught at approximately the same time of day as the music lessons, at a similar location, with similarly qualified instructors.

In the selective overview that follows, I first review studies with more-or-less optimal designs, followed by those with designs that are less than optimal (i.e., passive controls, self-selection into music training).

Longitudinal, Random Assignment, Active Controls

Let us first consider studies that included random assignment and an active control group. Schellenberg (2004) recruited 144 6-year-olds who were assigned randomly and individually to a year (36 weeks) of weekly keyboard, vocal (Kodály method), drama (active control), or no lessons (passive control). All lessons were provided free of charge and taught in groups of six children, at the same location, with similarly qualified instructors. Attrition over the course of the study was moderate (8.3%), leaving 132 children for the data analysis. Pre- to post-test improvements in IQ were greater for the children in the two music groups, who did not differ, compared to children in the two control groups, who did not differ. More detailed analyses revealed that the two music groups had larger improvements than children in the no-lessons group, but direct comparisons with the drama group led to inconsistent results (i.e., null, marginal, or significant), depending on the analysis (Schellenberg, 2005–2006). At post-test, it became apparent from parent reports that the children practiced minimally between lessons, which raises questions of ecological validity. The same children were invited back to take a test of their ability to decode the emotions conveyed by prosody in speech (Thompson, Schellenberg, & Husain, 2004). For one comparison (anger vs. fear), the keyboard and drama children outperformed the control children. It is unclear why the keyboard and vocal group performed differently, but attrition was substantial (only 30% of the original 144 participated) so the findings are equivocal.

In a large-scale attempt to replicate and extend the original Schellenberg (2004) findings to academic achievement (mathematics and literacy), 909 2nd-graders from 19 different schools in the UK were assigned randomly to string lessons (violin or cello), singing lessons based on the Kodály method, or drama lessons (Haywood et al., 2015). Children were pretested with standardized tests at the end of 1st grade, and post-tested a year later after taking 32 weeks of weekly, 45-min lessons, in groups of approximately 10 children. Attrition was modest (10.5%), leaving 814 children in the sample at post-test. Children from all three groups performed similarly at post-test (controlling for pre-test scores), and neither music group had larger improvements in mathematics or literacy compared to the drama group. In fact, effect sizes were close to 0 ($ds < .05$), even when the two music groups were collapsed and compared to the drama group. The findings were identical when the analyses were limited to children from low-SES families. Unfortunately, details of the study were published in an "evaluation report and executive summary"[1], but not in an academic journal. Nevertheless, the information provided in the report suggests that the design, method, and analysis were meticulous. Although one can never prove the null hypothesis, the power afforded by the large sample size implies that if music confers nonmusical, cognitive benefits that extend to academic achievement, such effects are very small indeed.

Besson and her colleagues assigned children individually to music or painting training. Instead of true randomization, the authors used pseudo-randomization, to ensure that the two groups were equivalent at pre-test on the measures of interest. In the first study, after 6 months of two 75-min lessons per week, 8-year-olds in the music group could read irregularly spelled words better than children in the painting group, but on two other reading tests, the groups had similar improvement (Moreno et al., 2009). The music group was also better at detecting subtle pitch anomalies in speech (one word in a sentence shifted in pitch), but not in music (one note in a melody shifted in pitch). Finally, the music group had stronger electrophysiological (ERP) responses to pitch anomalies in speech and music. Because the music and speech tasks involved changes in pitch, these results are best considered as examples of near transfer. The reading result appears to provide evidence of far transfer, but the findings are far from conclusive because of the small sample sizes (n = 16 per group).

In a second study, the design was similar except that 8-year-olds took music or painting lessons for two years, six months per year. At the end of the study, the children in the music group had larger mismatch negativity (MMN) responses to syllables that were altered in duration or voice-onset time, but not in vowel frequency (i.e., pitch), which seems counter-intuitive (Chobert, François, Velay, & Besson, 2014). After the first year, the music group was also better at a task that required them to identify whether sequences of three syllables were similar to those heard during an exposure phase (François, Chobert, Besson, & Schön, 2013). This advantage was even greater by the end of the second year, and ERP responses paralleled the behavioral results. During the exposure phase of the task, however, individual syllables were matched one-to-one with different tones, which likely provided a better learning cue for the music group than for the painting group. In other words, the data provide no behavioral evidence for far transfer, and the electrophysiological data are confusing. As in the first study, the sample sizes were small (n = 12 per group).

Another pair of studies tested whether six weeks of child-centered music or visual-arts training leads to cognitive benefits among 4-year-olds (Mehr, Schachner, Katz, & Spelke, 2013). Lessons were provided to groups of 7–8 children, each of whom was accompanied by a parent. In the first study, children in the music group (n = 15) had marginally higher performance at post-test on one measure of spatial abilities (map use/navigation), whereas children in the visual-arts group (n = 14) had marginally higher performance on a second measure (visual form analysis). The second study was the same except that children in the music group (n = 23) were compared to a passive control group (n = 22), and no effects were found. Null findings also emerged when children from the two studies were combined. The null result could be due to the small sample sizes, or because children had only 4.5 hours of training in total. Nevertheless, if there is an effect of music training on nonmusical cognitive abilities, it appears to be relatively small.

Two other studies used pedagogies that were markedly different from those of typical music lessons. Degé and Schwarzer (2011) asked whether phonological awareness could be improved by music training. Phonological awareness is an important prerequisite for learning to read. The authors assigned 5- and 6-year-olds to 20 weeks of daily 10-minute training in music (primarily listening), explicit training in phonological awareness, or sports (participant numbers per group, ns = 13–14). Improvement from pre- to post-test was virtually identical for the music and phonological-awareness groups, but no improvement was evident for the sports group. These results are some of the most clear-cut in the literature, but the samples were small, and attrition was substantial (25%). Nevertheless, the authors successfully replicated the findings with a new sample of children from immigrant families (Patscheke, Degé, & Schwarzer, 2016).

Finally, Moreno et al. (2011a) assigned preschoolers to computer-based training in music listening or visual arts, five days per week for four weeks. Children were pre- and post-tested on measures of vocabulary, spatial ability (block design), and attention/inhibition (go/no-go). Improvements were evident for only the music group on the measures of vocabulary and attention/inhibition. In the latter case, ERPs were also correspondingly larger for the music group. Another test that required children to match arbitrary symbols with words showed inconsistent results: The music group had larger improvements in one analysis (ANCOVA) but not in another (mixed-design ANOVA; Moreno, Friesen, & Bialystok, 2011b). In a follow-up study, the visual-art (control) program was replaced with a second language (French) program (Janus, Lee, Moreno, & Bialystok, 2016). Both groups showed similar improvements over the four weeks on tests of verbal and nonverbal executive functions. In other words, the French-language control program was as beneficial as the music program.

Other results suggest that phonological awareness and early reading skills can be enhanced among atypically developing children—children with dyslexia—after they take music lessons that focus specifically on rhythm. A core deficit in dyslexia appears to be one of temporal processing (Goswami, 2011), such that the deficit in reading ability is predicted by temporal-processing difficulties in speech (Leong & Goswami, 2014) and in music (Flaugnacco et al., 2014; Goswami, Huss, Mead, Fosker, & Verney, 2013; Huss, Verney, Fosker, Mead, & Goswami, 2011). Flaugnacco et al. (2015) assigned 8- to 11-year-old children with dyslexia to seven months of training in music or painting for two hours per week. The music training was based on the Kodály method, but modified to focus on rhythm and temporal processing. After the intervention, the music group had larger improvements on tests of rhythm skills, as one would expect. More importantly, the music group also had larger improvements in phonological awareness and on tests that required them to read aloud text or pseudo-words.

If we consider these "best designed" studies as a whole, what can we conclude? The Schellenberg (2004) results are weak, without successful replication for almost 15 years. The null results from the large UK study are particularly disheartening (Haywood et al., 2015). If music lessons cause increases in nonmusical cognitive ability, the effect appears to be very small. Besson's studies (Chobert et al., 2014; François et al., 2013; Moreno et al., 2009) suggest that electrophysiological responses to speech become stronger and more reliable as a consequence of music lessons, but the behavioral results are weak, perhaps because of small samples. The most reliable results come from studies of rhythm-based training, which appear to improve phonological awareness among young children who are learning to read, and among children with dyslexia who have difficulty reading. Such improvements may, in turn, lead to improvements in reading.

It remains unclear, however, just how "musical" the music training has to be in order to see these effects. For example, Thomson, Leong, and Goswami (2013) compared a seven-week, rhythm-based intervention to one that used commercial software specifically designed to improve phonological awareness. A third group was a passive control group. Both interventions improved phonological awareness relative to controls. The most musical components of the rhythm intervention involved (1) copying a rhythm on a drum as a warm-up activity, and (2) moving the middle tone of a three-tone sequence forward or backward in time to make the sequence isochronous. In short, music per se may not be necessary to see beneficial effects of rhythm training on phonological awareness, although incorporating music into the training regimen may make the experience more enjoyable.

Finally, some findings stand out as anomalies. For example, one would expect that better phonological awareness leads to improvements in reading aloud nonwords, for which grapheme-phoneme matching is regular, but not necessarily to reading irregularly spelled words (e.g., thyme, cello; Moreno et al., 2009). Moreover, there is no obvious mechanistic explanation that would motivate one to predict that short-term but relatively intense music-listening training improves vocabulary (Moreno et al., 2011a).

Longitudinal, Random Assignment, Passive Controls

The next group of studies included random assignment, which eliminates the role of self-selection, but passive control groups, which make the findings impossible to interpret unequivocally. In one such study, Iranian 5-year-olds were assigned randomly to 13 weeks of music lessons (Orff method) or to no lessons (Kaviani, Mirbaha, Pournaseh, & Sagan, 2014). Both groups ($ns = 30$) were matched for age, gender, and SES, and they took the Farsi version of the Stanford-Binet IQ test before and after the intervention. The children in the music group had larger increases in IQ compared to the control group, which stemmed from greater improvement in visual/abstract and verbal reasoning. Although these results parallel the findings of Schellenberg (2004), the increases in performance cannot be attributed without doubt to music training. Other interventions could have the same effect.

In another study of low-income Hispanic children living in Los Angeles, Kraus and her colleagues recruited families of 6- to 9-year-olds, who were on a waiting list for a community-based music program. Enrollment in the study guaranteed a place in the program either right away (Group 1) or a year later (Group 2), with group assignment determined pseudo-randomly. Thus, Group 2 served as a passive control group during the first year. At the end of the year, Group 2 exhibited a *decline* in age-normed reading level, which is normal in this population, but Group 1 did not (Slater et al., 2014). After the second year, Group 1 had larger improvements in speech-in-noise perception compared to Group 2 (Slater et al., 2015). The authors concluded that music training causes improvement in the perception of speech in noise after two years of training but not after one year. In other words, more training was associated with better performance.

The results are less than compelling, however, because in a sample of low-SES children, the structure and routine of being involved in any extra-curricular activity could improve motivation, self-esteem, and performance on many tests. This perspective helps to explain the widespread popularity of *El Sistema*, and why children who were more engaged in the music program (i.e., with the best attendance and participation) also tended to show the largest increases in reading ability and strongest neural encoding of speech at the end of the study (Kraus, Hornickel, Strait, Slater, & Thompson, 2014). The very small sample sizes (n = 19 per group at the end of the second year in Slater et al., 2015) and the data analysis are also problematic. Instead of using multi-level modeling for the speech-in-noise data, the authors used repeated-measures analysis of covariance, which leads to interpretive problems (i.e., distorted estimates of the within-subject variable, increased Type I error, or reduced power), particularly if the covariates are not centered (Schneider, Avivi-Reich, & Mozuraitis, 2015). Finally, of the 80 participants who were tested at the beginning of the study, fewer than half (47.5%) were included in the final data analyses.

A group of Spanish researchers compared the development of phonological awareness among 4-year-olds, who were randomly assigned to eight weeks of phonological training, combined phonological *and* music training, or no training (Herrera, Lorenzo, Defior, Fernandez-Smith, & Costa-Giomi, 2011). Improvements in phonological awareness were greater in the two intervention groups than in the control group. The group with phonological and music training, however, had the best performance on tasks that required rapid naming or identifying word-final sounds. In this instance, incorporation of music into the intervention may have made the phonological training more engaging. Thus, nonmusical pedagogical improvements could have a similar effect.

Longitudinal, Self-selection

Another longitudinal design involves following children from families who choose to begin taking music lessons at some point in time. In one study of this sort, researchers from the Boston area recruited 70 5- to 7-year-old children, approximately half of whom were just beginning to take weekly, private music lessons. The children were tested twice: once at the beginning of the study (Time 1) and again 15 months later (Time 2). The testing battery included a variety of cognitive tests, tests of listening ability and music aptitude, and structural MRI scans. At Time 1, the children in the music group came from higher-SES families compared to children in the control group, and they were also slightly older (Norton et al., 2005). After controlling for age and SES, the children did not differ on any other measure, and the groups were matched for handedness and gender. Nevertheless, the means were higher in absolute terms for the music group for all seven of the behavioral tests (Table 16.2), which is significant with a two-tailed binomial test (p = .016). As one might expect, music aptitude was correlated with measures of general cognitive ability and with phonological awareness.

At Time 2, fewer than half of the original children (31 of 70) were included in the analyses (Hyde et al., 2009). Structural brain differences now distinguished the two groups, and these were correlated with changes in motor skills and music aptitude. Although the authors attributed these results to experience-dependent plasticity, it is also possible that pre-existing group differences, which were evident at Time 1, became exaggerated over a period of 15 months, such that they became evident in the brain scans. At the very least, the results highlight the interpretive problems that arise from longitudinal designs when groups are formed naturally.

In a similar study conducted in Los Angeles, researchers compared the development of 5- to 6-year-olds who enrolled in a community music program modeled on El Sistema (music group), to same-age children who registered for swimming or soccer classes (sports group). A third, control group did not have any intensive extra-curricular activity. All children were recruited from low-SES areas of the city. At the beginning, the three groups did not differ on a variety of cognitive, neural, or social measures (Habibi et al., 2014). After one year, near transfer was evident in the sense that the music group had improved pitch perception and production ability, but the control group showed *poorer* singing and pitch discrimination, which is difficult to interpret (Ilari, Keller, Damasio, & Habibi, 2016). After two years, the music group had structurally different brains than the other children (Habibi et al., 2017), which the authors attributed to the different training experiences. The music group was also better than the sports group at detecting an altered tone in a melody, but only marginally different from the control group (Habibi, Cahn, Damasio, & Damasio, 2016). Electrophysiological responses (ERPs) to musical notes were also more mature among the music group. In short, in the absence of clear behavioral evidence, even for near transfer, it is impossible to interpret structural and functional changes in the brain. The small samples sizes at the end of two years (ns ≤ 13 and 20 in Habibi et al., 2016, 2017, respectively) undoubtedly contribute to this interpretive difficulty. Moreover, the different sample sizes across four reports from the same study are disconcerting.

In a study of 66 Finnish 5- to 6-year-olds, children were recruited from 26 different kindergartens that also functioned as daycare centers (Linnavalli, Putkinen, Lipsanen, Huotilainen, & Tervaniemi, 2018). Some of the kindergartens offered music playschool classes during daycare hours, others offered dance lessons, and some offered neither music nor dance training. All of the children in the control group (no music, no dance) came from kindergartens that offered neither program, which meant that the intervention was confounded with the specific kindergarten. Children were tested four times over a two-year period on measures of phonological awareness, vocabulary, perceptual reasoning (block design and matrix reasoning), and inhibition. Because children could enter and leave the programs at will, or take private music or dance lessons outside of school, these predictors were treated as con-tinuous variables (i.e., duration of time in music or dance classes). As noted earlier, duration of music training is correlated with SES, cognitive abilities, and personality (Corrigall et al., 2013).

Improvement over time on the measures of phonological awareness and vocabulary were larger as duration of music training (compared to no music training) increased, but there was no association with perceptional reasoning or inhibition. Other findings indicated that children from high-SES families with higher vocabulary scores—across time points—were more likely to take dance lessons for longer durations of time. Similarly, high-SES children with higher perceptual reasoning scores—across time points—were also more likely to take music *and* dance training for longer periods of time. These data clarify that self-selection into arts lessons plays a major role in the outcomes, despite the authors conclusion that "music playschool *enhances* children's linguistic skills" (emphasis added).

Kraus and her colleagues used a similar design to study 68 high-school fresh-men in low-SES areas in Chicago (Tierney et al., 2015; Tierney, Krizman, Skoe, Johnston, & Kraus, 2013). As part of the curriculum, students were required to choose between taking a music course (band or choir) or enroll-ing in the Junior Reserve Officers Training Corps (JROTC), which focused primarily on fitness. The students were tested at the beginning of high school and again two and three years later, but only 43 (after 2 years) and 40 (after 3 years) of 68 were included in the analyses (e.g., many students had moved from music to JROTC or vice versa). After two years, neural encoding of a speech sound presented in noise was more rapid in the music group (Tierney et al., 2013). After three years, outcome measures included subcortical and cortical neural responses to a repeating consonant-vowel syllable, as well as behavioral measures of phonological awareness, rapid naming, and phonologi-cal memory. The music group had larger and more adult-like cortical responses at the end of the study, whereas the JROTC group had smaller subcortical responses. The music group also improved more on the test of phonologi-cal awareness, but the two groups did not differ at either time on any of the measures. In short, music training may have caused changes in brain develop-ment that were more or less independent of behavior. Alternatively, neural-developmental trajectories may have differed between students who chose one program or the other.

In a similar design, Degé and her colleagues examined memory develop-ment among German 9- to 11-year-olds, some of whom opted to take an extended music curriculum in school (Degé, Wehrum, Stark, & Schwarzer, 2011). The children were tested when the program began and again two years later. Outcome variables included measures of short-term visual and auditory memory. Unlike children in the control group, children in the music group exhibited improvement on both memory tests over the course of two years. These findings remained evident when confounding variables such as general intelligence, SES, motivation, and music aptitude were held constant, even though the sample comprised only 34 children in total.

Kreutz and his colleagues examined whether an extended music curriculum taught in primary schools influences cognitive development. The program (JeKI—*Jedem Kind ein Instrument*, An Instrument for Every Child) offered German 7- to 8-year-olds a musical instrument and weekly 45-minute lessons. Families chose whether to enroll, so self-selection was an issue, as was finding an appropriate control group. The author's solution to these problems was to measure and control for as many extraneous variables as possible, and to compare children with counterparts who self-selected into extended training in the natural sciences at different schools in another state. Even before the intervention began, however, the children in the music group had higher IQ scores.

The first two studies had small samples ($ns = 25$) and tested children three times over 18 months. In one, the music group had larger improvements in short-term and long-term verbal memory, but not in short-term visuospatial memory, even after controlling for IQ (Roden, Kreutz, & Bongard, 2012). In a second report, visuospatial short-term and working memory were tested, as well as auditory short-term memory (Roden, Grube, Bongard, & Kreutz, 2014). The music group had greater improvement that the natural-sciences group on the auditory tests (i.e., immediate recall of a list of words, or a multisyllabic nonword), and on three measures of visuospatial working memory (span tasks). As in the 2012 paper, the group differences were evident after controlling for IQ, and the groups performed similarly on the tests of short-term visuospatial memory.

In a subsequent paper (Roden, Könen et al., 2014), the same design was used but the authors recruited and tested much larger samples of children (music: $n = 192$, natural sciences: $n = 153$). The outcome variables for tests of far transfer were measures of visual attention and processing speed. Both were paper-and-pencil tasks that required children to cross out items selectively, or to connect consecutive digits, respectively. As with the smaller samples, the music group had higher IQ scores at the beginning of the study. The additional power meant that the groups also differed significantly in SES: Children in the music group came from higher-SES families. For the visual attention task, both groups improved over time but the natural sciences group had larger improvements, with performance exceeding the music group at the end of the study. SES was unrelated to performance or to the rate of change. By contrast, IQ was related to performance but it did not account for improvements across time. For processing speed, both groups again improved over the 18 months. Although the music group had larger improvements from the second to the third testing session, the groups did not differ at any point in time. As with the attention task, SES had no association with performance but IQ did, although IQ could not account for improved speed over time.

Roden, Könen et al. (2014) also included measures of near transfer—performance on a test of music aptitude that included melody and rhythm subtests. For the rhythm subtest, the music group had greater improvements from Time 1 to Time 2, and performance exceeded that of the natural sciences children at Time 2 and Time 3. For the melody subtest (administered only at Times 2 and 3), the music group had higher scores at both time points, but improvement over time was similar between groups. SES differences between groups were unrelated to the findings, but IQ predicted performance on both subtests, and could explain a small proportion of the improvements in performance. In short, when the researchers tested large samples of children from the JeKI program, there was evidence of inconsistent near transfer, but no evidence of far transfer.

Finally, researchers in China used a *retrospective* longitudinal design to study whether private music training could predict 250 children's past academic performance, focusing on native-language (L1) ability, foreign language (L2) ability, and mathematics (Yang, Ma, Gong, Hu, & Yao, 2014). All of the children entered the same school when they were 6.5 years old on average. Eleven semesters (5.5 years) later, they were asked whether they had taken private music lessons—or private painting lessons—since they started. The researchers then compared students with or without music (or painting) training, using scores from standardized tests that each student took at the end of each semester. An interaction between testing time and group indicated that musically trained children improved more than untrained children in L2 development, but not in L1 performance or mathematics. Moreover, although the music group exhibited an advantage at the end of the eleventh semester on all three tests, the group difference disappeared for L1 and mathematics (but not for L2) when IQ and SES were held constant. Painting training had no association with academic performance. It is unclear why there was a "selective" partial association between music training and L2 ability, but personality (e.g., conscientiousness, motivation) could have played a role.

In short, my review of these natural but longitudinal experiments highlights that children who take music lessons are not a random sample but rather a select group who are likely to differ from other children in terms of general cognitive ability, SES, music aptitude, and personality variables. Whether they are similar to (or not significantly different from) other children at the beginning of a longitudinal study on music training does not mean that group differences, which may be observed later on, can be attributed unequivocally to the music training. It is also clear the natural longitudinal studies with low-SES populations are very difficult to conduct, with attrition being a major problem. My hunch is that interpersonal dynamics within small groups also make the data noisier than they would be otherwise. Moreover, in my own experience of dealing with children in El Sistema, which typically runs every day for hours after school, low-income families are eager for after-school childcare that is both free and safe.

Meta-analysis of Longitudinal Studies

In a recent meta-analysis, Sala and Gobet (2017b) reviewed all of the available longitudinal studies that examined whether music training is associated with cognitive and academic skills. Inclusion criteria included (1) participants who were typically developing children or adolescents with no history of formal music training, (2) a control group, and (3) an outcome variable that measured an academic or cognitive skill, which was not music related. They considered four moderator variables, which might influence whether a positive result emerged. These included age, random assignment, whether the control group was active or passive, and the particular outcome variable (e.g., literacy, mathematics, intelligence).

When all studies were considered jointly, the average effect size was small ($d = 0.16$), but statistically significant, and slightly larger for studies that tested intelligence or memory. Nevertheless, moderator analysis revealed that effects tended to be larger for studies with less than optimal designs, specifically a passive control group or no random assignment. By contrast, 95% confidence intervals for the mean effect size for better designs (i.e., active control group *or* random assignment) included 0. In fact, the mean effect size for studies with an active control group *and* random assignment was −0.12; for studies with a passive control group and no random assignment it was 0.33. The authors concluded that "music training does not reliably enhance children and young adolescents' cognitive or academic skills, and that previous positive findings were probably due to confounding variables" (Sala & Gobet, 2017b, p. 55).

Correlation, Causation, Context, and Conclusion

Although many studies have reported that music training is associated with a variety of nonmusical cognitive abilities (for review see Schellenberg & Weiss, 2013), evidence indicating that music training causes the observed associations is very weak. Alternative interpretations include (1) individual differences, including those in cognitive ability, influence who takes music lessons, or (2) unidentified variables are causing cognitive abilities and music training to co-vary in tandem. In my view, the second alternative could only be describing genetic or demographic factors, which contribute to the individual differences in the first alternative. In short, the two alternatives are describing the same thing. Nevertheless, there is an overwhelming bias in the psychology and neuroscience research communities to interpret positive correlations as evidence for a causal role of music training. Even when researchers acknowledge that causation cannot be inferred, a clear bias for interpreting the results remains evident, even though this requires turning a blind eye to the research on genetics and far transfer. This section of the chapter focuses on delineating this problem and trying to explain it.

Consider one example: an article entitled "Music and words in the visual cortex: The impact of musical expertise" (Mongelli et al., 2017). The title infers causation even though the design was quasi-experimental. The justification for this inference appears to be that the musically trained and untrained groups did not differ significantly in terms of age, education, or gender. Consider another example: an article entitled "Different neural activities support auditory working memory in musician and bilinguals" (Alain et al., 2018). Although the title is neutral with respect the role of causation, the first and last sentences of the abstract are not: "Musical training and bilingualism benefit executive functioning and working memory," and "These findings indicate that the auditory WM advantage in musicians and bilinguals is mediated by different neural networks specific to each life experience." In addition to inferring causation, the sentences are problematic because they equate music training with bilingualism. The sample of bilinguals recruited for the study comprised immigrants to Toronto who came from many different countries. Thus, there is no reason to think that these "forced" bilinguals, who needed to speak English in an English-speaking city, had anything in common other than being bilingual, or that they differed systematically from other Torontonians, except for their native tongue and country of birth. The fact that they successfully immigrated to Canada may be a marker of relatively high SES and cognitive ability compared to compatriots in their home country, but many immigrants in Canada are economic refugees, to which this point is less likely to apply. People with music training, by contrast, differ from musically untrained individuals in many ways, even before the training begins.

Table 16.1 provides examples of 16 articles published since 2013. Each has a title that infers causation from correlational designs that were not longitudinal

Table 16.1 Titles of Example Journal Articles, Published since 2013, That Inferred Causation From Correlation (causal terminology in **bold**)

Title	Year
Pitch and Time Processing in Speech and Tones: The **Effects** of Musical Training and Attention	2018
Musical literacy **shifts** asymmetries in the ventral visual cortex	2017
Music training **enhances** the automatic neural processing of foreign speech sounds	2017
Musical training **shapes** neural responses to melodic and prosodic expectation	2016
Tuning the mind: Exploring the connections between musical ability and executive functions	2016
Bilingualism and Musicianship **Enhance** Cognitive Control	2016
Investigating the **effects** of musical training on functional brain development with a novel melodic MMN paradigm	2014
Inhibitory control in bilinguals and musicians: Event related potential (ERP) evidence for experience-specific **effects**.	2014
Degree of musical expertise **modulates** higher order brain functioning	2013
Biological **impact** of preschool music classes on processing speech in noise	2013
Effects of music learning and piano practice on cognitive function, mood and quality of life in older adults	2013
Musical expertise **modulates** early processing of syntactic violations in language	2013
Musical training **heightens** auditory brainstem function during sensitive periods in development	2013
Early musical training and white matter **plasticity** in the corpus callosum: evidence for a sensitive period	2013
Musical training **enhances** neural processing of binaural sounds	2013
Musical experience **influences** statistical learning of a novel language	2013

and had no random assignment. The table is not meant to be exhaustive or even representative. Rather, the articles were selected solely because the title displayed a logical failure, and to document that the problem is common. Note, however, that the problem appears to be particularly acute in neuroscience, perhaps because neuroscientists believe that they are looking at the underlying mechanism for an "established" phenomenon, which blinds them to the limitations of their correlational data. This speculation led to the formation of a hypothesis that I tested recently (Schellenberg, 2018), specifically that *in the published literature on music training, inferring causation from correlation is more common among neuroscientists than it is among psychologists.* The sample included 114 published articles (in English) that reported results from correlational or quasi-experimental studies, each of which examined associations between music training and nonmusical abilities (including brain structure/function). Raters who were blind to the hypothesis analyzed the titles and abstracts for causal language. Inferring causation from correlation was notably high in general, evident in 64% of the articles across disciplines, which was particularly notable because each instance represented a fundamental error in scientific reasoning. As expected, the odds of inferring causation were two to four times greater among neuroscientists than among psychologists, depending on the particular analysis.

Why do many of us believe, or want to believe, that music has transformative powers beyond the pleasure it gives the listener, the feeling of connectedness to others it provides, the happy and sad memories it evokes, and the sense of wonder and awe that listeners often experience? For one thing, scholars and arts advocates complain that music is not taken seriously as a school subject, and that when budget-tightening is the rule of the day, music courses suffer more than math, science, and English courses. The National Endowment for the Arts (NEA) notes, moreover, that music and visual-arts education in schools has declined since the 1970s, and that studying the arts in school predicts subsequent participation in the arts, such as going to the ballet, the opera, the theatre, or to concerts that feature classical or jazz music (Rabkin & Hedberg, 2011). One has to wonder, though, why the NEA did not consider concerts by popular contemporary artists (e.g., Beyoncé, Kanye West, Rihanna). One could also argue that music education and participation have not declined, but simply changed, as consumers now have access to an infinite amount of music via smart phones and the internet, and individuals with no formal training can make professional-sounding recordings in the comfort of their homes, with relatively inexpensive software, a personal computer, and no musical instruments.

In my view, government support for music and other art forms is always going to be lukewarm (or cold) when compared to its support for STEM subjects (science, technology, engineering, and mathematics) and core subjects in the humanities such as English and history. Reports from neuroscience and psychology, which claim that music has beneficial, nonmusical side effects, are unlikely to change things. Moreover, justifying support for music based on nonmusical benefits implies, with just a little slippage, that without such benefits, music is unimportant. In short, science and advocacy make strange bedfellows.

434   E. Glenn Schellenberg

Another explanation of the radical environmentalism that has taken over this research area is that it is much easier to receive funding for research programs that seek to document positive findings, rather than null results, about links between music training and nonmusical abilities. The same argument applies to publications in peer-reviewed journals. Recent evidence suggests, however, that instead of making you smarter, playing music in groups facilitates social bonding and social behavior (Kirschner & Tomasello, 2010; Schellenberg, Corrigall, Dys, & Malti, 2015), a view that is consistent with some evolutionary accounts of music's universality (e.g., Dunbar, 2012; Tarr, Launay, & Dunbar, 2014). Moving in synchrony appears to play a central role in the effect. For example, toddlers who are bounced in synchrony to music with an experimenter are more likely to be helpful to the same experimenter (Cirelli, Einarson, & Trainor, 2014), or to her friend (Cirelli, Wan, & Trainor, 2016), than they are to a stranger, or to someone who bounced out-of-sync with the toddler. Similar but smaller effects of synchrony are evident even without the music (Cirelli, Wan, Spinelli, & Trainor, 2017). In other words, music with a beat is likely to promote synchronous movement, which in turn facilitates social bonding. More generally, music listening often makes us feel good, and making music often makes us feel good together. Isn't that enough?

Overview

What has neuroscience added to our understanding of the nonmusical consequences of music training, over and above psychology? The reviewed findings are largely negative. In my opinion, neuroscience has detracted from research because neuroscientists routinely impute causality from correlation, even more so than psychologists do. The lack of behavioral evidence for far-transfer effects—in the case of music training and otherwise—means that the search for neural mechanistic explanations is unwarranted.

What are the concrete implications of research in this area, and opportunities for translation to education? Music training improves *musical* skills, which should be enough.

How can the reader learn more about the topic? Overviews of the available literature are provided by a recent meta-analysis of music training in particular (Sala & Gobet, 2017b), and by an article that provides a concise review of the lack of evidence for far transfer in general (Sala & Gobet, 2017a).

Note

1. https://files.eric.ed.gov/fulltext/ED581247.pdf

References

Alain, C., Khatamian, Y., He, Y., Lee, Y., Moreno, S., Leung, A. W. S., & Bialystok, E. (2018). Different neural activities support auditory working memory in musician and bilinguals. *Annals of the New York Academy of Sciences, 1423*, 435–446.

Au, J., Sheehan, E., Tsai, N., Duncan, G. J., Buschkuehl, M., & Jaeggi, S. M. (2015). Improving fluid intelligence with training on working memory: A meta-analysis. *Psychonomic Bulletin & Review, 22*, 366–377.

Benz, S., Sellaro, R., Hommel, B., & Colzato, L. S. (2016). Music makes the world go round: The impact of musical training on non-musical cognitive functions—a review. *Frontiers in Psychology, 6.* doi:10.3389/fpsyg.2015.02023

Bouchard, T. J. Jr., & McGue, M. (2003). Genetic and environmental influences on human psychological differences. *Journal of Neurobiology, 54*, 4–45.

Butkovic, A., Ullén, F., & Mosing, M. A. (2015). Personality related traits as predictors of music practice: Underlying environmental and genetic influences. *Personality and Individual Differences, 74*, 133–138.

Chobert, J., François, C., Velay, J.-L., & Besson, M. (2014). Twelve months of active musical training in 8- to 10-year-old children enhances the preattentive processing of syllabic duration and voice onset time. *Cerebral Cortex, 24*, 956–967.

Cirelli, L. K., Einarson, K. M., & Trainor, L. J. (2014). Interpersonal synchrony increases prosocial behavior in infants. *Developmental Science, 17*, 1003–1011.

Cirelli, L. K., Wan, S. J., Spinelli, C., & Trainor, L. J. (2017). Effects of interpersonal movement synchrony on helping behaviors: Is music necessary? *Music Perception, 34*, 319–326.

Cirelli, L. K., Wan, S. J., & Trainor, L. J. (2016). Social effects of movement synchrony: Increased infant helpfulness only transfer to affiliates of synchronously moving partners. *Infancy, 21*, 807–821.

Corrigall, K. A., Schellenberg, E. G., & Misura, N. M. (2013). Music training, cognition, and personality. *Frontiers in Psychology, 4.* doi:10.3389/fpsyg.2013.00222

Costa-Giomi, E. (2012). Music instruction and children's intellectual development: The educational context of music participation. In R. A. R. MacDonald, G. Kreutz, & L. Mitchell (Eds.), *Music, health & wellbeing* (pp. 339–355). Oxford: Oxford University Press.

Costa-Giomi, E. (2015). The long-term effects of childhood music instruction on intelligence and general cognitive abilities. *Update: Applications of Research in Music Education, 33*, 20–26.

Deary, I. J., Yang, J., Davies, G., Harris, S. E., Tenesa, A., Liewald, D., . . . Visscher, P. M. (2012). Genetic contribution to stability and change in intelligence from childhood to old age. *Nature, 482*, 212–215.

Degé, F., & Schwarzer, G. (2011). The effect of a music program on phonological awareness in preschoolers. *Frontiers in Psychology, 2*, 124. doi:10.3389/fpsyg.2011.00124(2011).

Degé, F., Wehrum, S., Stark, R., & Schwarzer, G. (2011). The influence of two years of school music training in secondary school on visual and auditory memory. *European Journal of Developmental Psychology, 8*, 608–623.

Doidge, N. (2007). *The brain that changes itself.* New York: Viking.

Dumont, E., Syurina, E. V., Feron, F. J. M., & van Hooren, S. (2017). Music interventions and child development: A critical review and further directions. *Frontiers in Psychology, 8.* doi:10.3389/fpsyg.2017.01694

Dunbar, R. I. M. (2012). On the evolutionary function of song and dance. In N. Bannan & S. Mithen (Eds.), *Music, language and human evolution* (pp. 201–214). Oxford: Oxford University Press.

Ericsson, K. A., Krampe, R. T., & Tesch-Römer, C. (1993). The role of deliberate practice in the acquisition of expert performance. *Psychological Review, 100*, 363–406.

Flaugnacco, E., Lopez, L., Terribili, C., Montico, M., Zoia, S., & Schön, D. (2015). Music training increases phonological awareness and reading skills in developmental dyslexia: A randomized control trial. *PLoS One, 10*(9), e0138715. doi:10.1371/journal.pone.0138715

Flaugnacco, E., Lopez, L., Terribili, C., Zoia, S., Buda, S., Tilli, S., . . . Schön, D. (2014). Rhythm perception and production predict reading abilities in developmental dyslexia. *Frontiers in Human Neuroscience, 8*, 392. doi:10.3389/fnhum.2014.00392

Foster, J. L., Harrison, T. L., Hicks, K. L., Draheim, C., Redick, T. S., & Engle, R. W. (2017). Do the effects of working memory training depend on baseline ability level? *Journal of Experimental Psychology: Learning, Memory, and Cognition, 43*, 1677–1689.

François, C., Chobert, J., Besson, M., & Schön, D. (2013). Music training for the development of speech segmentation. *Cerebral Cortex, 23*, 2038–2043.

Goswami, U. (2011). A temporal sampling framework for developmental dyslexia. *Trends in Cognitive Sciences, 15*, 3–10.

Goswami, U., Huss, M., Mead, N., Fosker, T., & Verney, J. P. (2013). Perception of patterns of musical beat distribution in phonological developmental dyslexia: Significant longitudinal relations with word reading and reading comprehension. *Cortex, 49*, 1363–1376.

Gromko, J. E. (2005). The effect of music instruction on phonemic awareness in beginning readers. *Journal of Research in Music Education, 53*, 199–209.

Habibi, A., Cahn, B. R., Damasio, A., & Damasio, H. (2016). Neural correlates of accelerated auditory processing in children engaged in music training. *Developmental Cognitive Neuroscience, 21*, 1–14.

Habibi, A., Damasio, A., Ilari, B., Veiga, R., Joshi, A. A., Leahy, R. M., . . . Damasio, H. (2017). Childhood music training induces change in micro and macroscopic brain structure: Results from a longitudinal study. *Cerebral Cortex.* Advance online publication. doi:10.1093/cercor/bhx286

Habibi, A., Ilari, B., Crimi, K., Metke, M., Kaplan, J. T., Joshi, A. A., . . . Damasio, H. (2014). An equal start: Absence of group differences in cognitive, social, and neural measures prior to music or sports training in children. *Frontiers in Human Neuroscience, 8*. doi:10.3389/fnhum.2014.00690

Hambrick, D. Z., & Tucker-Drob, E. M. (2015). The genetics of music accomplishment: Evidence for gene-environment correlation and interaction. *Psychonomic Bulletin & Review, 22*, 112–120.

Haywood, S., Griggs, J., Lloyd, C., Morris, S., Kiss, Z., & Skipp, A. (2015). *Creative futures: Act, sing, play. Evaluation report and executive summary.* London: Educational Endowment Foundation.

Herholz, S. C., & Zatorre, R. J. (2012). Musical training as a framework for brain plasticity: Behavior, function, and structure. *Neuron, 76*, 486–502.

Herrera, L., Lorenzo, O., Defior, S., Fernandez-Smith, G., & Costa-Giomi, E. (2011). Effects of phonological and musical training on the reading awareness of native and foreign-Spanish-speaking children. *Psychology of Music, 39*, 68–81.

Howe, M. J. A., Davidson, J. W., & Sloboda, J. A. (1998). Innate talents: Reality or myth? *Behavioral & Brain Sciences, 21*, 399–442.

Huss, M., Verney, J. P., Fosker, T., Mead, N., & Goswami, U. (2011). Music, rhythm, rise time perception and developmental dyslexia: Perception of musical meter predicts reading and phonology. *Cortex, 47*, 674–689.

Hyde, K. L., Lerch, J., Norton, A., Forgeard, M., Winner, E., Evans, A. C., & Schlaug, G. (2009). Musical training shapes structural brain development. *Journal of Neuroscience, 29*, 3019–3025.

Ilari, B. S., Keller, P., Damasio, H., & Habibi, A. (2016). The development of musical skills of underprivileged children over the course of 1 year: A study in the context of an El Sistema-inspired program. *Frontiers in Psychology, 7.* doi:10.3389/fpsyg.2016.00062

Jaeggi, S. M., Buschkuehl, M., Jonides, J., & Perrig, W. J. (2008). Improving fluid intelligence with training on working memory. *Proceedings of the National Academy of Sciences of the United States of America, 105,* 6829–6833.

Jaeggi, S. M., Buschkuehl, M., Jonides, J., & Shah, P. (2011). Short- and long-term benefits of cognitive training. *Proceedings of the National Academy of Sciences of the United States of America, 108,* 10081–10086.

Jäncke, L. (2009). The plastic human brain. *Restorative Neurology and Neuroscience, 27,* 521–538. doi:10.3233/RNN-2009-519

Janus, M., Lee, Y., Moreno, S., & Bialystok, E. (2016). Effects of short term music and second language training on executive control. *Journal of Experimental Child Psychology, 144,* 84–97.

Jaschke, A. C., Honing, H., & Scherder, E. J. A. (2018). Longitudinal analysis of music education on executive functions in primary school children. *Frontiers in Neuroscience, 12.* doi:10.3389/fnins.2018.00103

Kaviani, H., Mirbaha, H., Pournaseh, M., & Sagan, O. (2014). Can music lessons increase the performance of preschool children in IQ tests? *Cognitive Processing, 15,* 77–84.

Kirschner, S., & Tomasello, M. (2010). Joint music making promotes prosocial behavior in 4-year-old children. *Evolution & Human Behavior, 31,* 354–364.

Kraus, N., Hornickel, J., Strait, D. L., Slater, J., & Thompson, E. (2014). Engagement in community music classes sparks neuroplasticity and language development in children from disadvantaged backgrounds. *Frontiers in Psychology, 5.* doi:10.3389/fpsyg.2014.01403

Leong, V., & Goswami, U. (2014). Impaired extraction of speech rhythm from temporal modulation patterns in speech in developmental dyslexia. *Frontiers in Human Neuroscience, 8.* doi:10.3389/fnhum.2014.00096

Linnavalli, T., Putkinen, V., Lipsanen, J., Huotilainen, M., & Tervaniemi, M. (2018). Music playschool enhances children's linguistic skills. *Scientific Reports, 8,* 8767. doi:10.1038/s41598-018-27126-5

Love, J. M., Chazan-Cohen, R., Raikes, H., & Brookes-Gunn, J. (2013). What makes a difference: Early head start evaluation findings in a developmental context. *Monographs of the Society for Research in Child Development, 78*(1).

Mackintosh, N. J. (2011). *IQ and human intelligence* (2nd ed.). Oxford: Oxford University Press.

Macnamara, B., Hambrick, D. Z., & Oswald, F. L. (2014). Deliberate practice and performance in music, games, sports, education, and professions: A meta-analysis. *Psychological Science, 25,* 1608–1618.

McClearn, G. E., Johansson, B., Berg, S., Pedersen, N. L., Ahern, F., Petrill, S. A., & Plomin, R. (1997). Substantial genetic influence on cognitive abilities in twins 80 or more years old. *Science, 276*(5318), 1560–1563.

Mehr, S. A., Schachner, A., Katz, R. C., & Spelke, E. S. (2013). Two randomized trials provide no consistent evidence for nonmusical cognitive benefits of brief preschool music enrichment. *PLoS One, 8*(12), e82007. doi:10.1371/journal.pone.0082007

Melby-Lervåg, M., Redick, T. S., & Hulme, C. (2016). Working memory training does not improve performance on measures of intelligence or other measures of "far transfer": Evidence from a meta-analytic review. *Perspectives on Psychological Science, 11,* 512–534.

Mongelli, V., Dehaene, S., Vinckier, F., Peretz, I., Bartolomeo, P., & Cohen, L. (2017). Music and words in the visual cortex: The impact of musical experience. *Cortex, 86*, 260–274.

Moreno, S., Bialystok, E., Barac, R., Schellenberg, E. G., Cepeda, N. J., & Chau, T. (2011a). Short-term music training enhances verbal intelligence and executive function. *Psychological Science, 22*, 1425–1433.

Moreno, S., Friesen, D., & Bialystok, E. (2011b). Effect of music training on promoting preliteracy skills: Preliminary causal evidence. *Music Perception, 29*, 165–172.

Moreno, S., Marques, C., Santos, A., Santos, M., Castro, S. L., & Besson, M. (2009). Musical training influences linguistic abilities in 8-year-old children: More evidence of brain plasticity. *Cerebral Cortex, 19*, 712–723.

Mosing, M. A., Madison, G., Pedersen, N. L., Kuja-Halkola, R., & Ullén, F. (2014). Practice does not make perfect: No causal effect of musical practice on musical ability. *Psychological Science, 25*, 1795–1803.

Mosing, M. A., Madison, G., Pedersen, N. L., & Ullén, F. (2016). Investigating cognitive transfer within the framework of music practice: Genetic pleiotropy rather than causality. *Developmental Science, 19*, 504–512.

Mosing, M. A., Pedersen, N. L., Madison, G., & Ullén, F. (2014). Genetic pleiotropy explains associations between musical auditory discrimination and intelligence. *PLoS One, 9*(11), e113874. doi:10.1371/journal.pone.0113874

Mosing, M. A., & Ullén, F. (2018). Genetic influence on musical specialization: A twin study on choice of instrument and music genre. *Annals of the New York Academy of Sciences, 1423*, 427–434.

Münte, T. F., Altenmüller, E., & Jäncke, L. (2002). The musician's brain as a model of neuroplasticity. *Nature Reviews Neuroscience, 3*, 473–478.

Norton, A., Winner, E., Cronin, K., Overy, K., Lee, D. J., & Schlaug, G. (2005). Are there pre-existing neural, cognitive, or motoric markers for musical ability? *Brain and Cognition, 59*, 124–134.

Patscheke, H., Degé, F., & Schwarzer, G. (2016). The effects of training in music and phonological skills on phonological awareness in 4- to 6-year-old children of immigrant families. *Frontiers in Psychology, 7*. doi:10.3389/fpsyg.2016.01647

Plomin, R., & DeFries, J. C. (1985). *Origins of individual differences in infancy: The Colorado adoption project*. Orlando, FL: Academic Press.

Plomin, R., DeFries, J. C., Knopik, V. S., & Neiderhiser, J. M. (2016). Top 10 replicated findings from behavioral genetics. *Perspectives in Psychological Science, 11*, 3–23.

Plomin, R., & von Stumm, S. (2018). The new genetics of intelligence. *Nature Reviews Genetics, 19*, 148–159.

Portowitz, A., Lichtenstein, O., Egorova, L., & Brand, E. (2009). Underlying mechanisms linking music education and cognitive modifiability. *Research Studies in Music Education, 31*, 107–128.

Power, R. A., & Pluess, M. (2015). Heritability estimates of the big five personality traits based on common genetic variants. *Translational Psychiatry, 5*, e604. doi:10.1038/tp.2015.96

Rabkin, N., & Hedberg, E. C. (2011). *Arts education in America: What the declines mean for arts participation*. Washington, DC: National Endowment for the Arts.

Rauscher, F. H., & Zupan, M. A. (2000). Classroom keyboard instruction improves kindergarten children's spatial-temporal performance: A field experiment. *Early Childhood Research Quarterly, 15*, 215–228.

Roden, I., Grube, D., Bongard, S., & Kreutz, G. (2014). Does music training enhance working memory performance? Findings from a quasi-experimental longitudinal study. *Psychology of Music, 42*, 284–298.

Roden, I., Könen, T., Bongard, S., Frankenberg, E., Friedrich, E. K., & Kreutz, G. (2014). Effects of music training on attention, processing speed and cognitive music abilities—findings from a longitudinal study. *Applied Cognitive Psychology, 28*, 545–557.

Roden, I., Kreutz, G., & Bongard, S. (2012). Effects of a school-based instrumental music program on verbal and visual memory in primary school children: A longitudinal study. *Frontiers in Psychology, 3*. doi:10.3389/fpsyg.2012.00572

Sala, G., & Gobet, F. (2017a). Does far transfer exist? Negative evidence from chess, music, and working memory training. *Current Directions in Psychological Science, 26*, 515–520.

Sala, G., & Gobet, F. (2017b). When the music's over. Does musical skill transfer to children's and young adolescents' cognitive and academic skills? A meta-analysis. *Educational Research Review, 20*, 55–67.

Sala, G., & Gobet, F. (2017c). Working memory training in typically developing children: A meta-analysis of the available evidence. *Developmental Psychology, 53*, 671–685.

Scarr, S., & McCartney. K. (1983). How people make their own environments: A theory of genotype → environmental effects. *Child Development, 54*, 424–435.

Schellenberg, E. G. (2004). Music lessons enhance IQ. *Psychological Science, 15*, 511–514.

Schellenberg, E. G. (2005–2006). Music lessons enhance IQ: A reply to Black (2005) and Steele (2005). *Scientific Review of Mental Health Practice, 4*(2), 10–13.

Schellenberg, E. G. (2016). Music training and nonmusical abilities. In S. Hallam, I. Cross, & M. Thaut (Eds.), *The Oxford handbook of music psychology* (2nd ed., pp. 415–429). Oxford: Oxford University Press.

Schellenberg, E. G. (2018). *Correlation = causation: The case of music training, psychology, and neuroscience*. Manuscript submitted for publication.

Schellenberg, E. G., Corrigall, K. A., Dys, S. P., & Malti, T. (2015). Group music training and children's prosocial skills. *PLoS One, 10*(10), e0141449. doi:10.1371/journal.pone.0141449

Schellenberg, E. G., & Weiss, M. W. (2013). Music and cognitive abilities. In D. Deutsch (Ed.), *The psychology of music* (3rd ed., pp. 499–550). Amsterdam: Elsevier Academic Press.

Schlaug, G. (2001). The brain of musicians: A model for functional and structural adaptation. *Annals of the New York Academy of Sciences, 930*, 281–299.

Schneider, B. A., Avivi-Reich, M., & Mozuraitis, M. (2015). A cautionary note on the use of the analysis of covariance (ANCOVA) in classification designs with and without within-subject factors. *Frontiers in Psychology, 6*. doi:10.3389/fpsyg.2015.00474

Simons, D. J., Boot, W. R., Charness, N., Gathercole, S. E., Chabris, C. F., Hambrick, D. Z., & Stine-Morrow, E. A. L. (2016). Do "brain-training" programs work? *Psychological Science in the Public Interest, 17*, 103–186.

Slater, J., Skoe, E., Strait, D. L., O'Connell, S., Thompson, E., & Kraus, N. (2015). Music training improves speech-in-noise perception: Longitudinal evidence from a community-based music program. *Behavioural Brain Research, 291*, 244–252.

Slater, J., Strait, D. L., Skoe, E., O'Connell, S., Thompson, E., & Kraus, N. (2014). Longitudinal effects of group music instruction on literacy skills in low-income children. *PLoS One, 9*(11), e113383. doi:10.1371/journal.pone.0113383

Soveri, A., Antfolk, J., Karlsson, L., Salo, B., & Laine, M. (2017). Working memory training revisited: A multi-level meta-analysis of n-back training studies. *Psychonomic Bulletin & Review, 24*, 1077–1096.

Strait, D. L., & Kraus, N. (2014). Biological impact of auditory expertise across the life span: Musicians as a model of auditory learning. *Hearing Research, 308,* 109–121.

Swaminathan, S., & Schellenberg, E. G. (2016). Music training. In T. Strobach & J. Karbach (Eds.), *Cognitive training: An overview of features and applications* (pp. 137–144). New York: Springer.

Swaminathan, S., & Schellenberg, E. G. (2018a). Musical competence is predicted by music training, cognitive abilities, and personality. *Scientific Reports.* doi:10.1038/s41598-018-27571-2

Swaminathan, S., & Schellenberg, E. G. (2018b). Music training and cognitive abilities: Associations, causes, and consequences. In M. H. Thaut & D. A. Hodges (Eds.), *The Oxford handbook of music and neuroscience.* Advance online publication. doi:10.1093/oxfordhb/9780198804123.013.26

Swaminathan, S., Schellenberg, E. G., & Khalil, S. (2017). Revisiting the association between music lessons and intelligence: Training effects or music aptitude? *Intelligence, 62,* 119–124.

Swaminathan, S., Schellenberg, E. G., & Venkatesan, K. (2018). Explaining the association between music training and reading in adults. *Journal of Experimental Psychology: Learning, Memory, and Cognition.* Advance online publication. doi:10.1037/xlm0000493

Tarr, B., Launay, J., & Dunbar, R. I. (2014). Music and social bonding: "Self-other" merging and neurohormonal mechanisms. *Frontiers in Psychology, 5.* doi:10.3389/fpsyg.2014.01096

Thompson, W. F., Schellenberg, E. G., & Husain, G. (2004). Decoding speech prosody: Do music lessons help? *Emotion, 4,* 46–64.

Thomson, J. M., Leong, V., & Goswami, U. (2013). Auditory processing interventions and developmental dyslexia: A comparison of phonemic and rhythmic approaches. *Reading and Writing, 26,* 139–161.

Thorndike, E. L., & Woodworth, R. S. (1901). The influence of improvement in one mental function upon the efficiency of other functions (I). *Psychological Review, 8,* 247–261.

Tierney, A. T., Krizman, J., & Kraus, N. (2015). Music training alters the course of adolescent auditory development. *Proceedings of the National Academy of Sciences of the United States of America, 112,* 10062–10067.

Tierney, A., Krizman, J., Skoe, E., Johnston, K., & Kraus, N. (2013). High school music classes enhance the neural processing of speech. *Frontiers in Psychology, 4,* 855. doi:10.3389/fpsyg.2013.00855

Ullén, F., Hambrick, D. Z., & Mosing, M. A. (2016). Rethinking expertise: A multifactorial gene-environment interaction model of expert performance. *Psychological Bulletin, 142,* 426–446.

Ullén, F., Mosing, M. A., Holm, L., Eriksson, H., & Madison, G. (2014). Psychometric properties and heritability of a new online test for musicality, the Swedish musical discrimination test. *Personality and Individual Differences, 63,* 87–93.

U.S. Department of Health and Human Services & Administration for Children and Families. (2010). *Head start impact study: Final report.* Washington, DC. Retrieved from www.acf.hhs.gov/opre/resource/head-start-impact-study-final-report-executive-summary

Vernon, P. A., Martin, R. A., Schermer, J. A., & Mackie, A. (2008). A behavioral genetic investigation of humor styles and their correlations with the big-5 personality dimensions. *Personality and Individual Differences, 44,* 1116–1125.

Wai, J., Worrell, F. C., & Chabris, C. F. (2017). The consistent influence of general cognitive ability in college, career, and lifetime achievement. In K. L. McClarty, K. D. Mattern, & M. N. Gaertner (Eds.), *Preparing students for college and careers: Theory, measurement, and educational practice* (pp. 46–56). New York: Routledge.

Yang, H., Ma, W., Gong, D., Hu, J., & Yao, D. (2014). A longitudinal study on children's music training experience and academic development. *Scientific Reports, 4.* doi:10.1038/srep05854

Section 5

Into the Classroom

17 Towards a Science of Teaching and Learning for Teacher Education

Paul Howard-Jones, Konstantina Ioannou, Ruth Bailey, Jayne Prior, Tim Jay and Shu Yau

Teachers are a significant factor contributing to individual differences in the educational achievement, school behaviour and well-being of their students (Blazar & Kraft, 2017; Gershenson, 2016; Vanwynsberghe, Vanlaar, Van Damme, & De Fraine, 2017). It appears reasonable to suggest that a scientific understanding of the processes underlying teaching and learning might inform teachers' practice, and so positively influence outcomes in these areas. Here we consider the potential for teacher effectiveness to be improved by an understanding of learning that is informed by cognitive neuroscience. We argue that the identification and communication of concepts from cognitive neuroscience should focus on providing an insightful understanding of the processes underlying "everyday" effective instruction in the classroom, and by way of exemplification, we present and critique a selection of such concepts that we have introduced into the Post-Graduate Certificate in Education (PGCE) at the University of Bristol.

Quality of Teaching Is Important

The relation between teaching quality and learner outcome has been confirmed by efforts in the US and elsewhere to measure the value that an individual teacher adds to their students' achievement. For example, a teacher in the top 16% of effectiveness, compared with an average teacher, has been estimated to produce students whose level of achievement is, on average, somewhere between 0.2 and 0.3 standard deviations higher by the end of the school year (Hanushek, 2011). Such data confirm a long-held view amongst policy makers, parents and educators that teacher quality is a very important determinant of individual differences in educational outcome (Hanushek, 2011). Although the data converge clearly on the importance of teacher quality, the research is less clear as to what characteristics comprise a quality teacher (Coe, Aloisi, Higgins, & Major, 2014).

The Value of a Teacher Knowing How Learning Works Rather Than Just What Works

Good teaching appears to be more than just the arbitrary application of recommended practices. Teachers who are effective in helping their students to learn tend to employ practices that have, in general terms, been identified by educational researchers as effective. However, attempts to identify effective teaching using a checklist of desirable observed behaviours have low predictive power (Brown, Roediger III, & McDaniel, 2014; Strong, Gargani, & Hacifazlioglu, 2011). Therefore, such practices may be important or even necessary, but they are not sufficient in themselves to assure the best possible levels of learning will be achieved. This may be because teachers require an understanding of why, when and how each practice can be effective, and exactly what it means to use them in a way that is optimal for their students (Coe et al., 2014). The possession of a set of beliefs justifying the use of different approaches has been identified as one factor that helps differentiate effective teachers (Askew, Brown, Rhodes, Wiliam, & Johnson, 1997). Pre-service teachers bring with them many beliefs in relation to education and teaching, including beliefs about how learning occurs, that are subject to change during their training (Bramald, Hardman, & Leat, 1995; Buitink, 2009). The importance of attending to teachers' ideas about learning has also been highlighted by Timperley, Wilson, Barrar, and Fung (2007) who, in a review of professional development programmes, found that those programmes which benefited learners generally included engagement with teachers' existing theories, values and beliefs. This evidence resonates with the common-sense argument that a teacher must constantly orchestrate their skills and knowledge when attending to the very specific individuals and contexts they encounter. In adapting their teaching to the learner and the context, a teacher must apply some theory about their students' mental processes and consider how they can influence these processes and so scaffold learning (Mevorach & Strauss, 2012). On this basis, one might also expect an association between beliefs about learning and educational practice. This was borne out in a large OECD survey, where "constructivist" beliefs about how learning occurs were correlated with student-oriented practices and/or enhanced learning activities in 20 of the 23 countries surveyed (OECD, 2009).

The suggestion follows, therefore, that an important way in which the sciences of mind and brain can enrich education is to inform the processes by which teachers critically reflect upon and develop an understanding of their own practice. Such a notion is aligned with a growing awareness of the many unscientific beliefs held by teachers that are linked to poor practice (Howard-Jones, 2014), and calls for a scientific understanding of learning to become part of initial teacher education and teacher professional development (e.g., Ansari & Coch, 2006; Dehaene, 2009; Royal Society, 2011).

An Education-first Approach to Identifying Core Concepts From the Science of Learning

Addressing the aim of helping teachers gain insight into their everyday work requires selection of core scientific concepts based on their relation to established educational practices. This leads naturally to a strongly education-centred approach to developing a curriculum. This contrasts with some previous attempts to incorporate neuroscience into teacher development. For example, "Brain-U" was a 3-year series of intensive summer teacher professional development workshops combining inquiry-based pedagogy with delivery of neuroscience. These workshops succeeded in improving teachers' knowledge of neuroscience and implementation of student-centred reform and inquiry-based pedagogy, but did not aim to provide teachers with an understanding of their classroom practice informed by neuroscience (Dubinsky, 2010; Dubinsky, Roehrig, & Varma, 2013; Roehrig, Michlin, Schmitt, MacNabb, & Dubinsky, 2012). In developing core concepts for these workshops, the authors argue that "Tailoring a message specifically for teachers requires an approach that emphasizes the big ideas in neuroscience" (Dubinsky, 2010). Here, however, we take a different approach. We believe that the tailoring of messages should emphasise ideas from neuroscience that are considered (by educators) as useful for understanding their "everyday" teaching and learning in the classroom. In other words, it should be about the "big" priorities and needs of the learners in the classroom—not necessarily the big ideas in neuroscience. Such an approach is closer to a previous small-scale attempt to include neuroscience in teacher training focused on creativity in drama education. This employed exploratory workshops with teacher educators and student teachers to identify concepts useful for deepening reflection on practice (Howard-Jones, 2009; Howard-Jones, Winfield, & Crimmins, 2008, 2009).

Initial Concerns When Devising Core Concepts to Support Classroom Practice

The core concepts from the science of learning, and the ways in which these should be presented, were identified and developed through discussion between the authors and lecturers on the PGCE (secondary education) team at the School of Education, University of Bristol, UK. From the outset, several concerns impacted on this process in addition to the relevance of concepts to everyday teaching practice. These included the need for parsimony and to avoid any sense that teaching approaches were being prescribed that would be suitable for all classes and students.

It also seemed important to anticipate misconceptions wherever possible and, as far we were able, to "inoculate" student teachers against these. It was never assumed that introducing good science would necessarily and automatically lead to improved classroom practice, or even improved ideas about classroom practice. The dangers of such assumptions are highlighted by the study of common neuromyths (Howard-Jones, 2014). In the absence of a broader scientific understanding of how learning proceeds, an initial scientific fact can develop into something fanciful and deleterious to effective practice, often guided more by wishful thinking than by evidence from science or education. For example, teachers cannot be expected to know that the right and left hemispheres are joined by the corpus callosum, or how the cortical activity recruited by creativity and scientific reasoning is distributed across hemispheres. Without due attention to such facts, introducing the idea of lateralisation (e.g., discussing how language is lateralised to the left hemisphere) might feasibly encourage left-brain/right-brain ideas that are associated with poor practice in the classroom.

In terms of "future-proofing", we sought concepts with explanatory value across curriculum areas but which also offered a foundation for further studies. These further studies might, for example, focus on understanding that is emerging around particular curriculum content such as mathematics and reading, or be focused more on infant development and early years education. In these respects, we ensured our introduction included concepts such as attention and control of attention, memory and working memory, the reward system, fear responding, plasticity and individual differences.

It also seemed helpful to consider how student teachers might align concepts from cognitive neuroscience with the well-established learning theories they would encounter during training. The Vygotskian tradition is particularly influential amongst educational researchers and the ideas of Vygotsky underlie much educational thinking. Vygotsky discussed learning as a process of knowledge construction and promoted the idea that old knowledge provides a critical role in the processes by which new knowledge is acquired. This concept of learning is not at odds with modern scientific understanding of the learning process and, indeed, some have considered the possibility of synthesising neuroscientific and Vygotskian frameworks (Ghassemzadeh, Posner, & Rothbart, 2013). This reflection on current and traditional ideas about learning was the beginning of a discussion that would focus on how best to organise scientific insights in a way that would support their mapping to classroom practice.

Organising Scientific Insights Into Learning Processes Into Three Categories

The traditional learning model of Vygotsky is concerned chiefly with the processes underlying those critical moments when new knowledge is understood for the first time. However, the concerns of educators now include those parts of the learning experience that precede and follow these moments of construction. Over recent decades, there has been increasing interest in the pedagogic improvement of children's motivation and readiness to learn, as well as classroom practices that lead to the retention and mastery of learning following initial knowledge acquisition. Such considerations suggested to us three categories of insight that were particularly meaningful for classroom learning. We organised insights into those relevant to processes underlying 1) engagement with learning, 2) the building of new knowledge and understanding and 3) the consolidation of learning. It is proposed here that these three categories are helpful in organising the scientific concepts in a way that supports their interrelation with educational practice.

That said, there is no 3-stage model of pedagogy being suggested here and we emphasise to our student teachers that the categories "engage, build, consolidate" should not be used to conveniently partition a lesson. Such partitioning would over-simplify the learning experiences encountered in a classroom. In everyday teaching and learning, all three types of process might occur simultaneously, or at least in such quick succession that attempting a one-to-one mapping between category and classroom activity is unhelpful. For example, consider the situation in which a teacher uses a game to introduce a new topic, using examples that link the new topic to what was covered in yesterday's learning. Based on a scientific understanding of emotional processing, the teacher has developed a game that encourages the children to **engage** and the game-like context might reasonably reduce the effects of anxiety on their mental abilities. Neuroscience has also revealed how those regions required for making links to prior knowledge are still developing in children. This prompts the teacher to verbally scaffold the children's efforts to **build** their knowledge and consciously link the new learning content to old. Neuroscience has also shown how knowledge becomes more variably represented in the brain after questioning—making it more accessible and useful. In response to this, the teacher has designed the questions to encourage the students to apply their old knowledge in different ways and in different contexts. This helps to **consolidate** their learning. So, this short lesson introduction includes all three categories of learning process.

"Engage, build, consolidate" are broad headings that order and present the scientific concepts and findings in a way that is broadly aligned with recognisable aspects of classroom practice. They are intended to encourage educators' reflection on processes beyond the instance of initial knowledge construction, to include readiness for learning and the need to revisit it. By aiding the interrelation of classroom learning behaviour and the putative underlying processes, these headings help initiate and support an analysis beyond whether learning is occurring or not, to include how and why this may be the case. Under each of these headings that follow, we outline some of the concepts we are choosing to introduce to our student teachers.

Engagement

In education, engagement is associated with emotions (interest and enthusiasm, lack of anger, anxiety, and boredom) and effortful thinking processes (such as use of active self-regulation and more sophisticated learning strategies). In the classroom, engagement may also be observed in behaviours that include on-task attention and persistence in completing a task. The term "engagement" can be applied very broadly in education, and can mean simply a general involvement with school (Hidi, Renninger, & Krapp, 2004; Schiefele, 2001). Here, however, it is used more narrowly to refer to the state of being "caught and held" in a learning opportunity (Skinner, Kindermann, & Furrer, 2009).

There is a large range of strategies used routinely by teachers to engage their students in this sense (Guilloteaux & Dornyei, 2008). Very few of these strategies have themselves been the subject of focused scientific investigation in terms of their underlying neurocognitive processes. However, some have included types of stimuli found in studies investigating "approach motivation" in the brain. For example, praise is a social reward commonly used as an effective means to reinforce classroom behaviours conducive to learning (Becker, Madsen, Arnold, & Thomas, 1967; Dufrene, Lestremau, & Zoder-Martell, 2014; Reinke, Lewis-Palmer, & Merrell, 2008; Sutherland, Wehby, & Copeland, 2000). Social reward appears to stimulate some similar regions of the brain's reward system to those activated by physical/concrete rewards such as when we receive money (Izuma, Saito, & Sadato, 2008; Knutson, Adams, Fong, & Hommer, 2001), anticipate food (Farooqi et al., 2007) or play video games (Koepp et al., 1998). Educational learning, in conditions that favour engagement through the offering of points, can also stimulate these regions (Howard-Jones, Jay, Mason, & Jones, 2016).

Other strategies thought to improve engagement in the classroom include the use of novelty, the stimulation of curiosity and working with peers. In a recent study, novelty has been shown to orient our attention, releasing neuromodulators in the brain that can increase engagement and promote learning (Schomaker & Meeter, 2015). Curiosity, which can be aroused by novelty, tends to generate a similar neural response (Min Jeong et al., 2009). Another way that teachers can engage students using "social reward" is to make the process of education more social and "personable" or emotionally relevant, in order to harness our natural social tendencies (Lieberman, 2012). Encouraging peer collaboration can help create a more social environment for learning, and this involves the sharing of attention. When self-initiated, shared attention also involves activation of reward-related brain areas (Schilbach et al., 2010), attesting to the desirable nature of successfully prompting someone else to share attention with you. This may help explain how asking students to communicate their ideas in different ways to each other can engage their interest in their learning, whether through addressing the class or through helping one another in pairs to master skills. However, while we can assume the functioning of the reward system is key to understanding many classroom engagement strategies, there have been relatively few studies of its role in educational learning. The challenges to be addressed in providing such data include balancing ecological validity with experimental control, and the limits of current neurocomputational models of the reward system. In the future, it seems likely that addressing these challenges will lead to a more complete understanding of how classroom learning is impacted by the type and scheduling of reward, and the likely timescales of the associated effects (Howard-Jones & Jay, 2016). Already, however, it seems reasonable that a neurobiological model of educational engagement should refer to the response of the brain to reward and the reward-related modulation of networks for attention and memory.

In contrast to features of an educational experience that encourage an "approach" response, anxiety can produce avoidance of a topic and so prevent engagement. For example, avoidance is a well-established characteristic of maths anxiety. Maths-anxious students generate additional activity in regions of their amygdala associated with negative emotions and fearfulness (Young, Wu, & Menon, 2012). When students become anxious, studies have shown they become less able to sustain activity in frontal regions of the brain, suggesting less control over their working memory[1] and a struggle to maintain their attentional focus. In particular, students who are "rejection sensitive" can experience a strong and automatic anxiety response that disrupts learning (Mangels, Hoxha, Lane, Jarvis, & Downey, 2017). In their event-related potential study, Mangels et al. found that the attentional orienting network in the brains of women, but not men, was disrupted by feedback from perceived authority figures (males), which reduced recovery from mistakes and engagement with further learning opportunities.[2]

Unduly harsh or inconsistent approaches to maintaining order also have the potential to create anxiety. In contrast, effective teachers tend to use management techniques that positively maintain cooperation and engagement in interesting activities. Sometimes the source of the anxiety may be the teacher's own emotions. Observing an emotion in someone else activates some of the same brain regions involved with experiencing those emotions (Gallese, 2003; Gallese, Eagle, & Migone, 2007; Wicker et al., 2003). These unconscious workings of our brains help explain how easily negative emotions, such as anxiety about mathematics, can be transmitted from teacher to student (Beilock, Gunderson, Ramirez, & Levine, 2010), and how positive teacher attitudes can become linked to higher student achievement (Ker, 2016). This emphasises the importance of a teacher being able to present concepts and knowledge with confidence and enthusiasm, while considering individual differences when providing feedback on student work.

Emotion is distributed across the brain and an individual emotion should not be conceptualised as located in just one region. Nevertheless, whether it is the desire to approach a learning opportunity or to avoid it, the workings of our sub-cortical regions such as those involved with the processing of reward and fear, have a major impact on our readiness to learn. When discussing the concept of engagement with student teachers, we have been referring to the two-way connectivity between sub-cortical structures and those frontal regions that support working memory and attention. We indicate this bidirectional influence with a two-headed arrow linking frontal cortical regions to subcortical structures (see Figure 17.1).

While much of the emotional processing that impacts on engagement may be largely unconscious, the building of new knowledge is always likely to involve a significant degree of conscious, effortful processing of internal and/ or external information. Also under the heading of engagement, we have considered a scientific understanding of ideas such as "grit" and so-called "growth mindset", including how the latter can be prompted by interventions that

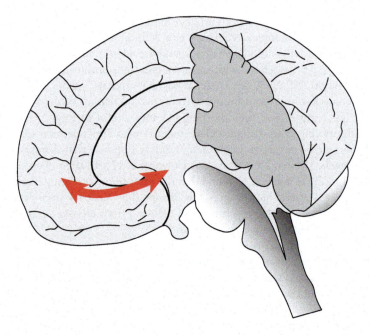

Figure 17.1 Schematic Representation of Processes of Engagement. Engagement with a learning opportunity can rely on an interaction between subcortical limbic and mesolimbic structures (which are important for processing emotion) and frontal networks (which are involved with attention and working memory).

emphasise brain plasticity. Student resilience may benefit from both teachers and students understanding their important role in constructing the brain's functionality, connectivity and structure. Promoting such understanding has been revealed as potentially helpful for nudging students towards an incremental theory of intelligence and for improving their self-concept and academic achievement (Blackwell, Trzesniewski, & Dweck, 2007; Paunesku et al., 2015).

Building of Knowledge

Once a student is engaged with a learning opportunity, which might include an explanation or other type of stimulus provided by the teacher, a channel of curriculum-relevant communication may open that can lead to learning—although much depends on the quality of this communication. Effective teachers communicate clearly and concisely, with little unnecessary information. Consideration of how to use the different senses when communicating is important here. There is some evidence that redundant multisensory information can support learning amongst the youngest of primary school children

(Kirkham, Rea, Osborne, White, & Mareschal, 2019), but generally there appears little evidence for the effectiveness of teaching to a student's preferred modality or for the use of all modalities indiscriminately. Instead, it is the use of modalities to represent the same concept in different ways (e.g., auditorily and visually) that that can help students gain understanding of that concept, when they are encouraged and supported to make links between these representations (Mayer & Anderson, 1991). On the other hand, attempts to present information in a multisensory way can sometimes also go wrong too. Reading text and listening to speech might be thought of as essentially visual and auditory forms of communication, but reading employs much of the circuitry we use for understanding speech (Buchweitz, Mason, Tomitch, & Just, 2009). This means that presenting verbal explanations alongside a lot of text (e.g., on a Powerpoint slide) is similar to asking the learner to process two explanations at the same time—making it difficult to understand either (Horvath, 2014). Issues of communication also have relevance for engagement. If the communication is not effective, this increases the likelihood that students will disengage from a learning opportunity. More subtly, when teachers communicate verbally to their classes, they may communicate information about the concepts and their own emotional responses. The processes by which such information can be unconsciously transmitted and received have been studied in terms of brain function and the recruitment of the so-called mirror neuron system. We activate particular brain regions when we make a gesture but, surprisingly perhaps, this activates some of the same regions in the brain of anyone who observes us (Filimon, Nelson, Hagler, & Sereno, 2007; Rizzolatti & Craighero, 2004). This so-called Mirror Neuron System is thought to help learning through imitation and may also help transmit attitudes and emotional responses. Observing an emotion in someone else (e.g., through their expression) activates brain mechanisms involved with experiencing similar emotions (Gallese, 2003; Gallese et al., 2007; Wicker et al., 2003). Such unconscious workings of our brains can, therefore, help explain how easily negative emotions, such as anxiety about mathematics, can be transmitted from teacher to student (Beilock et al., 2010) and how positive teacher attitudes can become linked to higher student achievement (e.g., Ker, 2016). Rather than an innate system of dedicated neurons, the mirror neuron system is likely acquired early in our development through simple associative learning processes (Catmur et al., 2008). Nevertheless, the early acquisition of this system emphasises the potential importance of teachers feeling confident and enthusiastic about the content they teach.

Although the incoming information may be accurately received by the student, its future usefulness will also depend on how it connects to what is already known. Studies suggest the medial part of the prefrontal cortex (PFC) is involved in detecting fit or congruency between new information and prior knowledge (van Kesteren, Ruiter, Fernandez, & Henson, 2012). Where the fit is good, this part of the brain helps us use the information to generalise existing schemas,[3] directly connecting to representations of prior knowledge already stored elsewhere in the cortex. Where the fit with potentially relevant schemas is less good, this lack of fit with prior knowledge may initiate the forming of new connections between concepts, resulting in the making of new memories with the aid of the hippocampus. Learning is jeopardised when this comparing of new with old fails to occur—e.g., when no relevant schema can be found that are either congruent or clearly incongruent with the new. In this case, neither generalisation nor new memory formation is likely to occur, leading to poor memory for the new information (Brod, Lindenberger, Werkle-Bergner, & Shing, 2015). So, if some associated prior knowledge is not activated—irrespective of whether this conflicts with, or is aligned with the new information—the likelihood is that this new information will just get lost. In schoolchildren, prefrontal regions are known to be relatively immature (Brod, Werkle-Bergner, & Shing, 2013), and this may help explain the difficulties of younger children in making use of prior knowledge even when they possess it. It can be important, therefore, that children are prompted to consciously re-activate appropriate prior knowledge (e.g., through question-and-answer or other revision strategies) before new information is presented, and that they are encouraged to make connections between the new information and their existing knowledge. Differentiation may be helpful here, although according to developmental status rather than age, due to individual differences in the protracted development of the PFC (Shing & Brod, 2016).

Learning how to apply the new information will also require transforming, organizing, or elaborating the new input alongside what is already known. These conscious effortful processes that characterise so much of educational learning activate the so-called "working memory" network in the brain. In particular, the PFC has been implicated in several effortful and conscious processes that can be critical for first applying new information pertinent to a curriculum, including controlling attention, selecting strategies, and manipulating information in working memory (Kane & Engle, 2002). The critical involvement of working memory networks in the building of knowledge and understanding led us to represent these processes schematically by indicating activity in the PFC (see Figure 17.2).

Consolidation of Learning

The term "consolidation" in education is applied broadly to indicate the reinforcement of learning, usually through repeated revision, application and active processing of the content. In scientific reports, "consolidation" is defined more narrowly and refers to the progressive post-acquisition stabilization of long-term memory (Dudai, 2004). However, in both disciplines, the usage of the term acknowledges that new learning can be vulnerable and requires further processing to enable it to become more permanent and durable.

The shift towards greater permanency in accessing and applying new knowledge can be accompanied by greater processing speed, a decrease in the conscious effort required and greater automaticity (Tham, Lindsay, & Gaskell,

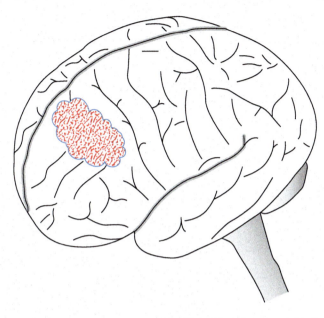

Figure 17.2 Schematic Representation of Building Knowledge and Understanding. Building new knowledge and understanding requires effortful conscious processing and activation of a working memory network that includes prefrontal regions of the cortex.

2015). Accordingly, there can be a decrease in the type of PFC activity associated with the working memory network. Practice and rehearsal of the new knowledge can help consolidate it, and the associated neural changes have been neatly illustrated in a study of adults practising new complex mathematical routines (Delazer et al., 2003). After a week of practising 25 minutes a day, activity when carrying out the routines had shifted away from working memory regions (in the front of the brain) to more posterior regions that have been identified in other studies with more automatic unconscious processing, including the angular gyrus (a region that is not domain specific in its involvement with automatic processing of information (Gonzalez-Garrido, Barrios, Gomez-Velazquez, & Zarabozo-Hurtado, 2017; Simon, Mangin, Cohen, Le Bihan, & Dehaene, 2002; Stanescu-Cosson et al., 2000)), and the inferior temporal gyrus and cerebellum (regions that can be activated by rapid forms of processing (Lesage, Nailer, & Miall, 2016; Menon, Rivera, White, Glover, & Reiss, 2000; Zago et al., 2001)). This led us to represent this category of processes as a shift away from PFC activity towards activity in other regions of the brain (see Figure 17.3).

Carrying out a task that requires you to process the fuller meaning of new knowledge in different contexts is a double bonus. It can not only help you

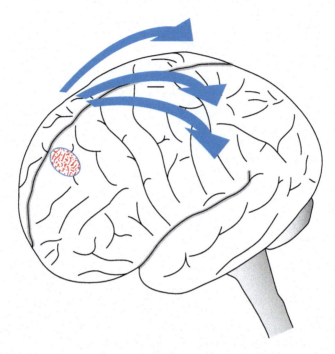

Figure 17.3 Schematic Representation of the Consolidation of Learning. Consolidation of knowledge and understanding results in a shift in activation away from frontal regions—freeing up working memory for more learning.

understand the knowledge better but will also help you remember it longer (Craik, 2002; Craik & Lockhart, 1972). Testing[4] is often used only to evaluate student knowledge but it is an effective way of ensuring this deeper processing occurs and for accelerating the rate at which learning becomes consolidated. Being tested on material makes it more likely to be remembered in the final test, and more so than simply rereading the material (McDaniel, Roediger, & McDermott, 2007). There is also evidence that testing slows the rate of forgetting in the longer term (Roediger & Karpicke, 2006). It works well for learning a diverse range of topics, over a wide range of education levels and for many different age groups (Campbell & Mayer, 2009; Johnson & Mayer, 2009; Karpicke & Blunt, 2011; McDaniel, Agarwal, Huelser, McDermott, & Roediger, 2011; Rohrer & Pashler, 2010). All of this points towards the need to provide engaging opportunities for students to test their knowledge, but in low-risk tasks that are free of anxiety (unlike exams or formal assessments). Recent neuroimaging research suggests that repeatedly retrieving information causes it to become represented in the brain in different ways—essentially connecting it with different meanings and making it easier to retrieve in the future (Wirebring et al., 2015).

Research has revealed that sleep also plays an important role in making memories more permanent. Indeed, sleep is so fundamental to learning, that it has been described as "the price we pay for brain plasticity" (Tononi & Cirelli, 2014). While we are awake, memories of what happens during the day are first encoded into representations in the hippocampus but, during sleep, these fresh representations are then replayed and reorganised as longer lasting memories stored in our cerebral cortex. This reactivation of fresh memories is thought to happen during deep sleep, when the brain produces slow waves (less than one per second) of synchronised electrical brain activity. The consolidation provided by slow-wave sleep can improve memory of the context, but it also helps generalise and extract the gist of the memory. In this way, sleep helps us store and later recall the memory in a form that is more ready to be used in new situations, with the unhelpful detail edited out. These processes have been explored in human neuroimaging studies (see Stickgold, 2005 for a review; also Marshall & Born, 2007). One of these revealed how, during REM sleep, the brain reproduced neural traces that were similar to those experienced in preceding hours of wakefulness, where participants were learning a task (Maquet et al., 2000).

The Cognitive Neuroscience of Effective Instruction

The aforementioned concepts were co-selected through discussion amongst the co-authors, based on their scientific validity and educational relevance. In terms of educational relevance, they offer insight into some familiar classroom practices whose general effectiveness has been established. Here are three examples to illustrate this. In each case, key considerations are whether (1) the practice can be explained with reference to the identified scientific concepts and (2) whether the concepts might potentially contribute to effective implementation of the practice. It is not suggested here that the science can provide a prescription for successful implementation. Rather, its potential benefit is in supporting adaptation of the practice to a specific context, through prompting critical and scientific reflection on why the practice may or may not work within this context and prompting an informed revision of approach as appropriate. Examples are drawn from two issues of the IAE-IBE Educational Practices Series, where practices are often referred to as "principles" (Pekrun, 2014; Rosenshine, 2010). These concepts are general in respect of their potential relevance to the school curriculum, (i.e., they were not tied to specific topics such as literacy or numeracy but could be considered relevant to any subject area).

Example 1 Classroom Instruction and Teacher Emotions

The seventh principle provided in IAE-IBE's "Emotion and Learning" in the Educational Practices Series (Pekrun, 2014) is "Provide high-quality lessons and make use of the positive emotions you experience as a teacher." This is justified on the basis that the "motivational quality of instruction influences the

perceived value of learning, thereby promoting enjoyment and reducing boredom" (p. 20). In respect of teacher emotions, the report advises that "teachers should take care to show the positive emotions they feel about teaching
and the subject matter, and make sure that they share positive emotions and
enthusiasm with their students" (p. 21).

Scientific insights into processes whereby we communicate emotion offer
a slightly different explanatory emphasis that has implications for practice.
They suggest the likely transmission of the teacher's genuine emotion irrespective of their careful effort. This highlights the need for the teacher to
maintain an active interest in the topics they teach, to make communication
of genuine competence and enthusiasm more likely. In terms of modelling,
this is more suggestive of "Think/feel as I think/feel" than simply "do as I do".

Example 2 Guide Student Practice

The fifth principle of instruction provided in IAE-IBE's "Principles of instruction" in the Educational Practices Series (Rosenshine, 2010) is "Successful
teachers spent more time guiding the students' practice of new material". The
IAE-IBE review points out that more successful teachers check for student
understanding, offer additional explanations and examples and provide sufficient instruction for students to learn to practice independently without difficulty. Implicit here is the concept of building knowledge, and the importance
of prior knowledge in informing the guidance provided by teachers. This can
be understood in terms of the difficulties children have in making use of prior
knowledge, which recruits regions of the PFC that are still developing. This
understanding emphasises the need to consider individual progress and differences in the rate of progress, and that, accordingly, different students will
require scaffolding to different degrees.

Example 3 Daily Review

The first principle of instruction provided in IAE-IBE's "Principles of instruction" in the Educational Practices Series (Rosenshine, 2010) is "Daily review
can strengthen previous learning and can lead to fluent recall". It is pointed
out that the most effective teachers understand the importance of practice and
begin their lessons with a five- to eight-minute review of previously covered
material. The report explains that the practice helps us recall concepts and
procedures effortlessly and automatically, freeing up our working memory. This
echoes our discussion in the previous section on consolidation, but this discussion also extended the explanation to consider how expressing knowledge in
new forms helps it become stored in different ways—making it easier to recall
and apply it. This draws attention to the likely value of using novel contexts
and examples when encouraging the class to rehearse their new knowledge.
The scientific insights regarding engagement and building of knowledge may
also help a teacher to implement daily review more effectively. Understanding

of the role of prior knowledge in constructing new understanding can prompt a teacher to pay particular attention to students' demonstration of that knowledge soon be built upon, which can inform the scaffolding the teacher aims to provide. An understanding of engagement may be helpful in considering the best environment for motivating students and diminishing anxiety during a daily review. Finally, the consolidating effects of sleep can provide insight when comparing outcomes of a morning review of yesterday's learning compared with an end-of-day review of today's learning.

Mapping the Extent to Which Science Concepts Can Underpin Teaching Principles

A mapping exercise was undertaken to evaluate more systematically the extent to which the identified scientific concepts were relevant and potentially insightful for implementation of the full set of teaching principles identified in Rosenshine (2010) and Pekrun (2014). Science concepts were mapped to each of the 10 principles identified in "Principles of Instruction" and "Emotions and Learning". A scientific concept was considered to have relation to the principle when it provided insight into how/why the principle works and/ or might be implemented (see Table 17.1). This mapping was not carried out in order to identify potentially unscientific teaching practices. As discussed in Rosenshine (2010) and Pekrun (2014), these practices have already established their potential educational effectiveness through classroom-based research. Instead, the intention was to evaluate the effectiveness of the scientific concepts outlined earlier in providing insight into underlying processes.

The mapping in Table 17.1 was based on discussion amongst the authors regarding the extent and nature of the relevance of each concept to each principle. A mapping was made when a scientific concept provided educational insight. That does not mean that *all* aspects of the principles were necessarily explained by the scientific concepts identified. Inevitably, such judgements also involve some interpretation, and we accept an element of subjectivity here. We would encourage scientists and educators from other institutions to carry out this exercise as a means to initiate dialogue across disciplines and identify concepts most relevant to their own classroom contexts. Such discussions may well produce mappings that differ in some respects from each other.

The overall outcome of the mapping appears encouraging for efforts to build dialogue between education and the sciences of mind and brain. We found that all the core scientific concepts and all principles could be mapped. This supports the basic thrust of arguments that the underlying science can deepen insight into everyday teaching practice. However, the mapping also identified some weaknesses in the interrelation across the science and the educational principles, which may also point the way towards some valuable avenues for future interdisciplinary enterprise. For example, Principle 4 in "Principles of Instruction" was "Provide models". Discussion of the principle in the IAE-IBE text refers to guiding the student and encouraging independent practice.

Table 17.1 Mapping of Core Scientific Concepts (Identified in Main Text) to Teaching Principles (as Identified in Pekrun, 2014; Rosenshine, 2010)

Principles of instruction (Rosenshine, 2010):
1. Daily review
2. Present new material in small steps
3. Ask questions
4. Provide models
5. Guide student practice
6. Check for student understanding
7. Obtain a high success rate
8. Provide scaffolds for difficult tasks
9. Independent practice
10. Weekly and monthly review

Principles for Emotion and Learning (Pekrun, 2014):
1. Understanding emotions
2. Individual and cultural differences
3. Positive emotions and learning
4. Negative emotions and learning
5. Self-confidence, task values and emotions
6. Emotion regulation
7. Classroom instruction and teacher emotions
8. Goal structures and achievement standards
9. Test-taking and feedback
10. Families, peers and school reform

Scientific concepts explaining underlying processes:

Group	Concept	R1	R2	R3	R4	R5	R6	R7	R8	R9	R10	P1	P2	P3	P4	P5	P6	P7	P8	P9	P10
ENGAGE	Individual differences in engagement							X				X	X	X	X	X	X		X	X	X
ENGAGE	Approach response		X		X	X		X				X	X	X	X	X	X	X	X	X	X
ENGAGE	Fearfulness and anxiety				X	X		X	X			X		X	X	X	X	X	X	X	X
ENGAGE	Understanding plasticity																				
BUILD	Prior knowledge	X	X	X			X				X										
BUILD	Connection-making brain development	X	X	X	X	X															
BUILD	Multimodal/multisensory representation					X			X												
CONSOLIDATE	Unconscious communication, MNS													X	X			X			X
CONSOLIDATE	Practice, working memory, automatisation	X		X			X		X	X	X										
CONSOLIDATE	Variable representation of knowledge in brain	X								X	X										
CONSOLIDATE	Sleep	X								X	X										

These two ideas could be supported by the scientific principles identified, but we had difficulty in identifying a scientific basis for understanding the underlying processes involved with some forms of modelling (such as worked examples) despite clear evidence for their effectiveness (Bentley & Yates, 2017; van Gog & Kester, 2012; van Loon-Hillen, van Gog, & Brand-Gruwel, 2012). The type of mapping exercise carried here may, therefore, be useful in exposing areas where further scientific research might reveal some scientifically interesting and educationally valuable insight.

Critique of Scientific Concepts

In the future, we hope that every teacher will embark on a journey of reflection on their classroom practice in terms of the brain, as might be expressed by a teacher training curriculum that includes in-depth scientific understanding of learning and its detailed relation to classroom practice. The problem we have focused on here is how to start such a journey. What should be the first concepts that a teacher should encounter about the brain? It can be assumed that while some students may acquire and be influenced by only these initial concepts, others will venture further and embrace the fuller complexity of the scientific understanding of learning. These first concepts should, therefore, be "core" in the sense that they have prime relevance to a teacher's everyday experience, while also providing a foundation suitable for exploring and embracing the fuller complexity of knowledge regarding how the brain learns. More specifically, they should provide insight into established classroom educational practices, while having the potential for development into a finer-grain understanding of brain structure and function. In respect of the latter issue, it may be helpful to critique the major differences between the very simplified version of brain function expressed in our concepts and current understanding from cognitive neuroscience. For example, we believe the schematics representing engage, build and consolidate categories of the learning process provide a visual, accessible and memorable way to discuss the core concepts we have identified. They promote the idea of bidirectional connectivity between the cortex and subcortical structures, and that activation of the working memory network in relation to fresh learning can be diminished as that learning is consolidated. However, an awareness of the scientific limitations of our curriculum and schematics may help sensitise teacher educators to detect and avoid misunderstandings. Here, we deliberately draw attention to the distance between these explanations and a more sophisticated scientific understanding because we believe this may prove helpful when monitoring and assuring appropriate interpretation and usage of our core concepts in teacher education.

In respect of engagement, there is an established body of animal and human findings that help explain the motivation to approach a stimulus in terms of the brain's reward system. However, the relation between reward and learning has predominantly been studied in detail at the brain level chiefly in terms of reinforcement and reward learning. These typically involve learning to carry out simple actions, such as pressing buttons or pulling levers, in ways that opti-mise the receipt of reward. There is still much work to be done in elucidating the role of the reward system in the classroom and in relation to forms of learn-ing that are directly relevant to education. While researchers have explored the role of the reward system in economic decisions (e.g., Genevsky & Knut-son, 2015; Kühn, Strelow, & Gallinat, 2016; Venkatraman et al., 2015), only in recent years have studies considered its role in relation to anything like educational learning. Existing examples of such studies include identification of adult ventral striatal activation when learning facts and concepts in gami-fied contexts as opposed to just reading notes (Howard-Jones et al., 2016) and behavioural studies of the effects on educational learning of manipulating reward schedule (Devonshire et al., 2014; Ozcelik, Cagiltay, & Ozcelik, 2013). More circumstantial evidence arises from data showing increased functional connectivity between the ventral striatum and those bilateral prefrontal net-works thought to be important for cognitive-behavioural control measures ("grit" and "growth mindset") associated with academic performance (Myers, Wang, Black, Bugescu, & Hoeft, 2016). Otherwise, the potential educational relevance of the functioning of the brain's reward system depends on studies relating reward to declarative memory formation (for reviews see Howard-Jones & Jay, 2016; Miendlarzewska, Bavelier, & Schwartz, 2016). Addition-ally, human data in this area are constrained by an overwhelming focus on adult participants, with only a few studies addressing the development of the reward system during childhood (e.g., Fareri et al., 2015; Van Leijenhorst et al., 2010). In terms of pupils responding to the teachers' emotions, the neural response of watching emotion in others has been confined to basic emotions such as disgust. The enthusiasm displayed towards a curriculum topic has not been studied in this way. Behavioural evidence exists for the transfer of maths anxiety from female teachers to their young female students (Beilock et al., 2010) but, although our understanding of implicit communication of emo-tions offers insights that *might* explain these data, the transfer of maths anxiety has not been studied at the neural level. In many cases, the cognitive neuro-science can deepen our understanding of the *potential* mechanisms but stops short of providing data directly from learning contexts recognisable by educa-tors. Similarly, understanding of the Mirror Neuron System (MNS) alerts us to mechanisms by which emotions and ideas *may* be unconsciously communicated or picked up on. However, although advances in Functional Near-Infrared Spectroscopy (fNIRS) show promise, we do not currently have technology that is cheap, portable and sensitive enough to study such phenomena in the classroom. Our schematic of engagement includes the bidirectional nature of the interaction between PFC and subcortical regions, but it clumps all subcor-tical regions and their pathways to the cortex together. Research over the last three to four decades has revealed loops interconnecting the "higher" cortical brain functions and "lower" subcortical structures, and emphasise the role of these loops in vigilance, attention, emotion, memory and learning (Parvizi, 2009). Our arrow is intended to suggest a bidirectional flow of information between cortex and subcortical structures. The simple point that our arrow makes is that a student's "higher" cortical brain function influences, and is influenced by, those "lower" subcortical structures that are critical for our emotional responding. This supports simple explanations about, e.g., the effects of anxiety and approach motivation on working memory and attention, while being sufficiently aligned with current scientific understanding to later support construction of a more sophisticated concept brain connectivity. At the same time, however, it is important to acknowledge that this is a gross simplification of current understanding, since pathways back to the cortex from each subcortical structure are known to travel either upwards via the thalamus or descend downwards via the brain stem, contacting sites in the latter case that comprise ascending projection systems involving a broad range of neurotransmitters (Pessoa, 2017).

In terms of building on prior knowledge, studies suggest the involvement of medial and lateral prefrontal cortex in the detection of fit with prior knowledge and in making connection with it. It was proposed earlier that the lack of maturity of these regions in children suggests a need for teachers to support students in making links to what they have already learnt. However, we currently have no studies that directly link maturity of these regions to difficulties in using prior knowledge, or studies showing the impact on connection making, learning or brain function when such support is provided for children with less developed function in these regions. Also, it should be noted that the theoretical model proposing schema-linked interactions between medial prefrontal and medial temporal regions is not without its competitors. This model proposes that the medial PFC detects a fit with prior knowledge and so an opportunity to generalise to an existing schema, and helps to suppress the involvement of the hippocampus in creating a new schema. Other models prefer adding emphasis to the role of the hippocampus in relating new events to prior knowledge (Gilboa & Marlatte, 2017). The schematic indicating activation of working memory networks during the building of new knowledge also focuses on dorsolateral PFC. More precisely, neuroimaging studies have indicated that storage of working memory contents is distributed across multiple regions from sensory to parietal and prefrontal cortex (e.g., Brahmbhatt, White, & Barch, 2010; Siffredi et al., 2017). However, working memory activity associated with abstractness and generalizability has been linked more to prefrontal cortex than other brain regions (Christophel, Klink, Spitzer, Roelfsema, & Haynes, 2017), suggesting it is the prefrontal cortex that is most involved in maintaining the flexible representations suitable for transformation and the generation of new knowledge. As student teachers develop their knowledge in this area, they may come to understand that the focus on PFC in our simple explanation has been applied in a somewhat constrained manner, i.e., on the capacity to maintain those types of representations that precede learning. Their understanding of the term working memory may then develop to include the temporary representation of lower-level sensory information that is more associated with regions beyond the PFC.

In scientific terms, consolidation may refer to two types of process: synaptic consolidation, which is accomplished within the first minutes to hours after any type of learning; and system consolidation, in which new memories that initially depend upon the hippocampus are reorganised to become more hippocampal-independent. The first type of consolidation may be relevant to the effectiveness of spaced or distributed learning, since scientists have speculated that this strategy supports long-term memory consolidation by differentially mediating the spacing of memory reactivation (Litman & Davachi, 2008). However, studying the consolidation of episodic memory in intact human populations at the neuronal level presents many difficulties and so the educational link is likely to remain speculative for some time. On the other hand, there are more human studies relating a reduction in effortful processing to increased automaticity and reduced recruitment of prefrontal networks, and some have been carried out with educational types of learning such as second language acquisition (Saidi et al., 2013) and learning complex multiplication (Delazer et al., 2003). The schematic we have used for consolidation indicates activity shifting away from PFC and becoming more distributed across the brain. Again, this is a simplistic representation compared with our current understanding. For example, it ignores the role of the hippocampus in indirectly associating cortical representational areas activated by new experiences and thoughts encountered during learning, and the various putative roles of these different areas in long-term memory formation. The schematic is intended merely to highlight that a stage of learning exists beyond the initial representation of new knowledge that reduces the burden on working memory networks. Although the schematics for "engage, build, consolidate" are simplified, these are carefully considered simplifications aimed at communicating educationally relevant explanations that are essentially aligned with current scientific understanding.

Conclusion

What Neuroscience Has Added to Our Understanding Over and Above Psychology

The dearth of imaging studies employing educational-like tasks means that, in almost all cases, the relevance of cognitive neuroscience to classroom practice is a reasoned hypothesis that would benefit from further research. However, although this scientific understanding of classroom learning is incomplete, we believe it is already sufficient as a basis for critically considering classroom learning processes and that this basis should be guided chiefly by cognitive neuroscience. Cognitive neuroscience is framed by an established brain-mind-behaviour model of explanation (Morton & Frith, 1995) and, although concerned with biological processes, also has psychology, quite literally, at the centre of its theorising (Bruer, 1997). The additional preoccupation of cognitive neuroscience with biological processes adds value because 1) most importantly, a scientific learning concept may be judged as more established when it rests upon convergent evidence that includes both observable behavioural data and also measurable biological data; 2) the inclusion of explanations informed by cognitive neuroscience allow for the dispelling of students' existing myths about the brain and can provide some "inoculation" against acquiring these; and 3) explanations couched in terms of brain function allow a visual, accessible and engaging means by which to communicate about learning processes.

Concrete Implications of Research and Opportunities for Translation

We have presented concepts from the science of learning that we are currently introducing into the Post-Graduate Certificate in Education (PGCE) at the University of Bristol. However, as suggested at the beginning of this chapter, the practical implementation of these concepts requires them to become part of the reflective processes of the students. We are doing this in a number of ways.

Firstly, we scaffold students as they work collaboratively to initially apply the concepts to classroom practice. In lectures, we ask them to critique different teaching approaches communicated through vignettes describing fictional lessons. This generates discussion around how the concepts should be applied, and what constraints on interpretation should be considered, so allowing misconceptions to be corrected. Secondly, we encourage students to make links between the concepts from cognitive neuroscience and the traditional perspectives on learning offered by Piaget and Vygotsky. Here, we offer opportunities to consider a lesson plan and ask student teachers to explain, from a Vygotskian, Piagetian and cognitive neuroscience perspective, why different parts of the lesson might have gone well or poorly in terms of student learning. This encourages discussion of the value added by concepts from cognitive neuroscience and where these may complement insights from other perspectives. Thirdly, when planning lessons, we ask the student teachers to indicate where a scientific rationale can be provided for their planning decisions and identify which scientific concepts are relevant. This helps provide prompts for observations during the teaching of the lesson—so providing a richer and scientifically informed basis for reflecting on how some parts of their lesson appeared effective in promoting engagement and learning, while other parts appeared not to be.

Further Resources for the Reader to Learn More About the Topic

At the time of writing, guidelines are being prepared to support teachers, schools, and institutions involved with teacher training wishing to introduce concepts from the sciences of mind and brain into classroom practice (www. edneuro.net). An article for practitioners outlines some of the concepts discussed in this chapter (Howard-Jones et al., 2018) and a MOOC has been completed that also provides further exploration of this area for teachers:

www.futurelearn.com/courses/science-of-learning.

Notes

1. Working memory is our ability to keep information in mind and manipulate it—and it is very limited.
2. For women, but not men, higher rejection sensitivity predicted poorer error correction in the social condition. A path analysis suggested that, for women, high rejection sensitivity disrupted attentional orienting to the social-evaluative performance feedback, which affected subsequent memory for the correct answer by reducing engagement with learning opportunities. These results suggest a mechanism for how social feedback may impede learning among women who are high in rejection sensitivity.
3. The mental structures that link multiple representations of ideas (Piaget, 1923).
4. When presenting these concepts to student teachers, we referred to "responding to questions" rather than "testing" due to the strong association of testing with summative assessment, government tests and examinations, rather than the support of learning processes.

References

Ansari, D., & Coch, D. (2006). Bridges over troubled waters: Education and cognitive neuroscience. *Trends in Cognitive Sciences*, 10(4), 146–149.

Askew, M., Brown, M., Rhodes, V., Wiliam, D., & Johnson, D. (1997). *Effective teachers of numeracy: Report of a study carried out for the teacher training agency*. London: King's College, University of London.

Becker, W. C., Madsen, C. H., Arnold, C. R., & Thomas, D. R. (1967). Contingent use of teacher attention and praise in reducing classroom behavior problems. *Journal of Special Education*, 1(3), 287–307. doi:10.1177/002246696700100307

Beilock, S. L., Gunderson, E. A., Ramirez, G., & Levine, S. C. (2010). Female teachers' math anxiety affects girls' math achievement. *Proceedings of the National Academy of Sciences of the United States of America*, 107(5), 1860–1863. doi:10.1073/pnas. 0910967107

Bentley, B., & Yates, G. C. R. (2017). Facilitating proportional reasoning through worked examples: Two classroom-based experiments. *Cogent Education*, 4, 14. doi:10. 1080/2331186x.2017.1297213

Blackwell, L. S., Trzesniewski, K. H., & Dweck, C. S. (2007). Implicit theories of intelligence predict achievement across an adolescent transition: A longitudinal study and an intervention. *Child Development*, 78(1), 246–263.

Blazar, D., & Kraft, M. A. (2017). Teacher and teaching effects on students' attitudes and behaviors. *Educational Evaluation and Policy Analysis*, 39(1), 146–170. doi:10.3102/0162373716670260

Brahmbhatt, S. B., White, D. A., & Barch, D. M. (2010). Developmental differences in sustained and transient activity underlying working memory. *Brain Research*, 1354, 140–151. doi:10.1016/j.brainres.2010.07.055

Bramald, R., Hardman, F., & Leat, D. (1995). Initial teacher trainees and their views of teaching and learning. *Teaching and Teacher Education, 11*(1), 23–31. doi:10.1016/0742-051x(94)e0009-t

Brod, G., Lindenberger, U., Werkle-Bergner, M., & Shing, Y. L. (2015). Differences in the neural signature of remembering schema-congruent and schema-incongruent events. *Neuroimage, 117*, 358–366. doi:10.1016/j.neuroimage.2015.05.086

Brod, G., Werkle-Bergner, M., & Shing, Y. L. (2013). The influence of prior knowledge on memory: A developmental cognitive neuroscience perspective. *Frontiers in Behavioral Neuroscience, 7*, 13. doi:10.3389/fnbeh.2013.00139

Brown, P. C., Roediger III, H. L., & McDaniel, M. A. (2014). *Make it stick: The science of successful learning*. Cambridge, MA: Harvard University Press.

Bruer, J. (1997). Education and the brain: A bridge too far. *Educational Researcher, 26*(8), 4–16.

Buchweitz, A., Mason, R. A., Tomitch, L. M. B., & Just, M. A. (2009). Brain activation for reading and listening comprehension: An fMRI study of modality effects and individual differences in language comprehension. *Psychology & Neuroscience, 2*(2), 111–123.

Buitink, J. (2009). What and how do student teachers learn during school-based teacher education. *Teaching and Teacher Education, 25*(1), 118–127. doi:10.1016/j.tate.2008.07.009

Campbell, J., & Mayer, R. E. (2009). Questioning as an instructional method: Does it affect learning from lectures? *Applied Cognitive Psychology, 23*(6), 747–759. doi:10.1002/acp.1513

Catmur, C., Gillmeister, H., Bird, G., Liepelt, R., Brass, M., & Heyes, C. (2008). Through the looking glass: Counter-mirror activation following incompatible sensorimotor learning. *European Journal of Neuroscience, 28*(6), 1208–1215. doi:10.1111/j.1460-9568.2008.06419.x

Christophel, T. B., Klink, P. C., Spitzer, B., Roelfsema, P. R., & Haynes, J.-D. (2017). The distributed nature of working memory. *Trends in Cognitive Sciences, 21*(2), 111–124. https://doi.org/10.1016/j.tics.2016.12.007

Coe, R., Aloisi, C., Higgins, S., & Major, L. E. (2014). *What makes great teaching? Review of the underpinning research*. London: Sutton Trust.

Craik, F. I. M. (2002). Levels of processing: Past, present . . . and future? *Memory, 10*(5–6), 305–318. doi:10.1080/09658210244000135

Craik, F. I. M., & Lockhart, R. S. (1972). Levels of processing—framework for memory research. *Journal of Verbal Learning and Verbal Behavior, 11*(6), 671–684. doi:10.1016/s0022-5371(72)80001-x

Dehaene, S. (2009). *Reading in the brain*. London: Viking Penguin.

Delazer, M., Domahs, F., Bartha, L., Brenneis, C., Lochy, A., Trieb, T., & Benke, T. (2003). Learning complex arithmetic—an fMRI study. *Cognitive Brain Research, 18*, 76–88.

Devonshire, I. M., Davis, J., Fairweather, S., Highfield, L., Thaker, C., Walsh, A., . . . Hathway, G. J. (2014). Risk-based learning games improve long-term retention of information among school pupils. *PLoS One, 9*(7), 9. doi:10.1371/journal.pone.0103640

Dubinsky, J. M. (2010). Neuroscience education for prekindergarten-12 teachers. *Journal of Neuroscience, 30*(24), 8057–8060. doi:10.1523/jneurosci.2322-10.2010

Dubinsky, J. M., Roehrig, G., & Varma, S. (2013). Infusing neuroscience into teacher professional development. *Educational Researcher, 42*(6), 317–329. doi:10.3102/0013189x13499403

Dudai, Y. (2004). The neurobiology of consolidations, or, how stable is the engram? *Annual Review of Psychology*, 55, 51–86. doi:10.1146/annurev.psych.55.090902. 142050

Dufrene, B. A., Lestremau, L., & Zoder-Martell, K. (2014). Direct behavioral consultation: Effects on teachers' praise and student disruptive behavior. *Psychology in the Schools*, 51(6), 567–580. doi:10.1002/pits.21768

Fareri, D. S., Gabard-Durnama, L., Goff, B., Flannery, J., Gee, D. G., Lumian, D. S., . . . Tottenham, N. (2015). Normative development of ventral striatal resting state connectivity in humans. *Neuroimage*, 118, 422–437. doi:10.1016/j.neuroimage.2015.06.022

Farooqi, I. S., Bullmore, E., Keogh, J., Gillard, J., O'Rahilly, S., & Fletcher, P. C. (2007). Leptin regulates striatal regions and human eating behavior. *Science*, 317(5843), 1355–1355. doi:10.1126/science.1144599

Filimon, F., Nelson, J. D., Hagler, D. J., & Sereno, M. I. (2007). Human cortical representations for reaching: Mirror neurons for execution, observation, and imagery. *Neuroimage*, 37(4), 1315–1328. http://dx.doi.org/10.1016/j.neuroimage.2007.06.008

Gallese, V. (2003). The roots of empathy: The shared manifold hypothesis and the neural basis of intersubjectivity. *Psychopathology*, 36(4), 171–180. doi:10.1159/000072786

Gallese, V., Eagle, M. N., & Migone, P. (2007). Intentional attunement: Mirror neurons and the neural underpinnings of interpersonal relations. *Journal of the American Psychoanalytic Association*, 55(1), 131–176.

Genevsky, A., & Knutson, B. (2015). Neural affective mechanisms predict market-level microlending. *Psychological Science*, 26(9), 1411–1422. doi:10.1177/095679 7615588467

Gershenson, S. (2016). Linking teacher quality, student attendance, and student achievement. *Education Finance and Policy*, 11(2), 125–149. doi:10.1162/EDFP_a_00180

Ghassemzadeh, H., Posner, M. I., & Rothbart, M. K. (2013). Contributions of Hebb and Vygotsky to an integrated science of mind. *J Hist Neurosci*, 22(3), 292–306. doi: 10.1080/0964704x.2012.761071

Gilboa, A., & Marlatte, H. (2017). Neurobiology of schemas and schema-mediated memory. *Trends in Cognitive Sciences*, 21(8), 618–631. https://doi.org/10.1016/j.tics.2017.04.013

Gonzalez-Garrido, A. A., Barrios, F. A., Gomez-Velazquez, F. R., & Zarabozo-Hurtado, D. (2017). The supramarginal and angular gyri underlie orthographic competence in Spanish language. *Brain and Language*, 175, 1–10. doi:10.1016/j.bandl.2017.08.005

Guilloteaux, M. J., & Dornyei, Z. (2008). Motivating language learners: A classroom-oriented investigation of the effects of motivational strategies on student motivation. *Tesol Quarterly*, 42(1), 55–77. doi:10.2307/40264425

Hanushek, E. (2011). Valuing teachers: How much is a good teacher worth? *Education Next*, 11(3), 40–45.

Hidi, S., Renninger, K. A., & Krapp, A. (2004). Interest, a motivational variable that combines affective and cognitive functioning. In D. Y. Dai & R. J. Sternberg (Eds.), *Motivation, emotion, and cognition: Integrative perspectives on intellectual functioning and development* (pp. 89–115). Mahwah, NJ: Lawrence Erlbaum Associates Publishers.

Horvath, J. C. (2014). The neuroscience of powerpoint (TM). *Mind Brain and Education*, 8(3), 137–143. doi:10.1111/mbe.12052

Howard-Jones, P. A. (2009). Creativity, the mind and drama: Studying links between brain activity and creativity. *Teaching Drama*, 23(4).

Howard-Jones, P. A. (2014). Neuroscience and education: Myths and messages. *Nature Reviews Neuroscience, 15*(12), 817–824.

Howard-Jones, P. A., Ioannou, C., Bailey, R., Prior, J., Yau, S. H., & Jay, T. (2018). Applying the science of learning in the classroom. *Impact (The Journal of the Chartered College of Teaching), 2*, 9–12.

Howard-Jones, P. A., & Jay, T. (2016). Reward, learning and games. *Current Opinion in Behavioral Sciences,* (10), 65–72.

Howard-Jones, P. A., Jay, T., Mason, A., & Jones, H. (2016). Gamification of learning deactivates the default mode network. *Frontiers in Psychology, 6,* 16. doi:10.3389/fpsyg.2015.01891

Howard-Jones, P. A., Winfield, M., & Crimmins, G. (2008). Co-constructing an understanding of creativity in the fostering of drama education that draws on neuropsychological concepts. *Educational Research, 50*(2), 187–201.

Howard-Jones, P. A., Winfield, M., & Crimmins, G. (2009). Fostering creative thinking. *The Journal for Drama in Education, 25*(2), 8–22.

Izuma, K., Saito, D. N., & Sadato, N. (2008). Processing of social and monetary rewards in the human striatum. *Neuron, 58*(2), 284–294. doi:10.1016/j.neuron.2008.03.020

Johnson, C. I., & Mayer, R. E. (2009). A testing effect with multimedia learning. *Journal of Educational Psychology, 101*(3), 621–629. doi:10.1037/a0015183

Kane, M. J., & Engle, R. W. (2002). The role of prefrontal cortex in working-memory capacity, executive attention, and general fluid intelligence: An individual-differences perspective. *Psychonomic Bulletin & Review, 9*(4), 637–671. doi:10.3758/bf03196323

Karpicke, J. D., & Blunt, J. R. (2011). Retrieval practice produces more learning than elaborative studying with concept mapping. *Science, 331*(6018), 772–775. doi:10.1126/science.1199327

Ker, H. W. (2016). The impacts of student-, teacher- and school-level factors on mathematics achievement: An exploratory comparative investigation of Singaporean students and the USA students. *Educational Psychology, 36*(2), 254–276. doi:10.1080/01443410.2015.1026801

Kirkham, N. Z., Rea, M., Osborne, T., White, H., & Mareschal, D. (2019). Do cues from multiple modalities support quicker learning in primary schoolchildren? *Developmental Psychology, 55*(10), 2048–2059. doi:10.1037/dev0000778

Knutson, B., Adams, C. M., Fong, G. W., & Hommer, D. (2001). Anticipation of monetary reward selectively recruits nucleus accumbens. *Journal of Neuroscience, 21*(RC159), 1–5.

Koepp, M. J., Gunn, R. N., Lawrence, A. D., Cunningham, V. J., Dagher, A., Jones, T., . . . Grasby, P. M. (1998). Evidence for striatal dopamine release during a video game. *Nature, 393*(6682), 266–268.

Kühn, S., Strelow, E., & Gallinat, J. (2016). Multiple "buy buttons" in the brain: Forecasting chocolate sales at point-of-sale based on functional brain activation using fMRI. *Neuroimage, 136,* 122–128. https://doi.org/10.1016/j.neuroimage.2016.05.021

Lesage, E., Nailer, E. L., & Miall, R. C. (2016). Cerebellar BOLD signal during the acquisition of a new lexicon predicts its early consolidation. *Brain and Language, 161,* 33–44. https://doi.org/10.1016/j.bandl.2015.07.005

Lieberman, M. D. (2012). Education and the social brain. *Trends in Neuroscience and Education, 1*(1), 3–9. doi:https://doi.org/10.1016/j.tine.2012.07.003

Litman, L., & Davachi, L. (2008). Distributed learning enhances relational memory consolidation. *Learning & Memory, 15*(9), 711–716. doi:10.1101/lm.1132008

Mangels, J. A., Hoxha, O., Lane, S. P., Jarvis, S. N., & Downey, G. (2017). Evidence that disrupted orienting to evaluative social feedback undermines error correction in rejection sensitive women. *Social Neuroscience*, 1–20.

Maquet, P., Laureys, S., Peigneux, P., Fuchs, S., Petiau, C., Phillips, C., . . . Cleermans, A. (2000). Experience dependent changes in cerebral activation during human REM sleep. *Nature Neuroscience*, 3(8), 831–836.

Marshall, U., & Born, J. (2007). The contribution of sleep to hippocampus-dependent memory consolidation. *Trends in Cognitive Sciences*, 11(10), 442–450. doi:10.1016/j.tics.2007.09.001

Mayer, R. E., & Anderson, R. B. (1991). Animations need narrations—an experimental test of a dual-coding hypothesis. *Journal of Educational Psychology*, 83(4), 484–490. doi:10.1037//0022-0663.83.4.484

McDaniel, M. A., Agarwal, P. K., Huelser, B. J., McDermott, K. B., & Roediger, H. L. (2011). Test-enhanced learning in a middle school science classroom: The effects of quiz frequency and placement. *Journal of Educational Psychology*, 103(2), 399–414. doi:10.1037/a0021782

McDaniel, M. A., Roediger, H. L., & McDermott, K. B. (2007). Generalizing test-enhanced learning from the laboratory to the classroom. *Psychonomic Bulletin & Review*, 14(2), 200–206. doi:10.3758/bf03194052

Menon, V., Rivera, S. M., White, C. D., Glover, G. H., & Reiss, A. L. (2000). Dissociating prefrontal and parietal cortex activation during arithmetic processing. *Neuroimage*, 12(4), 357–365. doi:10.1006/nimg.2000.0613

Mevorach, M., & Strauss, S. (2012). Teacher educators' in-action mental models in different teaching situations. *Teachers and Teaching*, 18(1), 25–41. doi:10.1080/135 40602.2011.622551

Miendlarzewska, E. A., Bavelier, D., & Schwartz, S. (2016). Influence of reward motivation on human declarative memory. *Neuroscience and Biobehavioral Reviews*, 61, 156–176. doi:10.1016/j.neubiorev.2015.11.015

Min Jeong, K., Ming, H., Krajbich, I. M., Loewenstein, G., McClure, S. M., Wang, J. T.-Y., & Camerer, C. F. (2009). The wick in the candle of learning: Epistemic curiosity activates reward circuitry and enhances memory. *Psychological Science (0956–7976)*, 20(8), 963–973. doi:10.1111/j.1467-9280.2009.02402.x

Morton, J., & Frith, U. (1995). Causal modelling: A structural approach to developmental psychopathology. In D. Cicchetti & D. J. Cohen (Eds.), *Manual of developmental psychopathology* (Vol. 1, pp. 357–390). New York: Wiley.

Myers, C. A., Wang, C., Black, J. M., Bugescu, N., & Hoeft, F. (2016). The matter of motivation: Striatal resting-state connectivity is dissociable between grit and growth mindset. *Social Cognitive and Affective Neuroscience*, 11(10), 1521–1527. doi:10.1093/scan/nsw065

OECD. (2009). *Creating effective teaching and learning environments: First results from TALIS*. Paris: OECD.

Ozcelik, E., Cagiltay, N. E., & Ozcelik, N. S. (2013). The effect of uncertainty on learning in game-like environments. *Computers & Education*, 67, 12–20. http://dx.doi.org/10.1016/j.compedu.2013.02.009

Parvizi, J. (2009). Corticocentric myopia: Old bias in new cognitive sciences. *Trends in Cognitive Sciences*, 13(8), 354–359. doi:10.1016/j.tics.2009.04.008

Paunesku, D., Walton, G. M., Romero, C., Smith, E. N., Yeager, D. S., & Dweck, C. S. (2015). Mind-set interventions are a scalable treatment for academic underachievement. *Psychological Science*, 26(6), 784–793. doi:10.1177/0956797615571017

Pekrun, R. (2014). *Emotions and learning.* Brussels and Geneva: International Academy of Education (IAE) and International Bureau of Education (IBE).

Pessoa, L. (2017). A network model of the emotional brain. *Trends in Cognitive Sciences, 21*(5), 357–371. https://doi.org/10.1016/j.tics.2017.03.002

Piaget, J. (1923). *Langage et pensée chez l'enfant* (3rd ed.). Neuchâtel: Delachaux et Niestlé.

Reinke, W. M., Lewis-Palmer, T., & Merrell, K. (2008). The classroom check-up: A classwide teacher consultation model for increasing praise and decreasing disruptive behavior. *School Psychology Review, 37*(3), 315–332.

Rizzolatti, G., & Craighero, L. (2004). The mirror neuron system. *Annual Review of Neuroscience, 27,* 169–192.

Roediger, H. L., & Karpicke, J. D. (2006). Test-enhanced learning—taking memory tests improves long-term retention. *Psychological Science, 17*(3), 249–255. doi:10.1111/j.1467-9280.2006.01693.x

Roehrig, G. H., Michlin, M., Schmitt, L., MacNabb, C., & Dubinsky, J. M. (2012). Teaching neuroscience to science teachers: Facilitating the translation of inquiry-based teaching instruction to the classroom. *Cbe-Life Sciences Education, 11*(4), 413–424. doi:10.1187/cbe.12-04-0045

Rohrer, D., & Pashler, H. (2010). Recent research on human learning challenges conventional instructional strategies. *Educational Researcher, 39*(5), 406–412. doi:10.3102/0013189x10374770

Rosenshine, B. (2010). *Principles of instruction.* Brussels and Geneva: International Academy of Education (IAE) and International Bureau of Education (IBE).

Royal Society. (2011). *Brain waves module 2: Neuroscience: Implications for education and lifelong learning.* London: Royal Society.

Saidi, L. G., Perlbarg, V., Marrelec, G., Pelegrini-Issac, M., Benali, H., & Ansaldo, A. I. (2013). Functional connectivity changes in second language vocabulary learning. *Brain and Language, 124*(1), 56–65. doi:10.1016/j.bandl.2012.11.008

Schiefele, U. (2001). The role of interest in motivation and learning. In J. M. Collis & S. Messick (Eds.), *Intelligence and personality. Bridging the gap in theory and measurement* (pp. 163–193). Mahwah, NJ: Lawrence Erlbaum Associates.

Schilbach, L., Wilms, M., Eickhoff, S. B., Romanzetti, S., Tepest, R., Bente, G., . . . Vogeley, K. (2010). Minds made for sharing: Initiating joint attention recruits reward-related neurocircuitry. *Journal of Cognitive Neuroscience, 22*(12), 2702–2715. doi:10.1162/jocn.2009.21401

Schomaker, J., & Meeter, M. (2015). Short- and long-lasting consequences of novelty, deviance and surprise on brain and cognition. *Neuroscience and Biobehavioral Reviews, 55,* 268–279. doi:10.1016/j.neubiorev.2015.05.002

Shing, Y. L., & Brod, G. (2016). Effects of prior knowledge on memory: Implications for education. *Mind, Brain, and Education, 10*(3), 153–161. doi:10.1111/mbe.12110

Siffredi, V., Barrouillet, P., Spencer-Smith, M., Vaessen, M., Anderson, V., & Vuilleumier, P. (2017). Examining distinct working memory processes in children and adolescents using fMRI: Results and validation of a modified Brown-Peterson paradigm. *PLoS One, 12*(7), 22. doi:10.1371/journal.pone.0179959

Simon, O., Mangin, J. F., Cohen, L., Le Bihan, D., & Dehaene, S. (2002). Topographical layout of hand, eye, calculation, and language-related areas in the human parietal lobe. *Neuron, 33*(3), 475–487. doi:10.1016/s0896-6273(02)00575-5

Skinner, E. A., Kindermann, T. A., & Furrer, C. J. (2009). A motivational perspective on engagement and disaffection conceptualization and assessment of children's behavioral

472   Paul Howard-Jones et al.

and emotional participation in academic activities in the classroom. *Educational and Psychological Measurement*, 69(3), 493–525. doi:10.1177/0013164408323233

Stanescu-Cosson, R., Pinel, P., van de Moortele, P. F., Le Bihan, D., Cohen, L., & Dehaene, S. (2000). Understanding dissociations in dyscalculia—a brain imaging study of the impact of number size on the cerebral networks for exact and approximate calculation. *Brain, 123,* 2240–2255. doi:10.1093/brain/123.11.2240

Stickgold, R. (2005). Sleep-dependent memory consolidation. *Nature, 437*(7063), 1272–1278. doi:10.1038/nature04286

Strong, M., Gargani, J., & Hacifazlioglu, O. (2011). Do we know a successful teacher when we see one? Experiments in the identification of effective teachers. *Journal of Teacher Education, 62*(4), 367–382.

Sutherland, K. S., Wehby, J. H., & Copeland, S. R. (2000). Effect of varying rates of behavior-specific praise on the on-task behavior of students with EBD. *Journal of Emotional and Behavioral Disorders, 8*(1), 2. doi:10.1177/106342660000800101

Tham, E. K. H., Lindsay, S., & Gaskell, M. G. (2015). Markers of automaticity in sleep-associated consolidation of novel words. *Neuropsychologia, 71,* 146–157. doi:10.1016/j.neuropsychologia.2015.03.025

Timperley, H., Wilson, A., Barrar, H., & Fung, I. (2007). *Teacher professional learning and development: Best evidence synthesis iteration.* Wellington, New Zealand. Retrieved from www.educationcounts.govt.nz/publications/series/2515/15341

Tononi, G., & Cirelli, C. (2014). Sleep and the price of plasticity: From synaptic and cellular homeostasis to memory consolidation and integration. *Neuron, 81*(1), 12–34. doi:10.1016/j.neuron.2013.12.025

van Gog, T., & Kester, L. (2012). A test of the testing effect: Acquiring problem-solving skills from worked examples. *Cognitive Science, 36*(8), 1532–1541. doi:10.1111/cogs.12002

van Kesteren, M. T. R., Ruiter, D. J., Fernandez, G., & Henson, R. N. (2012). How schema and novelty augment memory formation. *Trends in Neurosciences, 35*(4), 211–219. doi:10.1016/j.tins.2012.02.001

Van Leijenhorst, L., Moor, B. G., de Macks, Z. A. O., Rombouts, S. A. R. B., West-enberg, P. M., & Crone, E. A. (2010). Adolescent risky decision-making: Neuro-cognitive development of reward and control regions. *Neuroimage, 51*(1), 345–355. doi:10.1016/j.neuroimage.2010.02.038

van Loon-Hillen, N., van Gog, T., & Brand-Gruwel, S. (2012). Effects of worked examples in a primary school mathematics curriculum. *Interactive Learning Environments, 20*(1), 89–99. doi:10.1080/10494821003755510

Vanwynsberghe, G., Vanlaar, G., Van Damme, J., & De Fraine, B. (2017). Long-term effects of primary schools on mathematics achievement of students at age 17. *British Educational Research Journal, 43*(6), 1131–1148. doi:10.1002/berj.3311

Venkatraman, V., Dimoka, A., Pavlou, P. A., Vo, K., Hampton, W., Bollinger, B., . . . Winer, R. S. (2015). Predicting advertising success beyond traditional measures: New insights from neurophysiological methods and market response modeling. *Journal of Marketing Research, 52*(4), 436–452. doi:10.1509/jmr.13.0593

Wicker, B., Keysers, C., Plailly, J., Royet, J.-P., Gallese, V., & Rizzolatti, G. (2003). Both of us disgusted in my insula: The common neural basis of seeing and feeling disgust. *Neuron, 40*(3), 655–664. http://dx.doi.org/10.1016/S0896-6273(03)00679-2

Wirebring, L. K., Wiklund-Hornqvist, C., Eriksson, J., Andersson, M., Jonsson, B., & Nyberg, L. (2015). Lesser neural pattern similarity across repeated tests is associated with better long-term memory retention. *Journal of Neuroscience*, 35(26), 9595–9602. doi:10.1523/jneurosci.3550-14.2015

Young, C. B., Wu, S. S., & Menon, V. (2012). The neurodevelopmental basis of math anxiety. *Psychological Science*, 23(5), 492–501. doi:10.1177/0956797611429134

Zago, L., Pesenti, M., Mellet, E., Crivello, F., Mazoyer, B., & Tzourio-Mazoyer, N. (2001). Neural correlates of simple and complex mental calculation. *Neuroimage*, 13(2), 314–327. doi:10.1006/nimg.2000.0697

18 Educational Neuroscience
Ethical Perspectives

Victoria Knowland

The ethics of educational neuroscience, or *educational neuroethics* (Lalancette & Campbell, 2012), is an ongoing dialogue between researchers, educationalists and ethicists about the principles and practice of educational neuroscience research. We can define two distinct strands of educational neuroethics. The first is responding to specific issues that arise during the everyday running of a research project. Many of the ethical issues encountered during educational neuroscience research are common to research in areas such as developmental psychology, cognitive neuroscience and genetics, but arguably some are unique and deserve consideration in their own right (Fischer, Goswami, Geake, & Task Force on the Future of Educational Neuroscience, 2010; Howard-Jones & Fenton, 2012); for example, obtaining informed consent from all parties involved in large-scale school intervention studies, or dealing with incidental educationally relevant findings from cognitive assessments. These issues must be properly addressed whilst ensuring research remains practically viable. In reality, much of educational neuroscience is about small changes in classroom practice or lifestyle (health and fitness), where the practical ethical issues are relatively uncontroversial.

The second strand of educational neuroethics is about guiding the path of research: what educational neuroscience is trying to achieve, what are deemed useful and valid topics of study, and how the field may impact upon children, teachers, parents, funders, and ultimately society at large. It is this second strand that we consider here.

Educational neuroscience takes the tools of neuroscience and applies them to understanding and optimising learning in the classroom, to enhance cognition; in the process, it presents an interesting ethical challenge. We can draw an important distinction here between two types of learning: *experience-expectant* learning refers to the kind of learning all human brains can expect as a result of experiences in a typically stimulating environment; for example, learning the sounds of speech, how to walk or how to catch an object. By contrast, *experience-dependent* learning is anything beyond that universal learning: things which individuals learn as a result of their own personal experiences (Bruer & Greenough, 2001). Learning in school (and, by extension, what educational neuroscience aims to boost) comes under the experience-dependent umbrella. Purposefully making experience-dependent changes to the developing brain presupposes that those changes will benefit that individual over their lifespan, so the ethical problem is how to ensure that new teaching techniques and interventions confer that benefit. Children are, by virtue of being at school anyway, required to participate in activities prescribed by an authority figure with the express goal of changing their brains, so arguably the issues we discuss here could be applied to education in general (Bostrom & Sandberg, 2009).

We take the example of neuromodulation. Neuromodulation refers to the artificial enhancement of the human brain, typically for non-therapeutic purposes. Although this may seem like an extreme example, techniques for neuromodulation are already in use, and research into use with healthy children is beginning to happen. Society's flirtation with neuromodulation provides us with an opportunity to interrogate what we are asking of, and for, our children. Indeed, it demands that we ask these questions. Many of the issues we consider can be applied to more familiar forms of cognitive enhancement, such as waking up with a cup of coffee, or going for a run to clear the head. Similarly, children are taught relaxation and meditation techniques in schools, to help them approach their work and behaviour with a new focus. If these less controversial strategies have the potential to change cognition, then they need cost-benefit analyses and ethical consideration in just the same way that neuromodulation techniques do: Taking the more extreme examples serves to bring the issues into starker relief. In the course of this chapter we also draw out some of the ethical issues raised by neuromodulation that bear relevance to the field of educational neuroscience more broadly.

Although this volume considers learning across the lifespan, there is considerably more literature on the ethics of neuromodulation in adults (e.g., Davis, 2017; Greely et al., 2008; Savulescu, 2006; Savulescu, Meulen, & Kahane, 2011), so here we will constrain our discussion to school-aged children.

What Is Neuromodulation and Does It Work?

Artificial enhancement may seem like science fiction, but it's already part of education. Slow-acting psychostimulants such as methylphenidate (e.g., Ritalin™) are a common prescription for children with Attention Deficit Hyperactivity Disorder (ADHD), but are also known to be used illicitly by healthy college students to help them study (Farah et al., 2004; Hall, 2003; Maier, Ferris, & Winstock, 2018; Singh, Bard, & Jackson, 2014). Non-therapeutic enhancement by prescription psychostimulants is one of the two forms of neuromodulation we consider in this chapter. The other is non-invasive brain stimulation using Transcranial Electrical Stimulation (tES). Both techniques have the potential to be used in the classroom, as they are portable, relatively inexpensive and arguably non-invasive (although see Davis & van Koningsbruggen, 2013). Compared to psychostimulants, the mechanisms by which brain stimulation operate are not well understood, and while there is some experimental evidence as to efficacy, it is not a generally accepted part of the clinical toolkit. This is a timely point at which to discuss the two together as they contribute slightly different perspectives to the debate but have fundamentally similar goals.

Slow-acting prescription psychostimulants, most notably methylphenidate (e.g., Ritalin™), amphetamine salts (e.g., Adderall™) and modafinil (e.g., Provigil™) are sometimes described as 'smart pills' (nootropics) due to the belief that they enhance cognition and performance in healthy individuals, releasing the potential of the human brain. These three types of stimulant have slightly different mechanisms of action, but all are thought to increase arousal by increasing concentrations of the neurotransmitters/neuromodulators dopamine and norepinephrine in certain parts of the brain (Wood, Sage, & Anagnostaras, 2014). For individuals with pathologically low levels of dopamine, as is believed to be the case in ADHD (e.g., Volkow et al., 2009), boosting levels of available dopamine is associated with an improvement in neuropsychological functioning in adults (Boonstra, Kooij, Oosterlaan, Sergeant, & Buitelaar, 2005). In the UK, 0.5% of under-16s have been prescribed psychostimulants, according to NHS records (Beau-Lejdstrom, Douglas, Evans, & Smeeth, 2016; also see McCarthy et al., 2012), and in the USA 8.4% of children are diagnosed with ADHD (Danielson et al., 2018), the majority of whom are prescribed psychostimulants. Although psychostimulants cannot be legally purchased over the counter, prescriptions are open to abuse and some doctors in the USA have reported prescribing medications for non-therapeutic cognitive enhancement (Hotze, Shah, Anderson, & Wynia, 2011). Estimates of the prevalence of psychostimulant use in the college population in America vary from 5.3%–55.0% (Smith & Farah, 2011), with the most common reason for non-prescription use being to help students stay awake to study (DeSantis, Noar, & Webb, 2009). Usage significantly increases during times of stress, including exams (Moore, Burgand, Larson, & Ferm, 2014). Although non-therapeutic use among college students is most common in the USA, it is documented in other countries (Castaldi et al., 2012; Eslami et al., 2014; Forlini, Schildmann, Roser, Beranek, & Vollmann, 2015; Singh et al., 2014) and a recent survey indicates a surge in use in European countries over the last few years (Maier et al., 2018).

In healthy young adults, low doses of slow-acting psychostimulants have been found to have a small positive effect on inhibitory control, working memory ($g = 0.13$), short-term episodic memory ($g = 0.20$; Ilieva, Hook, & Farah, 2015), and processing speed ($g = 0.28$; Marraccini, Weyandt, Rossi, & Gudmundsdottir, 2016), and a medium-sized positive effect on delayed episodic memory ($g = 0.45$; Ilieva et al., 2015). In adults they also result in an enhanced willingness to exert effort, particularly when a small reward is on offer (Wardle, Treadway, Mayo, Zald, & de Wit, 2011). However, at higher doses, rather than having a calming, focusing effect, psychostimulants act to substantially impair aspects of cognition reliant on the prefrontal cortex, rendering users distractible, inattentive and hyperactive (see Urban & Gao, 2014). At the time of writing, we are not aware of any studies that have explored the effects of psychostimulants on cognition in healthy children. That being said, psychostimulants are used by teenagers to support their school studies, in at least the USA (McCabe, Teter, & Boyd, 2004) and Canada (Poulin, 2001), suggesting (though not definitively) that there is at least a self-perceived efficacy in healthy children.

Non-invasive brain stimulation refers to directly altering the electrical activity of the brain using electrical or magnetic energy. This broad description encompasses quite a wide range of techniques, but for the purposes of talking about educational goals, the most relevant ones fall under the umbrella of transcranial electrical stimulation (tES; see Guleyupoglu, 2013 for a classification); specifically, transcranial direct current stimulation (tDCS). During tDCS, two or more electrodes are placed on the participating individual: one is positioned on the head over the area of brain that is of interest, while the other is placed elsewhere on the body contralaterally to complete the circuit; a constant low current is then passed between the electrodes. The effect of tDCS is tailored by altering the placement of the scalp electrode, the length of the stimulation session and the intensity and polarity of the current. The aim of tDCS is to change the excitability of neurons underlying the scalp electrode. Stimulation is not strong enough to induce neuronal firing, but is believed to alter the resting state of neurons (Nitsche, Fricke, & Henschke, 2003) such that either a stronger or weaker input is required to induce an action potential. Evidence for this mechanism of action comes from studies which measure the excitability of motor cortex as a function of tDCS by then applying transcranial magnetic stimulation (TMS) and measuring the resultant motor evoked potentials with electroencephalography (EEG; Nitsche & Paulus, 2000). Cortical excitability in adults has been repeatedly shown to be sensitive to modulation by tDCS in this way, with the duration, strength and polarity of the current determining how the motor cortex responds.

In theory, brain stimulation could alter the extent to which neurons are ready to fire in any area of cortex to which it is applied (Polanía, Paulus, Antal, & Nitsche, 2011): More ready firing allows more neurons to be recruited into plastic changes in the brain to increase performance on target behaviour in the future. The possibility of altering plasticity in this way has huge implications for educational neuroscience: If you set a goal for learning in the classroom and then alter your students' neural plasticity, it could improve learning times and possibly alter other outcomes such as degree or depth of learning, or how easily information is integrated into existing knowledge.

Currently, the potential of altered plasticity is largely speculative, but nonetheless intriguing. Evidence for changing cognition and performance in typically developing adults (see Buch et al., 2017 for a review) and to a much lesser extent, children (Cienchanski & Kirton, 2017) has certainly been seen. However, effects are neither consistent (Horvath, Forte, & Carter, 2015a, 2015b) nor well understood (Horvath et al., 2015a). In the context of non-therapeutic enhancement, we should also bear in mind that behavioural ceiling effects have been found to prevent a benefit of stimulation in skilled musicians (Furuya, Klaus, Nitsche, Paulus, & Altenmüller, 2014), reminding us that not everybody is likely to benefit from interventions to improve performance.

Broadly speaking then, neuromodulation by psychostimulant drugs or electrical stimulation have an effect, to some degree, in adults, but there is currently very little research considering empirical effects in healthy children. Before this line of research gathers pace unchecked, it is imperative that we take a step back and open the debate about the ethical implications of pursuing it. In order to inform this debate, the issue of publication bias should be considered. Publication bias refers to the preferential publication of positive findings and those with large effect sizes. This is something which has been specifically demonstrated with respect to the effects of psychostimulants on executive function (Ilieva et al., 2015), such that even the modest effects outlined here may be overestimations. Educational neuroscience is a field where practical changes can be rapidly made in the classroom by engaged and caring teachers. The research community therefore has a duty to take particular care to publish, discuss and communicate all findings which may inform teaching practice, be they in line with hypotheses or not.

Weighing Benefits and Risks

For the purpose of this chapter, we will use the term *stimulation* to refer to electrical brain stimulation, *nootropics* to talk about psychostimulants, and *neuromodulation* to talk about either. These techniques share the potential to alter performance in the classroom, but they also have important differences. Stimulation (tDCS in this context, but the arguments apply equally to other forms of tES) aims to alter cortical excitability and hence neural plasticity in targeted regions of the brain, while pills primarily affect attention and motivation: these commonalities and distinctions will guide our discussion.

We will take as our underlying premise that an ethically acceptable line of research has the potential to engender great benefits to individuals with minimal risks to health, wellbeing, personal identity and dignity. This is immediately problematic in the case of neuromodulation, because the available research in healthy adults suggests that the cognitive benefits an individual might expect to reap are small; in fact, they are equivalent to the effects of much more familiar enhancers like caffeine, exercise and sleep (Caviola & Faber, 2015). However, small benefits in cognitive performance could result in a step change if they push performance up just enough to get an A grade, or allow clearer focus in a job interview. Furthermore, neuromodulation is relatively new; future techniques are likely to be considerably more effective than the stimulation and nootropic options available today. For argument's sake, we will assume that the academic performance of healthy children could, in theory, be improved with the use of neuromodulation.

Boosting the cognitive ability and behavioural performance of children in schools could result in substantial rewards for an individual: for example, we know that academic performance is clearly linked to life outcomes such as employability and earnings (e.g., Current Population Surveys, 2004). The Welfarist argument (see Savulescu et al., 2011) runs that parents have a moral duty to maximise their children's welfare, and that more cognitive ability leads to enhanced welfare, such that parents have a moral obligation to enhance their children's cognition. The assumption that to enhance cognition improves something for the children who are enhanced is what drives research into neuromodulation. Arguably, many parents take a Welfarist view of cognitive enhancement every day when they feed fish oil supplements to their children: there's no good evidence to show that fish oil supplements enhance cognitive performance in healthy children with a varied diet, but children are given supplements because parents want to provide them with the best possible chance of success, in a safe, acceptable way. Although those who advocate the Welfarist argument have not practically defined welfare or shown that improved cognition contributes to it (Krutzinna, 2016), both researchers and parents often take the general line that a cognitive boost is a good thing.

Risks to Cognitive Performance

Unexpected Outcomes

If we accept that neuromodulation has (or will have) the power to result in positive changes in the brain, then we must also accept that it has the power to result in negative changes, or at least unanticipated changes. Just because a child receives neuromodulation to improve their maths skills does not mean that the only consequence of that modulation protocol will be a change to maths ability. One obvious example in the case of psychostimulants like methylphenidate are the known physical side effects, which range from the largely innocuous (like tingling in the extremities) to the more concerning (like anxiety, vomiting, psychosis and heart problems). Methylphenidate is also known to interact harmfully with other common drugs, including the decongestant phenylephrine found in cold medicines (Nevels, Weiss, Killebrew, & Gontkovsky, 2013). These non-desired effects have been deemed acceptable by medical regulators when the drugs are used in their intended way to combat disease or disorder, but not for use in healthy populations (Drabiak-Siad, 2011). Cognitive trade-offs are also emerging; for example, in a study of chess performance in adults, the benefits of nootropics with respect to reflective decision making was balanced by the increased time that players took to make a move (Franke et al., 2017). It may be difficult to predict such cognitive trade-offs in children and adolescents based on research in adults given that a low dosage of methylphenidate in adolescent rats has the opposite effect on neuronal activity in the prefrontal cortex compared to adult rats (Urban,

Waterhouse, & Gao, 2012), suggesting that optimal nootropic doses are critically age-dependent. Similarly, the effect of tDCS on the excitability of the motor system differs in children and adolescents compared to adults (Moliadze et al., 2018).

In the case of electrical stimulation, it would not be unreasonable to expect cognitive 'side effects', especially given that most stimulation protocols are currently not very topographically focused (see Davis & Koningsbruggen, 2013). This is somewhat akin to the effects of pain killers, which do not target pain in just the part of the body they are intended for. For example, stimulation over Broca's area may well affect cognitive functions known to be subserved by that area, such as verbal fluency (as has been shown: Bashir & Howell, 2017). However, Broca's area is intimately interconnected with much of the language network as well as its homologue in the opposite hemisphere, and any of these areas may show unpredicted changes in function if tested. Moreover, brain regions typically do more than one thing: The dorsolateral prefrontal cortex is often targeted in stimulation research, which can show positive outcomes for mathematics ability (Looi et al., 2017; Sarkar, Dowker, & Cohen Kadosh, 2014) and working memory ability (Ruf, Fallgatter, & Plewia, 2017). However, stimulation of this area has also been found to alter the likelihood of making high-risk, high-gain decisions (Zheng et al., 2017). This means that stimulation targeting one sort of behaviour, for example maths ability, could inadvertently alter children's behaviour in other, unexpected ways, influencing not just cognitive performance but judgement. We should perhaps be especially cautious here. Transfer effects, which refer to the impact of training in one cognitive domain on another, have been all too elusive in the cognitive training literature (e.g., Guye & von Bastian, 2017), but have been shown when tDCS is combined with more traditional training paradigms in healthy adults (Ruf et al., 2017; Trumbo et al., 2016; Yen Looi et al., 2016).

Critical to understanding the potential consequences of neuromodulation in childhood is the idea of neuroplasticity: The ability of the brain to change, usually in response to the environment. Plasticity is a feature of the human brain throughout life, but the nature and extent of that plasticity is dynamic, with high plasticity being a hallmark of the immature brain (see Power & Schlaggar, 2017 for a review). This is no coincidence: Plasticity is fundamental to the learning that babies and children must do to become culturally adapted adults. As the environment becomes more predictable in later life, a plastic brain is less critical to functioning. The majority of research into brain stimulation, which is thought to manipulate local plasticity, has been done with healthy young adults, so the short and long-term consequences of manipulating plasticity in an immature brain are not yet understood. The brain is in a delicate balance of stability and plasticity throughout life so that it can learn new information without disrupting the old. In manipulating one half of the balancing act, you risk encoding overly specific information and interfering with existing knowledge. A similar balance has been found in the case of methylphenidate, which is thought to directly manipulate the plasticity of the prefrontal cortex. Manipulating plasticity in this region has been hypothesised to increase long-term memory at the cost of behavioural flexibility (Urban & Gao, 2014). Changes to the developing system, which in the case of the prefrontal cortex means any time up to early adulthood, may well have lasting effects. For example, one study with rats found that adult animals show increased anxiety behaviours in response to stressful situations if they were exposed to methylphenidate in adolescence (Bolaños, Barrot, Berton, Wallace-Black, & Nestler, 2003). In making decisions about the modulation of children's brains then we may unintentionally be making decisions about the neural functioning of those individuals much later in life.

Predicting the consequences of neuromodulation arguably becomes a more acute problem if we think about the *when* of intervention. One of the areas of greatest potential for educational neuroscience is predicting which children may go on to show educational difficulties before they start school. One example of this is the use of electrophysiological measures in infancy to predict which children are at risk of poor reading skills later in childhood (Guttorm, Leppänen, Hämäläinen, Eklund, & Lyytinen, 2010). There is currently very little research seriously considering early versus later intervention, but the underlying assumption is that if the plasticity of the brain diminishes over time then, theoretically, earlier prediction and intervention stands a better chance of success. If non-therapeutic neuromodulation becomes an acceptable part of the educational landscape, does that therefore mean it should be considered in infancy? Earlier implementation could bring greater positive, but also potentially negative, results. This may seem a little implausible given that neuromodulation is often intended to increase the infant-like properties of the brain. However, the point for educational neuroscience is that the field should consider what level of intervention is acceptable, at what age, and given what degree of certainty that an educational issue will become apparent later in childhood. Indeed, are the pre-school years within the remit of educational neuroscience at all?

Individual Differences

The ethical implications of cognitive enhancement protocols are not just a question of what happens at the group level: Different individuals respond differently to the same interventions, just as people differ in their metabolism of, and preferences around, caffeine consumption (see Nehlig, 2018). Even the robust effect of brain stimulation on the excitability of the motor cortex shows substantial variability, with up to 50% of healthy adults showing a minor or no response to stimulation (Wiethoff, Hamada, & Rothwell, 2014; and see Li, Uehara, & Hanakawa, 2015). This means that a risk-benefit analysis done at the group level may only be pertinent to some individuals. An educationally relevant example of this individual variability is provided by Sarkar et al. (2014), who studied the effects of stimulation in the prefrontal cortex during a maths training task in adults and found improved reaction times and lowered cortisol in those with high maths anxiety, but slowed reaction times and no decrease in cortisol compared to sham stimulation in individuals with low maths anxiety. Notably, both groups showed impaired executive control alongside the maths-specific changes.

Other factors have also been found to drive variability in response to neuromodulation. These include: performance at baseline, with stimulation (Yen Looi et al., 2016) being more beneficial for those who start off with lower baseline scores; cognitive ability, with nootropics being more beneficial for individuals with lower IQ (Randall, Shneerson, & File, 2005); and genotype, with the COMT genotype (which determines how quickly a person can break down dopamine in the brain) influencing whether nootropics improve or degrade performance on certain tasks (Mattay et al., 2003). This suggests a massive amount of data need to be collected on the effects of neuromodulation techniques across individuals covering different behavioural, cognitive, genetic and contextual factors to effectively target intervention.

This point reflects a wider challenge in educational neuroscience: how to scale-up interventions in the face of massive individual variability. Just because an intervention has a positive effect at the group level doesn't mean that every individual in that group will benefit; indeed, some may show a negative response. Without sensitive measures to predict who is likely to benefit from an intervention, we run the risk of improving outcomes for some children at the cost of worsening outcomes for others. Looking forward, this kind of predictive power may be possible; for example, Hoeft et al. (2011) were able to use brain responses during a reading task to predict which children with dyslexia went on to benefit from an intervention.

The Context of the Classroom

So far, the work considering cognitive effects of enhancers have looked at individual performance on tasks in the lab, while educational neuroscience is concerned not with the lab, but with the classroom. Faber et al. (Faber, Häusser, & Kerr, 2017) have developed a framework for considering how the effects of neuromodulation might be modified by a group context: the "Effects of Grouping on Impairments and Enhancements" (GIE) framework. The framework was developed by asking how sleep deprivation and caffeine alter task performance when individuals work on their own, compared to when they work in a group. The authors show that, generally speaking, sleep deprivation has a greater negative effect when individuals are working as part of a group compared to working alone, and that a small-to-medium dose of caffeine has a greater benefit for individuals working in groups than for individuals working alone. The moderating effect of group context is thought to depend on changes in motivation, changes in individual capability as a result of input from other group members, and the ability of the group to co-ordinate their individual contributions. Although this research relates more directly to situations where a team has a specific goal in the context of the workplace, it should remind us that children learn and develop in a group setting in school, and that the consequences of any educational intervention, including neuro-modulation, must be evaluated in that group context. In classrooms children work together on the same material, they share ideas, they receive scaffolding from teaching staff and they encounter environmental noise; each of these factors will alter the performance of the individual, and we therefore cannot directly extrapolate the effects of neuromodulation in the lab to the noisy, co-operative classroom.

Not only do these potential cognitive risks make it very difficult to evaluate the real-world benefit of neuromodulation, it also makes consent in educational neuroscience a particularly tricky issue. Consent, and assent, should be given on the basis of 'adequate information' (British Psychological Society, 2014), yet the full effects of this class of interventions cannot reasonably be said to be known. Even the long-term consequences of commonly used psychostimulants in the developing brain are largely unknown; they are certainly complex and dependent on age, duration and dosage of drug use (see Berman, Kuczenski, McCracken, & London, 2009 for a thorough review). The idea that parents and adolescents could be capable of digesting this information to give informed consent, even if the data were available, is entirely unreasonable. This is an example of the kind of ethical question that scientists face in the everyday management of educational neuroscience research.

Risks to Psychological Well-being

The Child

The potential effects of neuromodulation on mental state are difficult to predict, though we can look at the limited data from children who take psychostimulants for ADHD and consider how neuromodulation may impact psychological traits known to influence academic and non-academic function.

Firstly, what might neuromodulation do to children's attitudes and how might that affect academic performance? To a degree, academic performance is predicted by how children approach their work. Achievement in school at various ages and stages has been found to be predicted by effort and perseverance (Lee, 2013), resilience in the face of failure (Martin & Marsh, 2006), and adaptability in the face of uncertainty and novelty (Martin, Nejad, Colmar, & Liem, 2013), though the predictive power of attitudes to schoolwork may be subsumed by the Big Five personality trait 'conscientiousness', which predicts 6% of the variance in GCSE grades (Rimfeld, Kovas, Dale, & Plomin, 2016). It is quite conceivable that if children receive neuromodulation and believe it will make learning easier, then that may reduce the determination and effort with which they approach their schoolwork. A further potential factor is the growth mindset: the tendency when faced with, for example, a difficult maths problem to think 'I can't do this maths problem because I haven't learned how to do it yet' rather than 'I can't do this maths problem because I'm bad at maths'. Although not an uncontroversial idea (see Sisk, Burgoyone, Sun, Butler, & Macnamara, 2018 for meta-analyses of growth mindset research), Carol Dweck and colleagues have found the growth mindset both to predict academic success (Claro, Paunesku, & Dweck, 2016) and to promote academic success (Paunescu et al., 2015). Conceivably, neuromodulation could disrupt a growth mindset, promoting the response 'I can't do this maths problem because I haven't taken my pill today'.

The psychological risks that neuromodulation engenders go beyond academic performance and extend to personality, personal identity and the notion of the self. Effects on personality have been frequently reported in studies on the side effects of psychostimulants in children with ADHD. Personality changes that result from methylphenidate are generally poorly described, but when reported the most common are 'irritability' (0%–80%), 'prone to crying' (1%–71%), 'staring' (21%–62%), and 'anxiety' (2%–61%); it is not clear if these symptoms persist after medication stops (Konrad-Bindl, Gresser, & Richartz, 2016). Children themselves report that personality changes contribute to negative feelings towards psychostimulant medication (Harpur, Thompson, Daley, Abikoff, & Sonuga-Barke, 2008). Similar effects have not yet been explored in response to stimulation but doing so will be important in understanding the risks of neuromodulation for healthy children.

Society

Societal response is a very practical consideration here, as attitudes may alter the effects of neuromodulation, and define how individuals who have used these techniques are treated in academic endeavours, employment and personal relationships. Faber, Douglas, Heise, and Hewstone (2015) explored how non-users in the general public perceive cognitive enhancement and motivation enhancement. A scenario was presented to participants based on a student taking either 'smart pills; to think faster and more clearly', or 'motivation pills; to be keener to study and overcome motivational problems'. Participants were then asked to make judgements about the student's exam success, giving ratings of how fair they thought success to be, how much the student deserved that success, how much effort they had put in, and overall how acceptable their cognitive enhancement was. Broadly, participants perceived any pharmacological enhancement to be morally unacceptable. The more participants judged effort to be necessary for an individual to deserve success, the more the use of enhancement was judged morally wrong and the less they deemed the enhancement-user to deserve success. If the student had taken a 'smart pill' they tended to be judged as being less deserving of praise and success, and the 'smart pill' was judged as more morally wrong, with success resulting from taking it to be more unfair than taking the 'motivation pill'. Judgements of unfairness were found to drive judgements of moral unacceptability of the smart pill (Faber, Savulescu, & Douglas, 2016). This suggests that the sort of neuromodulation that nootropics offer would be more morally acceptable to the public than brain stimulation, with the attribution of performance being a key factor in the negative appraisal of modulation (Faulmüller, Maslen, & de Sio, 2013). Other work suggests that the public are generally open to cognitive enhancement (Fitz, Nadler, Manogaran, Chong, & Reiner, 2014), but have concerns about medical safety, coercion, and fairness (Schelle, Faumüller, Caviola, & Hewstone, 2014).

Pharmacological enhancement is also seen as powerful by the public. Ilieva, Boland, and Farah (2013) explored the cognitive benefits of mixed amphetamine salts (Adderall™) in healthy adults. They show that while the drug did not result in any notable improvement on any cognitive task or on overall performance, participants did report an increased *belief* of cognitive enhancement, compared to those who took a placebo pill. Degree of perceived improvement was largely unrelated to actual improvement. Public ideas about the power of nootropics may result from the considerable media coverage of pharmacological enhancers (Partridge et al., 2011), including films such as *Limitless* (Dixon, Kroopf, Kavanaugh, & Burger, 2011) and *Lucy* (Besson-Silla & Besson, 2014), in which individuals become cognitive superheroes after taking drugs which 'release their potential'. Nootropics are also believed to reduce the self-esteem of users and make users appear more intelligent than they are (Forlini & Racine, 2010). Healthy young adults reported that they would be more reluctant to enhance traits which they felt were more fundamental to their self-identities (e.g., social comfort) compared with traits which they saw as less fundamental (e.g., concentration ability) (Riis, Simmons, & Goodwin, 2008). This speaks to the belief that neuromodulation has the power to fundamentally change who we are. It is interesting to note that, although nootropics and brain stimulation are only as effective as cognitive enhancers such as caffeine and exercise, they are viewed as fundamentally different with respect to acceptability and fairness (Caviola & Faber, 2015). In the classroom these attitudes could translate to under-acknowledgement of hard work, and a more competitive environment centred around the acquisition of neuromodulators.

A Question of Fairness

Socioeconomic Status

When considering a technique for cognitive enhancement which has the potential to make a difference to an individual's cognitive profile, there is an argument that it should be wielded to support education goals for the least advantaged members of society (Ray, 2016). There are currently strong socioeconomic gradients in educational opportunity and attainment, both within countries and between them. In developed countries such as the United States and Canada, low socioeconomic status predicts slow early cognitive development (Morgan, Farkas, Hillemeier, & Maczuga, 2009), lower rates of school readiness at age five (Thomas, 2006), poor achievement throughout school (Phipps & Lethbridge, 2007), higher secondary school drop-out rates

486   *Victoria Knowland*

(National Center for Education Statistics, 2008), fewer well-qualified teachers in the classroom (Clotfelter, Ladd, & Vigdo, 2006), and being less ready for the world of work at the end of school (Diemer & Ali, 2009). In the case where children are disadvantaged relative to their peers, substantial negative mental health outcomes have been observed (McLaughlin, Costello, Leblanc, Sampson, & Kessler, 2012). Education inequality sustains and widens achievement gaps between the wealthy and the poor.

Levelling the Playing Field

Currently, those using psychostimulants as a study aid in developed countries tend to be college students, who already have a substantial educational advantage and are more likely to come from advantaged backgrounds (U.S. Census Bureau, 2000). Around 80% of psychostimulants are consumed in the USA (Scheffler, Hinshaw, Modrek, & Levine, 2007), the wealthiest country in the world. If left unchecked, market forces will continue to drive this unequal distribution of nootropics. The question, then, is could neuromodulation be harnessed instead to close the educational achievement gap, instead of widening it?

All the research related to this question addresses nootropics but speaks equally well to brain stimulation. Before considering whether neuromodulation could be used to level the playing field in any given country, it first needs to be established that doing so is a key educational goal. Indeed, this is a question for the whole field of educational neuroscience: The provision of equal educational opportunities for all by boosting performance at the bottom of league tables is quite distinct from supporting a few individuals to perform at the peak of, or beyond, current species-typical ability by boosting performance at the top of league tables. Beyond the moral arguments, one clear incentive for a level field comes from a study of mathematics achievement in the 13-to14-year-olds around the world, which found a negative correlation between dispersion of test scores and median test score for that country (Freeman, Machin, & Viarengo, 2010). Countries are therefore likely to gain more in terms of overall educational outcome by improving scores at the bottom than by increasing scores at the top; and given that education outcomes predict a country's long-term economic growth (Lindahl & Krueger, 2001; Lutz, Creso Cuaresma, & Sanderson, 2008), equality is a wise policy decision. Notably though, neuromodulation may not lead to equal gains across countries. The value of boosting individual cognitive faculties may vary depending on what the constraining factors in educational achievement are. Nieto and Ramos (2015) explored the explanatory power of individual factors (e.g., motivation), school factors (e.g., resource availability), and teaching factors (e.g., training) in relation to science and reading achievement in two high-income countries and ten middle-income countries. The authors found that individual factors provided the most explanatory power for science achievement in the high-income countries, while for middle-income countries, and reading across the board, school factors were the best predictors of success. For the moment then, the question of whether neuromodulation can be harnessed to address educational inequality relates most clearly to the socioeconomic gradient within developed nations.

Enhancement or Treatment?

It has been argued that we not only have the option of addressing educational inequality with neuromodulation, but a moral duty to do so (Ray, 2016; Sandberg & Savulescu, 2011). Ray (2016) suggests that giving stimulants to less advantaged children could be thought of as 'opportunity maintenance', and that this could be a practical solution to the issue of educational inequality in the current social and political landscape. Ray argues that stimulants should be used to remedy social deficits that impact on well-being, given that educational opportunities result in a wider array of options later in life, freeing children from their social shackles.

The main ethical argument against this practice is that to provide neuromodulation as a 'treatment' for a cognitive issue of social origin would grossly misattribute the academic problems that children from disadvantaged backgrounds face, pathologising a non-pathological state. If we know that some children are falling behind because of environmental constraints, then trying to address that gap with anything other than environmental solutions could be seen to place both the blame and the impetus to remedy it on the children themselves. Stevenson (2016) suggests that a programme of neuromodulation would exacerbate students' tendency to self-pathologise by making them feel that they are not normal without that modulation, as well as making them feel that they are dependent on modulation to achieve their goals and overcome their environmental disadvantage. Sattler and Singh (2016) present further concerns over the risk to human dignity and the social exclusion that selective neuromodulation would result in. In addition, they point out that social inequality often goes hand in hand with racial inequality, and that selectively providing enhancement for a population over-represented by certain ethic or cultural groups is tacit racism.

Interactions Between Cognition and Context

The consequences of neuromodulation in the classroom could certainly interact with social context, and this could be true when we consider both enhanced plasticity and the effects of psychostimulants on attention. Consider a brain stimulation technique like tDCS, which increases the plasticity of some area of cortex. How long tDCS acts for depends on the length of each session and the number and frequency of sessions, but a single, ten-minute session can result in enhanced plasticity for up to an hour in adults (Nitsche et al., 2008). In that hour, a child may encounter all sorts of stimuli not directly related to the training paradigm, and the nature of those stimuli may well vary by socioeconomic status. If the susceptibility of the brain to change in response to environmental stimuli is changed, then experiences with potentially negative content or valance may have more of an impact on that child than they would have done without the brain stimulation. While it is not yet clear what the medium-term effects of brain stimulation might be, one possible mechanism of action is via changes in brain derived neurotrophic factor (BDNF) in the hippocampus. In mice BDNF has been shown to be elevated for a full week after a single 20-minute session of tDCS, resulting in increased long-term potentiation (Podda et al., 2016) and opening up the possibility of much longer-term vulnerability to negative experiences. In the case of an intervention working to improve focused attention in the classroom, neuromodulation could have a positive effect on academic attainment at school but be uniquely detrimental for children from deprived backgrounds. Low socioeconomic status is associated with a more stressful home environment, and children who are exposed to stressful home environments show greater levels of threat assessment (vigilance) (Chen & Matthews, 2001; and see Matthews, Gallo, & Taylor, 2010), and a tendency to process task-irrelevant auditory information (Stevens, Lauinger, & Neville, 2009). While targeting this 'failure' of selective attention might make sense in the context of the classroom, that manipulation could prove detrimental at home. Interactions between the potential cognitive risks of neuromodulation and factors such as stress, diet, and sleep deprivation, which vary systematically by socioeconomic status (Alkerwi, Vernier, Sauvageot, Crichton, & Elias, 2015; Jarrin, McGrath, & Quon, 2014), have not been studied.

Possible interactions between socioeconomic status and intervention are a good example of how our discussion of neuromodulation is directly relevant to more socially acceptable forms of cognitive enhancement in children. Mindfulness is a practice commonly taught in schools, in which children learn to reduce stress by focusing on bodily sensations and perceptions happening at that moment rather than allowing their mind to wander. As growing up in low socioeconomic circumstances has been associated with chronic stress (Vliegenthart et al., 2016), some have suggested that mindfulness techniques may be especially helpful for children from these backgrounds to help relieve that stress (Ortiz & Sibinga, 2017). However, mindfulness meditation has also been associated with negative effects such as depression and anxiety (Lustyk, Chawla, Nolan, & Marlatt, 2009), believed to result from a focus on internal states. Conceivably this negative effect could be moderated by children's socioeconomic status, and at least this possibility has not been considered thoroughly enough for the practice to be safely used universally in school-aged children.

Practicalities

Asking ethical questions in educational neuroscience means asking questions whose answers confer practical value (Stein & Fischer, 2011). Consider the

Welfarist stance that, as cognitive advantage amounts to social advantage and a better life, those who need a bigger dose of a better life need neuromodulation. Presumably this argument is predicated on there being a gap between potential and achievement; in the case of socioeconomic status, this gap is the result of environmental factors. Would neuromodulation then be provided to children who fall below a certain poverty line, or who demonstrate that their potential is not being realised? And if the latter, could any child receive neuromodulation on the grounds that they are not realising their potential for any number of reasons? Selective provision of neuromodulation may result in differences in how children perceive their own academic success and, far from closing a gap, would create a new one driven by differential treatment, which may cause social problems even greater than the ones the intervention seeks to solve.

For neuromodulation to be a useful tool in the fight against educational inequality, it would need to show not only a substantial cognitive benefit, but also a much larger benefit to those from disadvantaged backgrounds compared to their more advantaged peers. Beyond the cognitive effects though, neuromodulation would have to be equally available to all. Without this condition, the social disadvantages to selective neuromodulation would likely far outweigh any potential cognitive benefits.

Neurodevelopmental Disorders

Using neuromodulation to support cognitive development in children with neurodevelopmental disorders can be seen as fundamentally different to using it for children who have no identified needs. By neurodevelopmental disorders, we mean children who have a disorder of the development of the central nervous system, such as autism spectrum disorders, ADHD, or dyslexia. While the conversation around neuromodulation in typically developing children is about the enhancement of cognition, neuromodulation in the case of a child who has a specific cognitive deficit is a treatment. A focus group of parents, some of whose children had developmental disorders, was clear in the view that for children with disabilities, nootropics can be a valid treatment to bring children's performance up to an average level, so long as they are safe, while for typically developing children the benefits are not evident enough to outweigh the risks (Ball & Wolbring, 2014).

Neuromodulation techniques are showing some promise in the case of neurodevelopmental disorders; for example, tDCS has been shown to enhance the effectiveness of a reading intervention for a group of children with dyslexia (Costanzo et al., 2018). However, research in this area also illustrates a cautionary tale for educational neuroscience. Working at the level of the brain is not a shortcut to remediation, and trying to normalise the brain activity of individuals with neurodevelopmental disorders (e.g., Kang et al., 2018) without understanding links to behavioural functioning or the nature of compensatory mechanisms in the brain could have serious adverse implications for children.

In contrast to stimulation, which is at the beginning of a clinical journey, psychostimulants have already proven to be a valuable tool in supporting children with ADHD to manage their symptoms. Their widespread use has also offered valuable insight into the possible negative consequences of neuromodulation in childhood. Some risks are evident; for example, social stigma is a reality for many children taking psychostimulants. A literature review from 2012 (Mueller, Fuermaier, Koerts, & Tucha, 2012) highlights stigmatising beliefs about ADHD medication, including concerns about becoming addicted, not being in control and feeling different from peers. Analysis of parental and child responses to the Southampton ADHD Medication Behavior and Attitudes Scale showed that although parents perceived the benefits of medication over and above the risks, children themselves focused on the risks, including decreased levels of pleasure and activity and negative changes to personality, with perception of risks being related to perception of stigma (Harpur, Thompson, Daley, Abikoff, & Sonuga-Barke, 2008).

Conclusions

What Is the Unique Contribution of Neuroscience Here?

The primary focus of this chapter has been considering which factors could be important in an analysis of the potential benefits and costs inherent to the development of new types of classroom practice. Ethical intervention fundamentally comes down to this kind of analysis, and to inform it we need to both describe and explain the behavioural and cognitive consequences of new practices. Psychological studies have been highly informative in the *description* of these effects, but the power of neuroscience (and cognitive neuroscience) comes in *explaining* it. Studies of neurophysiological mechanisms allow us to map and predict what happens when different people receive a given intervention in different contexts. Neuroscience will also be crucial in the development of new neuromodulatory techniques and the optimisation of current ones. For example, understanding the genetic and neurobiological factors which drive change with modulation could lead to tailored programmes to maximise individual benefit in the classroom.

What Are the Practical Implications of This Research?

The work outlined here shows us the sort of considerations that should drive research in this area. There is nothing to say that research into cognitive enhancement shouldn't be done or that neuromodulation shouldn't be used— that's up to individuals and societies. As in the case of caffeine use, social conventions and expectations adjust over time to the use of new cognitive enhancers in adulthood, and trial and error by a large population can work through potential interactions and individual differences. People regulate their own caffeine intake well and there is little judgement from others about the way this is done. In time the range of acceptable cognitive enhancers may include not only off-prescription medications and at-home brain stimulation, but micro-doses of currently illegal substances such as LSD.

The fundamental question is how this relates to children. If educational neuroscience ultimately shares the same goals as education, then to direct research in this area we need to ask: What is it that we value about education? As Bostrom and Sandberg (2009) so aptly put it: 'If school is seen as being significantly about the acquisition of information and learning, then cognitive enhancements may have a legitimate and useful role to play'. However, school is also about grades and competition and going on to a place at university or a job. In which case, is education something that can only fulfil its purpose when pursued without artificial enhancement?

Neuromodulation is one of a small set of tools currently being developed and evaluated with a view to boosting general cognition. This set includes meditation, exercise, working memory training and chess. The fact that these techniques are popular tell us a bit about what we want from education—we want children to attend, be motivated, to explore, to be receptive to teaching. Educational neuroscience has an important role to play in the ethical development of these interventions by having available answers to the questions about risk and benefit that people are going to ask.

Further Resources

A number of excellent, thought-provoking articles have been written on this subject, including

- Hall, S. (2003). The quest for a smart pill. *Scientific American, 289*, 54–65.
- Sandel, M. (2004). The case against perfection. *The Atlantic Monthly, 293*(3), 51–62.
- Schwarz, A. (2012). Retrieved from www.nytimes.com/2012/10/09/health/attention-disorder-or-not-children-prescribed-pills-to-help-in-school.html

And for overviews of the academic literature, see:

- Davis, N. J. (2014). Transcranial stimulation of the developing brain: A plea for extreme caution. *Frontiers in Human Neuoscience, 8*, 600.
- Cohen Kadosh, R., Levy, N., O'Shea, J., & Savulescu, J. (2012). The neuroethics of non-invasive brain stimulation. *Current Biology, 22*(4), R108–R111.
- Maslen, H., Earp, B. D., Cohen Kadosh, R., & Savulescu, J. (2014). Brain stimulation for treatment and enhancement in children: an ethical analysis. *Frontiers in Human Neuroscience, 8*, 953.
- Urban, K. R., & Gao, W.-J. (2014). Performance enhancement at the cost of potential brain plasticity: Neural ramifications of nootropic drugs in the healthy developing brain. *Frontiers in Systems Neuroscience, 8*, 38.

References

Alkerwi, A., Vernier, C., Sauvageot, N., Crichton, G. E., & Elias, M. F. (2015). Demographic and socioeconomic disparity in nutrition: Application of a novel correlated component regression approach. *BMJ Open, 5*, e006814. doi 10.1136/bmjopen-2014-006814

Ball, N., & Wolbring, G. (2014). Cognitive enhancement: Perceptions among parents of children with disabilities. *Neuroethics, 7*, 345–364. doi:10.1007/s12152-014-9201-8

Bashir, N., & Howell, P. (2017). P198 tDCS stimulation of the left inferior frontal gyrus in a connected speech task with fluent speakers. *Clinical Neurophysiology, 128*(3), e111 doi:10.1016/j.clinph.2016.10.317

Beau-Lejdstrom, R., Douglas, I., Evans, S. J. W., & Smeeth, L. (2016). Latest trends in ADHD drug prescribing patterns in children in the UK: Prevalence, incidence and persistence. *BMJ Open, 6*, e010508. doi:10.1136/bmjopen-2015-010508

Berman, S. M., Kuczenski, R., McCracken, J. T., & London, E. D. (2009). Potential adverse effects of amphetamine treatment on brain and behaviour: A review. *Molecular Psychiatry, 14*(2), 123–142. doi:10.1038/mp.2008.90

Besson-Silla, V. (Producer) & Besson, L. (Director). (2014). *Lucy* [Motion Picture]. USA: TF1 Films.

Bolaños, C. A., Barrot, M., Berton, O., Wallace-Black, D., & Nestler, E. J. (2003). Methylphenidate alters behavioural responses to emotional stimuli at adulthood. *Biological Psychiatry, 54*(12), 1317–1329.

Boonstra, A. M., Kooij, J. J., Oosterlaan, J., Sergeant, J. A., & Buitelaar, J. K. (2005). Does methylphenidate improve inhibition and other cognitive abilities in adults with childhood-onset ADHD? *Journal of Clinical and Experimental Neuropsychology, 27*(3), 278–298.

Bostrom, N., & Sandberg, A. (2009). Cognitive enhancement: Methods, ethics, regulatory challenges. *Science and Engineering Ethics, 15*(3), 311–341.

British Psychological Society. (2014). *Code of human research ethics.* Leicester: The British Psychological Society.

Bruer, J. T., & Greenough, W. T. (2001). The subtle science of how experience affects the brain. In D. B. Bailey, J. T. Bruer, F. J. Symons, & J. W. Lichtman (Eds.), *Critical thinking about critical periods* (pp. 209–232). Baltimore: Brooks Publishing Co.

Buch, E. R., Santarnecchi, E., Antal, A., Born, J., Celnik, P. A., Classen, J., . . . Cohen, L. G. (2017). Effects of tDCS on motor learning and memory formation: A consensus and critical position paper. *Clinical Neurophysiology, 128*(4), 589–603.

Castaldi, S., Gelatti, U., Orizio, G., Hartung, U., Moreno-Londono, A. M., & Schultz, P. J. (2012). Use of cognitive enhancement medication among Northern Italian university students. *Journal of Addiction Medicine, 6*(2), 112–117.

Caviola, L., & Faber, N. S. (2015). Pills or push-ups? Effectiveness and public perception of pharmacological and non-pharmacological cognitive enhancement. *Frontiers in Psychology, 6*. doi:10.3389/fpsyg.2015.01852

Chen, E., & Matthews, K. A. (2001). Cognitive appraisal biases: An approach to understanding the relation between socioeconomic status and cardiovascular reactivity in children. *Annals of Behavioral Medicine, 23*(2), 101–111.

Cienchanski, P., & Kirton, Z. A. (2017). Neurophysiological mechanisms of transcranial direct-current stimulation-enhanced motor learning in healthy children. *Clinical Neurophysiology, 128*(3), e137. doi:10.1016/j.clinph.2016.10.367

Claro, S., Paunesku, D., & Dweck, C. (2016). Growth mindset tempers the effects of poverty on academic achievement. *PNAS, 113*(31), 8664–8668. doi:10.1073/pnas.168207113

Clotfelter, C. T., Ladd, H. F., & Vigdor, J. L. (2006). Teacher-student matching and the assessment of teacher effectiveness. *Journal of Human Resources, 41*, 778–820. doi:10.3368/jhr.XLI.4.778

Costanzo, F., Rossi, S., Varuzza, C., Varvara, P., Vicari, S., & Menghini, D. (2018). Long-lasting improvement following tDCS treatment combined with a training for reading in children and adolescents with dyslexia. *Neuropsychologia.* doi:10.1016/j.neuropsychologia.2018.03.016. [Epub ahead of print]

Danielson, M. L., Bitsko, R. M., Ghandour, J. R., Holbrook, M., Kogan, M. D., & Blumberg, S. J. (2018). Prevalence of parent-reported ADHD diagnosis and associated treatment among U.S. children and adolescents, 2016. *Journal of Clinical Child and Adolescent Psychiatry, 47*(2), 199–212.

Davis, N. J. (2017). A taxonomy of harms inherent in cognitive enhancement. *Frontiers in Human Neuroscience, 11*, 63. doi:10.3389/fnhum.2017.00063

Davis, N. J., & van Koningsbruggen, M. G. (2013). "Non-invasive" brain stimulation is not non-invasive. *Frontiers in Systems Neuroscience, 7*, 76. doi:10.3389/fnsys.2013.00076

DeSantis, A. D., Noar, S. M., & Webb, E. M. (2009). Non-medical ADHD stimulant use in fraternities. *Journal of Studies on Alcohol and Drugs, 70*, 952–954.

Diemer, M. A., & Ali, S. R. (2009). Integrating social class into vocational psychology: Theory and practice implications. *Journal of Career Assessment, 17*, 247–265. doi:10.1177/1069072708330462

Dixon, L., Kroopf, S., Kavanaugh, R. (Producers) & Burger, N. (Director). (2011). *Limitless* [Motion Picture]. USA: Virgin.

Drabiak-Siad, K. (2011). Physicians prescribing "medicine" for enhancement: Why we should not and cannot overlook safety concerns. *The American Journal of Bioethics, 11*(1), 17–19. doi:10.1080/15265161.2010.534535

Eslami, A. A., Jalilan, F., Ataee, M., Alavijeh, M. M., Mahboubi, M., Afsar, A., & Aghaei, A. (2014). Intention and willingness in understanding Ritilin misuse among Iranian medical college students: A cross-sectional study. *Global Journal of Health Science, 6*(6), 43–53. doi:10.5539/gjhs.v6n6p43

Faber, N. S., Douglas, T., Heise, F., & Hewstone, M. (2015). Cognitive enhancement and motivation enhancement: An empirical comparison of intuitive judgements. *AJOB Neuroscience.* doi:10.1080/215077.2014.991847

Faber, N. S., Häusser, J. A., & Kerr, N. L. (2017). Sleep deprivation impairs and caffeine enhances my performance, but not always our performance. *Personality and Social Psychology Review, 21*(1), 3–28. doi:10.1177/1088868315609487

Faber, N. S., Savulescu, J., & Douglas, T. (2016). Why is cognitive enhancement deemed unacceptable? The role of fairness, deservingness, and hollow achievements. *Frontiers in Psychology, 7*, Article number 232. doi:10.3389/fpsyg.2016.00232

Farah, M. J., Illes, J., Cook-Deegan, R., Gardener, H., Kandel, E., King, P., . . . Root Wolpe, P. (2004). Neurocognitive enhancement: What can we do and what should we do? *Nature Reviews Neuroscience, 5*, 421–425.

Faulmüller, N., Maslen, H., & de Sio, F. S. (2013). The indirect psychological costs of cognitive enhancement. *American Journal of Bioethics, 13*(7), 45–47. doi:10.1080/15265161.2013.794880

Fischer, K. W., Goswami, U., Geake, J., & Task Force on the Future of Educational Neuroscience. (2010). The future of educational neuroscience. *Mind, Brain, and Education, 4*, 68–80.

Fitz, N. S., Nadler, R., Manogaran, P., Chong, E. W., & Reiner, P. B. (2014). Public attitudes toward cognitive enhancement. *Neuroethics, 7*(2), 173–188.

Forlini, C., & Racine, E. (2010). Stakeholder perspectives and reactions to "academic" cognitive enhancement: Unsuspected meaning of ambivalence and analogies. *Public Understanding of Science, 21*, 606–625. doi:10.1177/0963662510385062

Forlini, C., Schildmann, J., Roser, P., Beranek, R., & Vollmann, J. (2015). Knowledge, experiences and views of German university students toward neuroenhancement: An empirical-ethical analysis. *Neuroethics, 8*(2), 83–92.

Franke, A. G., Gränsmark, P., Agricola, A., Schühle, K, Rommel, T., Sebastian, A., . . . Lieb, K. (2017). Methylphenidate, modafinil, and caffeine for cognitive enhancement in chess: A double-blind randomised controlled trial. *European Neuropsychopharmacology, 27*, 248–260.

Freeman, R. B., Machin, S. J., & Viarengo, M. G. (2010). *Variation in educational outcomes and policies across countries and of schools within countries*. London: Centre for the Economics of Education.

Furuya, S., Klaus, M., Nitsche, M. A., Paulus, W., & Altenmüller, E. (2014). Ceiling effects prevent further improvement of transcranial stimulation in skilled musicians. *Journal of Neuroscience, 34*(41), 13834–13839. doi:10.1523/JNEUROSCI.1170-14.2014

Greely, H., Sahakian, B., Harris, J., Kessler, R. C., Gazzaniga, M., Campbell, P., & Farah, M. J. (2008). Towards responsible use of cognitive-enhancing drugs by the healthy. *Nature, 456*(7223), 702.

Guleyupoglu, B., Schestatsky, P., Edwards, D., Fregni, F., & Bikson, M. (2013). Classification of methods in transcranial electrical stimulation (tES) and evolving strategy from historical approaches to contemporary innovations. *Journal of Neuroscience Methods, 219*(2), 297–311. doi:10.1016/j.jneumeth.2013.07.016

Guttorm, T. K., Leppänen, P. H., Hämäläinen, J. A., Eklund, K. M., & Lyytinen, H. J. (2010). Newborn event-related potentials predict poorer pre-reading skills in children at risk for dyslexia. *Journal of Learning Disabilities, 43*(5), 391–401. doi:10.1177/0022219409345005

Guye, S., & von Bastian, C. (2017). Working memory training in older adults: Bayesian evidence supporting the absence of transfer. *Psychology and Aging, 32*(8), 732–746.

Hall, S. (2003). The quest for a smart pill. *Scientific American, 289*, 54–65.

Harpur, R. A., Thompson, M., Daley, D., Abikoff, H., & Sonuga-Barke, E. (2008). The attention-deficit/hyperactivity disorder medication-related attitudes of patients and their parents. *Journal of Child and Adolescent Psychopharmacology, 18*, 461–473. doi:10.1089/cap.2008.023

Hoeft, F., McCandliss, B. D., Black, J. M., Gantman, A., Zakerani, N., Hulme, C., . . . Gabrieli, J. D. E. (2011). Neural systems predicting long-term outcome in dyslexia. *Proceedings of the National Academy of Sciences of the United States of America, 108*(1), 361–366.

Horvath, J. C., Forte, J. D., & Carter, O. (2015a). Quantitative review finds no evidence of cognitive effects in healthy populations from single-session transcranial direct current stimulation (tDCS). *Brain Stimulation*, 535–550.

Horvath, J. C., Forte, J. D., & Carter, O. (2015b). Evidence that transcranial direct current stimulation (tDCS) generates little-to-no reliable neurophysiologic effect beyond MEP amplitude modulation in healthy human subjects: A systematic review. *Neuropsychologia, 66,* 213e36.

Hotze, T. D., Shah, K., Anderson, E. E., & Wynia, M. K. (2011). "Doctor, would you prescribe a pill to help me . . .?" A national survey of physicians on using medicine for human enhancement. *The American Journal of Bioethics, 11*(1), 3–13.

Howard-Jones, P. A., & Fenton, K. D. (2012). The need for interdisciplinary dialogue in developing ethical approaches to neuroeducational research. *Neuroethics.* doi:10.1007/s12152-011-9101-0

Ilieva, I., Boland, J., & Farah, M. J. (2013). Objective and subjective cognitive enhancing effects of mixed amphetamine salts in healthy people. *Neuropharmacology, 64,* 496–505. doi:10.1016/j.neuropharm.2012.07.021

Ilieva, I. P., Hook, C. J., & Farah, M. J. (2015). Prescription stimulants' effects on healthy inhibitory control, working memory, and episodic memory: A meta-analysis. *Journal of Cognitive Neuroscience, 27*(6), 1069–1089. doi:10.1162/jocn_a_00776

Jarrin, D. C., McGrath, J. J., & Quon, E. C. (2014). Objective and subjective socioeconomic gradients exist for sleep in children and adolescents. *Health Psychology, 33*(3), 301–305. doi:10.1037/a0032924

Kang, J., Cai, E., Han, J., Tong, Z., Li, X., Sokhadze, E. M., . . . Li, X. (2018). Transcranial direct current stimulation (tDCS) can modulate EEG complexity of children with autism spectrum disorder. *Frontiers in Neuroscience.* https://doi.org/10.3389/fnins.2018.00201

Konrad-Bindl, D. S., Gresser, U., & Richartz, B. M. (2016). Changes in behavior as side effects in methylphenidate treatment: Review of the literature. *Neuropsychiatric Disease and Treatment, 12,* 2635–2647. doi:10.2147/NDT.S114185

Krutzinna, J. (2016). Can a welfarist approach be used to justify a moral duty to cognitively enhance children? *Bioethics.* doi:10.1111/bioe.12244

Lalancette, H., & Campbell, S. R. (2012). Educational neuroscience: Neuroethical considerations. *International Journal of Environmental & Science Education, 7*(1), 37–52.

Lee, J.-S. (2013). The relationship between student engagement and academic performance: Is it a myth or reality? *The Journal of Educational Research, 107*(3), 177–185. doi:10.1080/00220671.2013.807491

Li, L. M., Uehara, K., & Hanakawa, T. (2015). The contribution of interindividual factors to variability of response in transcranial direct current stimulation studies. *Frontiers in Cellular Neuroscience, 12*(9), 181. eCollection 2015. doi:10.3389/fncel.2015.00181

Lindahl, M., & Krueger, A. B. (2001). Education for growth: Why and for whom? *Journal of Economic Literature, 39*(4), 1101–1136.

Looi, C. Y., Lim, J., Sella, F., Lolliot, S., Duta, M., Alexandrovich, A., & Cohen-Kadosh, R. (2017). Transcranial random noise stimulation and cognitive training to improve learning and cognition of the atypically developing brain: A pilot study. *Scientific Reports, 7,* 4633. doi:10.1038/s41598-017-04649-x

Lustyk, M. K. B., Chawla, N., Nolan, R. S., & Marlatt, G. A. (2009). Mindfulness meditation research: Issues of participant screening, safety procedures, and researcher training. *Advances in Mind Body Medicine, 24*(1), 20–30.

Lutz, W., Creso Cuaresma, J., & Sanderson, W. (2008). The demography of educational attainment and economic growth. *Science, 319*(5866), 1047–1048.

Maier, L. J., Ferris, J. A., & Winstock, A. R. (2018). Pharmacological enhancement among non-ADHD individuals- A cross sectional study in 15 countries. *International Journal of Drug Policy, 58,* 104–112.

Matthews, K. A., Gallo, L. C., & Taylor, S. E. (2010). Are psychosocial factors media-tors of socioeconomic status and health connections? A progress report and blue-print for the future. *Annals of the New York Academy of Sciences, 1186*, 146–173.

McCabe, S. E., Teter, C. J., & Boyd, C. J. (2004). The use, misuse and diversion of prescription stimulants among middle and high school students. *Substance Use & Misuse, 39*, 1095–1116. doi:10.1081/JA-120038031

McLaughlin, K. A., Costello, E. J., Leblanc, W., Sampson, N. A., & Kessler, R. C. (2012). Socioeconomic status and adolescent mental disorders. *American Journal of Public Health, 102*(9), 1742–1750. doi:10.2105/AJPH.2011.300477

Marraccini, M. E., Weyandt, L. L., Rossi, J. S., & Gudmundsdottir, B. G. (2016). Neu-rocognitive enhancement or impairment? A systematic meta-analysis of prescription stimulant effects on processing speed, decision-making, planning and cognitive per-severation. *Experimental Clinical Psychopharmacology, 24*(4), 269–284. doi:10.1037/pha0000079

Martin, A. J., & Marsh, H. W. (2006). Academic resilience and its psychological and educational correlates: A construct validity approach. *Psychology in the Schools, 43*(3), 267–281. doi:10.1002/pits.20149

Martin, A. J., Nejad, H. G., Colmar, S., & Liem, G. A. D. (2013). Adaptability: How students' responses to uncertainty and novelty predict their academic and non-academic outcomes. *Journal of Educational Psychology, 105*(3), 728–746. doi:10.1037/a0032794

Mattay, V. S., Goldberg, T. E., Fera, F., Hariri, A. R., Tessitore, A., Egan, M. F., . . . Weinberger, D. R. (2003). Catechol O-methyltransferase val158-met genotype and individual variation in the brain response to amphetamine. *PNAS, 100*, 6186–6191.

McCarthy, S., Wilton, L., Murray, M. L., Hodgkins, P., Asherson, P., & Wong, I. C. (2012). The epidemiology of pharmacologically treated attention deficit hyperactiv-ity disorder (ADHD) in children, adolescents and adults in UK primary care. *BMC Pediatrics, 19*, 12–78. doi:10.1186/1471-2431-12-78

Moliadze, V., Lyzhkoa, E., Schmanke, T., Andreas, S., Freitag, C. M., & Siniatchkina, M. (2018). 1mA cathodal tDCS shows excitatory effects in children and adolescents: Insights from TMS evoked N100 potential. *Brain Research Bulletin, 140*, 43–51.

Moore, D. R., Burgand, D. A., Larson, R. G., & Ferm, M. (2014). Psychostimulant use among college students during periods of high and low stress: An interdisciplinary approach utilizing both self-report and unobtrusive chemical sample data. *Addictive Behaviours, 39*(5), 987–993. doi:10.1016/j.addbeh.2014.01.021

Morgan, P. L., Farkas, G., Hillemeier, M. M., & Maczuga, S. (2009). Risk fac-tors for learning-related behavior problems at 24 months of age: Population-based estimates. *Journal of Abnormal Child Psychology, 37*, 401–413. doi:10.1007/s10802-008-9279-8

Mueller, A. K., Fuermaier, A. B. M., Koerts, J., & Tucha, L. (2012). Stigma in attention deficit hyperactivity disorder. *Attention Deficit Hyperactivity Disorder, 4*(3), 101–114. doi:10.1007/s12402-012-0085-3

National Center for Education Statistics. (2008). *Percentage of high school dropouts among persons 16 through 24 years old (status dropout rate), by income level, and percentage dis-tribution of status dropouts, by labor force status and educational attainment: 1970 through 2007.* Retrieved from http://nces.ed.gov/programs/digest/d08/tables/dt08_110.asp

Nehlig, A. (2018). Interindividual differences in caffeine metabolism and factors driv-ing caffeine consumption. *Pharmacological Review, 70*(2), 384–411. doi:10.1124/pr.117.014407

Nevels, R. M., Weiss, N. H., Killebrew, A. E., & Gontkovsky, S. T. (2013). Methylphenidate and its under-recognized, underexplained, and serious drug interactions: A review of the literature with heightened concerns. *German Journal of Psychiatry*, 16(1), 29–42.

Nieto, S., & Ramos, R. (2015). *Educational outcomes and socioeconomic status: A decomposition analysis for middle-income countries.* PROSPECTS 45. doi:10.1007/s11125-015-9357-y

Nitsche, M. A., Cohen, L. G., Wassermann, E. M., Priori, A., Lang, N., Antal, A., . . . Alvaro, P.-L. (2008). Transcranial direct current stimulation: State of the art 2008. *Brain Stimulation*, 1(3), 206–223. doi:10.1016/j.brs.2008.06.004

Nitsche, M. A., Fricke, K., & Henschke, U. (2003). Pharmacological modulation of cortical excitability shifts induced by transcranial direct current stimulation in humans. *Journal of Physiology*, 553(pt 1), 293–301. doi:10.1113/jphysiol.2003.049916

Nitsche, M. A., & Paulus, W. (2000). Excitability changes induced in the human motor cortex by weak transcranial direct current stimulation. *Journal of Physiology*, 527(3), 633–639. doi:10.1111/j.1469-7793.2000.t01-1-00633.x

Ortiz, R., & Sibinga, E. M. (2017). The role of mindfulness in reducing the adverse effects of childhood stress and trauma. *Children*, 4(3), 16. doi:10.3390/children4030016

Partridge, B. J., Bell, S. K., Lucke, J. C., Yeates, S., & Hall, W. D. (2011). Smart drugs "as common as coffee": Media hype about neuroenhancement. *PLoS One*, 6(11), e28416. doi:10.1371/journal.pone.0028416

Paunescu, D., Walton, G. M., Romero, C., Smith, E. N., Yeager, D. S., & Dweck, C. S. (2015). Mind-set interventions are a scalable treatment for academic underachievement. *Psychological Science*, 26(6), 784–793. doi:10.1177/0956797615571017

Phipps, S., & Lethbridge, L. (2007). *Income and the outcomes of children.* Business and Labour Market Analysis Division, Analytical Studies Branch Research Paper Series, No. 281. Statistics Canada, Ottawa, Ontario.

Podda, M. V., Cocco, S., Mastrodonato, A., Fusco, S., Leone, L., Barbati, S. A., . . . Grassi, C. (2016). Anodal transcranial direct current stimulation boosts synaptic plasticity and memory in mice via epigenetic regulation of BDNF expression. *Scientific Reports*, 6. doi:10.1038/srep22180

Polanía, R., Paulus, W., Antal, A., & Nitsche, M. A. (2011). Introducing graph theory to track for neuroplastic alterations in the resting human brain: A transcranial direct current stimulation study. *Neuroimage*, 54(3), 2287–2296. doi:10.1016/j.neuroimage.2010.09.085

Poulin, C. (2001). Medical and nonmedical stimulant use among adolescents: From sanctioned to unsanctioned use. *CMAJ: Canadian Medical Association Journal/Journal de l'Association Medicale Canadienne*, 165, 1039–1044.

Power, J. D., & Schlaggar, B. L. (2017). Neural plasticity across the lifespan. *Developmental Biology*, 6, e216. doi:10.1002/wdev.216

Randall, D. C., Shneerson, J. M., & File, S. E. (2005). Cognitive effects of modafinil in student volunteers may depend on IQ. *Pharmacology, Biochemistry and Behaviour*, 82(1), 133–139.

Ray, K. S. (2016). Not just "study drugs" for the rich: Stimulants as moral tools for creating opportunities for socially disadvantaged students. *The American Journal of Bioethics*, 16(6), 29–38. doi:10.1080/15265161.2016.1170231

Riis, J., Simmons, J. P., & Goodwin, G. P. (2008). Preferences for enhancement pharmaceuticals: The reluctance to enhance fundamental traits. *Journal of Consumer Research*, 35, 495–508. doi:10.1086/588746

Rimfeld, K., Kovas, Y., Dale, P., & Plomin, R. (2016). True grit and genetics: Predicting academic achievement from personality. *Journal of Personality and Social Psychology*, *111*(5), 780–789. doi:10.1037/pspp0000089

Ruf, S. P., Fallgatter, A. J., & Plewia, C. (2017). Augmentation of working memory training by transcranial direct current stimulation (tDCS). *Scientific Reports 7*, Article number 876. doi:10.1038/s41598-017-01055-1

Sandberg, A., & Savulescu, J. (2011). The social and economic impacts of cognitive enhancements. In J. Savulescu, R. ter Meulen, & G. Kahane (Eds.), *Enhancing human capacities* (pp. 93–112). Oxford: Wiley-Blackwell.

Sarkar, A., Dowker, A., & Cohen Kadosh, R. (2014). Cognitive enhancement or cognitive cost: Trait specific outcomes of brain stimulation in the case of maths anxiety. *Journal of Neuroscience*, *34*(50), 16605–16610. doi:10.1523/JNEUROSCI.3129-14.2014

Sattler, S., & Singh, I. (2016). Cognitive enhancement in healthy children will not close the achievement gap in education. *The American Journal of Bioethics*, *16*(6), 39–41. doi:10.1080/15265161.2016.1170240

Savulescu, J. (2006). Justice, fairness, and enhancement. *Annals of the New York Academy of Sciences*, *1093*(1), 321–338.

Savulescu, J., & Kahane, G. (2009). The moral obligation to create children with the best chance of the best life. *Bioethics*, *23*(5), 274–290. doi:10.1111/j.1467-8519.2008.00687.x

Savulescu, J., Meulen, R. T., & Kahane, G. (2011). *Enhancing human capabilities*. Oxford: Wiley-Blackwell.

Scheffler, R. M., Hinshaw, S. P., Modrek, S., & Levine, P. (2007). The global market for ADHD medications. *Health Affairs*, *26*, 450–457.

Schelle, K. J., Faumüller, N., Caviola, L., & Hewstone, M. (2014). Attitudes toward pharmacological cognitive enhancement- a review. *Frontiers in Systems Neuroscience*, *8*, 53. doi:10.3389/fnsys.2014.00053

Singh, I., Bard, I., & Jackson, J. (2014). Robust resilience and substantial interest: A survey of pharmacological cognitive enhancement among university students in the UK and Ireland. *PLoS One*, *9*(10), e105969. doi:10.1371/journal.pone.0105969

Sisk, V., Burgoyone, A. P., Sun, J., Butler, J. L., & Macnamara, B. N. (2018). To what extent and under what circumstances are growth mindsets important to academic achievement? Two meta-analyses. *Psychological Science*, *29*(4), 549–571. doi: 10.1177/0956797617739704

Smith, M. E., & Farah, M. J. (2011). Are prescription stimulants "smart pills"? The epidemiology and cognitive neuroscience of prescription stimulant use by normal healthy individuals. *Psychological Bulletin*, *137*(5), 717–741. doi:10.1037/a0023825

Stein, Z., & Fischer, K. W. (2011). Directions for mind, brain, and education: Methods, models and morality. *Educational Philosophy and Theory*, *43*(1), 56–66.

Stevens, C., Lauinger, B., & Neville, H. (2009). Differences in the neural mechanisms of selective attention in children from different socioeconomic backgrounds: An event-related potential study. *Developmental Science*, *12*(4), 634–644. doi:10.1111/j.1467-7687.2009.00807.x

Stevenson, C. (2016). Self-pathologizing and the perception of necessity: Two major risks of providing stimulants to educationally underprivileged students. *The American Journal of Bioethics*, *16*(6), 54–56. doi:10.1080/15265161.2016.1170233

Thomas, E. M. (2006). *Children and youth research paper series readiness to learn at school among five-year-old children in Canada*. Statistics Canada, Ottawa, Ontario.

Trumbo, M. C., Matzen, L. E., Coffman, B. A., Hunter, M. A., Jones, A. P., Robinson, C. S. H., & Clark, V. P. (2016). Enhanced working memory performance via transcranial direct current stimulation: The possibility of near and far transfer. *Neuropsychologia*, 93(A), 85–96. doi:10.1016/j.neuropsychologia.2016.10.011

Urban, K. R., & Gao, W.-J. (2014). Performance enhancement at the cost of potential brain plasticity: Neural ramifications of nootropic drugs in the healthy developing brain. *Frontiers in Systems Neuroscience*, 8, 38.

Urban, K. R., Waterhouse, B. D., & Gao, W. J. (2012). Distinct age-dependent effects of methylphenidate on developing and adult prefrontal neurons. *Biological Psychiatry*, 72, 880–888. doi:10.1016/j.biopsych.2012.04.018

U.S. Census Bureau. (2000). *Current population survey: Design and methodology.* Retrieved from www.census.gov/hhes/socdemo/education/index.html

Vliegenthart, J., Noppe, G., van Rossum, E. F. C., Koper, J. W., Raat, H., & van den Akker, E. L. T. (2016). Socioeconomic status in children is associated with hair cortisol levels as a biological measure of chronic stress. *Psychoneuroendochrinology*, 65, 9–14. https://doi.org/10.1016/j.psyneuen.2015.11.022

Volkow, N. D., Wang, G.-J., Kollins, S. H., Wigal, T. L., Newcorn, J. H., Telang, F., . . . Swanson, J. M. (2009). Evaluating dopamine reward pathway in ADHD. *JAMA*, 302(10), 1084–1091. doi:10.1001/jama.1308

Wardle, M. C., Treadway, M. T., Mayo, L. M., Zald, D. H., & de Wit, H. (2011). Amping up effort: Effects of d-amphetamine on human effort-based decision making. *Journal of Neuroscience*, 31(46), 16597–16602. doi:10.1523/JNEUROSCI.4387-11.2011

Wiethoff, S., Hamada, M., & Rothwell, J. C. (2014). Variability in response to transcranial direct current stimulation of the motor cortex. *Brain Stimulation*, 7(3), 468–475. doi:10.1016/j.brs.2014.02.003

Wood, S., Sage, J. R., & Anagnostaras, S. G. (2014). Psychostimulants and cognition: A continuum of behavioural and cognitive action. *Pharmacological Review*, 66(1), 193–221. doi:10.1124/pr.112.007054

Yen Looi, C., Duta, M., Brem, A.-K., Huber, S., Nuerk, H.-C., & Cohen Kadosh, R. (2016). *Scientific reports* 6, Article number 22003. doi:10.1038/srep22003

Zheng, H., Wang, S., Guo, W., Chen, S., Luo, J., Ye, H., & Huang, D. (2017). Enhancing the activity of the DLPFC with tDCS alters risk preference without changing interpersonal trust. *Frontiers in Neuroscience*, 11, 52. doi:10.3389/fnins.2017.00052

19 Educational Neuroscience
So What Does It Mean in the Classroom?

Derek Bell and Helen M. Darlington

Let us start by clarifying four points in order to provide some context for what follows. The first point is to emphasise that by using the term 'classroom' in the title does not imply that we think learning and teaching only take place within the four walls of a classroom or even within the buildings that make up a school or college. On the contrary, we fully acknowledge that a significant proportion of learning takes place in other situations both formally (by which we mean some form of structured programme) and informally as part of everyday experiences and interactions with other people. Similarly, what and how people learn depends on a vast range of factors, which also act beyond the confines of the classroom. As teachers it is important for us to recognise that what happens outside the classroom can significantly impact on what happens inside it and *vice versa*.

As a corollary we would also note that the use of the term 'teacher' covers a range of individuals working in different settings with students of all ages (0 to 100+ years). Much of what follows tends to focus on the years of formal school-based education (e.g., from age 5 to 18 in the UK) and teachers in that sector. We recognise, however, that there are also implications for teaching in wider contexts. The important thing to emphasise is that, whilst there are some generalisations that can be made, each setting and age range requires approaches based on sound principles and evidence. Teachers modify their approach to align with their own beliefs and to suit the particular context in which they are working. Therefore understanding the developmental changes that take place across the lifespan potentially has differing implications for individual teachers at each stage of education.

The second point is to admit up front that we believe neuroscience has much to contribute to discussions about education, approaches to teaching and, ultimately, the learning that might, or might not, take place. We fully agree that the likelihood of direct links between neuroscience (defined as the study of the structure and function of the brain) and what goes on in the classroom is small. However, stepping back to look at the bigger picture and accepting that the field of "educational neuroscience" is a multi-disciplinary endeavour, we would argue that neuroscience has an important contribution to make. This builds, and depends, on the research and practice of other cognitive sciences in studying the brain, mind and behaviour. To these we would add evidence from educational studies which too often in the past have been isolated from findings in disciplines such as psychology. A major part of the challenge, having brought the evidence together, is the need to reflect on the findings and translate them so that they can inform the practice of individual teachers (which is the main focus of this chapter) as well as policy at both school and national level.

The third point is to state that we know of no 'silver bullet' which provides a single overarching answer as to how we, as teachers, can get students to learn; it is all much too complex. From our personal perspectives, the evidence indicates that there are potentially subtle but significant changes that we can consider introducing into our practice. Major changes, if any, will take longer and require further evidence and development work. The insights drawn from educational neuroscience have come about because neurological studies have begun to provide evidence that re-enforces some existing models of learning and to offer findings that indicate relationships, sometimes unexpected, between different behaviours. In particular, we feel that looking at education from an educational neuroscientific perspective provides the opportunity to take a more holistic approach to understanding learning and education. As the preceding chapters of this book amply demonstrate, learning depends on more than the instructions given by teachers.

The fourth point is really the purpose of this chapter which is to try to address the overarching question in its title, "So what does it mean in the classroom?" In effect, for us as teachers, this is where and when it really matters. Do we really need to know about the research that is reviewed in the preceding chapters? Will it make us better teachers if we do? How will it affect our practice as we plan schemes of work, 'teach', provide feedback and engage with our students? What difference will it make to their performance and achievements? The honest answer to questions such as these is 'We really do not know.' but, in reading the chapters, we have found much food for thought and insights that could inform and modify our practice.

Although most, if not all, of our thoughts are interlinked, we have tried to structure them by addressing three questions:

1. Why should we try to understand learning and teaching?
2. How might understanding learning better inform our practice?
   We consider this question from three perspectives: the environment and context for learning, the process of learning, and the emotional welfare and mental health of learners.
3. So what does educational neuroscience mean in the classroom?

We conclude the chapter by briefly addressing a fourth question:

4. What might be the over-arching issues that lie ahead for all of us?

Why Should We Try to Understand Learning?

Simplistically the answer to this question is that, as teachers, we are the professionals and understanding learning and the implications it has for our teaching should be the basis of our practice. Knowing what to teach and what students should learn are not, of themselves, sufficient to be an accomplished teacher who supports effective learning. Nor will having a set number of techniques for instruction ensure that learning will take place or, more importantly, that students will make progress by advancing, deepening and expanding their learning within and between disciplines. This is not to say that having a strong grounding in subject knowledge and pedagogical skills with the expertise to use them appropriately is not important. On the contrary, they are an essential foundation but they are not enough. While particular techniques may work in many situations there are some contexts in which they don't work as effectively as expected and others where they may not work at all to the detriment of both teachers and students.

Additional knowledge and a wider range of instructional techniques coupled with more experience will almost certainly improve matters. However, this raises questions such as: 'Which approach to use?', 'When to engage an alternative approach?' and, 'On what grounds should the choice be made?'

Answers to these questions, although not necessarily thought through explicitly, are used by teachers in the classroom to decide the next course of action. Such decisions will be based on existing knowledge and understanding of why some things might work in some situations but not in others. If the alternative approaches also fail to have the desired effect then, as teachers, we need to find a solution. Our experience and its outcomes add to our understanding of teaching and learning at some level. This might be purely pragmatic and practical or much deeper involving exploration of research evidence and further reflection on the learning process. Thus the next time a similar situation arises it is possible to tackle the issue in the light of our new knowledge and understanding. Of course, this doesn't guarantee that other challenges will not arise. They will, causing us to reflect further as part of a process of our own continued learning. In short the first reason for understanding learning and teaching, is that we are the professionals; the people who have responsibility for a significant part of children's education.

Just as we would expect doctors to understand how the body works and keep up to date with new techniques, for example in treating cancer, teachers need to understand how learning takes place. We also need to keep up to date with new evidence on ways of improving the learning experience for all students. Furthermore, we should recognise that our personal learning is an important part of our teaching. As Howard-Jones et al. (Chapter 17, p. x) remind us, "Teachers' beliefs about learning may play a significant role in their practice . . ." and ". . . that positive change in the quality of teachers' practice may require change in their personal beliefs about the processes by which learning is achieved." Thus it is important that, as teachers, we continue to build our personal understanding of learning, testing our ideas and practices against the best possible evidence available, not simply against our own preconceived beliefs and intuition. Rather than implementing new approaches based on hearsay we should do so knowing why they work and not simply that they worked elsewhere.

So what does educational neuroscience and, more specifically, the contents of this book add to the argument? First, it is worth noting that the debate about what educational neuroscience has to offer education has raised the profile of the mechanisms of learning and, more recently, teaching strategies that might be more effective than some current practices. This combined with the increasing demand for evidence-based and evidence-informed practice has challenged beliefs as to the effectiveness of some high-profile teaching strategies. Several of these, e.g., Brain-gym and Learning Styles, despite making claims that they are brain-based, are not supported by the evidence available. Developing an understanding of learning based on reliable evidence enables teachers to question the claims made, testing them against more reliable, substantiated knowledge about how the brain works and the potential implications for behaviour and learning.

This raises two questions: 'At what level does the neuroscience component need to be understood?' and 'When might it be possible to relate it to what actually takes place in the classroom?' These points are only partially addressed in the preceding chapters but reviewing the material in the light of a model offered elsewhere by Dommett, Devonshire, and Churches (2018) (see Figure 19.1) might help put this in perspective. Research in neuroscience

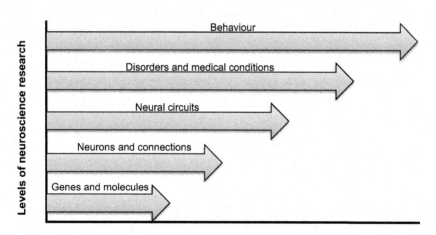

Figure 19.1 Levels of Research in Neuroscience and Degree of Direct Applicability to Education.

Source: Redrawn based on original by Dommett et al. (2018).

covers a large range of activities, some of which are far removed from direct application to education but other approaches which explore, for example, mechanisms of behaviour, are much closer. When the latter are combined with findings, often much older, drawn from other cognitive sciences including psychology, the evidence begins to offer more potential for informing what might take place in the classroom. This adds weight to the fact that there is no single bridge between neuroscience and education. Given the complexity of the relationship between brain, mind and education, stepping stones offering a series of alternative routes might be a better analogy. The multi-disciplinary approach adopted by educational neuroscience provides a helpful balance of evidence confirming the value of some existing strategies and techniques as well as offering potential insights for improving other areas of practice.

Understanding learning, as viewed through these chapters, also reminds us of three important issues that we need to take into account in planning our teaching and supporting the learning of our students.

- The first is the need to appreciate the students' perspective. Too often we look at learning from our perspective and focus on what we will do. We tend to plan lessons for our convenience (because we need to get through the syllabus!) and overlook the effect our actions might be having on students as learners. We often expect them to remember information and understand the ideas almost immediately, regardless of their pre-existing ideas or how they interpreted the phenomena in question. Furthermore, we assume they are able to transfer learning from one topic to another automatically. We get frustrated when they fail to do so and they become increasingly anxious which, in turn, can affect their capacity for learning.
- The second issue is the sheer complexity of learning. Identifying and unravelling neural pathways and networks are complicated enough but understanding learning is so much more. It requires wider knowledge about the way in which physiological changes, emotional reactions and behavioural responses impact on our cognitive processes. Establishing a link between factors is only the starting point in understanding the type of relationship between them. Thus to expect results quickly is unrealistic but there is much to build on.
- The third issue is the effect of growth and development, which is a particular focus of this book. As De Smedt (Chapter 7) points out, we cannot consider the brain of an infant to be simply a miniature version of an adult's. As pointed out in several chapters structural changes during the lifespan have an impact on how people respond to learning experiences. Whilst there are patterns of development that can be identified at the population level, we should remember that there are significant variations at the level of individuals. Children mature at different rates so they don't necessarily reach the same stage at the same age. We should also remind ourselves that for a given individual the different mechanisms that contribute to learning don't develop at the same rate, hence the compound

individual variation we see every day among our students and which, to a lesser or greater extent, we have to manage.

While it might be claimed that 'we know all of this', we need to step back and ask ourselves the question, 'If I know all of this, then how might a better understanding of learning affect what I do in my classroom?' This is not an easy question to answer at any level but, as a starting point, we offer some thoughts based on our experience and reflections on the content of the previous chapters.

How Might Understanding Learning Better Inform Our Practice?

Learning and teaching by definition are inextricably linked—two sides of the same coin. As our understanding of learning develops, our expertise as a teacher should improve and, in turn, so should the performance of our students. Fundamentally the learning that takes place, intended or otherwise, be it ours as teachers or that of our students, is the result of changes which take place in the brain. The new connections then become manifest as new knowledge and adjustments in our physical and mental capabilities. How learning takes place and what influences the process over our lifespan is influenced by several groups of factors that are reflected throughout the contributions to this book. We will consider these from three perspectives: the environment and context for learning, the process of learning, and emotional welfare and mental health of students.

The Environment and Context for Learning

It seems obvious to say that when, where and how learning takes place is not easily defined. We to our frustration recognise this when, at the end of what we considered to be a good lesson, some of our students do not seem to have grasped the ideas that were at the centre of the lesson. Yet occasionally those same students return a few days later, recall the material and, more importantly, are able to explain the ideas. There are also times when the reverse happens; students appear to have grasped the ideas but when questioned a little later appear to have misunderstood what was being taught. Similarly we experience situations when students appear to demonstrate learning which to us seems to have 'come from nowhere'. Anecdotally, we can recall such moments but fundamentally it raises the question, 'Why is knowing when, where and how learning has taken place so elusive?' In part the answer is that we simply don't understand the mechanisms of learning well enough and in part it is because of the sheer complexity of what is a very dynamic process. Although we can discuss and test the effects of different factors individually, it is essential to remember that the interaction between the various stimuli that are being processed by the brain plays a key role in influencing the learning that takes place. We will return to 'the learning process' in the next section but first we consider some of the environmental and contextual factors which might have an influence on learning. It is not possible to control all the potential factors and, inevitably, compromises have to be made. Thus in planning for learning it is worth considering the overall context in which the hoped-for learning will take place. We highlight four aspects here.

The first is to remind ourselves of the underlying 'nature-nurture' debate. As Meaburn (Chapter 3) explains, our understanding of the genetic basis of an individual's ability to learn is still in its infancy. Based on the evidence of twin studies, between 50% and 60% of the variation in achievement of students can be accounted for by inheritance; the level of heritability. DNA studies indicate a much lower figure but show that the genetic component comes from small contributions by a large number of genes rather than single genes controlling particular functions and capabilities. There is clearly a long way to go in terms of understanding the detail of the genetic control of learning. At this stage, we have to accept that ultimately academic performance, which remains the main focus of education systems world-wide, is genetically influenced. However, we must avoid allowing this to result in taking a deterministic view.

On the contrary, we need to pay greater attention to the environmental and social context of learning and those features which may act as 'limiting factors' preventing individuals from realising their potential. It is only when all the 'limiting factors' have been removed that the genetic element itself becomes limiting. To put it more positively, by mitigating the environmental limiting factors we are in fact enabling students to get closer to realising their full potential. Thus, as teachers, we should endeavour, through our teaching, to identify potential constraints on learning and do something to address them. Indeed, this would seem to have potential for collaborative studies between researchers and teachers. We suggest this because current understanding of brain plasticity is that the development of higher-level skills (such as reading, writing, and mathematics) is not limited to specific ages and can therefore continue to develop over the lifespan (Thomas, 2018). Working in joint teams has the potential not only to refine understanding of the impact of particular factors but also to test potential mitigating actions that teachers may be able to implement.

The second aspect we should consider is that of the physical environment in which learning takes place. Not a topic that has been addressed particularly by any of the authors here, it is interesting to note the marked difference between, for example, classrooms in primary schools (5- to 11-year-old children) and those in the vast majority of secondary schools (11- to 18-year-old students). In the former teachers go to great lengths to create 'displays' aimed at stimulating children's interest, celebrating their achievements and creating a lively environment which is perceived to be conducive to learning. As teachers who are committed to learning outdoors and 'in the field' we have personally experienced the effect that such experiences appear to have on individual students, but wonder to what extent and in what ways it affects their learning. Research into the classroom environment, for example, suggests that levels of auditory noise, temperature, lighting and ventilation impact on cognitive performance (e.g., Klatte, Bergström, & Lachmann, 2013; Knowland, 2018, pers. comm; Massonnié, Rogers, Mareschal, & Kirkham, 2019; Winterbottom & Wilkins, 2009). Optimising conditions appears to benefit all students but it seems to benefit those from lower socio-economic backgrounds disproportionately. Although some research exists, it is a perspective on learning which requires further attention and may also lend itself to collaborative projects between teachers and researchers.

The third aspect, the socio-economic context of learning, in contrast is one which has received significant levels of attention. In part this has been driven by a world-wide moral imperative to ensure that individuals, regardless of background, have the opportunities to progress and realise their potential. To this extent initiatives and interventions have been taken based on social and economic data, and political decisions. In England, for example, this has resulted in changes in policy such as an emphasis on the importance of 'early-years' education' (DfE, 2015) and the introduction of a funding stream, called 'Pupil Premium' (DfE, 2014), to provide additional support for students from disadvantaged backgrounds. While such policy initiatives are to be welcomed, especially if there is funding to support them, we have concerns as to the evidence base for them. In particular we worry about the effectiveness of some of the practices in schools and the wider community. There isn't the space to expand on the whole debate but using two initiatives referred to previously we will briefly try to illustrate our concerns.

By emphasising a particular stage of development as being important, in this case early years between 0 and 5 years (i.e., pre-school for the vast majority of children), risks giving the wrong impression. Undoubtedly children's experiences at this stage of their life are vital in terms of physical well-being, emotional and social security and their interaction with their immediate environment. However, as illustrated in the various chapters of this book, there is a great deal of development still to take place. This is especially so in relation to establishing and expanding higher cognitive abilities, advancing educational achievement and the potential benefits that brings. Hackman and Kraemer (Chapter 4, p. x), for example, in their discussion of the effects of socio-economic status (SES), emphasize that, "whereas *developmental timing is important, it is not deterministic—both earlier and later interventions may serve to reduce disparities* in neurocognitive development and academic success." (*Their emphasis*).

The Pupil Premium initiative recognised the gap in educational achievement between students from different backgrounds, in particular their socio-economic status (SES). Although much of the data used to justify the initiative was based on social studies, neuroscientific evidence contributed to the argument. As is more than amply discussed by Hackman and Kraemer (Chapter 4), establishing causal relationships is not straight forward but data overall support the underlying principle. Having accepted this, as teachers we are then faced with the more practical challenge of 'What do we spend the Pupil Premium money on?' We are considered accountable and expected to show improvements in the achievement of students from disadvantaged backgrounds relative to other students; i.e., we have to 'close the gap'. Inevitably this brings us back to the question of our practice in its widest sense. In particular we need to consider the question, 'What, if anything, should we do with such students that is different from what we do with our other students?' Reports (e.g., NGA, 2018) have indicated successful strategies adopted by schools but much needs to be done to understand better why some interventions have 'worked' and the mechanisms which underpin them.

The fourth aspect of learning we would highlight is that of the timing of when learning might take place: When should we introduce new ideas? When do we step back and allow students some time to think a problem through? When do we challenge their thinking? For a book which takes a developmental perspective in trying to understand learning, the question of timing is central. However, we must emphasize that the timing of stages of development is variable across individual students and there is little evidence to support the teaching of specific topics at particular ages. Perhaps more important is the need to understand the order of acquisition of concepts and skills so that they build on pre-existing ideas and capabilities. In short, as teachers, we need to give particular attention to understanding effective learning sequences and ensuring that students are prepared appropriately. This requires both sensitivity and some flexibility in order to accommodate the needs of individual students.

In terms of compulsory education, what is taught when is mainly determined by the school curriculum in the sense that it is 'done' in a particular year or grade. That does not mean to say it is the best time for the material to be covered in terms of individual students. We therefore have to be sensitive to the individual variation of students. At an instructional level this involves taking into consideration the pace at which new information is introduced; providing opportunities for students to 'think about' or 'respond to' questions; giving them time to assimilate new information and evidence and relating it to their pre-existing ideas. There are also occasions when we have to step back and accept that more time is needed for a pupil to grasp the idea and return to it at a later time. In doing so, we will be continually making our professional judgements as to when to 'push' a student, 'back off', repeat an activity or do something differently. Here an awareness of the idea of cognitive overload (e.g., De Jong, 2010) might help inform our decisions, recognising that, for all its capacity, brain pathways can become congested and time is required for information to be processed and stored. Thus strategies such as 'spaced-learning' (e.g., Smith & Scarf, 2017) may have something to offer in terms of consolidating learning. Planning for such an approach is helpful, as is the use of retrieval activities (e.g., Pastötter & Bäuml, 2014). We also have to be sensitive to shifts in students' responses and use our experience and, importantly, our understanding of the process of learning to adjust our approach rather than simply 'ploughing on' simply because it is in the lesson plan.

The Process of Learning

One of the challenges facing us as teachers when we try to engage with research in general is our understanding of how the findings of specific studies relate to the findings of other studies. Not surprisingly, this is particularly true when the evidence appears to be contradictory, which is often the case in a newly developing, multi-disciplinary field such as educational neuroscience. While each of the preceding chapters provides detailed reviews on the different aspects of the learning process it is not easy to construct an overall pattern of learning which can be used to inform day-to-day decisions in the classroom. As we have argued elsewhere, "To fully appreciate how the brain works it is necessary to consider not only the detail of the cells and the stages of development but also how the brain functions as an organ" (Bell & Darlington, 2018, p. 23). As we understand it, the brain makes multiple connections between neurones and groups of neurones creating multiple pathways and networks that transmit the signals controlling our actions, emotions, behaviours, and learning. Particular regions may be involved in more than one network and so may influence a wider range of activities than previously thought. Thus, unlike a computer which processes data sequentially through a central processing unit, the brain is involved in extensive parallel processing of information and pattern recognition. Thinking of the brain in this way can perhaps help us to understand better some of the behaviours we see in our students. At this almost simplistic level, it reminds us that there is more activity inside the heads of our students than just listening to us 'going on'. We also perceive other overarching principles that contribute to our understanding of the way the brain functions.

- The brain demonstrates neural plasticity which allows it to adapt to experiences and new ideas throughout life. This implies that there is the potential for learning at all ages but some activities, e.g., learning a second language (see Chapter 15) or to play a musical instrument (see Chapter 16), may require more effort at older ages.
- Neural plasticity does not suggest changes in the brain take place at a constant pace or at the same speed in any two individuals. In addition to natural variation, there appear to be times, often referred to as sensitive periods, during development when parts of the brain appear to be more susceptible to change than others. However, the current evidence suggests that sensitive periods in the brain mostly relate to low-level sensorimotor skills and not acquisition of the high-level cognitive skills relevant to education.
- Neural correlates show that particular behaviours are associated with specific pathways and areas in the brain. The most well known is the relationship between the prefrontal cortex and the executive functions

and the influence this has on adolescent behaviour. What is becoming more intriguing is evidence from neuroscience which indicates how some behaviours that were once thought to be independent are closely aligned or share the same neural correlates. For example, in her review on the role of rewards in motivation, Hidi (2016) argues that extrinsic and intrinsic motivation seem to activate "the same striatal areas of the reward circuitry."

- Emotions including stress and other stimuli not specific to the task or topic in hand interfere with learning and can prevent students from focussing on the relevant information. Once thought to be independent, we consider some implications of the important relationship between emotion and cognition in the next section.

We suggest that reflecting on our understanding of learning against the overall model of how the brain works and these principles can help to inform our classroom practice.

The vast majority of teachers work within a statutory or formal education system. It sets out the structures within which we work and determines how many years students are expected to attend school. The 'curriculum', often set nationally, outlines the learning objectives, against which the students' performance is measured, usually through written examinations. In many situations 'getting through the curriculum' and 'maximising students' examination performance' are considered to be major pressures for teachers. The associated stress is often, in turn, conveyed to the students. This introduces two dimensions that have an influence on learning: the emotional responses to pressure, which we reflect on in the following section; and the actual knowledge, skills and understanding that has to be 'taught' and students are expected to be 'learn', which we address now.

As teachers, we tend to see teaching through the lens of the subject being taught. From the beginning of the secondary phase of education, teachers are increasingly seen as 'experts in their discipline' who know about English literature, science, maths, geography, music etc. Most of our effort is focussed on how to 'teach' students the subject content and getting them to recall it in the examination. In contrast the majority of 'learning research' focusses on the generic processes and skills and mechanisms of how learning might take place. At one level such a situation is understandable but at another it is problematic in that it is another barrier between research and practice. At the very least, it sets up what is a superficial perception that the research has little relevance to the subject-teaching. This illustrates the need to introduce teachers to research that challenges such views. For example, recent behavioural genetics findings indicate that the principles of learning are not specific to particular academic content domains (e.g., Rimfeld, Kovas, Dale, & Plomin, 2015).

Being able to understand the relationship between the generic principles and processes of learning and subject-specific learning requires more research and development. This requires working with teachers in classrooms in order to tease out practices based on our understanding of, for example, how the executive functions can be used more effectively in order to maximise learning of particular types of subject content. Peters (Chapter 9), for example, focusses on the development of executive functions in adolescence. She reminds us that "in many cases educational programs are not well-tailored to the specific level of neural development and executive functions a child or adolescent possesses at that age" (p. x). She later suggests that, "The understanding that the brains of children and adolescents function differently from adults could inform changes in school curricula, as it underlines the importance of adjusting course programs to the specific skill level of students" (p. x). The challenge is to turn such claims into something that is recognisable and practical to help teachers in their day-to-day practice; attempts to do just that are rare.

Tolmie and Coecke (Chapter 8) go some way to trying to address the issue in the subject of science. They argue that learning science involves the development of *perceptual capacities*, which provide the sense of how things are; *conceptual understanding* putting in place frameworks for explicitly recognising causal relationships; and *abstract capacities* building towards the wider theories of science and being able to communicate them accurately. Elsewhere Tolmie (2016) argues that to do this teachers should engage students, regardless of age, in experiences and activities that:

- involve them in manipulating causal events;
- direct their attention to the exact sequences and components that make up the event or structure;
- link descriptions and explanations explicitly to the different elements of the events;
- connect their experiences to explanatory constructs and the bigger conceptual ideas of science.

While these ideas might never be taught explicitly, they should underpin the learning that is being encouraged. This would involve drawing students' attention to key features of the phenomena under investigation and checking that they are making appropriate links between events and ideas. Importantly, these principles should be continually strengthened as the scientific ideas and the treatment of topics becomes more sophisticated. One of the strengths of what Tolmie and Coecke do is to take the underlying principles of learning, ally them to the underpinning philosophy of the subject and then express the ideas in terms that can be applied in practice. It might be profitable to develop such sequences in more detail to take account of other educational neuroscience findings. This could provide a basis for planning and testing, for example, teaching sequences to tackle specific topics, or adopting more general approaches to improving executive functions through learning in a particular domain.

One of the reasons why the approach we have just illustrated is attractive is that investigations into executive functions show mixed evidence in relation to the transfer of skills from one context to another. There appears to be some near transfer but far transfer is much less likely (Sala & Gobet, 2017). This does not augur well for students being able to automatically transfer knowledge, ideas and skills they have learnt in one subject to the work they are doing in another. Without doubt this is a major frustration for many teachers but, rather than just getting angry, we should come to recognise this is not students 'just being difficult' and take appropriate actions to mitigate the problem. In essence the challenge is to enable students to develop metacognitive skills alongside the domain-specific knowledge and skills. The value of metacognition in the process of learning is supported by an extensive body of research (e.g., Hattie, 2009). Among other things this requires teachers to introduce and model suitable strategies for students, for example by providing example questions they might ask such as: What is it similar to? What kind of problem is it? This, of course, is easier said than done, but a first step is to be more explicit about linking ideas and to be as consistent as possible in the way in which they are addressed. Attempting to do this as an individual teacher is relatively straightforward but isn't enough. There needs to be school-wide consensus so that students are not exposed to conflicting approaches, risking unnecessary confusion. Helping students make links between ideas and the use of skills should contribute to strengthening the neural connections which are drawn on when faced with situations that have something in common.

Particularly important with regard to the transfer of ideas, as well as to learning more widely, is the use of language. The complexities of how language relates to conceptual understanding and development are beyond the scope of this chapter. However, from a teacher's perspective we acknowledge that the way we use language can result in misunderstandings, tensions and outright conflict. The language we use, and the way we use it conveys the meaning appropriate to the context. Further complications arise when the 'tone' of what is said varies such that a comment might be 'taken the wrong way'. However, having said that, more attention needs to be given to how language is used in the learning environment. Its role is multi-layered encompassing, among other things, expression of feelings and emotion, explaining and revealing levels of conceptual understanding, and, through dialogue with others, it becomes a powerful learning strategy.

One of the problems with language is that students do not always grasp the meaning of words used by teachers and vice versa, as teachers, we can misunderstand what students are trying to say. We therefore have to be highly sensitive and alert to the accuracy with which we use language and how this may change from context to context. Such underlying ideas have to be communicated to students; they often get a sense of how, for example, meanings shift but not before it has led to some degree of confusion. Again we need to take note of the way in which language and the use of language differs from subject to subject. For example, science demands specific and accurate use of terms while in, say, creative writing lessons students are encouraged to use diverse language in order to create images be they real or imaginary. We therefore need to keep checking what students mean and to keep reminding them of the way in which the language is being used. In some respects we add to the problem when, in order to get an idea across, we move into the area of metaphor and analogy as a basis for introducing concepts and types of problems. Using such approaches has many strengths but risks students developing misleading ideas which have to be 'deconstructed' at a later date. If we do not take this risk into account then we may leave students more confused than when they started!

Emotional Welfare and Mental Health

As Immordino and Gotlieb (Chapter 10, p. x) remind us "The way students feel affects how they learn"; we would argue that this is also true for teachers and how they teach. Despite the depth and breadth of research into the affective aspects of learning it is only relatively recently that interest in emotional welfare and mental health of both students and teachers has begun to receive the attention it deserves. In terms of practice it is probably fair to say that greater attention is given to how children feel in primary school contexts as compared with secondary. This is not to say that individual secondary teachers are uncaring, rather it is to some extent the result of a system which puts great emphasis on academic achievement. Pressures on schools, teachers and students to perform highly have been compounded in England, for example, by the publication of examination results and ranking of schools by their performance. This has, in turn, led to the development of a 'league table mentality' over the last 10–15 years as schools strive to improve their ranking position.

Reduction in mental health and wellbeing results from many factors that lead to changes in the behaviour of children and young people. Whilst some may be directly the result of actions in school, e.g., bullying or stress related to examination pressures, it is probably fair to say that the majority result from other aspects of students' lives. Regardless of the cause, teachers are often the people, after parents, who have to deal with the issues in the first instance. Many reports (e.g., Parkin, Long, & Bate, 2018) indicate the scale of the problem and highlight the immediate challenge as to how schools should respond to meet the immediate needs of their students. Perhaps even more important is the question of what actions should be taken in order to help the students take control and manage their own mental health more effectively. In the context of the developmental focus of this book, it should be noted that studies (e.g., see Blakemore, 2018) suggest in the region of 75% of all cases of mental illness start at some point before the age of 24. Adolescents are particularly vulnerable but recent reports (see e.g., Place2be & NAHT, 2018) suggest that more children in primary school are exhibiting signs of mental illness. The UK government has responded to these concerns about mental health by announcing proposals that the PSHE (Personal, Social and Health Education) curriculum in England should include students exploring the issue as part of a revision to be implemented from 2020. However, policy changes of this nature are only a start and require programmes to provide research along-side support and training for teachers if they are to make a difference.

The impact of mental illness on students is critical but maintaining teach-ers' own mental wellbeing is also important. This is not only for their own health, but also because it impacts their capacity to support students' mental health (Sisask, 2014). Teaching is a highly stressful occupation (see e.g., Edu-cation Support Partnership, 2018) and burnout has been associated with both academic adjustment and student mental health. Teachers who are able to build positive relationships are more likely to engender a sense of resilience amongst their students (Zee & Koomen, 2016). Further work investigating the relationship between students and their teachers is needed, however.

One of the major shortcomings in tackling the problems affecting learning has been the tendency to separate the cognitive and non-cognitive matters. This is not only in terms of research but also in terms of the way in which schools are organised with their academic structures and pastoral systems. Interestingly, one of the benefits of the introduction of the Pupil Premium has been for schools in England to look more holistically at student performance. It is now more common for schools to hold formal meetings to consider the progress of individual students by taking into account their attitudes towards school and learning, their behaviours in different contexts and their academic achievement across all subjects. The overall patterns are also considered against the student's social and cultural background. Evidence of the effec-tiveness of some practices is building (see e.g., Sutton Trust & EEF, 2015) but there is still much to do in order to understand why some approaches seem to work better than others. By examining the data across year groups, the whole school and other schools both locally and nationally, it should be possible to begin to identify general principles applicable to different contexts. It seems to us that, where there has been some success, there has been an effort to rec-ognise, explicitly, the interrelationship between cognitive and non-cognitive aspects of the learning. More specifically we would like to highlight areas that might influence and refine our practice.

Mindfulness, Resilience and Self-efficacy

Semenov et al. (Chapter 12), for example, emphasise the interaction between mindfulness and executive functions. They argue that, "The emerging evi-dence suggests that mindfulness practices may be beneficial for children, with concurrent as well as cascading benefits for academic and social success. (p. x)" They also remind us that emotional responses to events, images and other stimuli can interfere with the efficiency with which the executive func-tions process information. The impact of stress arising from different sources on both cognitive and non-cognitive outcomes is also increasingly acknowl-edged. In many situations the cause of stress is external to the school. Once again this underlines the importance of being aware of, and sensitive to, unex-pected changes in students' behaviour and progress.

For some students the source lies within school and maybe related specifically to their studies. Maths anxiety (Dowker, Sarkar, & Yen Lool, 2016) is perhaps the best-known example of stress resulting from a specific subject and affects about 25% of the population. The highest rates (35%) are found in students between 14 and 18 years old. It has been known for over fifty years and is a negative emotional reaction to mathematics, leading to varying degrees of helplessness, panic and mental disorganisation, when faced with a mathematical problem. Like many conditions it is multi-facetted and not well understood. In part it seems to be the result of general pressures and in part stress specifically related to maths. As teachers we need to be able to recognise possible signs, sometimes very subtle, that indicate someone might be inclined towards an anxiety of doing maths. This is an example of where we need the support of research to be able to recognise the signs of a problem and to develop potential interventions, both generic and specific, to address it.

Language development and disorders has been subject to a massive level of extremely detailed research. For example, as Goswami (Chapter 5) explains new brain research provides further evidence that dyslexia is a result of atypical brain activity. Tong and McBride (Chapter 6), exploring the problem from a different perspective, provide evidence that dyslexia is also affected by SES and other cultural factors. What isn't covered is the relationship between dyslexia and the stress and anxiety such a condition generates. Unwittingly many teachers may add to the stress levels of such students by suggesting, for example, that they find out how to spell something by looking it up in a dictionary. With greater awareness actions such as this can be addressed and familiarity with alternative strategies can be increased. However, in cases where high anxiety levels exist it is difficult to get students to adopt the specific approaches because the feeling of hopelessness gets in the way.

This is an example of a much wider problem—the need to build self-confidence and resilience in students. More specifically this incorporates developing the ability to cope and thrive in the face of negative events, challenges or adversity. The resilience of students is demonstrated through a combination of attributes including their social competence, a sense of agency and responsibility, optimism and sense of purpose, attachment to others, problem-solving skills, effective coping strategies and a sense of self-worth. Closely related to resilience is the concept of self-efficacy, first described by Bandura (1994), which relates to an individual's perception of their own ability to succeed in a specific area. This is closely linked with an individual's interest level and the feedback they receive from teachers. Self-efficacy can be developed through increasing students' awareness of their emotions (mindfulness) and developing coping strategies (resilience).

Addressing issues such as these have resulted in a wide variety of programmes, some of which are related specifically to mindfulness and others linked to other areas of social and emotional learning (SEL). This raises many challenges for teachers of which we highlight two. The first is being able to decide which programme(s) to adopt in the plethora of material that exists.

Mindfulness has support and the early evidence is encouraging but there is much still to learn. The second challenge is how we can implement the intervention for most gain. Is it something that needs to run as a stand-alone programme or is it something that can, and should, be incorporated into our day-to-day practice?

Interest, Curiosity and Rewards

Experience tells us that getting students interested in, and curious about, what is being taught is a key component in learning. As teachers we have our own activities and strategies which we use on a daily basis. We try to make it relevant to student experience, link it to previous ideas, or generate a surprise or 'wow' moment. Such techniques certainly have their place but they sometimes only result in 'passing interest'. The challenge is much greater to develop a sustained, deeper level of interest not only in the topic in question but also for the subject more widely and ultimately learning as a lifelong process.

In their model Hidi and Renninger (2006) propose four stages in the process of interest development, essentially moving from what they refer to as situational interest to individual interest. The former involves engaging students in the material but may be short lived. The later develops over time and becomes more sustained and robust. Such a shift involves an emotional connection and commitment such that a student's interest goes beyond 'learning it for the exam'. An important element appears to be students having a sense of some control (Darlington, 2017) in the learning process. Interest appears to be closely related to self-efficacy and is developed through allowing students increasing levels of autonomy, mastery experiences and social support.

Closely linked to building the interest of students is the use of rewards as a form of motivation. Rewarding students for good performance in some form through praise or physical items (e.g., money) has long been part of encouraging students to learn. While these are undoubtedly important 'weapons' for teachers and appear to be a 'good thing' at first glance, the overuse of extrinsic rewards may be counter-productive. Hidi (2016) reviewed evidence from both psychology and neuroscience and revealed a complex situation. She draws attention to the idea that responses to rewards vary from individual to individual and reactions may depend on context. Furthermore neuroscience evidence suggests that the neural triggers and pathways for extrinsic and intrinsic motivation are closely aligned, not independent as was once thought. This introduces questions as to the relationship between external rewards (e.g., money) and internal feelings such as of satisfaction. In practical terms for us as teachers this boils down to the questions, such as 'When and to what extent do we use external rewards?' and 'How do we know when such rewards become counter-productive?'

The use of rewards and indeed sanctions in order to encourage appropriate behaviour and attitudes in students is a wide field of study which, as evidence is becoming available, is challenging existing practices. Much more work and development trials are required but there are indications that, for example, adolescents tend to be influenced more by reward than by punishment and are less inclined to wait for long-term gains (Blakemore, 2018, p. 154). Reviewing practices in the light of such evidence is challenging as it would require a major shift in beliefs on the part of many teachers as well as school policies. Currently the majority of schools have systems based primarily on a range of sanctions rather than on degrees of rewards. Developing alternatives needs to be explored further and more widely but that requires more clarity in the evidence if such a major shift is to become widespread.

We are very aware that there are many more issues, e.g., the way in which students respond to risk, that we have not considered. Nor have we more than touched on specific behavioural and cognitive conditions, each of which has its substantial body of research. This does not mean that these issues are not important but we have focussed on issues that are applicable to the general classroom situation and ones we have used to inform our consideration of the final question, as follows.

So What Does Educational Neuroscience Mean in the Classroom?

Not surprisingly we were very much attracted to Chapter 17 by Howard-Jones et al. As teachers, we are looking for guidance on how an understanding of learning, informed by educational neuroscience, might change our teaching practice. We share many of the views expressed and agree with their conclusion that, "in teacher training and development, we now have sufficient knowledge to begin explaining and promoting evidence-based classroom learning practices using scientifically informed concepts of learning. (p. x)" In the light of what we have already said and in the spirit of taking the discussion further we would argue for further exploration of the "engage, knowledge-building, and consolidation" framework presented in Chapter 17.

As teachers we very much identify with the three elements proposed but would argue that there is a place for a fourth component. We would characterise this as the 'application and transfer of learning'. Whilst acknowledging Howard-Jones et al. refer to this under the 'consolidation' element, we propose the additional component for two main reasons. One, on pragmatic grounds, is that in England from 2018 amendments to the specifications for GCSE examination (taken by students at age 16) have raised the profile of the application of knowledge. Students have found responding to the resulting changes in examination questions more difficult. The second is more fundamental. It is based on the evidence indicating the tendency for learning to be developed in specific domains and that the degree of transfer to new contexts is limited. Similarly, as argued earlier, transfer of skills, both cognitive and practical, is not necessarily something that comes automatically. By making linkages across and between contexts and disciplines explicit, we can expand the learning of our students. This helps them make progress by widening their experience of the concepts in question rather than restricting them to a narrowly framed set of activities.

In addition, by taking a developmental perspective, we venture to suggest that the framework might be developed even further as illustrated in Figure 19.2. Here we have introduced a time dimension which can be used to influence our thinking at different levels. Although Howard-Jones et al. state the framework is not sequential, at different points in time each of the components will have a particular contribution to make. However, the emphasis placed on the individual components will vary depending on the phase of learning. In the early stages of a new topic engagement would be a significant, perhaps the major, focus of the activities and the start of knowledge building. Consolidation and application/transfer of learning will be smaller components. As learning proceeds the engagement component reduces, although it must be maintained at a level which avoids disengagement by the learner, and knowledge building expands. The consolidation and application/transfer components begin to expand as the knowledge base develops. An important step in the knowledge building element is the shift towards accommodating the formal structures of the discipline into the learning. Further consolidation of knowledge reinforces not only the subject knowledge but increasingly supports the application/transfer of learning to different contexts and relationships with other ideas, topics and disciplines.

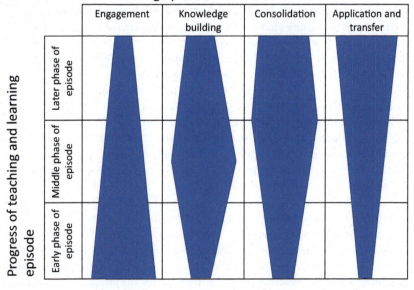

Shifts in emphasis between strands during a teaching and learning episode

Figure 19.2 Strands in Teaching and Learning: An Extension of Howard-Jones et al. (Chapter 17).

The framework could also be used to inform the selection of activities and experiences when planning schemes of work and lessons. In part, this could be as a check that each of the components are catered for and, in part, as a way of building progression, in its widest sense, into the learning experience. Taking a more long-term view, the framework might be used to inform the overall process of learning of students through their lifelong education. For example, in the early years, engagement with the environment and embryonic ideas of language, objects, sensations, number, events etc. is high and knowledge begins to accumulate. Repeating actions and phrases, alongside 'testing' the names of colours for example, introduce consolidation of the knowledge and initiation of application/transfer. From late childhood through adolescence engagement remains important but there is increasing emphasis on the building of both formalised and more general knowledge making greater use of powers of reasoning and other executive functions. Consolidation and the application/transfer of knowledge and learning, in turn, become more and more significant, supporting both depth and breadth of learning.

Translating such a framework into day-to-day practice is the challenge for teachers and we have offered some examples to consider in Table 19.1.

Our understanding of learning and thus our teaching is the result of our own experiences of teaching and being taught, our understanding and interpretation of the knowledge and skills we have built up over our careers. This all comes together when we take our classes on a day-to-day basis and translate all of the material into our professional practice, planning for lessons, making on-the-spot judgements and changes, and reflecting on the impact and outcomes of our efforts on our students. It seems obvious that evidence from educational neuroscience has a contribution to make and can inform the development of improvements in practice. Making sense of this developing field of research and translating the most appropriate elements for the classroom is by no means straightforward; indeed, it may be too early to do so on a wide scale. However, as already outlined, we would argue that it can add value now for us as individual teachers.

Given the risks of adopting misleading information, as has happened in the past, it is important that we treat evidence of all types, not just that coming out of educational neuroscience, with caution; question and test it as far as possible. We also need to be aware that educational neuroscience is a developing field and therefore, as in any other area of study, new evidence may lead to modification of theories. However there are some overarching principles, such as those we highlighted previously, on which we can build our thinking. In addition, we now know a great deal about some of the factors that affect learning, including biological factors such as sleep and exercise (Chapters 13 and 14); socio-cultural factors such as SES background (Chapter 4); and emotional factors such as interest, curiosity, aspirations and resilience (Chapter 10). All of these are important and need to be addressed. A key message for us is that much can be done by individual teachers taking note of findings supported by the evidence that arises from studies conducted across the cognitive

Table 19.1 Teaching and Learning Strands and Some Classroom Actions to Consider

Teaching and Learning strand	Classroom actions
Engagement	• Introduce a degree of novelty or surprise in order to generate curiosity about the topic. • Establish an early sense of student ownership of the learning. • Take students' ideas seriously. • Relate to students' experiences and interests. • Encourage student questions. • Convey appropriate purpose for the learning in question. • Use of collaboration between peers and sense of common goal. • Pitch at appropriate level of challenge. • Sensitive use of social (e.g., praise) and tangible (e.g., points) rewards. • Sustain positive attitudes and relationships.
Knowledge building	• Relate explicitly to students' pre-existing ideas and knowledge. • Checking student interpretation of the knowledge. • Clarity of communication using range of senses. • Plan learning sequence but allow for some flexibility. • Effective use of questions from both teachers and students. • Careful use of models and analogies. • Minimise risk of sensory overload and information. • Develop student sense of control of their learning.
Consolidation	• Modelling and rehearsal of knowledge being developed. • Use of range of retrieval activities using the knowledge and ideas (NB 'tests' should be 'low stakes'). • Revisit the topic from time to time. • Consider strategies such as 'spaced learning' and 'interleaving'. • Develop students' awareness of their own learning including problem solving.
Application and transfer	• Make explicit links between situations to which the skills and knowledge apply. • Provide range of examples in which the skills and knowledge are used. • Challenge students to explore new contexts in which the skills and knowledge may be used. • Introduce and discuss the 'big ideas' to which the knowledge applies. • Continue to support students' investigation of their own questions and awareness of their own learning.

sciences. In Table 19.2 we suggest some features for consideration. We should note that some of the ideas are not new but were identified through older behavioural studies. However, more recent evidence such has brain imaging has provided further support for these ideas. Based on this we would argue that individual teachers can make a difference in their classrooms by making small and subtle changes to their practice leading to significant incremental effects on students' learning.

Table 19.2 Features of Learning and Examples of Questions for Teaching

Features of learning	*Some questions to consider for teaching*
Quality of the learning environment	• Is the physical environment conducive to learning? • Does the physical environment provide stimuli that encourage students to ask questions/reinforce ideas? • Do students feel safe in offering explanations, even if they turn out to be incorrect?
Importance of language and social interaction	• Do students understand the meaning of the words used? • Are students encouraged to use vocabulary precisely and in the correct contexts? • What opportunities are there for students to exchange and discuss ideas, and develop their arguments?
Influence of pre-existing ideas	• Are students' ideas and pre-existing knowledge taken seriously? • Are students given any time to think about their responses to questions or discuss them with peers before 'giving an answer'? • Are students encouraged to be explicit about their pre-existing ideas and examine them against new evidence and alternative explanations?
Use of multi-sensory approaches	• To what extent do learning activities involve a range of senses? • Are students challenged to evaluate different forms of evidence to support their explanations of phenomena? • Are students expected to communicate their ideas in through a variety of media and styles?
Need for scaffolding	• What types of support are used to help students extend their understanding of phenomena?
Making things explicit especially if transfer of learning is to be supported	• How do students get experience of a range of contexts in which the phenomena they are studying might apply? • To what extent are students encouraged to demonstrate links between cause and effect? • In what ways are linking ideas across topics and subjects made explicit? • To what extent are students challenged to solve problems that draw on knowledge and skills from several domains?

What Might Be the Over-arching Issues That Lie Ahead for All of Us?

Without doubt there remains much that warrants further research in order to understand better how, why and when learning takes place. In addition there is much to understand about how best to support learning with the associated implications for teaching. In reflecting on the content of the chapters we noted a number of themes—overarching questions—which, individually and collectively, could provide further insights to inform our practice as teachers.

- *What is the value and potential impact of information and communication technologies (ICT) including developments in artificial intelligence (AI)?*

    There already exists a massive volume of research in this area and teachers are being exhorted to make greater use of the materials that are available. However, from our perspective it remains difficult to distil what has positive effects and what actually inhibits learning. Although increasingly the development of such products is based on evidence of how learning takes place, too often it is the technology that leads. Greater understanding of the effects of using such technologies as illustrated by Bavelier et al. (Chapter 11) is required. Such insights combined with greater clarity as to the problems being faced by teachers could help to improve the impact of the use of ICT and AI on students' learning.

- *How can the benefits of personalised learning be maximised within the social context of the school and its environment?*

    Meeting the learning needs of individual students is a constant challenge for even the most accomplished teachers. They constantly have to balance the demands of a class of students with the needs of specific individuals. They also have to value the need to develop students' capabilities for working independently as well as part of a team and being a member of a more informal social group. The use of ICT is often proposed as a solution but clearly has its limitations. Putting aside the constraints imposed by lack of compatible equipment, there is a need to explore strategies, informed by the educational neuroscience, which would improve personalisation of learning.

- *How can the impact of interventions be maximised?*

    No intervention whatever its scale is perfect, the impact of each being reduced for a variety of reasons. Despite a positive effect being demonstrated in 'laboratory' or 'trial' conditions, when variables are highly controlled, many fail to translate the effects into practice. Ideally it would be helpful to understand what might be referred to as the tolerance limits of the intervention. For example, if the dosage is 15 minutes, 3 times per week for 10 weeks, what is the impact of only running it for 5 weeks? Clearly there are many factors that contribute but some guidance could be helpful. Beyond the actual features of the intervention further consideration needs to be given to the interactions between the different groups e.g., parents, of people who might impact on the learning of individual students.

- *To what extent is it ethical to 'test' things out on students?*

    Knowland (Chapter 18) makes the claim that educational neuroethics is, "the bedrock of educational neuroscience research (p. x)." Issues of ethics however go beyond the 'research' and apply to the introduction or testing of new practices which might include everything from an alternative teaching approach to performance enhancing drugs. Whilst in general researchers are aware of such matters, ethics is not something that is discussed frequently or explicitly in relation to classroom practice.

- *How can research findings inform practice more effectively?*

From our perspective, perhaps the biggest challenge is that of translating and implementing findings from research into our own practice, that of immediate colleagues and the wider profession. This needs to be considered more systematically in order to explore ways of improving the current situation. One model would start with teachers and researchers jointly identifying the problem and together derive the research questions and programme through to implementation. Alternative models are also required in order to take promising aspects of the current body of research through the various stages of development to full implementation.

Indeed all the preceding questions need to be addressed not by groups working in isolation but by researchers from different disciplines coming together with teachers in both the 'laboratory' and the 'classroom'. Only by working closely together will it be possible to close the gap between the various parties in terms of issues such as developing a shared language, jointly generating common research questions, and testing the impact of a range of approaches to teaching. It is unlikely that the outcomes will identify a single approach but those that emerge are more likely to be underpinned by the best evidence available. It is probably reasonable to say progress is being made, however slowly. In our view, it needs to continue because we would rather be able to teach by adopting approaches that are born out of evidence; not simply mimicking traditional practices or chasing the whims of fads and fashions. In short we wish to teach 'smarter' and not 'harder'.

References

Bandura, A. (1994). Self-efficacy. In V. S. Ramachaudran (Ed.), *Encyclopedia of human behavior* (Vol. 4, pp. 71–81). New York: Academic Press.

Bell, D., & Darlington, H. M. (2018). Educational neuroscience and the brain: Some implications or our understanding of learning and teaching. In N. Serret & S. Earle (Eds.), *ASE guide to primary science education*. Hatfield: Association for Science Education.

Blakemore, S.-J. (2018). *Inventing ourselves: The secret life of the teenage brain*. London: Doubleday.

Darlington, H. M. (2017). *Understanding and developing student interest in science: An Investigation of 14–16 year-old students in England* (Unpublished PhD thesis), UCL Institute of Education, London.

De Jong, T. (2010). Cognitive load theory, educational research, and instructional design: Some food for thought. *Instructional Science*, 38(2), 105–134.

DfE. (2014). *Pupil premium funding and accountability for schools.* Retrieved July 2018, from www.gov.uk/guidance/pupil-premium-information-for-schools-and-alternative-provision-settings

DfE. (2015). *2010–2015 government policy: Childcare and early years education.* Retrieved May 2015, from www.gov.uk/government/publications/2010-to-2015-government-policy-childcare-and-early-education/2010-to-2015-government-policy-childcare-and-early-education

Dommett, E., Devonshire, I., & Churches, R. (2018, Spring). Bridging the gap between evidence and classroom "clinical practice": The potential of teacher-led randomised controlled trials to advance the science of learning. *Impact, 2,* 64.

Dowker, A., Sarkar, A., & Yen Lool, C. (2016). Mathematics anxiety: What have we learned in 60 years? *Frontiers in Psychology, 7,* Article number 508, 1–16.

Education Support Partnership. (2018). *Teacher wellbeing index 2018.* Retrieved from www.educationsupportpartnership.org.uk/sites/default/files/teacher_wellbeing_index_2018.pdf

Hattie, J. (2009). *Visible learning: A synthesis of over 800 meta-analyses relating to achievement.* Oxon: Routledge.

Hidi, S. (2016). Revisiting the role of rewards in motivation and learning: Implications of neuroscientific research. *Educational Psychology Review, 28,* 61–93.

Hidi, S., & Renninger, K. A. (2006). The Four-Phase model of interest development. *Educational Psychologist, 41*(2), 111–127.

Klatte, M., Bergström, K., & Lachmann, T. (2013). Does noise affect learning? A short review on noise effects on cognitive performance in children. *Frontiers in Psychology, 4,* Article number 578.

Knowland, V. (2018). Personal communication, 25 September 2018.

Massonnié, J., Rogers, J., Mareschal, D., & Kirkham, N. Z. (2019). Is classroom noise always bad for children? The contribution of age and selective attention to creative performance in noise. *Frontiers in Psychology,* 26 February 2019. Retrieved from https://www.frontiersin.org/articles/10.3389/fpsyg.2019.00381/full

NGA. (2018). *Spotlight on disadvantage: The role and impact of governing boards in speeding, monitoring and evaluating the pupil premium.* Retrieved from www.nga.org.uk/About-Us/Campaigning/Spotlight-on-Disadvantage.aspx

Parkin, E., Long, R., & Bate, A. (2018). *Children and young people's mental health—policy, services, funding and education.* Briefing Paper Number 0719 House of Commons Library. Retrieved from http://researchbriefings.files.parliament.uk/documents/CBP-7196/CBP-7196.pdf

Pastötter, B., & Bäuml, K. T. (2014). Retrieval practice enhances new learning: The forward effect of testing. *Frontiers in Psychology, 5,* Article number 286, 1–5.

Place2Be & NAHT. (2018). *Children's mental health matters: Provision of primary school counselling.* Retrieved from www.place2be.org.uk/media/10046/Childrens_Mental_Health_Week_2016_report.pdf

Rimfeld, K., Kovas, Y., Dale, P. S., & Plomin, R. (2015). Pleiotropy across academic subjects at the end of compulsory education. *Scientific Reports, 5,* Article number 11713. Retrieved from www.nature.com/articles/srep11713

Sala, G., & Gobet, F. (2017). Does far transfer exist? Negative evidence from chess, music, and working memory training. *Current Directions in Psychological Science, 26*(6), 515–520. Retrieved from http://journals.sagepub.com/doi/full/10.1177/0963721417712760

Sisask, M. et al. (2014). Teacher satisfaction with school and psychological well-being affects their readiness to help children with mental health problems. *Health Education Journal*, 73, 382–393.

Smith, C. D., & Scarf, D. (2017). Spacing repetitions over long timescales: A review and reconsolidation explanation. *Frontiers in Psychology*, 8, Article number 962, 1–17.

Sutton Trust & EEF (Education Endowment Foundation). (2015). *The pupil premium: The next steps*. Retrieved from www.suttontrust.com/wp-content/uploads/2015/06/Pupil-Premium-Summit-Report-FINAL-EDIT.pdf

Thomas, M. S. C. (2018). *Education and brain plasticity*. Retrieved from www.educationalneuroscience.org.uk/2018/07/20/education-and-brain-plasticity/

Tolmie, A. (2016). Educational neuroscience and learning. In D. Wise, L. Hayward, & J. Pandya (Eds.), *The Sage handbook of curriculum, pedagogy and assessment* (Vol. 1). London: Sage Publications.

Winterbottom, M., & Wilkins, A. (2009). Lighting and discomfort in the classroom. *Journal of Environmental Psychology*, 29(1), 63–75.

Zee, M., & Koomen, H. M. Y. (2016). Teacher self-efficacy and its effects on classroom processes, student academic adjustment, and teacher well-being. A synthesis of 40 years of research. *Review of Educational Research*, 86(4), 981–1015.

Conclusion

20 Key Challenges in Advancing Educational Neuroscience

Michael S. C. Thomas, Iroise Dumontheil and Denis Mareschal

In this final chapter, we identify some of the themes that have emerged in this volume, as well as some challenges for the future.

What Should Teachers Know About Neuroscience?

The research covered in this volume shows how advances in neuroscience can give insights into learning in the classroom. But what do teachers need to know about neuroscience? Do they need to know how the brain functions or what methods neuroscience uses? How detailed should this knowledge be? Several views were offered in different chapters. Bell and Darlington saw the goal of understanding learning as a professional responsibility for teachers and the basis of their practice: they drew an analogy to the importance of doctors understanding how the body works and being up to date with the latest treatments. Howard-Jones and colleagues offered a simplified version of brain function that captures key cycles of the process of learning in the classroom: engage—build knowledge—consolidate—apply. For these authors, explanations couched in terms of brain functions permit a visual, accessible, and engaging means to communicate about the learning process, and a basis for teachers to reflect on their practice.

Many of the authors saw neuroscience as part of a wider approach of informing teaching by evidence of what works, for them implicating neural mechanisms of learning. The factors influencing educational outcomes are many and complex; where there is ambiguity and risk of fads and fashions in teaching methods, convergent evidence of mechanistic plausibility increases confidence and motivates investment in more rigorous testing. At the very least, as Howard-Jones and colleagues say, the inclusion of explanations of learning informed by cognitive neuroscience allows for the dispelling of teachers' and students' existing myths about the brain and inoculates them against acquiring new ones.

We believe that what teachers need to know about neuroscience, therefore, is threefold: a broad characterisation of how learning works in the brain, to generate intuitions about the factors that may harness it; an understanding of how their own brain function may influence their teaching skills; and an awareness of the importance of convergent evidence across disciplines in evaluating whether teaching methods work.

Development Versus Individual Differences

The volume had four areas of focus: individual differences, development across the lifespan, cognitive enhancement, and translation into the classroom. The individual differences perspective considered what makes children better or worse at learning, either in terms of their cross-disciplinary skills (executive functions, emotion regulation, engagement) or in terms of their discipline-specific skills (e.g., phonology for reading, symbolic magnitude understanding for arithmetic, perceptual and conceptual understanding of physical systems for science). The implication of differences is that children may need to be taught differently depending on their abilities or prior knowledge. By contrast, the developmental perspective considered how abilities change across the lifespan, for example that executive function skills are late maturing providing an early constraint on learning, or that adolescence provides both vulnerabilities (e.g., decision making in the presence of peers) and opportunities (elevated response to feedback) for educators. The implication is that teaching methods need to be appropriate to skills levels at each age.

Taken in isolation, both these perspectives have downsides. The individual differences approach draws focus to the limiting factors on a child's progress, at the expense of understanding the learning mechanisms and environments that are needed to learn a skill at all. Limiting factors can mask each other: if one limiting factor is removed, the next is revealed. Moreover, the approach is sometimes drawn to focusing on those limits and can pay insufficient attention to factors that produce strengths. The developmental approach risks averaging across children, prompting a one-size-fits-all approach that sacrifices the opportunity to personalise learning and build on strengths of the individual. The two perspectives can at times diverge. In the chapters of Donati and Meaburn, and Hackman and Kraemer respectively, we saw considerations of genetic and environmental influences on educational outcomes. It might be that the principal driver of development is the environment, but the principal driver of individual differences is genetics. For example, in reading, exposure to print is necessary to learn to read at all, but if reading experience is sufficient, the limiting factor can be genetically caused differences in phonological ability. The ultimate goal must be to integrate both variation and development within a common framework: to consider individual differences as variations in trajectories of development.

Although the relation of individual differences and development may appear a theoretical concern, it has echoes in policy. Is the goal of education to improve the performance of the whole population—say in literacy or numeracy—by moving the whole distribution of performance further up the scale? This would be a developmental concern. Or is it to change the gaps between children, ensuring no child is left behind? This would be an individual differences concern. In her chapter, Knowland identifies similar ethical implications in the context of enhancing cognition. If school is deemed primarily to concern the acquisition of skills and learning (the developmental perspective of improving everyone), then it is less controversial that cognitive enhancements should have a legitimate role in aiding those improvements; but if school is primarily deemed to be about grades and competing for jobs and places at university (individual differences perspective), artificial enhancement is more akin to cheating in the competition. An integration of development and individual differences would prompt a resolution of these kinds of policy and ethical ambiguities.

The focus on neural mechanisms can also de-emphasise some other important questions here: individual differences and development can be combined into a measure of 'mental age'—should children be taught according to their mental age, so that the same method is appropriate for a young very bright child and an older less bright child? Should classes be streamed by ability? Should group work combine children with mixed abilities or be similarly streamed?

What Works?

Educational neuroscience is consistent with the wider ambition of accumulating an evidence base of what works in education. Quotes from two chapters illustrate this view: 'the integration of different levels of analysis and data has the potential to generate a better explanatory model of mechanisms underlying a particular educational phenomenon [and thereby] constitute a better base for grounding diagnostic approaches and educational interventions' (De Smedt, p. 182); 'studies of neurophysiological mechanisms allow us to map and predict what happens when different people receive a given intervention in different contexts' (Knowland, p. 488). The goal is to identify what works and why.

Organisations within the US and the UK now list the growing evidence base for particular techniques, for example the What Works Clearing House[1] and the Education Endowment Foundation (EEF)[2] with its Teaching Toolkit[3]. The EEF funds large-scale randomised control trials. In a randomised control trial, individuals are allocated at random to receive one of several interventions. In addition to the target intervention, there are one or more control conditions to provide a standard of comparison. This could be no intervention/standard practice, or an alternative intervention that is similar in many respects to the target intervention but does not contain the proposed active agent—serving as a sort of placebo to check that any effects are not produced just by 'being in an intervention'. The EEF's trials combine pre-registered studies and independent evaluation of trial outcomes to give maximum confidence in the results, as well as a preference for teaching as normal (or 'business as usual') control groups to verify that the intervention is better than current practice.

There are a number of issues that arise in the use of randomised control trials (RCTs)—the gold standard method used to evaluate new treatments in medicine. First, a consensus is only beginning to emerge in the appropriate methodology for educational interventions that target cognitive abilities (Green et al., 2019). The consensus distinguishes different types of studies that provide a pathway to produce new interventions and understand how they work. The first is a *feasibility* study, a small-scale study to demonstrate that a method might work. The second is a study of *mechanism*, using appropriate experimental methods and active control groups to establish the mechanisms underlying the effect. The third is an *efficacy* study, evaluating the performance of an intervention on a larger scale but still under ideal and controlled circumstances. The fourth is an *effectiveness* study, investigating performance under real-world conditions. Good practice pursues these types of study in sequence, and the different study types require appropriate control groups and sample sizes.

The second issue is whether RCTs should have the equivalent 'gold standard' status for educational interventions as they do for medicine. One challenge is that, cases of deprivation apart, gains in educational achievement may be the consequence of many small influences. Most of the effect sizes of successful interventions listed by the Educational Endowment Foundation and the What Works Clearing House are moderate or small. Large-scale RCTs vary just one factor compared to a control group, against a background of large variation from all the other uncontrolled factors. This leads to a paradox. It may be hard to detect successful interventions because they represent small signals against a background of larger noise. Many RCTs may produce null results. A large body of null results could lead to despondence that educational outcomes can be improved. Yet if all the effects are added together (e.g., in nutrition, sleep, aerobic fitness, stress reduction, engagement/knowledge building/consolidation activities in the classroom, topic-specific focus on core cognitive abilities, topic-general training in executive function skills and emotion regulation, meta-cognitive training to support transfer, resilience training for mental health, specific training in socioemotional skills, increased parental support, reduction of social inequalities, to list a few) very large increases in educational outcomes may be possible. In short, it may be that large improvements in educational outcomes are possible but only by combining many small effects, each of which is hard to establish individually.

Related to this is the tension between *investigating how it works* versus *getting it to work* (Thomas et al., 2019). The objective of the researcher is to understand how each factor contributes to educational outcomes and understand the mechanisms underpinning the effect. They must distinguish causal effects from many naturally occurring correlations, by systematic manipulation of individual factors. However, for those who solely want to improve outcomes, the best strategy is to 'throw everything at it' that might work. While this gives the best chance of a good outcome, the disadvantage is that if there is an improvement, there will be no insight into what factors produced it.

The final issue with RCTs is that they risk producing prescriptive techniques. The researcher has demonstrated that a technique works under certain conditions. They then instruct educators to use the technique replicating these conditions (retaining the so-called *fidelity* of the intervention). However, prescription undermines the teachers' autonomy. It is at odds with the way teachers normally teach, by adapting materials and techniques to particular content and the children in front of them. Prescriptive techniques are less likely to have wide uptake. By the same token, if teachers vary the technique, they may inadvertently omit the key ingredient by which it operates, rendering it ineffective. And when teachers conclude that—in their own hands—the supposed scientifically verified techniques don't work, there is a risk that confidence in the enterprise of using RCTs to build an evidence base will fall away.

What is needed, as Bell and Darlington articulate, is for researchers to identify the *tolerance limits* of an intervention—how much it can be varied and in what ways, while still retaining its effect. In order to do so, researchers must include an active control condition in their RCT (that is, a control intervention that is similar in all ways to the target intervention except without including the proposed active agent)—in addition to a teaching as normal control. Successful interventions that show benefits compared to both control groups can then be used flexibly by teachers without destroying their effects. Techniques can be adapted to context and content by retaining the active agent.

Translation and Policy

Debate still lingers within educational neuroscience about what type of field it should be. Some researchers view it as primarily a basic science, amounting to a sort of cognitive neuroscience of skills that are relevant to education (e.g., Gabrieli, 2016). Perhaps the majority of researchers view it as more inherently translational, with the goal of informing actual practice in the classroom. We believe that most of the chapters in the volume accord with this latter view. It would certainly be somewhat of a waste not to attempt translation from the basic science, when so many children might gain from the insights that basic scientists gain.

However, translation is not straightforward. As De Smedt says,

the mere identification of a neural correlate or neurocognitive factor does not readily answer questions about effective teaching and curriculum design. This requires a nuanced translation and an integration of findings from neurocognitive studies with educational theories and frameworks of effective instructional design. (p. 184)

The heart of educational neuroscience must remain a dialogue between educators, policymakers, and those working in the learning sciences. The dialogue needs to involve teachers influencing the direction of research as much as researchers communicating science findings, and the translation of individual techniques into forms that are useful (but still effective) in the classroom is an enterprise that can only be achieved collaboratively. The field of educational neuroscience will gain from greater investment in infrastructure that can support the influence of educators on neuroscience. There is much to gain from practitioners identifying the questions, puzzles, obstacles, and challenges that impede educational achievement, so that neuroscientific approaches (amongst others) can be used to try to understand and overcome these; and from practitioners helping shape neuroscientific insights into practices that are robust and useful in the classroom.

Interaction with policymakers and influence on policy is a frequently stated goal of researchers working in educational neuroscience. This brings its own set of challenges. For example, the role of policymakers is often to mandate national or regional requirements (such as, say, the phonics screening check given to six-year-olds in the UK, based on psychological research identifying early behavioural markers for future literacy problems). Researchers have to be clear on whether that is the goal of their research, or whether it is to provide a wider set of tools for teachers to (optionally) use in the classroom.

Engagement with policymakers also requires a communication strategy. There is usually debate in scientific fields, but a consensus position needs to be established among scientists prior to communication based on the balance of probabilities. To present dissenting scientific voices to policymakers risks undermining confidence in the maturity of the field and encourages the view that translation is premature.

Policymakers are often keen to have their policies informed by evidence and can be enthusiastic about neuroscience. This represents a dilemma. If educational neuroscientists 'hold their fire' until they feel the science is more certain, policymakers will be listening to others (lobbyists, interested parties) whose views may be less evidence based. Should researchers go ahead and offer 'best guesses' based on existing science? In the past, educational neuroscience has been criticised for offering policy advice because the science was deemed too immature (e.g., in Bruer's 1999 book, *The Myth of the First Three Years*). Then there is the risk that policymakers will cherry pick neuroscience evidence to fit pre-existing political agendas. Caught between the urge to say something, but not say something on which we are not yet certain, the educational neuroscientist is in a difficult situation. Researchers need to find a balance where they do not overstate the current state of the basic science and the maturity of translation, but do not understate the importance of the science of learning in supporting an evidence-informed approach to policymaking in education.

Can Cognition Be Enhanced?

This volume uniquely brought together in one place chapters evaluating diverse methods proposed to enhance cognition. Education as a whole can be viewed as a form of cognitive enhancement (Ritchie & Tucker-Drob, 2018; though see Cigman & Davis, 2009, for a counter view). The concern here was with more specific methods that might have general benefits for cognition, perhaps even to raise IQ. What conclusions can be drawn from this section as a whole?

First, the general pattern appears to be that cognitive training leads to near transfer—improvements are for the abilities that have been trained, or very similar ones. Far transfer to very different skills (or cognition as a whole) appears to be the exception. Far transfer may require interventions that operate on the functioning of the brain as a whole at a biological level, such as in nutrition, energy supply, or levels of stress hormones, rather than regimes of behavioural training. Or, as suggested by Semenov and colleagues, it may require specific training *in* far transfer, that is, explicit strategies in identifying what pre-existing skills and abilities may be applicable to new situations.

The lure of far transfer is perhaps that it would be *so efficient*. One would only have to undergo a single training regime to see benefits across other skills, rather than complete separate training in all the individual skills. Despite the many proposals for techniques giving general cognitive benefits, the suspicion is that we will not find this panacea. However, near transfer is not to be scoffed at. Improvements are readily available in individual skills, testament to the brain's enduring plasticity. And as a guiding principle, near transfer can be used to design interventions. For example, Wilkinson et al. (2019) designed a mathematics and science intervention for 8- and 10-year-olds that targeted inhibitory control in learning counter-intuitive concepts. By the principle of near transfer, the training for this executive function skill was embedded in the content of the domain in which it was required (the age-appropriate mathematics and science syllabuses). Improvements were then observed in subsequent achievement tests.

We might briefly reflect on what the pervasive lack of far transfer in cognitive training tells us about how the brain/cognitive system works. The most obvious conclusion is that the brain mostly comprises content-specific processing systems, rather than general 'jack-of-all-trades' processing mechanisms. This is at odds with much of traditional cognitive psychology, which has invoked general mechanisms such as working memory and attention (see Thomas, Ansari, & Knowland, 2019, for discussion). If those domain-general mechanisms really existed and were trainable, far transfer should be much more apparent than it is.

The chapters in this volume highlighted one key challenge in evaluating cognitive enhancement techniques—that of random allocation to condition. Unless the experimental design randomly assigns participants to intervention versus control conditions, any advantage for the intervention condition could be due to other pre-existing group differences rather than the intervention itself. So in a given time and region, bilinguals might be systematically different to monolinguals (say, in socioeconomic status [SES]); teenagers who ended up playing action video games throughout their teenage years might be systematically different to those who did not (say in their motor dexterity or sensitivity to reward structures); children who get to learn a musical instrument and put in a lot of practice may be systematically different to those who never had the opportunity or completed the practice (say in their SES or conscientiousness). Without random allocation, systematic group differences can only be suggestive and must be complemented by properly designed intervention studies. But such studies can rarely replicate the size of the dosages (in our examples, of language learning, of video game playing, and of instrument learning, respectively) that may have had the effect.

Of the interventions we saw in these chapters, aerobic exercise appeared to offer benefits for executive functions (and of course, health benefits), with primary age children perhaps most able to benefit (Wheatley and colleagues); action video games yielded benefits, though more narrowly to top-down attentional control of visual processing—putting aside issues around violent content[4] (Altarelli and colleagues); mindfulness offered benefits for executive function skills, particularly around emotion regulation, though the evidence from younger children was still thin (Semenov and colleagues); learning a musical instrument appeared not to offer wider cognitive benefits (Schellenberg) (see also a similar story with learning chess; Sala & Gobet, 2017; Sala, Foley, & Gobet, 2017); bilingualism improves language skills at some temporary cost to early vocabulary development, but the jury is still out on wider cognitive benefits (Phelps and Filippi); sleep deprivation is bad for learning, and may be a particular current issue for adolescents, but getting more than normal amounts of sleep does not produce particular cognitive benefits (Sharman and colleagues).

Because expectation and novelty can produce temporary illusions of cognitive benefits of an intervention, and because commercial organisations are motivated to promote brain training for financial gain, it remains important for educational neuroscientists to investigate the mechanisms that underpin purported training effects. That is, for each of the putative generally beneficial activities, it is desirable for investigators to propose and evaluate the cognitive and brain structures that mediate the transfer from training task to other cognitive skills. The less plausible the underlying mechanistic basis for the transfer, the more critically the published evidence in favour of the transfer must be examined.

What Is the Added Value of Neuroscience for Education?

Critics of educational neuroscience have sometimes portrayed neuroscience and psychology as being in competition for which discipline should inform education (e.g., Bowers, 2016). In our view, this is a nonsensical position. Neuroscience and psychology are complimentary approaches to studying the same system (the mind/brain), operating at different levels of description and employing different methods. The goal is to have convergent and consistent accounts (see Howard-Jones et al., 2016; Thomas, 2019). In our view, interdisciplinary research is the best way to improve learning outcomes in the classroom—that is, cooperation rather than competition. Moreover, terms like 'neurocognitive' and 'cognitive neuroscience' reveal how the disciplines are blending, so that the contribution of each is not easily discerned. Nevertheless, it is worth attempting to emphasise what particular value neuroscience can add for education, and we therefore requested each of our sets of authors to include a section on this point at the end of their chapters.

There were many different answers to this question, and readers might like to revisit these sections across the different chapters. Here, we pick out a few themes. Some authors pointed to the impact that neuroscience evidence could have both on researchers and policymakers—if something can be seen in the brain, it seems more real. The effect of SES on cognitive development (Hackman and Kraemer), the immaturity of certain aspects of executive function in adolescence (Peters), and the complex interactions between emotion and cognition (Immordino-Yang & Gotlieb) are some examples. Relatedly, some authors pointed to the role of neuroscience in adding convergent, independent evidence that effects observed in behaviour were real, rather than the product of measurement error or artefacts (for example, cognitive differences in bilinguals, Phelps & Filippi; or confirming the structure and function of the reading system, Tong & McBride-Chang. See also Ramsden et al., 2011, for a striking demonstration of how structural brain imaging data supported ambiguous behavioural evidence that intelligence is still changing across the teenage years).

Some authors identified new ideas that had emerged from neuroscience, such as a new sensory basis for dyslexia in rhythm processing (Goswami); symbolic magnitude as a key constraint on mathematical concept learning (De Smedt); adolescence as a period of risk and opportunity based on the neural systems maturing in those years (Peters); that shared biology partly underpins the observed relationships between educational performance and a diverse array of social, economic, and physical and mental health outcomes[5] (Donati and Meaburn); and that science education involves the construction of fragmented mental representations, built on top of each other rather than replacing each other, differentially activated according to task and context, and integrated only through the organising role of language-based concepts (Tolmie and Dündar-Coecke).

Other authors pointed to the opportunity neuroscience offers to understand *why* interventions work. For example, action video game playing improves reading speed in dyslexics because it enhances cortical top-down visual attention, although it leaves subcortical extrinsic orienting systems unaffected (Altarelli and colleagues). Mindfulness training produces effects through automatizing the screening out of environmental and emotional distractors (Semenov and colleagues). Peters suggested that if training results in enhanced recruitment of the same neural network that was active before training, this could indicate that capacity is increased by training, while if new brain regions are recruited after training, this may point to a different strategy being employed (see Thomas et al., 2019, for detailed discussion of neurocognitive mechanisms underlying interventions). Peters additionally argued that neuroscience might also lead to predictions of whom interventions will work better for: 'neuroscientific measures could eventually be used to tailor interventions to individual students. Understanding which strategies and neural networks a student currently uses during a cognitive task, could potentially indicate which type of intervention may work to bring their performance to a higher level' (p. 236).

While neuroscience can add value, its contribution also carries some risk. Where structural or functional differences are observed in the brain, they can lead to the assumption that there is nothing we can do about them, such as in genetic differences or those caused by SES. But this assumption would be wrong: the brain's plasticity across the lifespan supports plentiful behavioural change in response to training. Schellenberg, in his review of associations between music training and intelligence, laments the error of inferring causation from correlation. For music and intelligence, he argues a common causal factor, largely genetic, is probably responsible for the correlation, rather than there being a direct cause of music training improving intelligence. But with supporting evidence, he also argues that educational neuroscientists are more at risk of making this error—in studying the brain, they mistakenly believe they are studying mechanisms, and therefore believe the correlations they observe are more likely to be causal. Lastly, Hackman and Kraemer argue that neuroscience in education can produce too great a focus on individual factors affecting educational outcomes, rather than societal, school, and family factors that may have more powerful effects.

What Are the Concrete Implications of Neuroscience for the Classroom?

We also asked our authors to comment on what they saw to be the concrete implications of neuroscience research for the classroom. Again, the answers were diverse, and we encourage readers to compare and contrast these concluding sections across chapters. Some authors remained cautious. Tong and McBride-Chang argued that there still exists a big gap between laboratory research and practice, such that results of neuroscience research have not been directly and commonly used in practice. Howard-Jones and colleagues said that the dearth of brain imaging studies employing educational-like tasks means that the relevance of cognitive neuroscience to classroom practice is more reasoned hypothesis.

Nevertheless, many concrete examples were offered. De Smedt pointed to the identification of core skills in domains like mathematics that would help detect children at risk of poor learning. Like others, he recognised the potential of neural markers of those skills that could be measured before the developmental emergence of the behaviours themselves, and so offer the scope for earlier intervention. However, he conceded that such markers need to meet appropriate thresholds of sensitivity and selectivity (not to mention cost and practicality) to be of use beyond the laboratory. Sharman and colleagues pointed to both neuroscience and behavioural level responses to the shift in circadian rhythm in adolescence and subsequent reduced amounts of sleep: the neuroscience-inspired response is to shift the start of the school day to match the teenagers' shifted body clocks; the behavioural intervention is to educate teenagers in good sleep practices so that, for example, they don't drink coffee in the evening or use screen devices in darkened bedrooms before going to sleep.

Hackman and Kraemer admitted that the concrete implications of cognitive neuroscience research on SES are as yet limited, but speculated that there may be variation in what predicts academic success both within and across SES levels—and thus a multiplicity of strategies may be most effective rather than specific tailored approaches. This is striking, because the more common narrative that stems from educational neuroscience is one of the personalisation of education. Notably, Hackman and Kraemer proposed that neurocognitive measures need to be considered in a broader context, and that neuroscience may be most useful when it helps guide more refined interventions that focus on social systems and processes rather than on curricula or on individuals.

Several authors identified unexpected potential avenues to remediate literacy difficulties, among them processing of rhythm (Goswami), action video game playing (Altarelli and colleagues) and learning a musical instrument (Schellenberg). Immordino-Yang and Gotlieb sketched out an agenda for the development of the 'intellectual virtues', based on their analysis of the role of emotion in learning. These virtues included interest, curiosity, intellectual humility, and intellectual agency. Howard-Jones and colleagues argued that neuroscience concepts could be powerful tools in driving the reflective processes of both students and teachers. Phelps and Filippi urged educators not to misidentify characteristics of bilingual language acquisition as indicative of developmental language disorder, arguing that in the UK at least, English as an Additional Language (EAL) status has acquired unwarranted negative connotations. Instead, educators should focus on the benefits of experience of multiple languages, both within the classroom and in the wider (global) community. Lastly, Schellenberg argued that even if music training does not raise intelligence, music training improves *musical* skills, which should be enough!

Future Directions

Most neuroscience is not relevant to education. It is too low level, concerning particular biological processes or neural mechanisms; or it utilises animal models unsuited to address the cultural practices of education. By the same token, much of education is beyond the reach of neuroscience, concerning societal structures and institutions, decisions about funding and curricula. This volume has demonstrated, however, that there are ideas from cognitive neuroscience that can contribute to education where the focus is on mechanisms of learning. At this interface, a dialogue must take place, to render research into a form useful in the classroom, and to allow educators to guide researchers towards the most pressing challenges. It is important, therefore, to be realistic about the scope of educational neuroscience. It is not the be all and end all.

Within this restricted scope, it is possible to discern some of the most productive avenues to advance research. The first is to continue to identify sources of individual differences in educational outcome, at multiple levels of analysis. We saw chapters on genetic influences and socioeconomic influences—there are opportunities to integrate these views into a single account of variations in academic achievement. Two crucial questions remained to be answered: how much of the variation (in a given society) stems from home factors versus school factors? The answer should influence policy. Within school factors, how many of these will concern optimising the conditions of brains to learn (and consolidate learning), versus identifying content-specific approaches that will improve outcomes for particular skills or topics, versus enhancing skills that are applicable across learning situations?

The direction of travel of much of educational neuroscience is to identify how to personalise learning—to offer a child the tailored educational environment to get the best achievement (and happiness). Neuroscience and genetic data can offer more information to complement traditional demographic and behavioural data. However, the practical challenge still remains of generating the different pedagogical practices to exploit these data, and of delivering personalised learning given the constraints on materials, skills, and resources within the classroom. We have seen some debates in our chapters—for example, Hackman and Kraemer speculating whether multiple strategies might be superior to tailoring, or Knowland wondering whether the early years (the oft-purported best opportunity for intervention) should fall within the remit of an educational neuroscience at all. Donati and Meaburn opined that the time was right for a societal debate about whether we want to generate genetic information about our children's educational potential and if so, how such data might be safely and ethically used.

Technology has been offered as a solution to personalisation, in that computer-based tutoring approaches (or learning environments curated by the teacher for the child's autonomous exploration) can be adaptive, tailored to the user. Such adaptive systems are underpinned by powerful new developments in artificial intelligence and machine learning. If Facebook can tailor advertisements and swing elections, surely such technology can tailor tuition and swing examinations? We are not there yet. In their review of action video games, Altarelli and colleagues offered tantalising clues about the dynamics of computer games that produce powerful changes in behaviour. Unfortunately, most educational games currently focus on content and do not deliver the relevant game dynamics to deliver equivalent engagement.

Technology itself is an important future direction for educational neuroscience, given the pervasiveness of smart phones and other screen devices. There will be reactionary responses to these changes in society, as they alter past times and ways that people relate to each other. We might ask, how do they modify learning and the potential for learning? No doubt they will alter brain structure and function, because brains are plastic and afford acquisition of new skills. But changes in reliance on external tools will change what we learn, and we may therefore need to alter what we teach. Moreover, changes in habits may have side effects—changes in sleep patterns or levels of physical exercise, changes in the social interactions that provide support or challenges to mental health—that need to be addressed. Understanding the neurocognitive mechanisms will, we believe, help in these endeavours.

We believe the new focus on the role of emotion in learning, outlined by Immordino-Yang and Gotlieb, also offers great potential. This approach can harness both teachers' and students' skills to best outcome. For example, Immordino-Yang and Gotlieb used this framework to characterise what they call *high-quality educational practices*. Such practices 'place the learners' subjective emotional and social experience at the forefront, and help people build scholarly and social identities that incorporate their new skills and knowledge. They help people to feel safe and purposeful, and to believe that their work is important, relevant, and valuable. They support age-appropriate exploration and discovery, followed by cognitive elaboration for deeper understanding. And, they support the learners in pacing themselves to iteratively and authentically move between these modes of engagement as they pursue meaningful learning goals . . . when students are working hard because they are steering toward intrinsic, problem-centered goals, and not primarily because they are trying to satisfy some relatively arbitrary milestone . . . deep thinking and transfer of knowledge are more likely to happen' (p. 259).

Paul Howard-Jones and colleagues identify the important area of the neuroscience of teaching. This pertains to the processes underlying teaching skills (where, say, it is useful for teachers to understand that their emotional state with respect to a topic can influence students' learning); and it pertains to the explicit knowledge teachers need about neuroscience that will help them with their practice (such as these authors' schematic of engage-build-consolidate and apply).

Finally, there are areas that were not covered in much depth in this volume and which we think are of importance. The development of an evidence-based pedagogy for Special Educational Needs—informed by an understanding of the basis of developmental deficits and the differential constraints on brain plasticity—is one important avenue. A second is a deeper focus on the neuroscience of adult learning, how it differs from learning in childhood, and how it alters in later lifespan during ageing (see, e.g., Thomas, Knowland, & Rogers, 2020, for a recent consideration of the neuroscience of adult learning in the context of adult literacy programs in the developing world).

Educational neuroscience is still a young discipline, with lessons to learn. As psychology demonstrates, translation can be as challenging as the basic science. This volume naturally focuses on the insights offered by neuroscience at the interfaces with psychology and education, but we remain committed to the broader belief that interdisciplinary research is the best way forward for education.

Notes

1. https://ies.ed.gov/ncee/wwc/
2. https://educationendowmentfoundation.org.uk/
3. https://educationendowmentfoundation.org.uk/evidence-summaries/teaching-learning-toolkit
4. See, e.g., www.educationalneuroscience.org.uk/resources/neuromyth-or-neurofact/violent-video-games-make-children-more-violent/ for discussion of this issue
5. See Selzam et al. (2019) for a recent detailed analysis of the extent to which environmental and genetic effects on variation in cognition are confounded.

References

Bowers, J. S. (2016). The practical and principled problems with educational neuroscience. *Psychological Review, 123,* 600–612.

Bruer, J. T. (1999). *The myth of the first three years.* New York: The Free Press.

Cigman, R., & Davis, A. (2009). The enhancement agenda. In R. Cigman & A. Davis (Eds.), *New philosophies of learning* (pp. 171–172). Oxford: Wiley-Blackwell.

Gabrieli, J. D. E. (2016). The promise of educational neuroscience: Comment on Bowers (2016). *Psychological Review, 123,* 613–619.

Green, C. S., Bavelier, D., Kramer, A. F. et al. (2019). Improving methodological standards in behavioral interventions for cognitive enhancement. *Journal of Cognitive Enhancement, 3,* 2. Published online 8 January 2019. https://doi.org/10.1007/s41 465-018-0115-y

Howard-Jones, P., Varma, S., Ansari, D., Butterworth, B., De Smedt, B., Goswami, U., . . . Thomas, M. S. C. (2016). The principles and practices of educational neuroscience: Commentary on Bowers. *Psychological Review, 123,* 620–627.

Ramsden, S., Richardson, F. M., Josse, G., Thomas, M. S. C., Ellis, C., Shakeshaft, C., . . . Price, C. J. (2011, November 3). Verbal and non-verbal intelligence changes in the teenage brain. *Nature, 479,* 113–116. doi:10.1038/nature10514

Ritchie, S. J., & Tucker-Drob, E. M. (2018). How much does education improve intelligence? A meta-analysis. *Psychological Science, 29*(8), 1358–1369. doi:10.1177/095 6797618774253

Sala, G., Foley, J. P., & Gobet, F. (2017). The effects of chess instruction on pupils' cognitive and academic skills: State of the art and theoretical challenges. *Front. Psychol., 8,* 238. doi:10.3389/fpsyg.2017.00238

Sala, G., & Gobet, F. (2017). Does far transfer exist? Negative evidence from chess, music, and working memory training. *Current Directions in Psychological Science, 26*(6), 515–520.

Selzam, S., Ritchie, S. J., Pingault, J. B., Reynolds, C. A., O'Reilly, P. F., & Plomin, R. (2019). *Comparing within- and between-family polygenic score prediction.* bioRxiv Preprint. Retrieved April 10, 2019, from http://dx.doi.org/10.1101/605006

Thomas, M. S. C. (2019). Response to Dougherty & Robey on neuroscience and education: Enough bridge metaphors—interdisciplinary research offers the best hope for progress. *Current Directions in Psychological Science, 28*(4), 337–340. https://doi.org/10.1177/0963721419838252

Thomas, M. S. C., Ansari, D., & Knowland, V. C. P. (2019). Annual research review: Educational neuroscience: Progress and prospects. *Journal of Child Psychology and Psychiatry, 60*(4), 477–492. doi:10.1111/jcpp.12973

Thomas, M. S. C., Fedor, A., Davis, R., Yang, J., Alireza, H., Charman, T., . . . Best, W. (2019, June 6). Computational modelling of interventions for developmental disorders. *Psychological Review*, *126*(5), 693–726. doi:http://dx.doi.org/10.1037/rev 0000151

Thomas, M. S. C., Knowland, V. C. P., & Rogers, C. (2020). *The Science of Adult Literacy*. Social Protection and Jobs Discussion Paper, No. 2001. World Bank, Washington, DC. © World Bank. https://openknowledge.worldbank.org/handle/10986/33278.

Wilkinson, H. R., Smid, C., Morris, S., Farran, E. K., Dumontheil, I., Mayer, S., . . . Thomas, M. S. C. (2019). Domain-specific inhibitory control training to improve children's learning of counterintuitive concepts in mathematics and science. *Journal of Cognitive Enhancement*. doi:10.1007/s41465-019-00161-4

Index

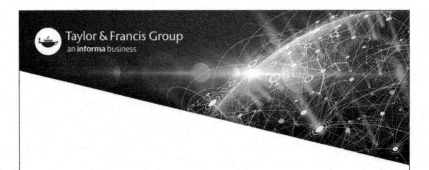